Teaching/Learning Package

For the Instructor

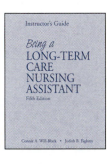

INSTRUCTOR'S GUIDE
(0-13-089433-8)
This invaluable tool contains complete lesson plans, supplemental materials on principles of adult learning, and teaching and clinical supervision strategies. It also includes the answer guide to all textbook learning objectives.

CUSTOM TEST MANAGER
The Test Manager is a comprehensive set of tools for testing and assessment. It allows instructors to create tests and exams tailored to their own needs, by allowing them to choose from approximately 500 questions.

- WIN PH Test Manager (0-13-031704-7)
- MAC PH Custom Test (0-13-040530-2)
- DOS PH Custom Test (0-13-040539-6)

TEST ITEM FILE
(0-13-028932-9)
Hard copy of test manager

CARE PROVIDER SKILLS VIDEOS *
These up-to-date and informative videos demonstrate skills the nursing assistant student needs for providing patient care. By demonstrating these procedures, this series will help students to carry out tasks with confidence. This video package is an essential tool for instructors that emphasizes the skills necessary for patient care.

Titles include:
- **Transfer and Ambulation**   (0-8359-5417-X)
- **Measuring Vital Signs**   (0-8359-5403-X)
- **Bed Bath**   (0-13-013924-6)
- **Age Specific Care**   (0-13-013925-4)
- **Body Mechanics**   (0-13-013928-9)
- **Personal Care**   (0-13-013919-X)
- **Transmission-Based Precautions**   (0-13-013931-9)
- **Dealing with Dementia**   (0-13-013918-1)
- **Patient Rights**   (0-13-013932-7)
- **Infection Control**   (0-13-013918-1)

* **Also available as a set, at a discounted price (0-13-015861-5)**

FOCUS ON PROFESSIONALISM
VIDEO (0-8359-5344-0)
Professionalism is a reflection of the nursing assistant as a person, and as a caring member of a profession that offers comfort to patients. This video clearly illustrates what professionalism is and gives contrasting examples of professional and unprofessional behavior. The "bring to life" concept of these demonstrations of professionalism will help students succeed as nursing assistants.

BEING A LONG-TERM CARE NURSING ASSISTANT

Fifth Edition

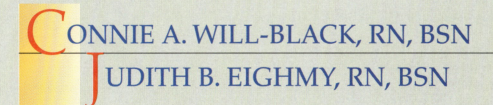

CONNIE A. WILL-BLACK, RN, BSN

JUDITH B. EIGHMY, RN, BSN

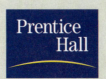

Prentice Hall

Upper Saddle River, New Jersey 07458

Library of Congress Cataloging-in-Publication Data

Eighmy, Judith B.
    Being a long-term care nursing assistant/
Connie A. Will-Black, Judith B. Eighmy,
—5th ed. update.
        p.; cm.
    Includes index.

    ISBN 0-13-089432-X

    1. Long-term care of the sick.   2. Nursing.
3. Nurses' aides. I. Will-Black, Connie, II.
Title.
    [DNLM: 1. Nurses' Aides—Nurses'
Instruction.   2. Long-Term Care—methods
—Nurses' Instruction. WY 18.2 E34b 2002]
RT120.L64 W54 2002
610.73'61—dc21200   1021467

NOTICE
The procedures described in this textbook are based on consultation with nursing assistant authorities. The author and publisher have taken care to make certain that these procedures reflect currently accepted clinical practice; however, they cannot be considered absolute recommendations.

The material in this textbook contains the most current information available at the time of publication. However, federal, state, and local guidelines concerning clinical practices, including, without limitation, those governing infection control and universal precautions, change rapidly. The reader should note, therefore, that new regulations may require changes in some procedures.

It is the responsibility of the reader to familiarize himself or herself with the policies set by federal, state, and local agencies, as well as the supplements written to accompany it, disclaim any liability, loss, or risk resulting directly or indirectly from the suggested procedures and theory, from any undetected errors, or from the reader's misunderstanding of the text. It is the reader's responsibility to stay informed of any new changes or recommendations made by any federal, state, and local agency as well as by his or her employing health care institution or agency.

Publisher: Julie Alexander
Executive Editor: Maura Connor
Acquisitions Editor: Barbara Krawiec
Managing Development Editor: Marilyn Meserve
Development Editor: Kathryn Kasturas
Director of Production and Manufacturing: Bruce Johnson
Managing Production Editor: Patrick Walsh
Production Editor: Linda Begley, Rainbow Graphics
Production Liaisons: Danielle Newhouse and Janet Bolton
Manufacturing Manager: Ilene Sanford
Design Director: Cheryl Asherman
Cover Design Coordinator: Maria Guglielmo
Cover Designer: Joseph Sengotta
Interior Designer: Amy Rosen
Marketing Manager: David Hough
Product Information Manager: Rachele Triano
Editorial Assistant: Michael Sirinides
Composition: Rainbow Graphics
Printing and Binding: Banta Book Group

Pearson Education LTD.
Pearson Education Australia PTY, Limited
Pearson Education Singapore, Pte. Ltd
Pearson Education North Asia Ltd
Pearson Education Canada, Ltd.
Pearson Educación de Mexico, S.A. de C.V.
Pearson Education—Japan
Pearson Education Malaysia, Pte. Ltd
Pearson Education, Upper Saddle River, New Jersey

10 9 8 7

ISBN 0-13-089432-X

This book is dedicated to my co-author and colleague, Connie Will-Black.

CONTENTS IN BRIEF

Chapter 7   The Skeletal System   194

SECTION

Chapter 8   The Muscular System   218

SECTION

Contents

Contents

PREFACE

Being a Long-Term Care Nursing Assistant, 5th edition, is filled with new features to enhance the learning of students preparing to become certified nursing assistants (CNAs). Written by two nurses involved in the day-to-day realities of long-term care, the text clearly demonstrates the many skills demanded of a competent CNA and explains other important aspects of care such as interpersonal relationships, communication and compassion.

These proven authors recognize not only the value of the caregivers but also the unique learning needs of today's adult learner. Learning objectives are realistic, understandable, measurable, and achievable, helping students and instructors zero in on what matters. Information is presented in short, manageable sections using a consistent format. The full-color, richly illustrated presentation and accessible reading level ensures that students of all ages and backgrounds can concentrate on information instead of struggling with the language.

EMPHASIS ON ESSENTIAL INFORMATION

This text focuses exclusively on "need-to-know" information about topics and procedures directly relevant to the job of the CNA in long-term care. Activities outside the scope of CNA practice have not been included. This is a text designed specifically for long-term care, not adapted from an acute care text.

CONSISTENT SYSTEMS APPROACH

The text is organized in a consistent body systems approach for easier learning. Each systems chapter introduces the normal anatomy and physiology of that system, followed by age-related changes and common symptoms, diseases, and conditions. Related guidelines for care and step-by-step procedures are integrated throughout, helping students recognize the direct relationship between the care provided and the rationale. Feedback from students and teachers alike has favored this approach.

KEY THEMES AND CONCEPTS REINFORCED THROUGHOUT

The authors have threaded key themes and concepts throughout the text, reinforcing their importance in quality care. Such themes and concepts include residents' rights, age-related changes, infection control, safety, cultural awareness, standard precautions, psychosocial needs, rehabilitation, documentation, age-specific competencies, and kind, compassionate care. Emphasis on the unique needs of the elderly and disabled contributes to improved job performance and client health and satisfaction.

UPDATED AND EXPANDED THROUGHOUT, INCLUDING TWO NEW CHAPTERS

This 5th edition has been updated and expanded with new content throughout, including:

- **New emphasis on pain management in the elderly.** New content helps students understand the importance of recognizing and treating pain in the elderly, whose pain tends to be undertreated nationwide.
- **The latest CDC guidelines for infection control.** Current Standard Precautions and Transmission-Based Precautions are included to keep students and clients healthy.
- **A new chapter on end-of-life care.** Research indicates that 20 percent of deaths each year occur in a long-term care facility. Chapter 19 discusses such topics as pain management, communication with dying patients and families, end-stage disease, and grief and bereavement, helping prepare students to offer compassionate care to these patients.
- **A new chapter on preparing for the certification examination.** Chapter 20 will help the student succeed on the competency examination and in finding employment.

A WEALTH OF HELPFUL LEARNING AIDS

This edition includes many learning aids:

- **Caring tips.** Quotations from nurses across America open each chapter and highlight practical ways the nursing assistant can deliver safe, effective care.
- **Marginal glossary.** Key terms highlighted in the text are listed and defined in the margin, avoiding the need to flip to the end-of-book glossary.
- **Cultural awareness.** A special cultural awareness icon alerts students to cultural issues related to each chapter, enhancing their sensitivity to clients' customs and beliefs related to their care.
- **Procedures.** Step-by-step procedures are highlighted in color for added emphasis.
- **OBRA highlights.** A special icon highlights OBRA regulations derived from the OBRA 1987 legislation as appropriate to the content of each chapter.
- **Chapter summary.** A new two-part summary concludes each chapter. Part 1 summarizes key points in the chapter. Part 2 helps students focus on key OBRA regulations to help them succeed on the exam and in the workplace.
- **Self-study multiple choice questions.** Students can test their understanding and retention of the chapter content to see if they need further study. These questions provide practice at test taking and preparation for the competency examination.
- **Case study.** Each chapter concludes with a case study or situation followed by related multiple-choice questions. This sharpens students' critical thinking skills and helps them apply the information learned from the chapter.

TEACHING/LEARNING PACKAGE

FOR THE STUDENT

- **New Companion Web Site.** Students can log on to *www.prenhall.com/will-black* and find an interactive learning guide with instant feedback, bulletin board questions, links to other interesting Web sites with additional content related to each chapter, and an audio glossary.
- **Prentice Hall Health's Survival Guide for Long-Term Care Nursing Assistants.** This is a new, free, 42-page quick-reference guide. This quick, convenient pocket guide (shrink-wrapped with the text) gives student instant on-the-job access to key facts.
- **Student Workbook.** This completely revised companion study guide has emphasis on the application of knowledge to work-related situations. Vocabulary and anatomy are emphasized. Critical thinking skills are incorporated both in multiple-choice and case-study questions. This excellent study tool will not only prepare students for the written competency evaluation, but also give them confidence in their knowledge of the course material.

FOR THE INSTRUCTOR

- **Instructor's Guide.** The complementary Instructor's Guide contains complete lesson plans, supplemental materials on principles of adult learning, teaching and clinical supervision strategies, and answers for all questions.
- **Test Manager.** Available in Windows, MAC, and DOS formats, as well as hard copy, Test Manager allows you to customize a test bank.

Being a Long-Term Care Nursing Assistant, 5th Edition, is intended for use in community colleges, vocational or technical schools, high schools, nursing care facilities, and other agencies educating tomorrow's nursing assistants. Your comments and suggestions will help us continue to improve this successful and respected text in the next edition.

ACKNOWLEDGMENTS

This book is dedicated to my co-author and colleague, Connie Will-Black. Although she did not participate in this edition, her impact is a visible presence throughout the text. This extraordinary woman continues to own and operate two outstanding skilled nursing facilities in California. Through her writing and teaching and her undying support of nursing education, she has improved the care of countless residents of long-term care facilities. In addition, Connie started a hospice program that improved end-of-life care in California.

With deepest gratitude, I acknowledge the contribution and support of family, friends, and professional associates. Elayne and Murray Nahman, my partners in my current consulting practice, have taken on additional burdens to allow me to spend time on this edition. Thank you!

It was an honor to work with photographer Bill Irwin for this edition. He is an incredible man, a friend, and a talented artist. Bill not only took the pictures; he shared his expertise in the medical world with a creative approach and precise attention to accuracy. His mother Wanda served as talent coordinator, calling on her friends and family to serve as models. Thank you, Bill and Wanda Irwin.

Special thanks are in order for the staff of West Anaheim Extended Care in Anaheim, California. Administrator Donna Meyer, Director of Nursing Mary Manson, and Director of Staff Development Jocelyn Cabrera, all went the extra mile to allow us to take pictures, to enlist the staff and residents in the process, and to keep us in coffee.

Grateful acknowledgment is made to the staff of Prentice Hall, including, of course, our acquisitions editor, Barbara Krawiec; production editors Janet Bolton, Danielle Newhouse, and Linda Begley (of Rainbow Graphics); and editorial assistants Melissa Kerian and Michael Sirinides. I know this was a difficult experience for all you. Thank you for your patience in the face of demanding deadlines and my busy schedule.

Judith B. Eighmy, RN, BSN, CHPN

REVIEWERS

Neva Babcock, BSN, RNC, CDONA, CIC
Performance Improvement/Infection Control Director
St. Thomas More Nursing & Rehab Center
Hyattsville, MD

Ron Bowser, MBA, EMTB
Regional Coordinator
Maryland Fire and Rescue Institute
University of Maryland
College Park, MD

Nancy Brown, RN, MS
Practical Nursing Program Director
San Juan Basin Technical School
Cortez, CO

Julie Capriola
Coordinator of Nurse Aide Program
Vance Granville Community College
Henderson, NC

Connie L. Davis, RN, MSN
Professor
Southwest Virginia Community College
Richlands, VA

Gail Diffley, RN
Inservice Educator
Wesley Health Care Center, Inc.
Saratoga Springs, NY

Patricia Edwards, RN, BA
Director of Education
Royal Park Care Center
Spokane, WA

Kathleen Gettrust, RN, MSN
Woukesh County Tech. College
Pewoukee, WI

Joe Nathan Gravely Jr.
Assistant Professor
Patrick Henry Community College
Martinsville, VA

Dr. Sheila Guidry, RN
Director/Chair LPN and NAS Program
Wallace Community College
Selma, AL

Susan Helmke, RNC
Coordinator, Allied Health
Pratt Community College
Pratt, KS

Christopher J. Le Baudour, BA, EMTI
Santa Rosa Community College
Santa Rosa, CA

Donna Mitchell, PhD, RN, CNS
Professor & Chair
University of Rio Grande
Rio Grande, OH 45674

Andrea B. O'Connor, EdD, RN
Professor of Nursing
Western Connecticut State University
Danbury, CT

Lori Popejoy, MSN, RN, CS, GCNS
Sinclair School of Nursing
University of Missouri
Columbia, MO

Mary Lou Roux, RN, BS
Program Coordinator
Fulton Montgomery Community College
Johnstown, NY

Joan Scribner
Affiliate Faculty
Penn Valley Community College
Kansas City, MO

Diane Weeks, RN
Certified Nursing Assistant Instructor
Cortland, NY

Dr. M. Anne Woodtli
University of Arizona
Tucson, AZ

ABOUT THE AUTHORS

Connie A. Will-Black, RN, BSN, PHN,
is a graduate of California State University at Long Beach and has been active in long-term care as a nursing consultant, educator, and owner for the past 25 years. Mrs. Black's teaching experience includes nursing education in both acute and long-term care settings as well as in community colleges. As CEO of Community Hospice Care, Mrs. Black created a large Medicare Certified Hospice program in Southern California. This program served thousands of terminally ill patients, both those who lived in their own homes, and those in retirement facilities and in long-term care facilities. Her commitment to education created a large group of professional staff with expertise in end-of-life care who continues to serve dying patients throughout Southern California. Although Connie did not participate in this 5th edition, her knowledge and philosophy of care are reflected throughout the book.

Judith B. Eighmy, RN, BSN, CHPN,
is a graduate of Texas Woman's University and has completed course work for her master's degree in nursing from California State University at Los Angeles. She is certified in hospice and palliative care nursing. Ms. Eighmy has been a nursing consultant and educator in long-term care and hospice for more than 25 years. In addition to teaching numerous continuing education courses for health care professionals in long-term care and hospice, she has taught in the acute care setting and in the university as well as in a school of nursing. She has developed quality assessment and improvement programs for long-term care facilities and hospice programs. Ms. Eighmy is active in her professional organization and widely recognized for her expertise in training and in care of the elderly and end-of-life care. She serves as an advisory board member and consultant to Medcom, Inc., of Cypress, California, in the development of education programs for long-term care. She is currently president of her consulting firm, Pacific Healthcare Consultants, Inc., where she and her partner Elayne Nahman, LCSW, serve hospice programs in California.

Procedures

The page number follows the Procedure title.

Guidelines

The page number follows the Guidelines title.

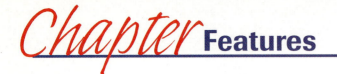

Chapter Features

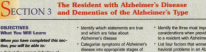

Key Terms

A list of key terms opens each chapter. Learning the meaning of these terms before reading the chapter helps you better understand and remember what you read.

SECTION 3 — The Resident with Alzheimer's Disease and Dementias of the Alzheimer's Type

OBJECTIVES
What You Will Learn
When you have completed this section, you will be able to:
• Select the correct definition of Alzheimer's disease
• Identify which statements are true and which are false about Alzheimer's disease
• Categorize symptoms of Alzheimer's disease into appropriate stages of the disease
• Identify the three most important considerations when providing care to a resident with Alzheimer's disease
• List four factors that worsen the behavioral problems in an Alzheimer's disease resident

KEY TERMS
alzheimer's disease
apathy
catastrophic reaction
dementia
reality orientation
reminiscence
validation

Alzheimer's disease (AD) is an incurable disease affecting the brain. It is the most common cause of progressive *dementia* in older adults. **Dementia** means deprived of reason, mentally deteriorated. Alzheimer's is the fourth leading cause of death in the United States of those over 75, and it affects an estimated 1.5 million Americans. Projections indicate that by the year 2040, one in every three families will be directly touched by this devastating disease. There is no cure and no way to slow the progress of the disease.

Several diseases can cause dementia besides Alzheimer's disease. They include:

• Huntington's disease
• Multi-infarct dementia
• AIDS-related dementia

These diseases of the brain may affect residents in different ways; however, loss of recent (short-term) memory, confusion, and lack of reasoning and poor judgment are the most common indicators (Figure 11-11).

The deterioration of the brain seen in the AD resident is not part of the normal aging process. AD usually begins after age 60, however it may occur as early as age 40. It is a terminal illness that affects more women than men and is more common in countries where the life expectancy is longer. It was first identified by a German pathologist, Dr. Alois Alzheimer, and bears his name.

Current research supports the theory that a *genetic* (inherited) mechanism is evident in the development of Alzheimer's disease. There are also, however, many cases of Alzheimer's disease in which there is no previous history of the disease within the family. There is no easy way to diagnose AD except by examining brain tissue after death, so diagnosis is done by excluding all other causes of curable and incurable memory loss.

During the course of the disease, the nerve cells in the brain that control memory, thinking, and judgment are damaged. There is disruption in the ability of nerve cells to transmit messages to one another, and one theory suggests that certain substances (called neurotransmitters) neces-

alzheimer's disease incurable disease affecting the brain that occurs predominantly in older adults and affects memory, thinking, and judgment

dementia deprived of reason; mentally deteriorated

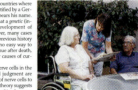
FIGURE 11-11
Residents in Alzheimer's unit.

Section 3 The Resident with Alzheimer's Diseases and Dementias of the Alzheimer's Type **321**

Margin Glossary

Key terms are defined in the margin next to the text where they are used. This timesaving feature avoids flipping to the end of the book each time you need a definition.

Cultural Awareness Icon

This icon points out ways you can show respect for residents' customs and beliefs as you care for them.

---

nor is everyone with epilepsy mentally retarded. In fact, ... with epilepsy are *not* retarded. (Chapter 11, "The Ner... formation on seizures and epilepsy; review that info... however, often present along with mental retardation... it may be caused by the same event that caused the ...

NORMALIZATION

A facility providing care to the developmentally dis... ciples or a philosophy of care that establishes not o... but also the kind of environment in which it will be ... cept is called normalization. **Normalization** means ... is as close as possible to the atmosphere provided ... mentally retarded (Figure 16-2). It means offering t... kind of treatment. Principles of normalization req... or qualities of the individual be emphasized while ... inated. For example, if a developmentally disabled r... ical abnormality such as crossed eyes that would mak... or abnormal, the crossed eyes should be corrected with surgery or special glasses. Great care should be taken in the grooming and dressing of your clients so that any negative physical traits are either disguised or offset by attractive, age-appropriate clothing and good grooming (based on chronological age, not mental or developmental age). With older clients, make special effort to select an appropriate hairstyle as well as clothing. For example, an older woman might look absurd in a ponytail with childlike bows or barrettes. There are, however, ways to pull the hair back that are more adult. A child's ponytail is placed high on the back of the head while an adult's is secured lower, at the back of the neck.

CULTURAL AWARENESS — One aspect of normalization is to recognize and to acknowledge the culture of the client. Each client brings an ethnic, racial, or cultural history. Even though the client cannot express his or her culture, the staff must keep it in mind. For example, if the family is Hispanic, it would be important to offer some Hispanic foods. If the family holds certain religious practices, the family may want the client to observe them too. Ask other staff and the family members what their practices and beliefs are so that you can help the client to follow them.

In order to create a normalized environment, it is essential that every staff member hold a particular belief: that all human beings are worthy of being treated with dignity and respect. If you believe that you are somehow "better" than those you serve, you will have difficulty treating your clients or residents as they deserve to be cared for.

Some of the ways you will know normalization when you see it are:

• Staff members treat people under their supervision with dignity and respect.
• Staff members do not exert undue power over the resident.
• Staff play the role of an associate or assistant, not a parent.
• Residents are encouraged ... themselves.
• Residents' rooms contain ...

normalization creating an atmosphere that is as close to normal as possible

FIGURE 16-2
Example of normalization.

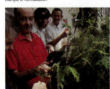

402 Chapter 16 Developmental Disabilities

Guidelines

This feature highlights important principles of care throughout the text to guide your care of the resident.

MEASURING FLUID INTAKE

• Obtain a list of the most commonly used fluid containers in your facility, along with a listing of how many ounces or cc's it will hold. If this is not available, you will need to measure the amount of liquid each container holds and make a list for yourself.
• Obtain the forms used for recording intake and output in your facility.
• Measure and record all fluids consumed by the resident during your shift of duty. (Calculate the difference between the full amount of the container and the amount left in the container.) Observe and record fluids consumed from the resident's meals, water pitchers, and between-meal snacks.
• Convert (change) amounts such as half a bowl of soup, half a glass of juice, or a quarter cup of coffee into cubic centimeters for recording. For example: Mrs. Jones's water pitcher contained 1

quart (liter), which equals 1000 cc. At the end of the shift, you would measure what remained (in this case, 250 cc) and subtract the difference: 1000 cc minus 250 cc equals 750 cc. In addition, Mrs. Jones drank half a glass of juice (4-ounce juice glass equals 120 cc) (120 cc divided by 2 equals 60 cc) and a quarter cup of coffee (8-ounce cup equals 240 cc) (240 cc divided by 4 equals 60 cc).

Water = 750 cc
Juice = 60 cc
Coffee = 60 cc
Total = 870 cc

• Record intake after each meal before the tray is removed.
• Record other intake as it is consumed.

Guidelines

Procedures

All procedures are highlighted in color and give you step-by-step guidance from preparation to follow-up for the most common procedures you will perform as a long-term care assistant.

PROCEDURE
Measuring Urinary Output

It is not possible to measure accurately the amount of fluid eliminated through the intestinal tract, the respiratory tract, or the skin. Therefore, the urinary output is the most reliable measurement of fluid output.

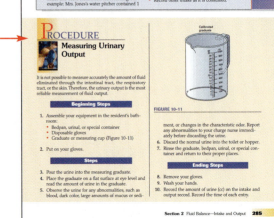
FIGURE 10-11

Beginning Steps

1. Assemble your equipment in the resident's bathroom:
   • Bedpan, urinal, or special container
   • Disposable gloves
   • Graduate or measuring cup (Figure 10-11)
2. Put on your gloves.

Steps

3. Pour the urine into the measuring graduate.
4. Place the graduate on a flat surface at eye level and read the amount of urine in the graduate.
5. Observe the urine for any abnormalities, such as blood, dark color, large amounts of mucus or sedi-

ment, or changes in the characteristic odor. Report any abnormalities to your charge nurse immediately before discarding the urine.
6. Discard the normal urine into the toilet or hopper.
7. Rinse the graduate, bedpan, urinal, or special container and return to their proper places.

Ending Steps

8. Remove your gloves.
9. Wash your hands.
10. Record the amount of urine (cc) on the intake and output record. Record the time of each entry.

Section 2 Fluid Balance—Intake and Output **285**

OBRA Highlights

A key OBRA training requirement is highlighted at the end of each chapter.

Self Study

Multiple-choice questions test your understanding of chapter content and help you prepare for the certification exam.

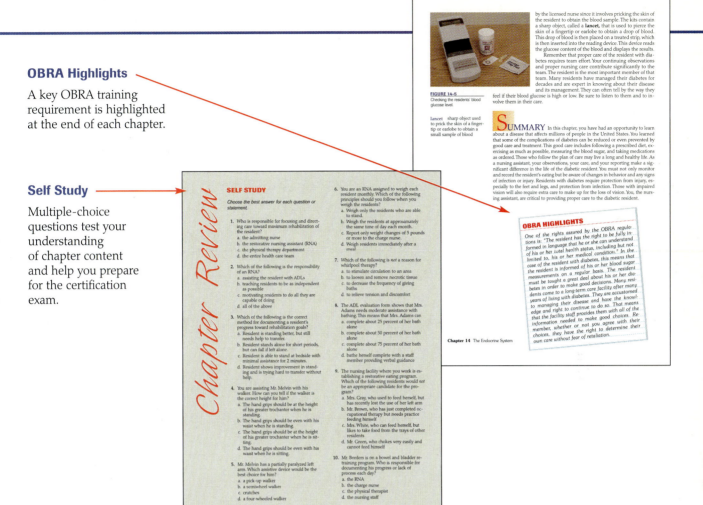

Getting Connected

Our free, interactive Companion Website **www.prenhall.com/will-black** provides you with more learning activities to use with this textbook. The interactive study guide gives you instant feedback, helpful hints, and textbook references to chapter-related multiple-choice questions. Our free audio glossary helps you learn how to pronounce key terms correctly. You can also link to other interesting websites with more information on chapter topics.

Video

Our *Care Provider Skills* video series shows you step-by-step how to perform procedures discussed in the chapter.

Case Studies

Each chapter concludes with a case study or situation followed by related multiple-choice questions. Each case study, and questions that follow, will help you sharpen your critical thinking skills and help you apply what you have learned.

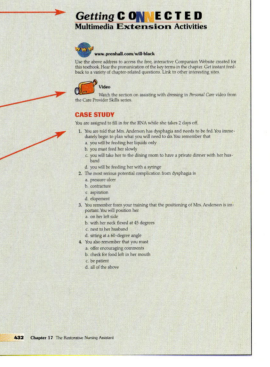

Chapter 1

INTRODUCTION TO LONG-TERM CARE

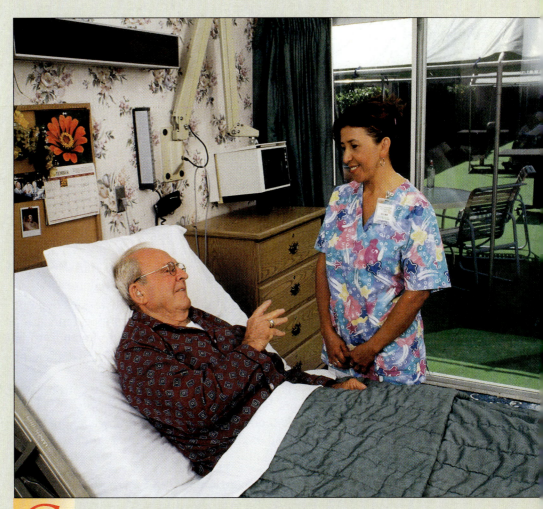

CARING TIP

Answering the call light promptly is one of the most important ways you can show a resident that you care!

Andrea O'Connor, EdD, JD, RN
Professor of Nursing
Western Connecticut State University
Danbury, CT

OBJECTIVES
What You Will Learn

When you have completed this section, you will be able to:

- Identify the functions and purposes of the long-term care facility
- List the three most common reasons residents require long-term care
- Identify three programs that pay for long-term care

KEY TERMS

activities of daily living (ADLs)

developmental disability

hospice

ICFMR facilities

long-term care (LTC) facility

LONG-TERM CARE FACILITIES

long-term care (LTC) facility a type of institution designed to provide care and services over a long period. Includes skilled nursing facility and rehabilitation centers. There is no age restriction

The **long-term care (LTC) facility** is an integral part of the nation's health care system. Census bureau statistics reflect the dramatic increase in the over-65 population and the expected continuing growth during the next decade (Figure 1-1). As life expectancy increases, the need for LTC services also increases— one out of every five persons over the age of 75 will require LTC services. After age 85, 23 percent will require LTC services.

The General Accounting Office has identified the three major reasons our elderly require LTC services:

activities of daily living (ADL) activities or tasks needed for daily living, such as eating, grooming, dressing, bathing, washing, and toileting

- Inability to perform **activities of daily living (ADL),** such as eating, bathing, toileting, and dressing (Figure 1-2)
- Decreased mental abilities with various dementias causing confusion and difficult behaviors as well as common medical problems, such as heart disease, stroke, hypertension, hip fracture, and arthritis
- Absence of a caregiver, spouse, immediate family member, or friend

The LTC facility is both a hospital with hospital-like services and the residents' home (Figure 1-3). The majority of people admitted to LTC facilities reside there permanently. The average length of stay in an LTC facility exceeds two and one-half years. Its primary functions are as follows:

Four Basic Functions and Purposes of the Long-Term Care Facility
1. To provide care to residents based on their identified needs
2. To utilize a multidisciplinary health care team to plan care and provide services
3. To prevent illness, injury, or loss of function
4. To promote recovery and health through maintaining existing abilities and restoring residents' former abilities

Some common terms used to describe LTC facilities are:

- Skilled nursing facility
- Nursing home
- Convalescent hospital
- Rehabilitation center
- Extended care hospital
- Nursing care center

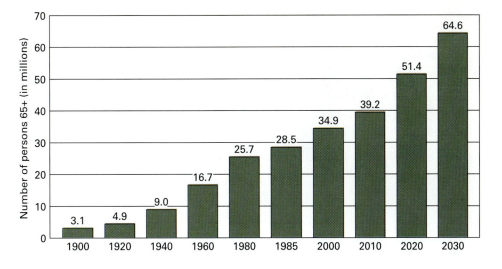

FIGURE 1-1

Increases in life expectancy, 1900 to 2030.

TYPES OF LTC FACILITIES

Some LTC facilities offer specialized care. They provide services to residents with special needs or problems, such as:

FACILITIES FOR THE DEVELOPMENTALLY DISABLED CLIENT

A **developmental disability** is a condition closely related to mental retardation—the client is often seriously handicapped. Clients who have cerebral palsy, autism, and seizure disorders may live in a special facility. These facilities are called intermediate care facilities for the mentally retarded **(ICFMR facilities).** There are federal regulations governing the care provided. Because of the vulnerability of the clients, the facilities are evaluated on an annual basis to ensure that good care is being provided. Most developmentally disabled (DD)

developmental disability a chronic condition related to or needing treatment similar to mental retardation

ICFMR facilities a type of facility designed to provide care for the developmentally disabled or mentally retarded

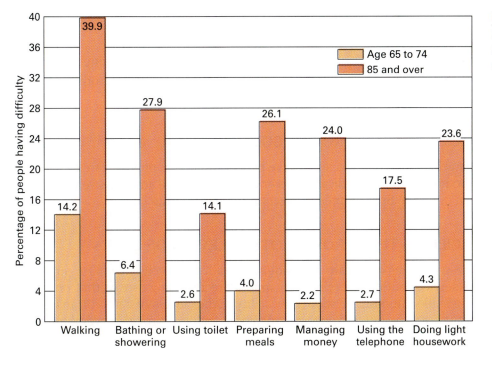

FIGURE 1-2

Percentage of elderly people who have difficulty performing seven ordinary tasks.

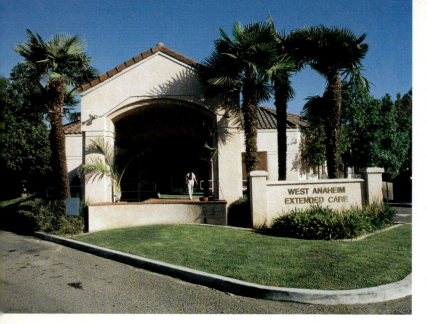

FIGURE 1-3

The long-term care facility.

clients continue to live in large, state-run institutions, although the goal is to move the clients to smaller, more homelike settings. There are common goals in providing care to the DD client:

- Maintaining good physical health (many DD clients have severe physical disabilities)
- Creating as normal and homelike an environment as possible while teaching the client to become as independent as possible
- Managing behavior and teaching the client to control unacceptable behaviors

Care of the DD individual requires unique knowledge and training. Chapter 16 is devoted to this subject.

FACILITIES THAT PROVIDE SPECIAL REHABILITATION SERVICES

This type of facility offers specialized care to assist residents in restoring normal levels of functioning following a stroke, fracture, or accident. There are physical therapists, speech therapists, occupational therapists, and licensed nurses available to provide specialized care and services on a daily basis. Residents in these facilities usually have a good potential for recovery and will remain in the facility only during the recovery phase of their illness.

FACILITIES THAT SPECIALIZE IN CARING FOR PATIENTS WITH THE SAME PROBLEMS

hospice a program of care for residents who have a limited life expectancy

- Alcoholic rehabilitation treatment centers
- Drug abuse units
- Psychiatric/mental health units
- **Hospice** inpatient centers (a facility that provides care to dying patients)
- Centers that care for residents with Alzheimer's disease and other kinds of dementia

FACILITIES THAT PROVIDE SUBACUTE CARE

Many long-term care facilities have opened units that provide care to patients who have complex medical needs and/or who require an intensive rehabilitation program. See Chapter 18, Section 1, The Subacute Unit.

FACILITIES THAT PROVIDE OTHER LEVELS OF CARE

These facilities offer care to residents who have special needs for supportive services but do not require as much direct nursing care as that provided by a skilled nursing or subacute facility. Other levels of care you may hear about are personal and supervisory. Some facilities provide several levels of care.

State and federal programs support more than 50 percent of the residents in LTC facilities through Medicare, Medicaid, or local programs. The payment system is directly related to the level of care that residents require.

ORGANIZATION OF THE LTC FACILITY

Most LTC facilities are organized in a similar way, and the easiest way to understand the lines of authority and responsibility is to understand the organizational chart of a typical facility (Figure 1-4). This helps establish appropriate lines of communication with facility management. Communication is always smoother when the chain of command is followed and understood.

THE PAYMENT SOURCES FOR LONG-TERM CARE

Paying for health care is a topic of national debate and interest. Health care reform is one of the nation's top priorities; many people do not have health care insurance coverage, and others have inadequate coverage to meet their medical needs. For these reasons, many people do not seek medical care soon enough or they go without other necessities. The elderly and indigent population are especially vulnerable.

People with private health care insurance may have most of their acute hospital costs covered, but not many programs cover the cost of long-term care. If long-term care is covered, there are many limitations related to eligibility, amount paid, and length of stay.

Medicare benefits are available to those age 65 and older; however, under special circumstances younger, disabled persons may also receive Medicare benefits. The Medicare program is administered by the Social Security Administration, a department of the federal government. Medicare benefits are provided under two programs:

- Part A pays for acute hospital costs up to a specified amount for a limited period of time. Home care costs and long-term care costs are covered only when certain eligibility requirements are met.
- Part B pays for certain medical expenses, such as some medical supplies and equipment, diagnostic tests, doctor visits, physical therapy, and language therapy.

FIGURE 1-4

Organization of a long-term care facility.

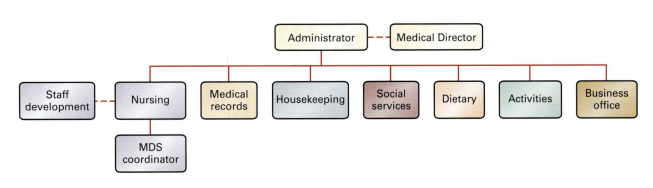

Understanding benefit programs under Medicare is not easy, and residents and families can seek assistance from knowledgeable facility staff members and/or their local Social Security office.

Medicaid benefits are provided jointly by the state and federal governments to eligible families and residents of long-term care facilities. Because the program is partially funded by the state, eligibility requirements and benefits vary. Medicaid benefits are to assist low-income families or those who are disabled. Medicaid pays a limited amount for each covered service: hospital services, doctor visits, diagnostic testing, home care, rehabilitation therapies, hospice care, family planning, immunizations, and dental and eye care. There is no insurance premium; however, the amount paid by families may be different based on their income level.

The long-term care facility is required by law to provide equally good care to all residents; it is never appropriate to discriminate because of payment status.

SECTION 2 The Nursing Assistant as an Employee

OBJECTIVES
What You Will Learn

When you have completed this section, you will be able to:

- Define the terms **policy, procedure,** and **job description**
- Explain where the employer's "rules" for employees can be found
- Compare your own job description with the sample job description provided in the Student Workbook

KEY TERMS

job description   policy   procedure

POLICIES, PROCEDURES, AND JOB DESCRIPTIONS

All LTC facilities must provide care and services according to established state and federal laws and regulations. The facilities are inspected regularly to ensure that these regulations are followed. If facilities fail to meet the established standards, they may lose their license to operate as well as state and federal payment for services.

As you learn about the LTC facility, you will become familiar with the specific state and federal regulations you will be expected to follow as you provide nursing care. Facilities establish written policies, procedures, and job descriptions to help them comply with regulations and to make their employees more efficient in the delivery of services to residents (Figure 1-5).

These policies, procedures, and job descriptions are very important "tools" you will need to help you become successful as a nursing assistant.

policy   describes what is to be done

- A **policy** describes what will be done.
- A **procedure** describes how something is to be done.
- A **job description** describes who is to do what.

procedure   description of how to do a task

job description   describes the duties of a particular job category

A sample job description for a nursing assistant is included in the student workbook. Review this job description carefully and make sure that you understand it. Compare it to your own job description and determine if it:

- Clearly describes your responsibilities
- Describes the duties or tasks you are expected to carry out
- Describes your relationships with other departments, as well as the department of nursing

PERSONNEL POLICIES

Personnel policies describe both the benefits provided to employees and the expectations of the employer. Included are guidelines for acceptable employee behavior. Just as we all must follow the "rules of the road" to avoid chaos on the streets, employees must follow the "rules to work by" to have order within a facility. Review the sample standards of conduct that follow.

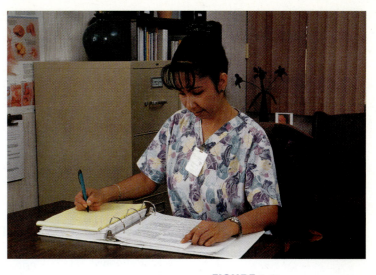

FIGURE 1-5
Using the Policy and Procedure manual.

STANDARDS OF CONDUCT

The following behaviors are not acceptable in facilities. They may result in disciplinary and/or legal action.

1. Verbal and/or physical abuse to a resident, visitor, or supervisory personnel
2. Inefficiency, inability, and/or gross or repeated negligence in performance of assigned duties
3. Stealing or willfully destroying or damaging any property of the facility, its residents, visitors, or other personnel
4. Disobedience or insubordination to supervisors
5. Disorderly, immoral, or indecent conduct
6. Reporting for work, or attempting to work, while under the influence of or addicted to alcohol, drugs, or narcotics
7. Borrowing money or other possessions from residents and/or accepting gratuities or tips from patients and/or their families
8. Unauthorized possession of firearms or other weapons on facility property
9. Absence without notifying the supervisor or administrator
10. Smoking in an unauthorized area
11. Selling tickets, pools, raffles, or soliciting of any kind on facility premises
12. Using the facility business phone for personal calls
13. Altering, falsifying, or making a willful misstatement of facts on any resident record or chart, job, or work report
14. Failure to provide care to residents in such a way as to guarantee them their right to be treated with respect and dignity
15. Failure to protect confidentiality of resident records, information, and so on, or disclosing anything of a personal nature concerning a resident at any time either inside or outside the facility
16. Punching another person's time card or requesting that another person punch your time card
17. Refusal to work where assigned

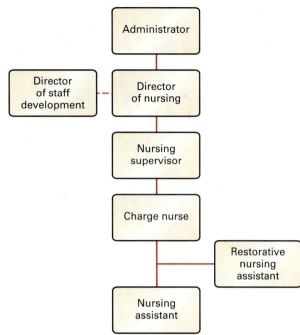

FIGURE 1-6

Organizational chart for the department of nursing.

ORGANIZATION OF THE DEPARTMENT OF NURSING

Generally, each department of the LTC facility will have additional policies and procedures specifically related to that department. Make sure you understand what these are and where they are located for the department of nursing.

The department of nursing is organized similarly in most LTC facilities (Figure 1-6). The lines of responsibility and authority are dictated by state and federal regulations.

- The director of nursing must be a registered nurse (RN). Most have specialized training and experience in caring for the elderly or the patient population served.
- The nursing supervisor is generally a registered nurse who is in charge of either an entire shift or a specific section of a facility.
- The charge nurse is responsible for or in charge of a specific unit on a specific shift. The charge nurse reports to the nursing supervisor. The charge nurse may be a registered nurse (RN), a licensed vocational nurse (LVN), or a licensed practical nurse (LPN).
- The director of inservice training or staff development is a licensed nurse (RN, LPN, LVN) who is responsible for orientation and training of nursing personnel. The director of inservice training or staff development may report to the director of nursing or to the facility administrator.
- The nursing assistant always works under the direct supervision of a licensed nurse (Figure 1-7). The nursing assistant usually reports to the charge nurse although some facilities use experienced certified nursing assistants (CNAs) as team leaders.

FIGURE 1-7

Nursing assistant working under the supervision of a licensed nurse.

Understanding the chain of command helps you to follow the lines of communication. Usually, you will give information about a resident directly to the charge nurse. If others need to know, it will be up to the charge nurse to tell them.

If you are not satisfied with a response you get, you can go to the next higher person on the organization chart. When a conflict with a person in another department arises, refer the problem to your immediate supervisor. Although "going all the way to the top" may bring faster results, the chain of communication is then broken and the entire structure of authority is undermined.

Providing care and service is a big responsibility, and doing a good job is often difficult. To be successful, a facility must have employees who work together and who are dedicated to their work. To become a valued member of the health care team, you need to thoroughly understand and accept the roles and responsibilities assigned to you as a nursing assistant.

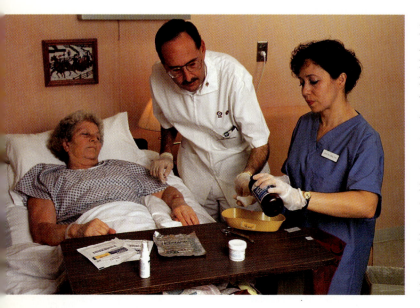

SECTION 3 Legal and Ethical Responsibilities

OBJECTIVES
What You Will Learn

When you have completed this section, you will be able to:

- Identify actions that are unethical or illegal
- Point out situations that show a resident's rights are being violated
- Define the terms **libel** and **slander**
- List three ways the nursing assistant can help prevent theft and loss

KEY TERMS

advance directives
assault
battery
chart
code of ethics
confidentiality

defamation of character
false imprisonment
gross negligence
invasion of privacy
legal
libel
negligence

ombudsman
Omnibus Budget Reconciliation Act (OBRA)
quality of life
residents' rights
slander

RESPONSIBILITIES AS A NURSING ASSISTANT

As a nursing assistant, you must acquire knowledge and demonstrate the ability to perform nursing skills competently. The skills you will be able to perform when you have completed your course of study are included in the table of contents and in the workbook. Review these skills in order to understand those tasks that are within the role of the nursing assistant. You may acquire additional training according to the specific requirements of the state in which you work.

In the performance of your duties as a nursing assistant, you have a legal obligation both to the residents you care for and to your employer. **Legal** means according to the laws of the community, state, or nation. The public expects that those providing care to residents in LTC facilities are qualified to do so. They have the right to expect that those providing care will behave in a way that does not cause the resident any harm, emotional or physical. You are legally responsible for your actions and for your failure to act.

legal   according to the laws of the community, state, or nation

REQUIREMENTS OF THE OMNIBUS RECONCILIATION ACT (OBRA) OF 1987

In 1987, the United States Congress passed legislation called the **Omnibus Budget Reconciliation Act (OBRA),** which addressed many issues concerning **quality of life** for residents of long-term care facilities. The law mandates that long-term care facilities must provide care and services that either maintain or improve each resident's quality of life, health, and safety. This new law expanded and strengthened the rights guaranteed all residents living in nursing care facilities (Figure 1-8). The **residents' rights** are granted under both federal and state laws. You will notice as you review these rights that many of them are the same rights you are guaranteed as a citizen of the United States.

Long-term care facilities must inform residents and families of their rights both orally and in writing in a language they understand upon admission to the facility. However, the most important requirement is that all care and services must be provided in such a way as to guarantee that these rights are not violated.

Omnibus Budget Reconciliation Act (OBRA)   a 1987 law passed by the U.S. Congress containing nursing home reform requirements

quality of life   a concept that includes all the aspects that make life worth living. Quality of life is best defined by the individual in the regulations

residents' rights   those aspects of care that the resident in a facility is entitled to have honored. There is a specific and detailed list identified in the regulations

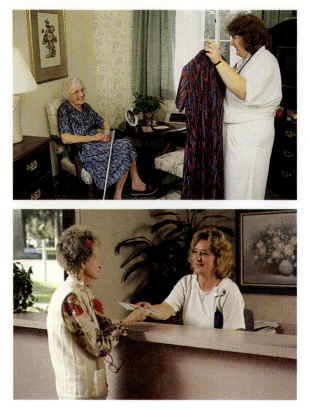

FIGURE 1-8
Residents' rights.

advance directives written documents that allow an adult with decision-making capacity to write their preferences regarding medical care and treatment. Some documents allow them to name a person to make decisions for them if they are unable

The nursing assistant must clearly understand what these rights are and learn how to provide care that safeguards these rights. (See the Student Workbook for a complete listing of the residents' rights.) Some states have adopted additional rights; be sure to review the resident rights applicable in the state in which you work. You will find specific references to residents' rights issues throughout the text.

In 1991, the Patient Self-Determination Act (PSDA) was enacted. This law required all health care facilities and agencies to notify clients/residents at time of admission of their rights to consent to or to refuse any medical treatment. The law applies to all persons receiving any kind of health care so it applies to you, too. It is particularly important when deciding what kind of care is wanted at the end of life. These decisions may be written down in advance in case the person is unable to decide or to communicate his or her choices. They are referred to as **advance directives.**

The advance directive is a written document (usually a Durable Power of Attorney for Health Care or a Living Will) that describes the individual's choices related to his or her medical treatment or identifies someone to make treatment decisions for the resident if they are unable to do so themselves.

Examples of decisions that might be made in advance include:

- Cardiopulmonary resuscitation (restarting the heart after it has stopped beating)
- Artificial ventilation (use of a machine for breathing)
- Artificial feeding (nasogastric or gastric tube feeding)
- Hospitalization (whether or not to go to the hospital)
- Medications (whether drugs such as antibiotics are to be given to prolong life)

End-of-life decisions made by the resident, the resident's family, or a legal guardian must be respected and care provided according to their wishes. There are times when others make decisions that may be in conflict with your own personal beliefs or value system, but it is important to remember that you are not responsible for the decisions of others and they have the legal right of self-determination.

CULTURAL AWARENESS Many cultures do not follow the concept of informed consent. They may surrender their choice and right to be informed to the physician or health care worker who is believed to know best. Some do not tell people what is wrong with them or how serious is their illness. Some of the Asian cultures never use the word "cancer" with their patients because they believe the patient will lose hope and will die sooner. This causes some conflict with the legal system in this country that requires informed consent. It is important to find out if there are cultural barriers or limits regarding informed consent.

In addition to resident rights, civil rights are guaranteed to all residents. Civil rights refer to the freedom from discrimination guaranteed to all citizens. This includes discrimination because of:

- Age
- Sex
- Religion
- Race
- Ethnic origin
- Physical handicap

Just as your employer may not discriminate in hiring practices, you may not discriminate in providing care or services to residents. LTC facilities provide services and care to residents of vastly different backgrounds, ethnic groups, religions, and economic levels. Regardless of whether a resident is wealthy, a private-paying resident, or a resident whose care is funded through state and federal assistance programs, *all residents must receive equally good care!*

Many facilities utilize the services of an **ombudsman** (an impartial person who investigates complaints and acts as an advocate for residents and/or families). The ombudsman is provided access to the resident, resident records, and facility personnel, as well as any other information needed to gather information or facts related to a complaint.

ombudsman an impartial person who investigates complaints and acts as an advocate for residents and/or families

LEGAL RESPONSIBILITIES

In addition to the residents' rights and civil rights, residents are protected by the laws that apply to everyone. Striking or handling a resident roughly or stealing from a resident are examples of crimes punishable by law.

As a nursing assistant, you also have legal responsibility regarding the accuracy or exactness of information you write in the resident's health record, which is a legal document.

A legal term related to providing care is **negligence.** This is the failure to act as an average nursing assistant would act under the same circumstances.

Gross negligence is more serious. Gross negligence occurs when the person responsible shows so little care that it appears that he or she is indifferent to the welfare of others.

Examples of negligence are:

negligence failure to act as an average nursing assistant would act under the same circumstances

gross negligence person responsible shows so little care that it appears that he or she is indifferent to the welfare of others

- A nursing assistant fails to raise the side rails on the resident's bed, and the resident falls out of bed.
- A nursing assistant leaves a helpless resident unattended in the bathtub.
- A nursing assistant fails to perform assigned nursing care, such as repositioning or feeding a helpless resident.
- A nursing assistant takes a resident outdoors on a sunny day. The resident is left out too long and receives a sunburn.

Other important legal terms and definitions you should know are:

- **Assault**—A threat or an unsuccessful attempt to commit bodily harm
- **Battery**—An assault that is actually carried out (the person is actually harmed in some way)
- **False imprisonment**—Detaining or restraining a person without proper consent (placing a resident in restraints without the order of a physician or using restraints for the wrong reasons)

assault threat or unsuccessful attempt to commit bodily harm

battery assault that is carried out, resulting in harm to another person

false imprisonment keeping or restraining a person without proper consent

Residents have the right under OBRA to be protected from neglect and abuse, whether verbal, physical, or sexual. They have the right to be protected from any mistreatment, including involuntary seclusion, which means that a resident is separated from others against his or her will.

State laws require that any actual or suspected abuse be reported by health care professionals as elder abuse. *No one* may abuse, neglect, or mistreat a resident, whether it be facility staff, volunteers, family, friends, legal guardians, or other residents. All long-term care facilities must have written policies and procedures for investigating reported or suspected cases of abuse.

As a nursing assistant, you have a legal responsibility to report to your charge nurse any events you observe or hear about that might be considered abuse.

You can protect yourself against legal actions by:

- Understanding and protecting the resident's rights
- Providing care in accordance with facility policies and procedures
- Documenting care provided promptly and accurately
- Observing and reporting changes in a resident's condition promptly
- Asking for help when you are not sure how to perform a task safely
- Providing care in accordance with the approved plan of care
- Reporting any suspected abuse of a resident by anyone

ETHICAL CODE OF CONDUCT

In addition to following legal guidelines, a nursing assistant must also follow a **code of ethics.** This is a code of conduct for a particular group, the do's and don'ts for group members.

Some examples of ethical behavior for nursing assistants are:

- Assisting any resident in need whether or not you are assigned to that resident
- Reporting to work as scheduled
- Doing your best every day
- Avoiding gossip about residents and their families (Figure 1-9)

Occasionally, a resident or family member may offer to pay or tip you to ensure special treatment for their loved one. It is unethical to accept money under these circumstances.

When situations arise that involve ethical behavior, ask yourself these questions to help you to make a decision. When you carefully consider your actions, you will make decisions that will not be harmful to yourself or others.

- How will my actions affect my residents?
- How will my actions affect my fellow workers?
- How will my actions affect my employer?
- How will my actions affect me?

CONFIDENTIALITY OF RESIDENT INFORMATION

An important legal and ethical responsibility is related to confidentiality of resident information. **Confidentiality** comes from two Latin words, *con* (with) and *fides* (faith or trust). Confidentiality, then, means "with trust."

Confidentiality guarantees the resident's right to privacy. It is based on the assumption that all personal and medical information will remain private and will be used only as nec-

code of ethics rules of conduct for a particular group

confidentiality not revealing private information to others

FIGURE 1-9

Avoid gossip about residents.

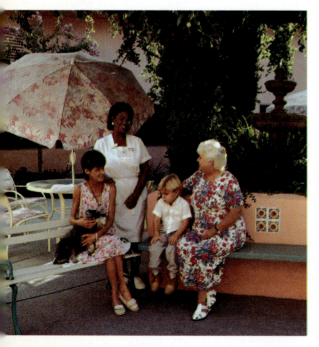

essary to provide care or treatment. It is unethical and sometimes illegal to violate a resident's right to privacy.

Invasion of privacy is a legal term used to describe circumstances when personal information is exposed publicly that violates an individual's right to privacy. An example of invasion of privacy would be as follows: A resident receives a letter stating that her son is in jail. The nursing assistant reads the letter without permission and relates this information to others in the facility. This is an invasion of privacy.

The resident's **chart** (health record) is a legal document. It is the property of the health care facility. As a nursing assistant, you are trusted to guard information contained in the chart. It is sometimes tempting to reveal information to your family or friends. This is always unethical and sometimes illegal and is punishable by law.

As a general rule, do not discuss personal information with:

- One resident about another resident
- Relatives and friends of the resident
- Visitors
- Representatives of news media
- Fellow workers, except when there is a need to know
- Your own relatives and friends

A legal and ethical problem closely related to confidentiality is **defamation of character,** which means to make false or damaging statements or misrepresentations about another person that defame or injure his or her reputation. There are two types of defamation of character: **slander** (a spoken statement) and **libel** (a written statement). Gossip is a type of slander.

THEFT AND LOSS

An important quality-of-life issue is the right of residents to keep and use their personal possessions. Residents often enter a long-term care center bringing with them their most treasured possessions. These personal items may not be replaceable. The resident's property must be treated with care and respect. The facility is responsible for safeguarding residents' personal belongings; however, residents and families are advised not to bring large amounts of cash or jewelry into the facility. The facility must investigate all reports of lost, stolen, or damaged personal possessions. It is your responsibility to observe and report any incidents or suspected incidents of theft to your supervisor immediately; doing so will help create an atmosphere in your facility making theft unacceptable. Residents of long-term care facilities have usually given up their homes and most of their personal belongings; those that they bring with them are often their most cherished possessions. It is an inhuman act to steal from those who have already given up so much!

Personal clothing items often become lost during the laundering processes. Be sure to remind visitors to clearly mark the resident's clothing upon admission and include all items in the admission inventory list. When new items are brought in, be sure to add them to the inventory list. Make every effort to place personal belongings in the appropriate closets and drawers; lost items become a source of great frustration to both residents and their families.

invasion of privacy when personal information is exposed publicly, violating an individual's right to privacy

chart written health or medical record, which is a legal document

defamation of character making false or damaging statements about another person which injure his or her reputation

slander a verbal type of defamation of character

libel a written type of defamation of character

SECTION 4 Personal Qualities

When you have completed this section, you will be able to:

- Evaluate yourself by completing the personal qualities assessment provided in the Student Workbook
- Determine if you are a good listener

- Explain how to tell the difference between information that should remain private and information that should be passed on to the charge nurse
- List five traits most beneficial in a helping relationship
- Give two examples of acceptable ways to control angry feelings

- Give three examples of what it means to be dependable
- Describe the signs that may indicate that the CNA is experiencing unusual stress
- List three ways of coping with stress in healthy ways

KEY TERMS

accuracy
caring
communication

courteously
empathy
genuineness
respect

tact
touch
warmth

DESIRABLE PERSONAL QUALITIES OF THE NURSING ASSISTANT

As you can see, fulfilling the many responsibilities of a nursing assistant takes a special kind of person. What kind of person makes a good nursing assistant?

That question was asked of over 400 nursing home residents in a recent nationwide study regarding what makes up quality care and a quality environment. The *staff* was named as the number one factor in determining quality care. The residents said that they need a caring staff who are well trained and skilled. Good staff give the residents help when they need it. They give this help in a kind, courteous, and respectful manner. Residents also want staff to be friendly, cheerful, and pleasant as well as being patient and interested and taking time. Finally, they want staff who listen, take their complaints seriously, and talk to them.

Certain traits, habits, and attitudes are seen in people of all occupations who are successful in their work. Some of these traits are a part of one's personality. In other words, you have always had them. Others can be learned through practice until they become part of your personality. It's important to reflect and decide how you see yourself. How you feel about yourself really influences how you feel about others.

Sit in a quiet place and review the Personal Qualities Assessment contained in your Student Workbook. Take time to think about these qualities and answer honestly. Place a check by the qualities you would like to develop further and describe in the space provided how you will begin. Set some time-limited goals. Review these each week and judge your progress. This is confidential information, so keep it in a private place where you can review and update it.

COMMUNICATION

In working through the Personal Qualities Assessment, did you notice how many elements dealt with some aspect of communication? One of the most important things you do as a nursing assistant is *communicate.* You communi-

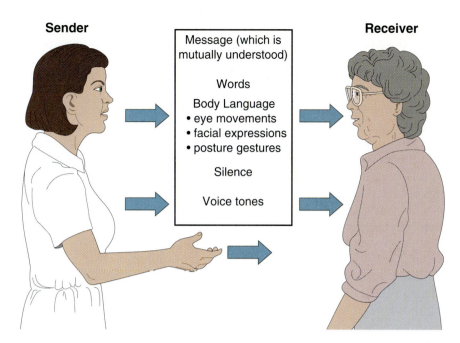

Sender

Receiver

Message (which is mutually understood)

Words

Body Language
• eye movements
• facial expressions
• posture gestures

Silence

Voice tones

FIGURE 1-10

Elements of communication.

cate with residents, families, visitors, and other members of the health care team. Most interpersonal problems that develop both at work and at home are due to a lack of communication. In order for communication to take place, three components are needed (Figure 1-10).

- A sender
- A message
- A receiver

If any of the three elements is missing, no communication can take place.

When communication takes place, the sender translates ideas into words. The sender also uses gestures, facial expressions, and body language to help the receiver understand the message. The receiver then translates the words and nonverbal observations back into ideas. Usually, the receiver understands what the sender wanted to convey.

Communication takes place with words as in speaking and writing or without words (nonverbal) through facial expressions, tone of voice, gestures, body position, and movement. We communicate all the time. Even as you read these words, you may be frowning with concentration, nodding with understanding, or yawning with boredom. In fact, it is generally felt that nonverbal communication is more accurate than communicating with words because we have less ability to control our nonverbal communications (Figure 1-11).

Touch is another important form of communication. In all cultures, gentle touching conveys friendliness and affection. Studies about touch show that

communication involves a sender, a message, and a receiver; it may take place in speaking or writing, or without words through facial expressions, tone of voice, gestures, body position, and movement

touch form of communication that conveys friendliness and affection

FIGURE 1-11

Facial expression is communication.

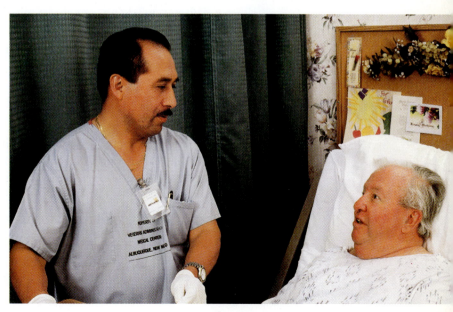

women are touched more than men and that the age group touched the least is persons aged 66 to 100. Other studies have proved that people need to be touched. Those who are not develop both physical and emotional problems.

There is some risk involved in touching unfamiliar people for the first time. For some, touch is a sign of intimacy and closeness that is reserved for certain people. For this reason, when first meeting a new resident, ask permission or find out how the person feels about being touched. For most people, though, a warm handshake or a pat on the shoulder or the back is an acceptable way of communicating your acceptance and caring.

Communication with words is important, too. Words are symbols of ideas, objects, feelings, and actions. Unfortunately, many words have several meanings or mean different things to different people. Common words that teenagers use, for example, are either often misunderstood or not understood at all by their parents.

In the medical profession, words are often used that the general public does not understand. You will be learning some of this special language or jargon. Medical terminology must be used with care when communicating with residents or in the presence of residents, family, and visitors. Misunderstanding could cause the resident unnecessary worry.

Another sensitive communication issue is talking in any language the resident does not understand. It is rude and improper for two staff members to speak another language in the presence or within the hearing range of a resident. When the resident speaks a language that the majority of the staff do not understand, it is important for the facility to locate a person who can translate and interpret for the resident.

Learn to communicate with your residents as you provide care. Avoid profanity or slang when you are in the health care setting. Remember that your goal is to understand and to be understood.

There are some "golden rules" to help you to be a better communicator. Practice these skills at home and with friends, as well as in your facility:

- Encourage the resident to express himself or herself more fully.
- Listen for the feelings being expressed, not just the words themselves.
- Avoid statements that negate the resident's feelings, such as "don't worry," "things aren't so bad," "you're really very lucky," and so on.
- Don't take away hope, but don't give false reassurance.
- When you are unsure about what a resident means, clarify by asking "Is this what you mean?" or "Do I understand you correctly?"
- Be courteous! Avoid rushing the resident, maintain good eye contact, and don't interrupt!

LISTENING SKILLS

Understanding requires good listening skills (Figure 1-12). In fact, communication can't take place without a listener or receiver. Test yourself with the questions that follow.

ARE YOU A GOOD LISTENER?

Ask yourself if these statements apply to you:

1. I never interrupt when another person is speaking.
2. While the other person is talking, I plan what I'm going to say next.

3. I try to nod, smile, and say, "Yes, tell me more."
4. I keep a "poker face" when listening.
5. I don't judge whether a person is good or bad, right or wrong.
6. I maintain eye contact when a person is talking to me.
7. I give my complete attention to the person who is talking.
8. I usually finish the sentence when a person is unable to find the right word.

If you answered yes to 1, 3, 5, 6, and 7, you are a good listener. If you aren't satisfied with your score, improve your listening skills by practicing. In addition to understanding how to communicate, the nursing assistant needs to know when and to whom to communicate.

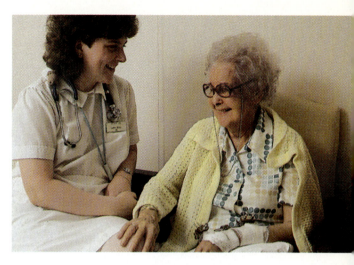

FIGURE 1-12
Are you a good listener?

DEALING WITH PERSONAL INFORMATION

As you provide care, you will learn many personal and private things about the residents. Some of these are written in their health records, and some the resident, family, or visitors will reveal to you.

In addition to the legal and ethical considerations associated with confidentiality, there is a need to treat private or personal information as a gift entrusted to your care. A good rule is not to pass on any information to other people unless they have a need to know. To determine if someone has the need to know, ask yourself:

- Does the information need to be passed on because it would have some bearing on the resident's care?
- Does the person to whom I'll relate this information need it in order to plan or provide care?

Some residents will communicate information to you that no one needs to know. Gossiping about residents or their families is unethical. If what is confided to you needs to be passed on, explain to the resident, "What you've told me is very important. I must tell the charge nurse." If what you are told has no bearing on a resident's care or treatment, you will of course keep it confidential.

The resident has the right under OBRA to privacy in his or her written communications, including the right to send and to receive mail that is unopened. The facility must assist a resident to have access to stationery, postage, and writing instruments. The resident also has the right to privacy while using the telephone, and facilities must ensure that residents are provided access to a telephone when requested.

Residents also have the right to visit with others in privacy; the facility must designate places for private visits to take place.

In an LTC facility, residents come to know each other very well. Frequently, one resident will ask you about the condition of another. Remember each resident's right to privacy and make only general comments. Do not discuss a resident's problems within hearing distance of other residents or visitors.

It is also unwise to share your personal or work-related problems with the residents. Complaints about co-workers, supervisors, or the employer are never appropriate. They may cause the resident needless worry, which affects his or her sense of safety and well-being.

COMMUNICATION WITH RESIDENTS WHO HAVE SPECIAL PROBLEMS

Some residents may seem not to hear or understand due to stroke, coma, deafness, or mental retardation, but never assume that you are not heard or understood. Treat all residents as if they can hear everything you say. Say nothing in the presence of a resident that you don't want to be heard. You may have to explain this tactfully to visitors also. Remember that at the time of death hearing is the last sense to leave the body and may even be intensified. People who describe a "near-death" experience can often repeat every word spoken during the attempts to revive them.

In addition to not saying things that you don't want the resident to hear, you must also communicate to each resident what you are going to do; for example, "I'm going to turn you on your right side now." Always explain what you are going to do, even when you aren't sure the resident understands. This may feel a little strange at first, but it's very important. You should talk to the resident as though he or she can understand and respond. In these situations, your tone of voice is also important. Never speak in a tone that would frighten the resident, and *never speak to the resident as though she or he were a child.* Terms such as "gramps," "pop," "mama," "baby," and the like should never be used unless the resident specifically asks to be addressed in that manner. All residents, regardless of their condition, need to feel that they are respected, valued members of society.

Even though the resident may not be able to communicate due to loss of hearing, stroke, or confusion, the need for communication still exists. There are some nursing measures designed to establish communication with residents who have these special problems, which you will study in another chapter.

ANSWERING THE CALL LIGHT

Answering the resident's call light is an important form of communication. It is a legal requirement that every resident have a mechanism that sends a signal, light, or bell to the nursing station. It is also necessary for residents to be able to reach the signal cord at all times. Most call systems operate so that when the button is pushed or the switch is turned on a light flashes above the door of the resident's room and at the nursing station. The flashing light is accompanied by a signal at the nursing station, such as a bell or buzzer.

FIGURE 1-13

Answering the call light.

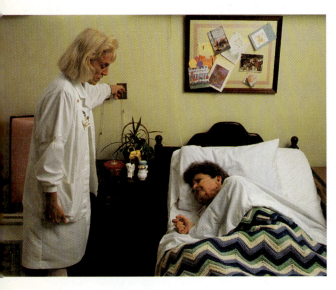

You must be alert and respond to the resident's call for help immediately (Figure 1-13). To a waiting resident, every minute seems like forever. Failure to respond promptly sends a negative message to the resident.

Residents often express the fear that no one will respond if they have an emergency. In the nursing home study conducted by interviewing nursing home residents, the most important indicator of quality care was getting help when they need it. Answering the call light promptly is one of the most important ways you can show a resident that you care!

Caution: Some residents are unable or unwilling to use the signal cord. These residents must be checked frequently to see if they need assistance. It is a good habit to check with the resident before leaving the room and ask, "Is there anything else I can do before I go?" Always be alert for cries of help or unusual sounds that would indicate that a resident is in trouble. Never ignore a cry for help.

Residents who have serious hearing or vision loss may use the signal cord differently. *Blind or visually handicapped residents always must be taught how to use the signal.* Help them locate the cord and assist them in practicing how to use it. If the signal is the kind that you push to turn on, you can call it a push button. If it works like a light switch, you can compare it to that.

Most facilities equip bathrooms and bathing areas with emergency call signals. These usually ring loudly and have a flashing red light. These indicate an emergency and must be answered *immediately* by any personnel in the area. Of course, you must never jeopardize the safety of one resident to respond to the call of another. Always leave the resident in a safe place or position if you must go.

Communication is the foundation of any relationship. Relating to people means making a connection between yourself and another human being. The relationship between yourself, residents, visitors, and fellow workers depends on your approach to them. If you have a kind, courteous, tactful, sympathetic, and open manner, you will find it easier to form positive, rather than negative, relationships.

THE HELPING RELATIONSHIP

Research has been done to determine which traits are most beneficial in a helping relationship. The traits include empathy, respect, genuineness, warmth, and caring (Figure 1-14).

Empathy is the ability to put yourself in another's place and to see things as he or she sees them.

Respect is recognition of the worth of another person. When you respect others, you recognize their right to make up their own minds and to make good decisions.

Genuineness is simply being yourself. When your actions match what you say, you are genuine. Remember, actions speak louder than words.

Warmth is shown by demonstrating concern and affection. A nursing assistant shows warmth by the way care is given, demonstrating kindness, patience, and a gentle touch.

Caring is understanding the fears, problems, and distress of another person combined with concern and a desire to help. Caring requires action. As a nursing assistant, you can demonstrate caring in many ways: answering the call bell promptly, offering fluids to the resident, and being sure that the resident is clean and well groomed. Caring is *doing*, not just feeling.

Other personal qualities that enhance relationships with residents, visitors, and staff are courtesy, emotional control, and tact.

Behaving **courteously** means putting the needs of others before your own. It means cooperating, sharing, and giving. Being polite and considerate of others shows that you care about them. Putting the needs of others first may mean toning down your cheerfulness around a person who is in pain, very ill, or depressed. Or it may mean putting aside your own gloomy feelings to be more cheerful and positive. It is never appropriate to burden the residents with your personal problems. As you gain more experience in nursing, you will learn to "read" the feelings of others and to judge how you should respond.

empathy   the ability to put oneself in another's place

respect   recognition of the worth of another person

genuineness   being yourself

warmth   demonstrating concern and affection

caring   compassion; understanding fears, problems, and distress of another

courteously   putting the needs of others before your own

FIGURE 1-14

The helping relationship.

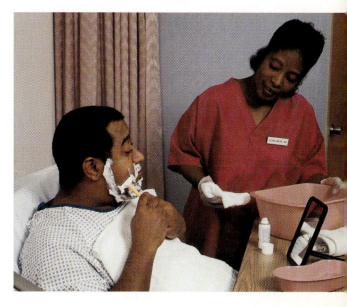

EMOTIONAL CONTROL

Sometimes a resident, another staff member, or a visitor can upset you so much that you get angry. You may feel like making a rude or unkind remark. *Don't!* Stop and think. The resident or visitor may be worried, nervous, or tense. Fellow workers may be under extra stress because of a problem at home or on the job. Try to be understanding, and your anger will fade. Feeling angry is natural, but you should control the way anger is expressed. You have a serious obligation to control your temper. You may have to remove yourself from the situation to "cool off."

We all have different ways of "cooling off," depending on what we were taught as children and what we saw others doing. Physical activity is a common way to cope with anger. Another way that people control their anger is by talking. Simply saying "I am angry" really gives a great sense of relief. Both are acceptable, appropriate ways to express anger.

A nursing assistant must learn to accept criticism and constructive suggestions without becoming hurt or defensive. When your supervisor criticizes you or tells you to do something, you may feel like saying, "That is not my job," or "Why do you pick on me?" Stop, think, and examine your attitude!

Frequently, your supervisor has information that you may not be aware of. Sometimes decisions have to be based on what is best overall, not on what is best for just one person. Your understanding of that fact, as well as a cooperative attitude, will be admired and appreciated.

TACT

tact the ability to say or do the right thing at the right time

Tact is the ability to say or do the right thing at the right time. Every resident sees her or his own problems as being most important. Listen to their concerns. Don't judge or give advice. Everyone has a right to his or her feelings. They shouldn't be judged as right or wrong. You will learn how to help residents to deal more effectively with their own feelings as you become more aware of residents' emotional needs.

All relationships are two sided. Even though you communicate well and employ all the traits essential to a helping relationship, you may not get the response you desire. Many things influence the residents' behavior—their personality, physical health, emotional health, and life experiences. Understanding why residents respond as they do will help you to accept their behavior and deal with it appropriately. You will learn more about dealing with difficult behavior in Chapter 3.

DEALING WITH FAMILIES AND VISITORS

Family and visitors often are the highlight of the day for residents. Knowing that one's family and friends are interested and concerned can relax tensions, ease feelings of loneliness and isolation, and reduce fears. Family members or visitors may be worried and upset over a resident's illness. They, too, need your kindness and patience.

You may find the following suggestions helpful when dealing with families and visitors:

- Listen to the visitor or family member. Whether it is a suggestion, a complaint, or just passing the time of day, listen! Some ideas or suggestions may be very helpful. Some complaints could be valid, others not. When a complaint is presented, try to obtain all the facts. Tell the visitor that you'll report it to the charge nurse. If it seems appropriate, take the visitor to the charge nurse so they can speak directly.

- Avoid involvement in family matters. Don't take sides in quarrels. Never give confidential information about the resident to family or visitors.
- Answer questions to the best of your ability. If you are unable or unsure of what to say, refer visitors to the charge nurse.

Generally, there are certain rules that family and visitors are asked to follow:

- Family and visitors are not allowed to remove any facility property.
- Family and visitors are not permitted to bring food, beverages, or smoking materials to the resident without checking with the charge nurse.
- Family and visitors are not permitted to provide technical nursing services for residents.

Residents and visitors often attribute their own feelings of helplessness, anger, or guilt to others. You may have these feelings projected toward you. Try to understand and be patient, courteous, and professional, even when others are not.

ESTABLISHING A GOOD EMPLOYEE–EMPLOYER RELATIONSHIP

When you do your job to the best of your ability and work cooperatively with your fellow workers, you have taken the most important steps in establishing a good relationship with your employer (Figure 1-15). All health-care facilities are organized to function efficiently with a certain number of people assigned to specific jobs. When employees are not dependable, everyone suffers, especially the residents.

Accuracy is part of being dependable. **Accuracy** means doing the right thing for the right resident at the right time in the right way. Always identify the resident before performing any nursing task. Check the resident's wrist band or photograph and verify accuracy by asking the resident his or her name. If there is no wrist band, notify the charge nurse immediately.

Make sure you know how to do what you are assigned to do. Follow established policies and procedures to reduce errors or mistakes while providing care. If you are unsure of what to do, ask for help. Never take chances when your work deals with the welfare and safety of others.

Should an error or mistake occur despite your best efforts, report the incident to your charge nurse immediately. No one is perfect, and mistakes do happen. An error becomes a serious legal issue if it is not reported and appropriate corrective actions are not taken.

REWARDS AND STRESSES OF THE CNA ROLE

After learning about the many demands on the nursing assistant to behave professionally at all times, you may have concerns about your ability to cope. A recent study was done to determine the sources of motivation in the job of the nursing assistant. The number one reason

accuracy factual or being correct

FIGURE 1-15

What being dependable means:

- Report to work on time
- Keep absence to a minimum
- Keep promises
- Do an assigned task as well as you can and finish it quickly, quietly, and efficiently
- Perform a task you know should be done without having to be told

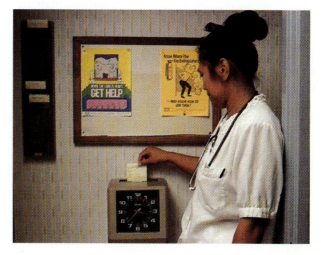

CNAs reported that they remain CNAs is the satisfaction of caring for others. While this is what motivates them and keeps them working, it does not always reduce the job stress. The stresses that most nursing assistants report include:

- Coping with residents' deaths
- Communication difficulties
- Conflict with family members
- Dealing with difficult behavior on the part of residents
- Balancing work and home life

Some of the things you will learn in your training will help you to cope by giving you skill in dealing with other staff and residents and their family members. It is important, however, to learn some techniques that help you to deal with stress. First, it is important to recognize stress when you are experiencing it. General signs of stress include:

- Difficulty relaxing or slowing down
- Overreacting to small events or problems
- Having trouble sleeping
- Increase in use of alcohol or drugs in order to "relax"
- Weight gain or weight loss
- Feeling very weak and tired
- Short attention span
- Having trouble getting out of bed and going to work
- Headaches and neck aches
- Friends and family complaining that you are "not yourself"

Sometimes grief over the deaths of residents looks like stress. It is important to recognize grief when it is occurring. Grief and its signs will be discussed in the chapter on end-of-life care. There are many ways of coping with stress. Most people have identified what works for them, but there may be a successful method that you have not thought of or tried. Remember that good health practices are necessary to cope with stress. That means getting adequate rest, eating three balanced meals per day, and obtaining regular exercise. Avoid smoking, drinking excess alcohol, and taking unnecessary drugs. Be sure you visit your physician or health clinic on a recommended basis. Follow the good hygiene practices that you will be learning to prevent acquiring or spreading diseases.

One strategy that is basic to all stress reduction is effective breathing. Learn to breathe slowly by inhaling through the nose and exhaling through the mouth. Count to five as you inhale, then exhale to a count of five. Breathe deeply using your abdominal muscles and try to blow out all the air in your lungs. To relax your muscles, first tighten or tense them, then release and relax. Some people start at the top of their head and work down to their toes while others begin with the toes and work their way up to the face and head, systematically tensing the muscles three times and relaxing. Other strategies include physical activity such as walking, biking, swimming, or playing sports. Some find talking, reading, taking a bubble bath, watching a movie, playing a musical instrument, or singing to be helpful. A popular method that may help you is writing in a journal. Books filled with blank pages are readily available at book and stationery stores. This journal allows you to express your thoughts and feelings in a private way. You can write anything you want without fear of judgment. It is always interesting and helpful to review what you wrote in the past and compare with your current feelings and thoughts.

SECTION 5 The Health Care Team

OBJECTIVES
What You Will Learn

When you have completed this section, you will be able to:

- Describe your goal for higher or continuing education and list the steps necessary to reach that goal
- Match the members of the health care team with their major responsibilities

KEY TERMS interdisciplinary

THE HEALTH CARE TEAM

The nursing assistant is an essential part of the health-care team (Figure 1-16). You actually will provide more direct care than all the other members of the team. Teamwork is essential. Teamwork means that everyone knows what is to be done and does it to the best of her or his ability with a spirit of cooperation.

The health care team is **interdisciplinary,** meaning that professionals with different educational backgrounds work together. They assess and evaluate the needs of the resident and together plan how to provide care and services that will meet these identified needs. The health care plan becomes a written source of all these collected facts.

Interdisciplinary a group of health care workers from different professions who work together to provide care to residents

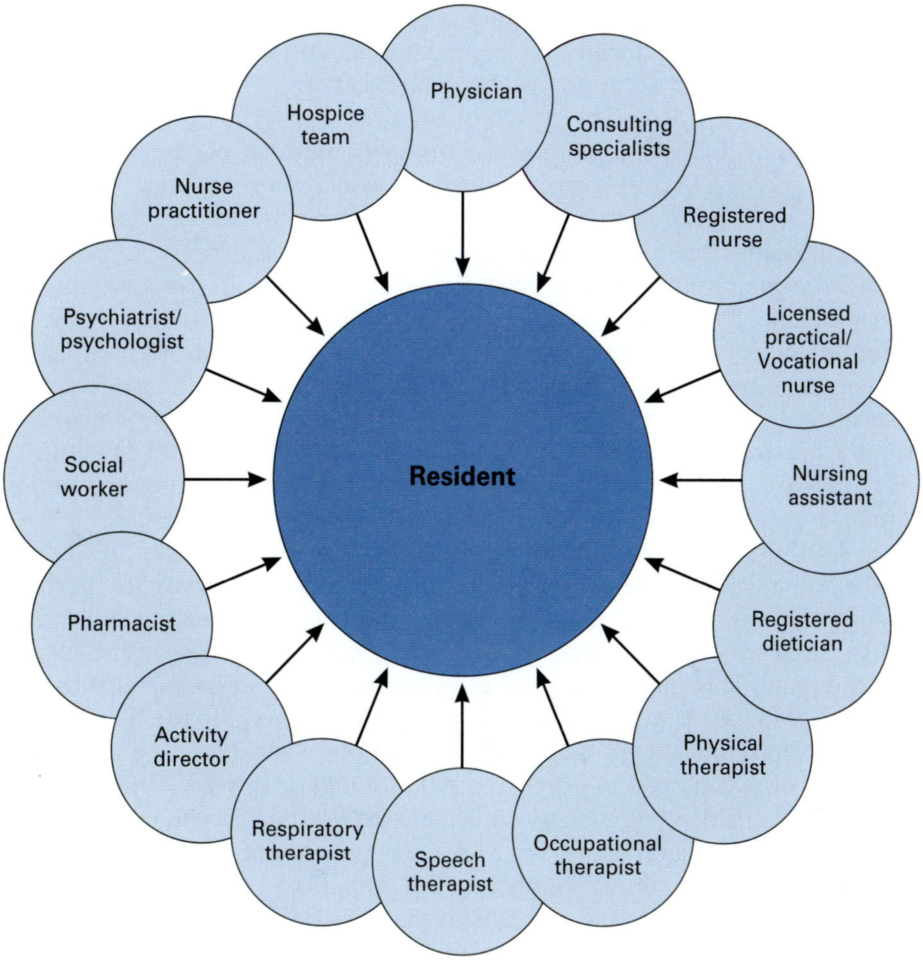

FIGURE 1-16
Health care team.

See the "Roles and Responsibilities of the Health Care Team" review chart provided in the Student Workbook. You may be interested in learning more about some of the different professions. You can obtain additional information regarding educational requirements, prerequisites, and locations of programs by writing to the professional organizations listed. Request information specifically for the state in which you plan to continue your education since programs differ from state to state.

Being a nursing assistant is an important job in itself. However, if you find your work enjoyable and rewarding, consider continuing your education in the field of nursing. If you do not have a high school diploma, that should be your first goal. Local high schools offer basic education programs that lead to a high school equivalency diploma.

LTC facilities also have organized inservice education or staff development programs. In general, this department is responsible for:

- Orientation of new employees
- Providing continuing education for licensed and nonlicensed nursing personnel (often called inservice)
- Organizing, planning, and implementing nursing assistant training programs
- Bedside teaching, demonstrating nursing care procedures, and supervising return demonstrations
- Classroom teaching and testing
- Providing instruction in the use of hospital equipment and supplies

Federal regulations now require special training for all nursing assistants employed in an LTC facility. Each state adopts and establishes its own nursing assistant certification program, which meets the requirements of the federal program (OBRA). The program requires a specific number of hours of classroom or theory attendance and a specific number of hours of clinical or bedside practice. Some programs allow you to take a test and demonstrate skills instead of requiring hours. Training may be offered by the LTC facilities, public educational institutions, and private vocational schools. The OBRA regulations that require nurse assistant training also require an examination or test to show that the training was effective. A competency examination or evaluation includes both a written and a skills test. The examinations are taken following completion of an approved course. For more information to help you successfully pass your test, refer to the Student Workbook. Some states also require nursing assistants to attend a certain number of hours of continuing education each year. Be sure that you know what your state requires, and plan time to seek out new learning experiences.

As a member of the health care team, you will be expected to work with others in a way that helps the team to reach the goal of good care for the resident. Being a member of a team means that you have a responsibility to the other members to help them, cooperate with them, and share in the successes of the team. This means that the team members are there to help you when you need it, too. Many duties of the nurse assistant require the help of others. If you help them, they'll help you. For example, a resident may need the assistance of two people in order to get out of bed or to walk. When you work effectively as a team, you show consideration for the other members by communicating ("I need help getting Mrs. Jones out of bed. What would be a good time for you?") and doing as much of the preparation as you can before seeking help. This prevents the other team member from wasting time waiting to help or from helping with tasks for which no help is really needed. Courtesy is an essential part of teamwork. When you need help, ask, don't demand. Be sure to thank team members for their help.

The job of the nursing assistant carries with it great responsibility for the health, safety, and comfort of other human beings. When you fulfill this responsibility, you enjoy many rewards. The satisfaction of giving your best, the appreciation of your employer, and the gratitude of the residents and their families all contribute to a positive feeling. It is a good feeling to help those who are sick, lonely, frightened, and confused toward a better quality of life. Knowing that even one person is better off because of your efforts means that you have fulfilled your role and responsibilities as a nursing assistant.

SUMMARY
In this chapter you have learned about the types of long-term care facilities and the conditions that bring the residents to them. You learned that facilities provide care for people who cannot care for themselves and care to help rehabilitate or restore previous abilities. There are many special facilities designed to meet the unique needs of all individuals who need care. These include subacute, Alzheimer's, ICFMR, and others. There are many regulations and laws that you must learn and follow, including the right of the residents to self-determination, the right to privacy and confidentiality, and the right to have their property respected.

Provision of long-term care requires a team of skilled health care workers including the nursing assistant. The staff must have not only skills but also personal characteristics in order to provide the highest quality of care. Many of these qualities can be learned, while others are traits that you bring to the job. The role of the nursing assistant is so important that behaving in a legal and ethically appropriate manner is a must. This includes always treating each and every resident with courtesy and respect. You also learned how to listen and communicate, as well as effective strategies for residents who have difficult behaviors.

Being a good nurse assistant and a good employee means learning how to care for you and to cope with the stresses of the job.

OBRA HIGHLIGHTS

The OBRA passed in 1991 addressed the rights of all patients to refuse unwanted medical care and to make decisions in advance. Some residents are fearful about refusing medical treatment because they fear the displeasure of their physician and health care team. They often believe that they must accept all treatments offered. It is common to hear residents state that the doctor wouldn't suggest a treatment if he or she didn't think it was helpful. The nursing assistant often knows more about what the resident is thinking than even his own family. He may share with you his hopes, fears, and concerns. You must share this information with the charge nurse so that those who need to know can be informed. In all cases, the resident's right to refuse treatment must be honored.

SELF STUDY

Choose the best answer for each question or statement.

1. Which of the following is **not** a type of long-term care facility?
   a. a facility for those with developmental disabilities
   b. ICFMR (intermediate care facility for the mentally retarded)
   c. a facility that provides acute and critical care
   d. a facility that provides rehabilitation services

2. Which of the following is true of Medicare payment for long-term care?
   a. Medicare covers long-term care only when certain eligibility requirements are met.
   b. Medicare covers long-term care for all people over the age of 65.
   c. Medicare covers only long-term care costs for very poor people.
   d. Medicare will pay 50 percent of the long-term care costs for those over 65.

3. What can happen if you are working as a certified nursing assistant and you are absent from work without notifying your supervisor?
   a. You could lose your nursing assistant certification.
   b. You could be disciplined or lose your job.
   c. You could be forced to work overtime.
   d. Nothing would happen; this occurs often.

4. You discover that someone in the housekeeping department has left a cleaning solution out where a resident could accidentally drink it. What should you do?
   a. Tell the housekeeper who made the error.
   b. Tell the head of the housekeeping department about the error.
   c. Tell the director of nursing about the error.
   d. Tell your immediate supervisor about the error.

5. A nursing assistant misunderstands his assignment and fails to provide care for a patient during his shift. Who is responsible for this failure?

   a. the charge nurse
   b. the director of nursing
   c. the nursing assistant
   d. no one; mistakes can happen

6. The Patient Self-Determination Act (PSDA) requires all health care facilities to notify residents and patients about which of the following?
   a. how to file a grievance about care received in the facility
   b. their right to consent to or to refuse any medical treatment
   c. residents' rights granted under both state and federal laws
   d. the number of deaths that occur in the facility each year

7. Which of the following are decisions that might be included in an advance directive?
   a. use of cardiopulmonary resuscitation
   b. use of artifical ventilation to breathe
   c. use of artificial feeding through a tube
   d. all of the above

8. Mrs. Marshall is a resident in a long-term care facility. She is often left in her room during activities because she is blind and cannot see to participate. This is an example of
   a. discrimination due to a physical handicap
   b. appropriate activity for physical disabilities
   c. respecting a resident's handicap
   d. a nonsocial resident

9. What should you do if you suspect that a resident's family may be physically abusing her?
   a. Accuse the family the next time they visit.
   b. Report your observations to the charge nurse.
   c. Notify the ombudsman to investigate the situation.
   d. Say nothing, because families all get along differently.

10. While on break, several nursing assistants discuss one of the residents. They discuss his temper and different incidents that have occurred when he was angry. Which of the following could the nursing assistants be guilty of?
    a. libel
    b. invasion of privacy

c. assault

d. negligence

11. Which of the following is **not** part of communication?

a. facial expressions

b. tone of voice

c. personal qualities

d. body position

12. A resident talks to you about her cancer diagnosis. Which of the following will you use to communicate effectively with her.

a. Listen for her feelings when she talks, not just her words.

b. Reassure the resident that everything will turn out all right.

c. Tell the resident about your aunt Sue, who was cured of cancer.

d. Keep a "poker face" while you listen to the resident talk.

13. A resident tells you about her daughter's financial problems. What should you do with this information?

a. Share it with the charge nurse because the resident has told it only to you.

b. Keep it to yourself since it does not affect the resident's care.

c. Mention it at break to see if other staff members are aware of the situation.

d. Tell the nursing assistant working with you in case the resident mentions it again.

14. The emergency light in Mr. Jay's bathroom starts to ring at the same time Mrs. Melvin's call light rings. You are assigned to care for Mrs. Melvin, but another CNA is assigned to Mr. Jay. You are near Mr. Jay's room. What will you do?

a. Answer Mr. Jay's light immediately since you are near his room.

b. Answer Mrs. Melvin's light and leave Mr. Jay's light for someone else.

c. Go find the nursing assistant assigned to Mr. Jay, then answer Mrs. Melvin's light.

d. Call loudly for more nursing assistants to help answer lights.

15. Which of the following actions would you take to be accurate when performing care?

a. Keep the side rails up at all times while giving care.

b. Ask the resident his or her name before you perform any care.

c. Identify the resident using a wrist band or photograph before giving care.

d. Make a photocopy of your assignment each day.

16. Which of the following is **not** a positive way to cope with your job stress?

a. Eat balanced meals and get regular exercise.

b. Write your thoughts and feelings about work in a journal.

c. Breathe slowly in through your nose and out through your mouth.

d. Have a few alcoholic drinks with friends after work to relax.

Getting C O NN E C T E D
Multimedia Extension Activities

 www.prenhall.com/will-black

Use the above address to access the free, interactive Companion Website created for this textbook. Hear the pronunciation of the key terms in the chapter. Get instant feedback to a variety of chapter-related questions. Link to other interesting sites.

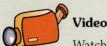 **Video**

Watch the *Patient Rights* video from the Care Provider Skills series and the *Focus on Professionalism* video.

CASE STUDY

Your neighbors just found out that you have started working in a skilled nursing facility. Their elderly mother lives with them and is losing her ability to care for herself. She is unable to feed, bathe, dress, or take herself to the bathroom. Her daughter has been caring for her but needs to have back surgery.

1. The neighbors ask you what kind of care is given in your facility. You tell them
   a. you provide rehabilitation and assistance in activities of daily living
   b. you provide classes for mentally ill
   c. you assist in performing surgical treatments
   d. you provide a nice environment but all the residents must care for themselves
2. Does their mother seem to you like an appropriate resident?
   a. yes
   b. no
3. The neighbors heard that another neighbor is a resident of the facility and ask you "What is wrong with George?" You reply
   a. "He is pretty much out of his mind. They brought him in because he wandered out of the house a few nights ago and they couldn't find him."
   b. "I can only tell what is wrong to his relatives."
   c. "We are not allowed to share any confidential information about our residents."
   d. "I don't know what is wrong with him but I would be happy to find out for you."
4. The family decides to admit their mother to the facility. They see you at work and give you $20 and say, "Please look out for mom. There is more where that came from." You respond by saying
   a. "Thank you, but I am not allowed to accept this. We look out for all of our residents."
   b. "You've given me lots of responsibility for just $20."
   c. "Thanks, I'll share it with my friend on the evening shift."
   d. "I'd prefer a check so I can deposit it."

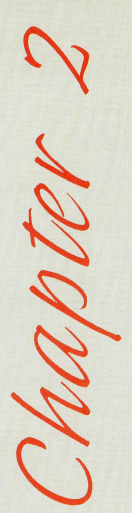

Chapter 2

YOUR WORKING
ENVIRONMENT

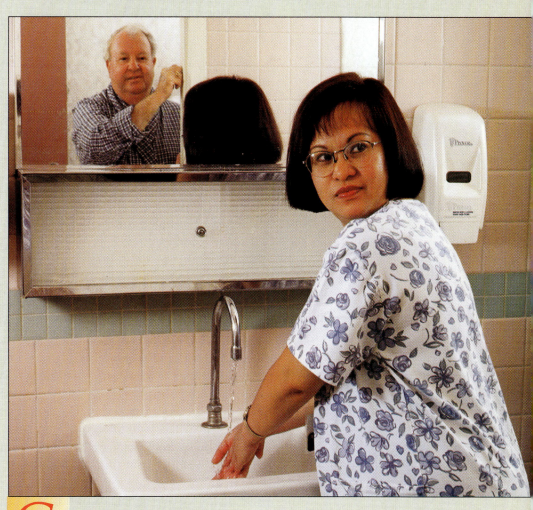

CARING TIP

A caring caregiver assures that the resident's living space is safe and free from obstacles.

Barbara Magrel, RN, MS
Horizon Career Center
Munster, IN

SECTION 1 Emergencies and Accident Prevention

When you have completed this section, you will be able to:

- Give four examples of the ways the nursing assistant helps to prevent residents from falling

- Select three ways the nursing assistant can help to prevent residents from being burned
- Demonstrate the application of a soft protective device
- Identify situations in which protective devices may be used

- Define **gravity, center of gravity, and base of support**
- Recognize safety hazards
- Demonstrate lifting an object using proper body mechanics

KEY TERMS

base of support
body mechanics

center of gravity
gatch
gravity

incident report
postural support

PROVIDING A SAFE ENVIRONMENT

Providing a safe environment is the responsibility of each facility employee. You must always protect the welfare and safety of each resident. To do this, you must be alert to potential hazards and take appropriate action as necessary to prevent accidents and injuries.

Falls in health care facilities account for almost 70 percent of all resident-related accidents! These falls occur most often at peak activity times such as mealtimes, bedtimes, and at change of shift. You can help prevent falls by:

- Answering the call light promptly so that residents who require assistance do not attempt to get out of bed without your help.
- Properly positioning residents in beds and wheelchairs, as well as using soft protective vests or seat belts when necessary.
- Following facility policies and procedures regarding the side rails. In general, side rails should be locked in the "up" position at night unless your charge nurse instructs you differently.
- Making sure that wheelchairs, beds, stretchers, and commodes have brakes locked when transferring residents.
- Keeping frequently needed articles within easy reach of the resident, such as water, bedpans, call signal cord, and TV control.

gatch handle or crank used to raise and lower the bed, head of bed, or foot of bed

- Making sure that the bed adjustment **gatch** (handle) is positioned "in" to avoid tripping over it.
- Removing any obstacle from floors and seeing that spills are wiped up immediately to prevent slipping (Figure 2-1).
- Reporting to your charge nurse your observations that a resident is prone to falling, unsteady, dizzy, slides out of a wheelchair, or climbs out of bed.
- Reporting any building hazards immediately, such as loose floor tiles or carpeting, loose or broken hand rails, and leaks in bathroom and shower areas.
- Reporting broken or malfunctioning equipment immediately. Always use facility equipment according to written policies and procedures.

PREVENTING BURNS

Burns are the second most common hazard to residents in a health care facility. Many residents have a decreased awareness of sensations of pain and temperature. The resident may not realize that the water is too hot. Some experience burns of the mouth from hot coffee without noticing. You can help prevent burns by:

- Checking water temperatures before placing residents in bath or shower.
- Reporting water temperatures that seem too hot in residents' rooms, showers, or bathing areas.
- Knowing the major causes of facility fires and practicing prevention.
- Monitoring residents, visitors, and other employees to ensure safe smoking practices. Report any violation of smoking rules to your licensed nurse immediately. Remember, smoking is permitted only in designated smoking areas.
- Providing necessary assistance to residents with meals to avoid spilling hot liquids.
- Reminding smokers not to smoke if the facility is a nonsmoking facility.
- Assisting the resident to a designated smoking area and providing supervision while the resident smokes.
- Using facility equipment (heating pads, heat lamps, hot packs, etc.) according to written policies.
- Protecting residents from overexposure to sunlight.

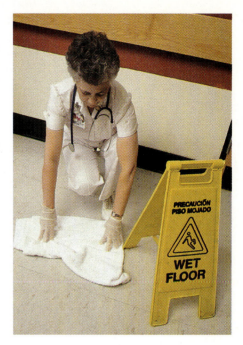

FIGURE 2-1
Being alert to potential hazards.

PREVENTING OTHER INJURIES

Residents of the LTC facility are frequently dependent on others for their care due to illness, confusion, disabilities, and even the effects of medication. For these reasons, you must be safety conscious at all times (Figure 2-2). You can help prevent other types of accidents or injuries by:

- Making sure no harmful substances are left where residents might ingest them, for example, cleaning solutions, lighter fluids, fingernail polish remover, unauthorized medications, insect sprays, or powders.

FIGURE 2-2
Being safety conscious at all times.

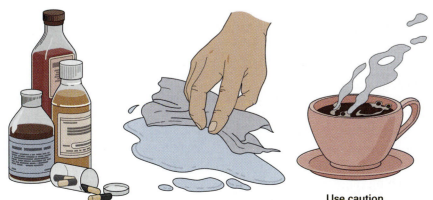

Keep harmful substances away from residents

Wipe up spills immediately

Use caution when serving hot foods or liquids

- Being alert to the potential hazards of swinging doors or doors opening into rooms or corridors.
- Moving equipment, wheelchairs, food carts, scales, and stretchers safely around corners.
- Being very careful of the feet when transporting residents in wheelchairs. Position feet on foot rests so that they are not in contact with the floor.
- Monitoring residents who may wander away. Special problems should be reported to the charge nurse immediately.
- Reporting immediately any observations that would lead you to believe that a resident is a danger to himself or others.
- Following the instructions of your charge nurse when providing care. Many times, the physician gives special orders that must be carried out or harm could come to the resident:

    No weight bearing

    Keep head of bed elevated at all times

    Do not position resident on right side

    May be out of bed with assistance only

Failure to follow physician orders has serious *legal consequences* and could cause harm to the resident.

USE OF PROTECTIVE DEVICES

postural support soft protective device or restraint used to protect a resident from injury

Many resident accidents can be avoided when soft protective devices are used and applied properly. You will need to practice the correct application of these devices. A soft protective device is often called a **postural support** or restraint. A restraint holds back or limits a resident's movements. When you restrain residents for any reason, you are infringing on their rights as individuals. For this reason, a protective device can be used *only under special conditions:*

- To protect residents from injury, such as falling from a wheelchair or out of bed
- To protect residents during treatment, such as tube feedings, intravenous therapy, or catheterization
- To keep residents from injuring themselves or others

Remember, when any type of protective device is used to restrain a resident, the physician must have given an order for its use. Postural supports include:

- Soft limb ties—used to keep a limb immobilized (Figure 2-3a).
- Vest support or crossover jacket—put on like a jacket to provide postural support in a wheelchair and limit mobility of upper body in bed (Figure 2-3b).
- Pelvic support—used between the thighs to keep a resident's hips from slipping forward. Special precautions must be used to prevent pressure on male genitalia.
- Soft cloth mittens—a mitt that limits mobility of hands and fingers. Used for residents who could harm themselves by pulling at dressings or scratching (Figure 2-3c).
- Seat belts—a belt around a resident's waist to prevent falls from a wheelchair (Figure 2-3d).

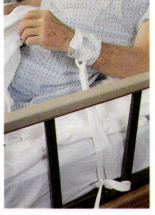
a

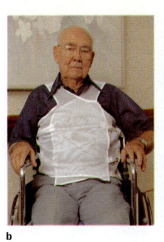
b

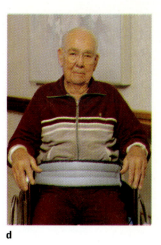
c

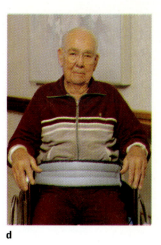
d

FIGURE 2-3

Soft protective devices: (a) soft limb tie, (b) safety vest, (c) soft cloth mitten, (d) seat belt.

Residents who require restraints must be observed at least once every 15 to 30 minutes. Check the restraint to be sure that it is not too tight and that proper circulation is maintained. Also check to see if the resident is comfortable and good body alignment is present. Make sure that the residents' special needs for hydration, toileting, and personal care are met.

A restraint *must* be released every 1 to 2 hours to allow a resident to change positions, exercise, and have periods of unrestricted movement. Gentle massage and application of lotion can help the resident relax before the restraint is reapplied.

No one likes to be confined or restrained! Restraints must be used *only as a last resort* to protect the welfare and safety of the resident or to protect others from a resident who poses a threat to them. Restraints must *never* be used as a form of punishment. Remember, use of a restraint takes away a resident's right to freedom and violates his or her right to be treated with respect and dignity.

CULTURAL AWARENESS There are some strong cultural and individual beliefs about use of restraints that may cause the resident or family to react strongly. Be aware that, for instance, a person who survived an experience of being captured or imprisoned during a war may have many strong fears about being restrained. By knowing the history of the resident and understanding their culture, you may develop a plan that is more appropriate.

ALTERNATIVES TO RESTRAINTS

When a resident is considered to be at high risk for falling or injury to self or others, various alternatives to the use of restraints need to be considered:

- Use of special devices such as wedge cushions, saddle cushions, and self-releasing safety belts. (See Figure 2-4.)
- Placing the resident in an area where he or she can be observed and monitored—near the nursing station or dining room.
- Encourage residents to participate in meaningful activities and social events.
- Pay close attention to residents' special needs and give them help when they need it (for example, answering the call light promptly).
- Establish a toileting routine for each resident, and follow it.
- Keep needed personal items within easy reach.

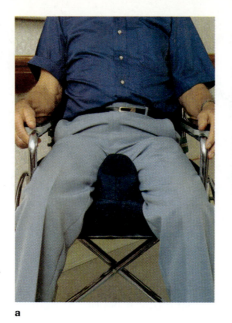 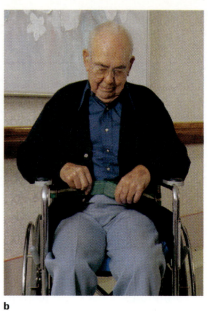

FIGURE 2-4

(a) Saddle cushion, which prevents sliding forward; (b) Self-releasing Velcro safety belt.

a   b

- Assist residents in changing positions and provide comfort measures often.
- Offer fluids and between-meal snacks and nourishments.
- Take extra time to give residents special attention.
- Encourage families and volunteers to take residents on outings.

Another way to help reduce falls is to assist residents with daily exercise designed to build muscle tone and increase strength—this will help with both walking balance and endurance. It is important to be sure that residents have properly fitted shoes with nonskid soles and that the environment is free of obstacles and spills.

REPORTING RESIDENT INCIDENTS

incident report written description of an accident involving resident, visitor, or staff member

Sometimes, despite our best efforts, accidents or incidents occur. Whenever an incident occurs involving a resident, an **incident report** must be written. An incident report is a written record of an accident involving a resident, visitor, or staff member. It is completed for insurance purposes and must be accurate and thorough. For that reason, the form is filled out as soon as possible after the event. This is true even if the resident was not injured. If you see a resident slip from a chair, find a resident on the floor, or observe any type of accident, you must report it to your charge nurse immediately so that emergency treatment and an incident report can be initiated.

BODY MECHANICS

body mechanics special ways of standing and moving one's body

Body mechanics refers to special ways of standing and moving one's body. The purpose of using good body mechanics is to maximize your strength, minimize fatigue, and, most important, avoid back strain and injury. When you understand basic principles of movement, you can make a conscious effort to use good body mechanics as you provide care.

gravity attraction that the earth has for an object on or near its surface

Gravity is the attraction that the earth has for an object on or near the earth's surface. It is the force of gravity that keeps us on the ground instead of floating in space.

APPLICATION OF SOFT PROTECTIVE DEVICES AND RESTRAINTS

When protective devices are used, follow these guidelines:

- Always approach the resident in a calm manner, regardless of his or her behavior.
- Explain to the resident (and family and visitors, if present) who you are and what you are going to do. Use terms that stress the protective nature of the restraint, such as *safety belt* and *postural support.* In the case of restraints used for certain treatments, say, "This wrist tie is to help remind you not to pull the catheter out."
- Residents should never be restrained in chairs without wheels. In the event of fire or other emergency, you must be able to move and transport residents quickly.
- When restraining a resident in a chair, tie the restraint under the chair, out of the reach of the resident, rather than tying elaborate knots that are difficult to untie in an emergency (Figure 2-5a).
- When you use any form of protective device, be sure the resident is properly aligned and comfortably positioned (see Chapter 8). Make sure

the resident is protected from pressure caused by knots, wrinkles, or buckles.

- Pad bony prominences under the device to reduce pressure and prevent trauma (see Chapter 6).
- Protective devices should be applied snugly without binding. (You should be able to slip two fingers under the edges of the device after tying.) Never restrict movement, and never impair or stop circulation (Figure 2-5b). Signs of restricted circulation include:

    Complaints of numbness or tingling
    Change in skin color (pale, blue)
    Change in skin temperature (cold)
    Swelling
    Complaints of pain

Note: Never use a "slip knot." It can tighten with movement and restrict circulation.

- Never tie restraints to side rails or a part of the bed that would cause tightening when the position of the head or foot of the bed is changed.
- Always make sure the resident can reach and use the call light when restraints are in place (Figure 2-5c).

Guidelines

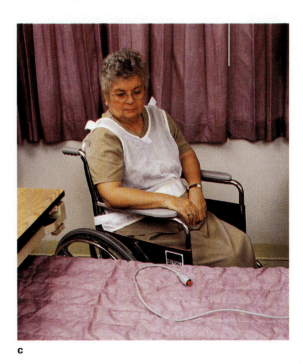

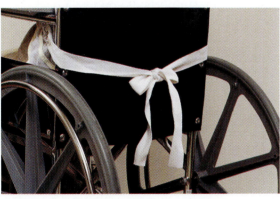

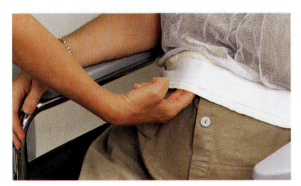

FIGURE 2-5
(a) Tie restraint out of reach; (b) slip two fingers under edge; (c) be sure call light is within reach.

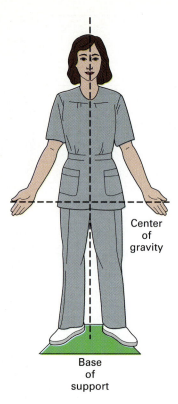

Center
of
gravity

Base
of
support

FIGURE 2-6

The line of gravity passes through the center of gravity and the base of support.

center of gravity place where the bulk or mass of an object is centered

base of support foundation of an object or person

Everything has a **center of gravity** where the mass or the bulk of the object is concentrated (Figure 2-6). Any object or person that is suspended from its center of gravity stays in balance without tipping or turning. The lower or closer the center of gravity is to earth, the more stable an object becomes.

Another term related to body mechanics is **base of support.** This is the base or foundation of an object or person. For example, when a person stands, the feet are the base of support. When the base of support is broadened, any object or person becomes better balanced and stabilized. If you stand with your feet very close together and someone tries to push you over, you can be pushed off balance very easily. As you spread your feet apart, your balance improves.

Rules to follow for good body mechanics are:

- When an action requires physical effort, try to use as many muscles or groups of muscles as possible. For example, use both hands rather than one hand to pick up a heavy object.
- Use good posture. Keep your body aligned properly. Keep your back straight. Have your knees bent. Keep your weight evenly balanced on both feet.
- Check your feet when you are going to lift something. They should be 12 inches apart. This will give you a broad base of support and good balance.
- When you have to move a heavy object, push or roll it rather than lifting and carrying it.
- Use your arms to support the object. The muscles of your legs actually do the job of lifting, not the muscles of your back.
- When you are doing work such as giving a back rub, making the bed, or moving the patient, work with the direction of your efforts. Avoid twisting your body as much as you can.
- Some organizations require use of back supports. If you use a back support you must tighten it immediately before lifting and loosen it after.
- Move your feet rather than twist your body.

LIFTING

When you lift an object, use good body mechanics (Figure 2-7):

- If you think you may not be able to lift the load or it seems too large or heavy, get help.
- Lift smoothly to avoid strain.
- Always count "one, two, three" with the person you are working with, or say "ready and go" so that you work together. Do this when lifting a resident or when helping other nursing assistants.

- Keep your feet 8–12 inches apart.
- Keep knees bent and back straight.
- Use the muscles of your thighs, not your back.
- Grip the object firmly with both hands.
- Hold the object close to your body.
- Turn your whole body; don't twist.
- Turn with short steps.
- Push or pull rather than twist.

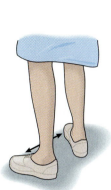
Feet 8–12
inches apart

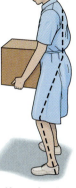
Knees bent,
back straight

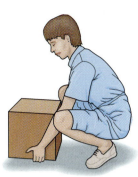
Use large muscles
of thighs to lift

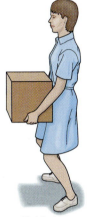
Hold object
close to body

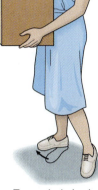
Turn whole body;
don't twist

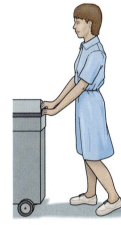
Push or pull
rather than twist

FIGURE 2-7

Correct body mechanics.

SECTION 2 Fire Safety and Disaster Preparedness

OBJECTIVES
What You Will Learn

When you have completed this section, you will be able to:

- List the three things necessary to start a fire

- List four major causes of fires in LTC facilities
- Complete a fire prevention inspection checklist for the facility where you are working or receiving clinical instruction

- Given a situation in which there is a fire, describe the correct sequence of steps to be taken
- Explain why a nursing assistant needs to know disaster plans before a disaster occurs

KEY TERM

spontaneous combustion

MAJOR CAUSES OF FIRE

Most people are aware of the dangers of fire, yet every year thousands die from fire-related causes. This occurs, to some extent, because people are not well informed regarding the causes of fire.

As a nursing assistant, you are responsible to see that residents, visitors, and employees follow the facility's smoking policies. Your facility has desig-

The Major Causes of Fire

- Smoking and matches
- Defects in heating systems
- Improper rubbish disposal
- Misuse of electricity
- Spontaneous ignition

nated smoking areas. Know where they are and politely explain to residents and visitors where smoking is permitted or is not permitted. If the rules are not followed, report these violations to your charge nurse immediately. Obviously, you and your fellow employees must always adhere to the smoking rules.

The best way to handle a fire is to prevent it! Fire prevention is aimed at keeping three elements from coming together at the same time or place. These elements are: fuel, heat, and oxygen (Figure 2-8). Because oxygen is always present, the other two elements must be controlled.

Ashtrays are potential fire hazards. A safe ashtray is made of a substance that will not burn. Never allow anyone to use paper cups or plates, trash containers, or plastic bags as ashtrays. Ashtrays must never be emptied into trash containers.

A resident's clothing may be ignited accidentally by a lighter, match, or hot ashes. Residents must be evaluated by licensed nurses to determine whether or not they are safely able to handle and keep smoking materials. For some residents, a "smoker's apron" may be needed. These fireproof aprons protect the resident and clothing from burns. Residents who are weak, confused, or taking certain medication may be dangerous to themselves and others and are not permitted to keep their own smoking materials. Sometimes families, visitors, or other residents will give smoking materials to residents. If the resident is not permitted to keep these items, explain politely, and ask them to give the materials to the charge nurse for safekeeping.

Misuse of electricity is the second most common cause of fire (Figure 2-9). You can help prevent electrical fires by:

- Checking appliances for frayed wires, loose connections, or defective plugs before use. Report problems immediately.
- Not overloading circuits or overheating equipment.
- Using extension cords safely. Never place extension cords under rugs or drapes where they can become worn and cause a spark.
- Checking plugs to ensure that they have three prongs; one is used for grounding.

FIGURE 2-8

The three elements needed to start a fire.

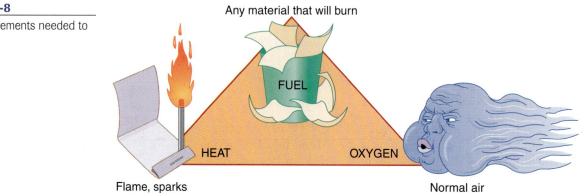

Any material that will burn

FUEL

HEAT   OXYGEN

Flame, sparks   Normal air

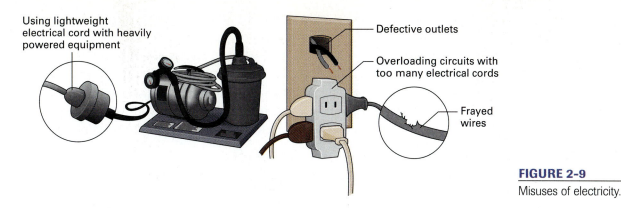

FIGURE 2-9
Misuses of electricity.

Defects in heating systems represent the third most common cause of fires. It is generally the responsibility of the maintenance department to ensure that the heating system is operating safely. However, you must be alert and report dirty heating outlets, vents, or smoke coming from any vent immediately.

Spontaneous combustion (ignition of burnable materials caused by a chemical reaction) may occur when dirty, oily rags are placed in poorly ventilated spaces or closets. Be alert. If you smell something burning, investigate! If the door to a closet or storage area is hot, never open it. This would cause the fire to spread. Report this potential fire immediately!

When trash and rubbish are not properly disposed of, a fire hazard is created. Aerosol cans require special handling as they can rupture and create flying metal if incinerated. Aerosol cans should never be sprayed in the presence of an open flame or lighted cigarette. Make sure that you understand how to dispose of trash in your facility.

spontaneous combustion ignition of burnable materials caused by a chemical reaction

OXYGEN SAFETY

Remember, oxygen is one of the three elements necessary to start a fire. Oxygen does not burn, but an oxygen-rich atmosphere will intensify the burning of ordinary combustibles. For this reason, smoking is *never* permitted where oxygen is being administered or stored. Some facilities use oxygen concentrators that take room air and deliver concentrated oxygen to the resident (Figure 2-10). It is best to follow the same guidelines regardless of whether an oxygen cylinder is used or wall oxygen is administered:

FIGURE 2-10
Use oxygen safely.

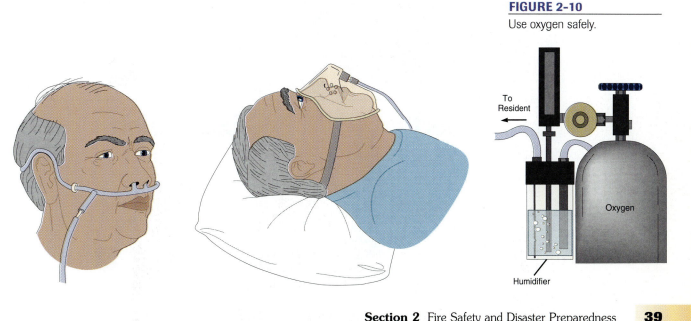

- Post "NO SMOKING, OXYGEN IN USE" signs on the resident's door and at the bedside.
- Check with your charge nurse before using any electrical equipment in the presence of oxygen. This includes electric razors, fans, radios, and TV sets.
- Never use flammable liquids such as alcohol, nail polish remover, or paint thinner in the oxygen-rich environment.
- Make sure the oxygen cylinder is secured with a chain to prevent it from falling to the floor.

As a nursing assistant, you have a serious responsibility to:

- Understand the nature of fire.
- Recognize fire hazards.
- Practice fire prevention as you provide care.

FIRE SAFETY PLANNING

When a fire occurs, you must act immediately. This is not the time to find out where the fire alarms are located or to learn how to use fire extinguishers or to review fire exit routes. You must be prepared through fire safety planning (Figure 2-11).

In case of fire, you must decide: Do I start rescue or set off the alarm first? Your first action is always to rescue anyone in danger. Then confine the fire, sound an alarm, and attempt to extinguish the fire if safe to do so.

In order to choose the proper type of fire extinguisher, fires are classified as Class "A," Class "B," or Class "C."

- Class "A" refers to a fire involving ordinary combustibles such as paper, wood, or cloth. The fire is extinguished by cooling. Usually, water is used.

FIGURE 2-11

Fire safety planning.

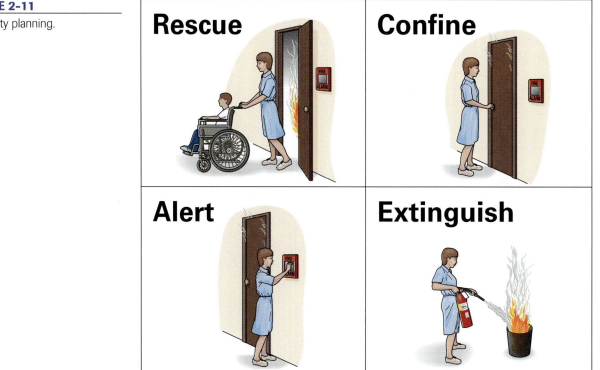

Rescue

Confine

Alert

Extinguish

DISASTER PREPAREDNESS

Facilities must always be prepared to cope with a disaster. A disaster is some type of catastrophe. It can be natural in origin, such as a flood, tornado, or earthquake, or it could be of human origin, such as an airplane crash, fire, or explosion. The threat of disaster is always present. Disasters don't just happen to others! Most facilities have disaster plans, and they practice disaster procedures on a regular basis. The most important points to remember in a disaster situation are:

- *First,* remove residents from immediate danger.
- Report to appropriate persons within the facility or other agencies, such as the fire department, police department, Red Cross, Civil Defense, nearest hospital, and so on.

- Follow the directions of the persons in charge.
- Evacuate the building, removing ambulatory, wheelchair, and bedfast residents, if instructed.
- Assist in organizing and monitoring residents when moving them to an appropriate shelter.
- Remove and secure necessary equipment, supplies, and records.
- Assist in the emergency record-keeping system.
- Think before you act. Make good use of your hands, feet, time, and energy. Don't be careless!
- Help lessen confusion by behaving in a calm, confident manner.

- Class "B" fires involve flammable liquids such as alcohol, gasoline, or oil. These fires are extinguished by smothering or by excluding the oxygen.
- Class "C" fires involve electrical equipment. These fires are also extinguished by smothering.

Fire extinguishers are classified as "A," "BC," and "ABC." It is important to use the proper fire extinguisher to fit the fire. Check your facility's fire extinguisher to determine the types available.

To operate all types of fire extinguishers, remember "PASS":

P—Pull the safety pin.
A—Aim toward the base of the flame.
S—Squeeze the trigger handle.
S—Sweep from side to side.

Follow your facility's emergency fire procedures in a calm, efficient manner. Panic worsens any emergency. Follow the direction of your charge nurse. Lives can be lost if staff members fail to respond quickly and efficiently! In addition:

- Know the floor plan of your facility.
- Know the exit routes.
- Know the location of fire alarms and fire extinguishing devices.
- Know how to report a fire.
- Know your facility's plan and your role in the plan.

Your facility will hold special classes in fire safety, and you will participate in practice drills. Complete the fire prevention checklist provided in your Student Workbook. Pay close attention so that if a fire emergency occurs, you will be prepared to respond appropriately.

The time to learn your facility's disaster plan is now. When a disaster occurs, it is too late! It is common to hear survivors of a disaster express regret and grief that they were not well enough prepared or informed to act efficiently. Every nursing assistant must know what to do in the event of a disaster!

SECTION 3 Infection Control

OBJECTIVES
What You Will Learn

When you have completed this section, you will be able to:

- Define the terms **organism, microorganism, pathogenic, nonpathogenic,** and **aseptic**
- List five ways that microorganisms are spread
- List four signs of infection
- Define the terms **isolation, disinfection,** and **sterilization**
- Identify which areas are considered clean and which are considered dirty
- Give two examples of materials that are considered infectious waste
- Demonstrate proper handwashing technique
- Demonstrate proper linen-handling procedures
- Explain when standard precautions are to be used
- List the three types of transmission precautions that are to be used in addition to standard precautions
- Explain when gloves are to be worn

KEY TERMS

aseptic
clean
cross-infection
culture
dirty
disinfection
environmental control

feces
incidence
infection
infectious objects
isolation
medical waste
microorganisms
nonpathogenic

organism
pathogenic
reinfection
standard precautions
sterilization
toxins
transmission-based precautions

INFECTION CONTROL

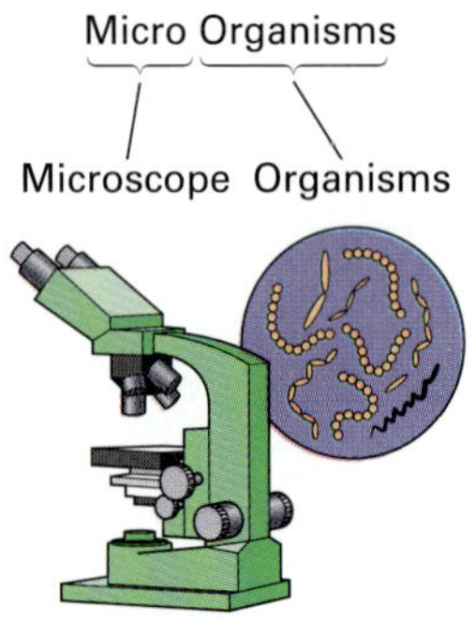

One of the most important aspects of environmental safety is infection control. All health care facilities must establish infection control programs. Each facility must have an infection control committee to write and approve policies and procedures and to monitor the infection control program. As a nursing assistant, you have responsibility to understand and to follow your facility's infection control policies and procedures. By doing so, you protect the residents, yourself and your family, and your fellow workers from the possibility of acquiring an infection.

Some important terms related to infection control are:

- **Organism**—any living thing
- **Microorganisms** (commonly called germs)—tiny living things seen only with a microscope (Figure 2-12)
- **Pathogenic**—causing disease
- **Nonpathogenic**—not capable of producing disease
- **Infection**—invasion of the body by a disease-producing (pathogenic) organism
- **Aseptic**—free of microorganisms

Microorganisms are everywhere—in the food we eat, the air we breathe, the water we drink, on objects we touch, and inside and outside our bodies. We are always in the presence of disease-producing microorganisms. Fortunately, the body has protective mechanisms to help us resist infection. The skin is one of the most important. If it is cut or injured, the person has a high risk of developing an infection. The mucous lining of the mouth and nose also helps to trap foreign substances and prevent infection. The body's immune system

Micro Organisms

Microscope Organisms

FIGURE 2-12
Microorganisms.

organism any living thing

microorganisms tiny living things seen only with a microscope

pathogenic causing disease

nonpathogenic not capable of producing disease

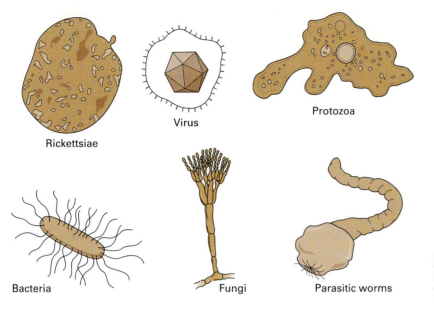

Rickettsiae

Virus

Protozoa

Bacteria

Fungi

Parasitic worms

FIGURE 2-13

Six major microorganisms known to cause diseases in humans.

is designed to fight the invasion. Despite the body's defense system, all of us have experienced illness related to an infection:

- Common cold
- Influenza (flu)
- Infection of a cut or wound
- Mumps, measles, chickenpox
- Skin eruptions
- Athlete's foot

infection invasion of the body by a disease-producing organism

aseptic free of micro-organisms

The microorganisms that produce disease in humans are classified as follows (Figure 2-13):

- Bacteria
- Viruses
- Fungi (including yeast and mold)
- Protozoa
- Rickettsia
- Parasitic worms

BACTERIA

The most important (according to the frequency of occurrence) are the bacteria and viruses. However, each classification has groups that can cause acute illness.

Two types of *harmful* bacteria that are present in health care facilities are *Staphylococcus* and *Streptococcus.* When these bacteria invade the body, they cause serious disease and illness. As a nursing assistant, you will come in contact with these and many other disease-producing microorganisms. When you understand how microorganisms are spread and what conditions affect the growth of bacteria, you will be better prepared to take special precautions (Figure 2-14).

You can help reduce the **incidence** (number of occurrences) of bacterial infections when you pay careful attention to the resident's personal hygiene and skin care needs and when you help keep the residents' units clean and free from the conditions that promote bacterial growth.

Bacteria are known to survive best in a warm, dark, and moist environment that contains both oxygen and nourishment (Figure 2-15). Nourishment may be living or dead matter.

incidence number of occurrences

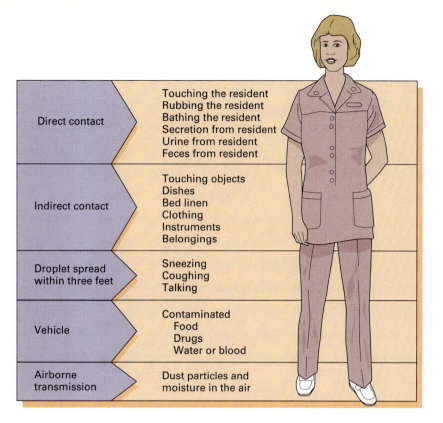

Direct contact	Touching the resident Rubbing the resident Bathing the resident Secretion from resident Urine from resident Feces from resident
Indirect contact	Touching objects Dishes Bed linen Clothing Instruments Belongings
Droplet spread within three feet	Sneezing Coughing Talking

Vehicle	Contaminated
	   Food
	   Drugs
	   Water or blood

Airborne transmission	Dust particles and moisture in the air

FIGURE 2-14

Ways that microorganisms are spread.

culture specimen of body tissue or fluids kept under special laboratory conditions to detect the presence of microorganisms

feces solid human waste

Specific drugs are known to kill specific bacteria. When infection occurs, physicians will order a sample of wound drainage or a scraping or swabbing of the infected area to be studied. This is called a **culture.** When a *bacterium* (singular of *bacteria*) is identified, physicians will order the proper drug known to kill that specific bacterium. These drugs are called *antibiotics.*

It is important to know that not all bacteria are harmful. For example, certain bacteria are responsible for the chemical changes that produce cheese, yogurt, sauerkraut, and alcohol. There are also "normal" or nonpathogenic bacteria that live and serve a necessary purpose in the human body. The bacterium called *Escherichia coli,* for example, is normally found in the intestinal tract. Here, it assists in breaking down unused food particles, turning them into stool or **feces** (solid human waste). *E. coli* is pathogenic (disease producing), however, when it enters other areas of the body such as the urinary tract, as can happen when an individual wipes or cleans himself improperly or when feces enter an open sore.

VIRUSES

Viruses generally are more difficult to treat because the drug must kill the virus without destroying the body cell in which the virus lives. For this reason, there are no drugs available to use against all viral infections. Vaccines have been developed that are effective against some specific viruses. Examples are measles, polio, and influenza vaccines.

FIGURE 2-15

Conditions that promote bacterial growth.

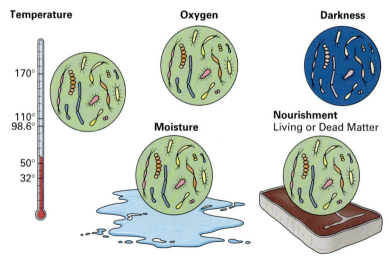

Most disease-producing microorganisms release waste products known as **toxins** that act like poison in the body. The body's immune system tries to fight the toxins. When this occurs, the common signs and symptoms associated with infection are present:

- Drainage from wounds, eyes, ears, nose
- Reddened or inflamed areas
- Increased heat in an area
- Fever or chills
- Pain
- Swelling

Be alert for these signs and symptoms in your residents and report them promptly to the charge nurse. Elderly residents differ from children and adults in that they may not have a fever even though a serious infection is present. It is important to act on the reported feelings and complaints of the resident.

toxins waste products released by disease-producing organisms

PRINCIPLES OF INFECTION CONTROL

All infection control programs are meant to:

- Protect residents, employees, families, and visitors from acquiring an infection from someone else (called **cross-infection**)
- Protect residents who have had an infection from becoming infected a second time (called **reinfection**)
- Provide residents, employees, and visitors with a safe environment that is as free as possible of pathogenic organisms (called **environmental control**)

cross-infection acquiring an infection from someone else

reinfection invasion of the body by a disease-producing organism

Some basic terms associated with an infection control program are:

- **Isolation**—to separate or set apart. Efforts are made to separate infectious residents and their belongings from others. Special procedures must be followed in handling these residents and their linen, trash, food trays, and personal belongings. There is a constant effort to avoid contact with infectious microorganisms by taking extra precautions. The kind of precautions necessary depend on the microorganisms causing the infection and how that type of infection is spread. For this reason, there are several different types of isolation called transmission-based precautions. You will learn about these precautions later in this chapter.
- **Disinfection**—the process of killing *most* microorganisms with a chemical substance. Some are not killed, but their growth and activity are slowed.
- **Sterilization**—the process of killing *all* microorganisms. There are several methods of sterilization, but the most commonly used is pressurized steam at a high temperature (called autoclaving). Special gases and chemical solutions are also used. An object is sterile when it is *free from all* microorganisms. An object is contaminated if it is not sterile. You contaminate a sterile object anytime you bring it into contact (touch) with a nonsterile object. The words clean and dirty have new meanings when discussing infection control.
- **Clean**—uncontaminated, free from pathogenic organisms (does not mean sterile).
- **Dirty**—contaminated, used, or exposed to persons or places where disease-producing organisms are present. Any object that has touched the floor is considered dirty or contaminated and should not be used.

environmental control means of providing a safe environment that is as free as possible of pathogenic organisms

isolation to separate or set apart

disinfection process of killing most microorganisms

sterilization process of killing all microorganisms

clean uncontaminated; free from known pathogenic organisms

dirty contaminated, used, or exposed to disease-producing organisms

You will notice that the utility rooms are designated as either "clean" or "dirty" rooms or divided into "clean" or "dirty" areas. The clean rooms or areas are used to store supplies and equipment that have not been used. The dirty rooms or areas are used to store supplies and equipment that have been used and are to be thrown away as rubbish or reprocessed to make them clean again (bedpans, urinals, thermometers, basins, etc.).

Remember this formula to help you follow good infection control practices:

$$\text{Clean} + \text{Clean} = \text{Clean}$$
$$\text{Clean} + \text{Dirty} = \text{Dirty}$$

PROPER LINEN HANDLING

Proper handling of linen is another important infection-control measure.

- Wash your hands before touching clean linen.
- Clean linen may be stored only in areas designated for clean linen.
- Carry linens away from your body. Avoid contact between your clothing and the linen. (In infection control, your uniform is considered contaminated.)
- Take only the necessary amount of clean linen into the room. Once linen is in the room, it may not be returned to the clean linen storage area.
- Any linen that falls to the floor is contaminated and may not be used.
- Avoid shaking or fluffing linens in the air. (This spreads microorganisms.)
- Soiled linen must be placed in covered containers, *never* on the floor, over-bed table, or chairs. The soiled linen is more contaminated than the floor, over-bed table, or chairs.
- Fill soiled linen containers so that they can be closed tightly. This prevents airborne contamination and reduces odor.
- Wash hands after handling soiled items.

Remember . . .

You must wash your hands before and after contact with each resident to prevent the spread of infection and disease.

Guidelines

HANDLING MEDICAL WASTE

Objects that have come in contact with a person who has an infection or communicable disease can carry or transmit the disease. For that reason, these objects are said to be **infectious objects.** Disposable items used by the resident and any body discharges (saliva, wound drainage, urine, feces) are called **medical waste.** These items require special handling by the nursing staff. There are laws regulating the handling of medical waste to protect the public health. Items classified as medical waste are usually placed in specially marked bags and stored in a locked area until they are picked up by a special disposal company, incinerated, or sterilized. Learn your facility's method for handling medical waste.

Items that might be considered medical waste include:

- Soiled wound dressings
- Used needles and syringes
- Used gloves
- Used urinary drainage bags
- Used colostomy bags
- Used facial tissues
- Soiled disposable diapers

In your work as a nursing assistant, you use your hands constantly. You can help reduce the chance of infection if you make it a habit to wash your hands *before* and *after* contact with any resident or unclean object.

The most effective way to control infection is to prevent it! The most important single principle of infection control is to practice *good handwashing.*

PROCEDURE

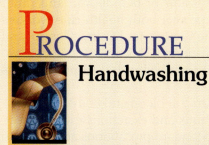

Handwashing

Preparation

1. Remove your watch and rings.
2. Do not let your clothing touch the sink.
3. Assemble your equipment or assure that it is available:
   - Soap or detergent
   - Paper towels
   - Wastepaper basket
4. Use a paper towel to turn the water on to a comfortable temperature.
5. Discard the paper towel.

Steps

6. Completely wet your hands and wrists. Keep your fingertips pointed downward.
7. Apply soap or detergent.
8. Work up a good lather. Spread it over the entire area of your hands and wrists. Get soap under your nails and between your fingers.
9. Wash the palms and backs of the hands (Figure 2-16a).
10. Clean under your nails by rubbing for 1 full minute.
    - Rub vigorously.
    - Rub one hand against the other hand and wrist.
    - Rub between your fingers by interlacing them (Figure 2-16b).
    - Rub up and down to reach all skin surfaces on your hands and between your fingers.
    - Rub the tips of your fingers against your palms to clean with friction around the nailbeds.
11. Hold your hands lower than your elbows with the fingertips down (Figure 2-16c).
12. Wash 3–4 inches above your wrists. Wash for 10–15 seconds.
13. Rinse well from above your wrists down to your fingertips using running water.

Ending Steps

14. Dry thoroughly with paper towels.
15. Turn off the faucet using a dry paper towel (Figure 2-16d). Do not touch the faucet.
16. Discard the paper towel into the wastepaper basket without touching the basket.

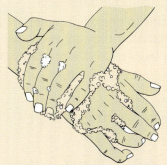

A. Wash the palms and backs of the hands

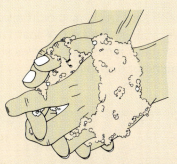

B. Interlace the fingers and thumbs and move the hands back and forth.

C. Keep your hands lower than your elbows with the fingertips down

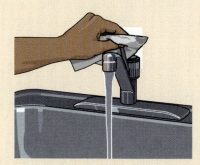

D. Use a dry paper towel to turn off the water faucet

FIGURE 2-16 a-d
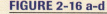

standard precautions a
system of precautions to be
used in the care of all residents in order to prevent
the spread of disease

**transmission-based pre-
cautions** a group of infection control methods based
on the way a particular disease is spread

In order to reduce the risk of transmission of bloodborne and other
pathogens in health care facilities and to protect both health care workers
and residents from the spread of disease, the Centers for Disease Control and
Prevention developed a new system of precautions. This new system has two
parts: (1) **standard precautions** and (2) **transmission-based precautions**
(isolation).

Standard precautions are directed primarily at blood and body fluid transmission of diseases. They include all secretions and excretions except sweat,
whether or not they contain visible blood. Standard precautions apply also to
nonintact skin and mucous membranes (Figure 2-17).

Standard precautions are to be used for the care of *all* residents regardless
of their infection status. Standard precautions are designed to reduce the risk
of transmission of bloodborne and other pathogens in health care facilities.
Standard precautions include the following:

1. Handwashing must always be performed after touching blood, body
   fluids, secretions, excretions, and contaminated items whether or not
   gloves are worn. Handwashing must take place after gloves are removed and between each resident contact.
2. Gloves must be worn when touching blood, body fluids, secretions, excretions (except sweat), mucous membranes, and contaminated items. Clean
   gloves are worn before touching mucous membranes and nonintact skin.
3. Masks, eye protection, and face shields are worn to protect mucous
   membranes of the eyes, nose, and mouth during activities likely to generate splashes of blood, body fluids, secretions, and excretions.
4. Gowns or aprons must be worn to protect the skin and prevent soiling
   of clothing during activities that are likely to generate splashes or sprays
   of blood, body fluids, secretions, or excretions.
5. Linen must be handled, transported, and processed in a manner that
   prevents exposure of skin and mucous membranes or contamination of
   clothing. Wet linen should be placed in plastic bags for transport.
6. All health care workers should take precautions to prevent injuries by
   needles, scalpels, and other sharp instruments. After they are used, disposable sharp items and needles should be placed in puncture-resistant
   containers for disposal.

Guidelines

USE OF GLOVES

- Gloves are to be worn any time you have a
  possibility of contact with blood, body fluids,
  nonintact skin, or mucous membranes. All of
  the procedures you are learning will indicate
  the need for gloves as part of the procedure but
  you will still have to use your judgment to decide. A good rule to follow is "When in doubt,
  wear gloves."
- You must wash your hands both before and
  after using gloves.
- Always check the gloves for tears or holes before putting them on.

- Knowing when to remove the gloves is as important as knowing when to put them on.
- They must be changed for each resident and
  for each task.
- They may not be worn outside the resident's
  room.
- Be aware that latex allergies exist.
- Report your allergy to your supervisor so you
  can be provided with nonlatex gloves.

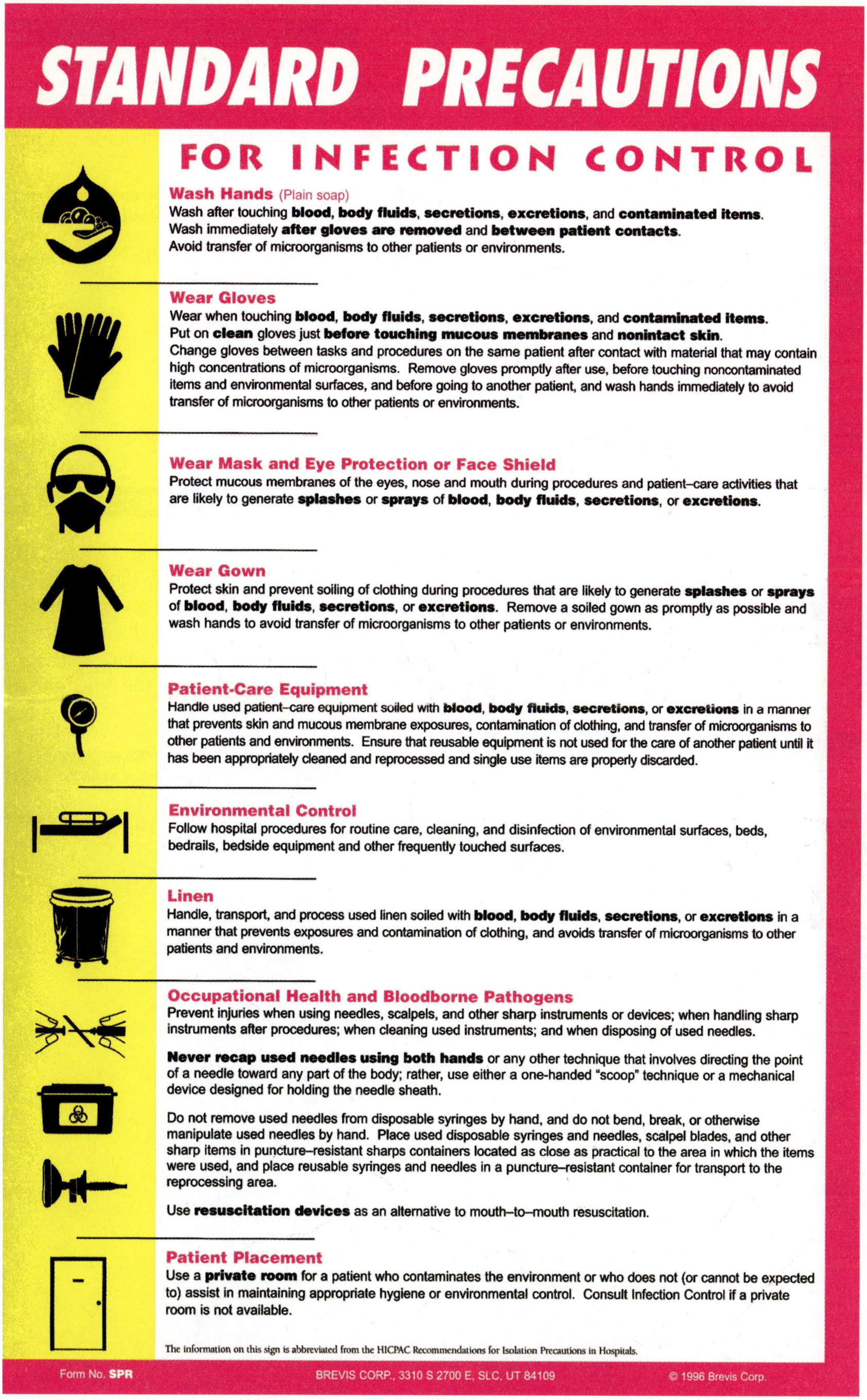

STANDARD PRECAUTIONS

FOR INFECTION CONTROL

Wash Hands (Plain soap)

Wash after touching **blood, body fluids, secretions, excretions**, and **contaminated items**. Wash immediately **after gloves are removed** and **between patient contacts**. Avoid transfer of microorganisms to other patients or environments.

Wear Gloves

Wear when touching **blood, body fluids, secretions, excretions**, and **contaminated items**. Put on **clean** gloves just **before touching mucous membranes** and **nonintact skin**. Change gloves between tasks and procedures on the same patient after contact with material that may contain high concentrations of microorganisms. Remove gloves promptly after use, before touching noncontaminated items and environmental surfaces, and before going to another patient, and wash hands immediately to avoid transfer of microorganisms to other patients or environments.

Wear Mask and Eye Protection or Face Shield

Protect mucous membranes of the eyes, nose and mouth during procedures and patient–care activities that are likely to generate **splashes** or **sprays** of **blood, body fluids, secretions**, or **excretions**.

Wear Gown

Protect skin and prevent soiling of clothing during procedures that are likely to generate **splashes** or **sprays** of **blood, body fluids, secretions**, or **excretions**. Remove a soiled gown as promptly as possible and wash hands to avoid transfer of microorganisms to other patients or environments.

Patient-Care Equipment

Handle used patient–care equipment soiled with **blood, body fluids, secretions**, or **excretions** in a manner that prevents skin and mucous membrane exposures, contamination of clothing, and transfer of microorganisms to other patients and environments. Ensure that reusable equipment is not used for the care of another patient until it has been appropriately cleaned and reprocessed and single use items are properly discarded.

Environmental Control

Follow hospital procedures for routine care, cleaning, and disinfection of environmental surfaces, beds, bedrails, bedside equipment and other frequently touched surfaces.

Linen

Handle, transport, and process used linen soiled with **blood, body fluids, secretions**, or **excretions** in a manner that prevents exposures and contamination of clothing, and avoids transfer of microorganisms to other patients and environments.

Occupational Health and Bloodborne Pathogens

Prevent injuries when using needles, scalpels, and other sharp instruments or devices; when handling sharp instruments after procedures; when cleaning used instruments; and when disposing of used needles.

Never recap used needles using both hands or any other technique that involves directing the point of a needle toward any part of the body; rather, use either a one-handed "scoop" technique or a mechanical device designed for holding the needle sheath.

Do not remove used needles from disposable syringes by hand, and do not bend, break, or otherwise manipulate used needles by hand. Place used disposable syringes and needles, scalpel blades, and other sharp items in puncture–resistant sharps containers located as close as practical to the area in which the items were used, and place reusable syringes and needles in a puncture–resistant container for transport to the reprocessing area.

Use **resuscitation devices** as an alternative to mouth–to–mouth resuscitation.

Patient Placement

Use a **private room** for a patient who contaminates the environment or who does not (or cannot be expected to) assist in maintaining appropriate hygiene or environmental control. Consult Infection Control if a private room is not available.

The information on this sign is abbreviated from the HICPAC Recommendations for Isolation Precautions in Hospitals.

Form No. **SPR**   BREVIS CORP., 3310 S 2700 E, SLC, UT 84109   © 1996 Brevis Corp.

FIGURE 2-17

Standard precautions. (Courtesy of BREVIS Corporation.)

PROCEDURE

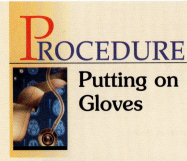

Putting on Gloves

Preparation

1. Gather supplies including two gloves.
2. Wash your hands.

Steps

3. Slip your hands into the gloves one hand at a time.
4. Work the gloves over your fingers so that they fit. They should neither be too loose nor too tight.

Ending Steps

5. Inspect the gloves for holes or tears and replace if damaged.

PROCEDURE

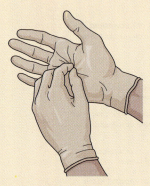

Removing Gloves

Preparation

1. Grasp the glove at the palm of the hand with the gloved fingers of the other hand (Figure 2-18a).

Steps

2. Pull the glove over your hand while turning the glove inside out (Figure 2-18b).
3. Place the ungloved index and middle fingers under the cuff of the remaining glove (Figure 2-18c).
4. Turn the cuff downward pulling it inside and out over your hand and over the other glove (Figure 2-18d).

Ending Steps

5. Discard the gloves in the appropriate container.
6. Wash your hands.

A. Grasp the glove at the palm of the hand with the gloved fingers of the other hand.

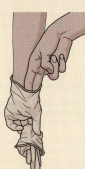

C. Place the ungloved index and middle fingers under the cuff of the remaining glove

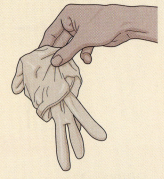

D. Turn the cuff downward, pulling it inside out over your hand and over the other glove

B. Pull the glove over your hand while turning the glove inside out.

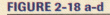

FIGURE 2-18 a-d

7. Although saliva has not been implicated to date in human immunodeficiency virus (HIV) transmission, to minimize the need for emergency mouth-to-mouth resuscitation, mouthpieces, resuscitation bags, or other ventilation devices should be used.

8. Health care workers who have open lesions or weeping dermatitis should avoid all direct resident care and handling of resident equipment until the condition is resolved.

Because gloves are such an important part of protection of the nursing assistant and the resident, you need to know when and how to use gloves properly.

Remember, standard precautions apply to all residents whether or not they have a known infection! This is the best way to protect yourself and your residents from the spread of disease.

SECTION 4 The Resident in Isolation

OBJECTIVES
What You Will Learn

When you have completed this section, you will be able to:

• Apply a mask and gown

• Describe how the nursing assistant can determine which type of isolation technique is required for a given resident

• List the ways AIDS is spread

• Describe the ways a nursing assistant can most effectively prevent the spread of any communicable disease, including AIDS

KEY TERMS

AIDS (acquired immune deficiency syndrome)
airborne transmission
communicable conditions

contact transmission
dermatologist
droplet transmission
exposure
isolation techniques

jaundice
opportunistic infections
scabies
transmission-based precautions
tuberculosis (TB)

COMMUNICABLE DISEASES AND INFECTIONS

In addition to handwashing, there are special methods the nursing assistant should use to prevent the spread of communicable diseases. The use of masks, gowns, gloves, and so on helps keep disease-producing germs away from equipment, residents, and personnel. Certain health care areas need extra precautions to prevent the spread of infection and disease.

Communicable diseases spread very quickly and easily from one person to another. Examples are *Staphylococcus* wound infections, *Shigella,* and other infectious diarrheas. Sometimes the more general term **communicable conditions** is used because it includes both diseases and infections. Ordinary cleanliness alone will not protect you and others from catching such diseases. When a patient has one of these diseases, special precautions are necessary. These safety measures are called **isolation techniques.** The resident is in isolation (separated) from other residents and personnel (Figure 2-19).

The major purpose of isolation techniques is to keep the germs that cause the disease inside the isolated resident's unit. Isolation techniques prevent germs from leaving the unit on your hands, arms, or on clothing or articles used in the unit. Another purpose of isolation techniques is to keep germs outside the iso-

communicable conditions
diseases and infections that spread from one person to another

isolation techniques
safety measure to prevent spread of communicable conditions

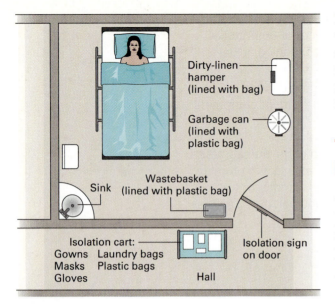

FIGURE 2-19

The isolation unit.

transmission-based precautions a group of infection control methods based on the way a particular disease is spread

lated resident's unit. This "protective" isolation is used to prevent infection in a resident who is very weak and susceptible to acquiring infections. Examples include residents being treated for cancer or those who have received some type of transplant. Their ability to fight infection is poor, so they require protective isolation.

TRANSMISSION-BASED PRECAUTIONS (ISOLATION)

A sign such as those shown in Figure 2-20 may be placed on the door of the isolated unit to identify the type of isolation and to give instructions to everyone entering. In an LTC facility, the types of precaution or isolation used are contact, airborne, and droplet. These are called **transmission-based precautions** and are used in addition to standard precautions. Always follow the instructions posted on the door of the resident's room.

There are three main ways that diseases are passed from one person to another. **Contact transmission** is the most frequent mode of transmission in the health care facility. This involves direct body-surface-to-body-surface touch with physical transfer of microorganisms between the infected person and another. It may also involve contact with contaminated objects such as linens, equipment, and gloves that were not changed between residents.

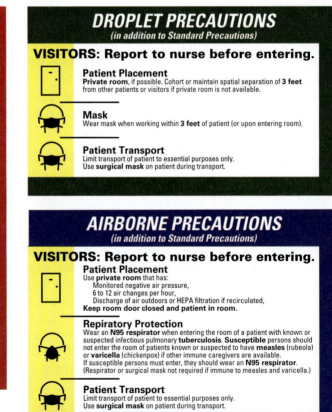

FIGURE 2-20

Isolation signs. (Courtesy of BREVIS Corporation.)

Another type of transmission is **droplet transmission.** Droplets can be produced by the resident during coughing, sneezing, talking, or during procedures such as suctioning. Transmission occurs when droplets are propelled short distances through the air and come into contact with mucous membranes of the eyes, nose, or mouth or an open area on the skin. Droplet transmission is a form of contact transmission.

Airborne transmission occurs when some particles of evaporated droplets containing microorganisms that remain suspended in the air are dispersed by air currents within a room or over a long distance. They are inhaled by the susceptible person.

Transmission-based precautions are designed to prevent the spread of disease by contact, droplets, and air.

When a resident's communicable condition can be spread by breathing, face masks are very important. Before you put on or take off a face mask, be sure that your hands are thoroughly clean. Face masks are effective for only 30 minutes, due to the moisture of normal respiration. If you stay in an isolated area longer, you must wash your hands and remove the old mask, then wash your hands again and put on a clean mask. Masks are used only once and then thrown away. If the mask becomes wet, it must be changed. Never let the face mask hang around your neck.

contact transmission
passing on microorganisms by touch; may be touching of objects or an infected person

droplet transmission
passing on microorganisms through droplets produced during activities like coughing, sneezing, and talking

airborne transmission
passing on microorganisms through the air

ISOLATION GOWNS

You will wear an isolation gown when you are caring for a resident in isolation. You will wear the gown if there is any possibility that your clothes could

Procedure

Putting on an Isolation Gown

Preparation

1. Wash your hands. If you are wearing a long-sleeved uniform, roll your sleeves above your elbows (Figure 2-21).

Steps

2. Unfold the isolation gown so that the opening is at the back.
3. Put your arms into the sleeves of the isolation gown.
4. Fit the gown at the neck, making sure your uniform is covered.
5. Reach behind and tie the neck back with a simple shoelace bow or fasten the adhesive strip.

Ending Steps

6. Grasp the edges of the gown and pull to back.
7. Overlap the edges and roll them together in back, closing the opening and covering your uniform completely.
8. Tie the waist tapes in a bow, or fasten the adhesive strip.

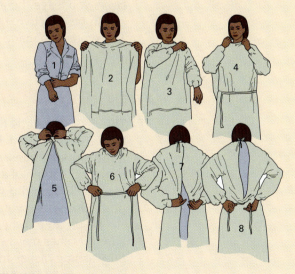

FIGURE 2-21

Putting on an isolation gown.

PROCEDURE

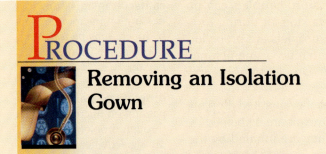

Removing an Isolation Gown

1. Remove the gloves and discard them in the trash container inside the resident's room.

Steps

2. Untie the gown and remove it by rolling it away from yourself into a ball.
3. Roll the gown with the contaminated portion inside.
4. If the gown is washable, put it in the dirty linen hamper inside the resident's room. If the gown is disposable, place it in the trash container inside the resident's room.
5. Wash your hands using paper towels to turn off the faucet.
6. Remove the face mask and discard.

Ending Steps

7. Wash your hands.
8. Use a paper towel to open the door to leave the room. Put the towel into the wastebasket inside the room as you leave.

A simple way to remember the process of gowning and ungowning whenever mask and gloves are worn is to gown from the top down (mask, gown, gloves) and ungown from the bottom up (gloves, gown, mask). Remember that your gloves are the dirtiest part of the isolation equipment. Handwashing is always indicated even when gloves are worn!

touch the resident or brush against any articles in the unit. Remember, all of this is considered *contaminated.* There are three types of isolation gown:

- Cotton twill (reusable after proper washing)
- Paper disposable gown (thrown away after one use)
- Plastic disposable apron (worn once and thrown away)

Individual gown technique means that a gown should be used only once. It is then discarded in the proper dirty linen hamper or trash can. This is done *before* you leave the isolation room.

To be effective, the isolation gown must cover your uniform completely. Therefore, it is made wide enough to overlap in back.

SERVING FOOD TO THE RESIDENT IN ISOLATION

The new standards for infection control may make it necessary to wear protective gear when delivering a food tray to a resident who is under one of the three forms of transmission precautions. For example, a gown would be worn to enter the room of a resident on contact precautions. A mask would be needed for droplet or airborne precaution cases. However, you must wear complete protective gear if you are staying to feed a resident.

Disposable dishes and utensils are not necessary for use in isolation situations. Dishes may be handled according to the institution's normal procedure for washing dishes in hot soapy water or in the dishwasher.

Generally, uneaten food is considered contaminated (Figure 2-22). Scraps are disposed of in a trash container *inside the resident's room.*

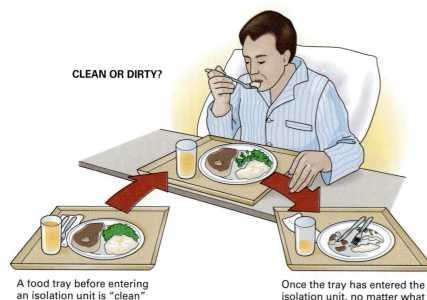

CLEAN OR DIRTY?

A food tray before entering an isolation unit is "clean" or uncontaminated

Once the tray has entered the isolation unit, no matter what the patient has eaten or touched, it is "dirty" or contaminated

FIGURE 2-22
Clean and dirty.

THE HANDLING OF SOILED LINEN

The double bagging of linen is no longer necessary, since all linen is considered infectious, and should be handled in a manner that prevents contamination. Linen that is wet should be placed in a plastic bag to prevent contamination of floors, linen chutes, or bins. Also, meltaway bags are unnecessary, again, since all linen is handled as infectious. Follow the policy of your long-term care facility.

THE HANDLING OF MEDICAL WASTE

Any medical waste must be handled in accordance with state and federal law. Follow the rules for medical waste management in your institution. Special procedures will include placing medical waste in color-coded or labeled bags and containers for special disposal. Waste from the isolation room should be treated as any medical waste. Double bagging is not necessary. Always follow the practices of your institution.

REVERSE ISOLATION PRACTICES

Reverse isolation has proved to be ineffective in preventing infection in those who have weak immune systems. These residents have difficulty in fighting disease. Their own bodily organisms have been found to be a major cause for infection. Limiting visitors, using good handwashing practices, and not providing uncooked food (such as fresh fruits and vegetables) have been found to be the most effective means to prevent infection. Even microorganisms found on fresh flowers can be cause for infection in this type of resident. Your institution may have additional practices.

Remember, diseases are caused by microorganisms, and the spread of disease is greatly reduced by keeping everything clean. Being extra careful to avoid contamination is a way of keeping the environment safe. The most important measures that you can take to reduce the chance of spreading disease and infection is to *wash your hands before and after contact with residents* and to *follow the isolation procedures carefully!*

SPECIAL NEEDS OF THE RESIDENT IN ISOLATION

The resident in isolation needs the same personal care as any other resident. It is very important to combine normal nursing care with good isolation technique. These tasks should be performed in your usual pleasant and supportive style. Make it clear that it is the disease-causing microorganisms that are unwanted, not the resident.

Residents in isolation may experience feelings of loneliness and anxiety. The entire staff must see that they are not deprived of contact with others. The need for touch, communication, and stimulation still exists. The resident should be provided with TV, radio, books, or magazines if appropriate. Visitors should be encouraged, although they must follow isolation techniques. Make a special effort to spend time with the isolated resident.

TUBERCULOSIS

tuberculosis (TB) an infectious disease that commonly attacks the lungs and is usually spread by contact with the sputum of an infected person

Tuberculosis (TB) is an infectious disease caused by *Mycobacterium tuberculosis.* Although this disease can affect any part of the body, it usually affects the lungs. Tuberculosis is increasing largely due to increases of TB among persons who are HIV positive or who have AIDS. Facility residents are considered at increased risk of becoming infected with tuberculosis, as are persons with other medical risk factors (diabetes, leukemia, Hodgkin's disease, end-stage renal disease, cancer, or those who are 10 percent below ideal body weight), foreign-born persons from countries where the incidence of TB is high (Asia, Africa, Latin America, and the Caribbean), populations with poor medical care, and alcoholics and IV drug abusers. Tuberculosis is transmitted by airborne droplets. Repeated and/or long exposures are usually required for infection to occur. A person may be "exposed," "infected," or have active tuberculosis. **Exposure** means that contaminated air has been inhaled, but without invasion of the tissue by the bacilli. Infection means:

exposure contact with microorganisms

- The bacilli are present.
- There are no symptoms.
- The person is not contagious.
- The person will test positively when a skin test is given.

A person who becomes infected with the TB bacillus remains infected for years. Usually, a person with a healthy immune system never develops active tuberculosis, although the infection remains present in the body. About 10 to 15 million persons in the United States are infected with *Mycobacterium tuberculosis.*

Symptoms of disease include fever, sweating, weight loss, productive cough, coughing up blood, and lung changes observable on an x-ray. In the elderly, changes in mental status or behavior may be the only symptoms noted. Usually, persons with AIDS are assumed to have the disease until proved otherwise.

Each long-term facility has a written plan to prevent the spread of tuberculosis among the residents and staff. This plan requires staff training about TB, including the causes, how it is spread, and how it is prevented. You will have opportunities to learn about it in your facility. In addition, staff and residents are tested at the time of hiring or time of admission and usually yearly after that for the presence of TB. Most of the time a skin test is used to detect whether the person has been exposed to the bacillus. If there is a positive reaction to the skin test or if the person has ever had a positive reaction, a chest x-ray is needed to find out if the disease is present. A sample of sputum may be required to test for the presence of *Mycobacterium tuberculosis.*

The facility plan must also include practices that prevent exposure of the employees and residents to the disease, including the use of masks. These special masks must be tested to be sure they fit properly in order to protect you from inhaling the infected material (Figure 2-23). The type of isolation used when a resident has been diagnosed with active tuberculosis is called airborne precautions and is described earlier in the chapter.

Residents with active tuberculosis must be taught to cover their mouths and noses with a tissue when coughing or sneezing, even while in isolation. Because the door must remain closed with the resident remaining in the room, efforts need to be made to provide for activities and for checking on the resident frequently. If a resident must be transported out of the isolation room, he or she should wear a mask that covers both mouth and nose during transport.

Tuberculosis is treated with multiple antituberculosis drugs that are usually given daily for at least 6 months. If the patient/resident does not take the medications for the full treatment period, the disease may not be cured and may recur. Sometimes this leads to the development of drug-resistant disease, which is difficult and expensive to treat.

Once persons are treated for 2 weeks, they are no longer able to transmit the disease to others. They may have their sputum tested and, if it is negative, the isolation precautions may be stopped.

If you are exposed to a person with TB, whether at home or at work, you must report the exposure to your employer so that your co-workers and the residents can be protected.

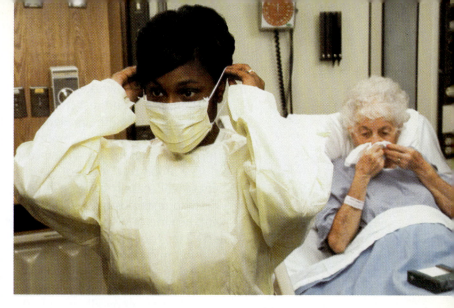

FIGURE 2-23

The face mask is worn over the mouth and nose to prevent infection from airborne microorganisms.

AIDS

One communicable disease that is a matter of great concern to the public and the health care field is **AIDS (acquired immune deficiency syndrome). AIDS** is a condition in which the body's immune system is damaged by attack from a virus (HIV). When the immune system is damaged, the body cannot fight infection. This creates an opportunity for many other microorganisms to survive in the body. These organisms take advantage of a diseased immune system, resulting in the development of **opportunistic infections.** Examples of opportunistic infections include pneumocystis pneumonia, candidiasis, cryptococcosis, herpes, and cancers such as Kaposi's sarcoma and lymphomas. AIDS is often first suspected because of the existence of one of these opportunistic infections.

AIDS is transmitted through sexual contact, needle and syringe sharing, from an infected mother to her unborn child, and blood transfusions (prior to the time the AIDS antibody test was developed and routinely used to screen blood). There must be some way for the virus to be passed from an infected person to the bloodstream of another person. AIDS is not transmitted through normal contact with strangers, family members, friends, or health care workers—except if there is sexual or needle contact with an infected person. Current research shows that AIDS cannot be contracted from coughing, sneezing, touching, or using dishes and utensils in common. Health care workers are considered to be at low risk for the disease. The only documented cases in

AIDS (acquired immune deficiency syndrome) a condition in which the body's immune system is damaged by attack from a virus (HIV)

opportunistic infections occurs when organisms take advantage of a diseased immune system

which health care workers who were not part of a high-risk group were infected involved exposure to infected blood combined with breaks in the skin of the health care worker.

There is a blood test that identifies those who have been exposed to the virus by measuring the presence of antibodies against the virus. Although the test is not 100 percent accurate, it has effectively protected the nation's blood supply by screening donors since 1985.

The blood test does not diagnose the disease itself or predict whether the person will actually develop AIDS. At present, it is not known whether everyone who tests positive will develop the disease. The time between infection with the virus and onset of the first symptoms of AIDS is thought to be as much as 5 years, though it may be less.

After infection (which is indicated by the presence of antibodies to the AIDS virus) some people do not develop AIDS, but they may develop a decreased immune response. This lowered immunity results in many different types of illness that are generally not life threatening; they may be called pre-AIDS or asymptomatic AIDS. These diseases often cause swollen lymph nodes lasting for a significant period of time and/or a lowered number of platelets involved in the blood-clotting process. Of those diagnosed with AIDS-related complex (ARC), many will experience no health problems, but they may be infectious.

Because the AIDS virus is not very strong, it is easily killed with a temperature of 140°F for 10 minutes or use of common chemicals like alcohol, Lysol, and a diluted solution of household bleach.

THE RESIDENT WITH AIDS

You may have the responsibility of providing care for a resident with AIDS in a hospice or a skilled nursing facility. The care required demands a concerned, committed, and knowledgeable approach. You must understand not only how to prevent the spread of the disease, but also how to protect the resident from opportunistic infections and to care for the psychosocial and physical needs of a dying person. Often, the resident will be younger (30 to 50 years old) than the usual long-term care resident, and you will need to cope with impending death at an age when it is not considered normal. Not only the resident but the resident's family and friends will need help and support as they grieve.

The person with AIDS has the same needs as any other resident and is entitled to the same good care. This resident needs recreation and social activities as well as comprehensive and competent medical and nursing care. Privacy is particularly important because of the fears of those who are uninformed and because of the attitudes toward those in the groups who are at highest risk for AIDS (homosexuals and intravenous drug abusers). Never reveal a resident's diagnosis of AIDS to anyone. The licensed nurse will inform anyone who needs to know.

The nursing needs of the resident with AIDS will vary greatly according to the disease or conditions present. Most will be thin and appear ill. They often have fevers and night sweats. Some have lesions or sores over their entire bodies. Chronic diarrhea is not uncommon. Some experience pain, confusion, memory loss, or unusual behavior when the nervous system is affected. Those with a type of cancer may be receiving chemotherapy, which causes side effects that must be managed or treated. If pneumonia is present, the resident may require oxygen or other types of respiratory treatment. Each is a unique individual whose care must be planned and carried out to meet the needs in the best way for that person.

If your facility is involved in care of residents with AIDS, the infection control committee will adopt special policies and procedures. You will be given specific, in-depth training in order to protect yourself and other residents from spread of the disease. Remember to use good infection control practices by treating all body fluids with caution at all times to avoid contracting any communicable disease.

HEPATITIS B

Another viral disease that is a concern for health care workers is hepatitis B (HBV). HBV infects about 300,000 people in the United States each year. Of those infected, about 7,000 will die. Hepatitis B is passed on in the same ways as HIV (AIDS).

Hepatitis is inflammation of the liver. The symptoms of hepatitis B occur only in some of those affected. Some may carry the disease and pass it on without knowing they have it. Some become gravely ill and die within days after the first symptoms appear. Symptoms include fatigue, fever, nausea, and loss of appetite. The person may experience pain in the abdomen and jaundice. **Jaundice** is a yellow coloring of the skin and the white portion of the eye. Jaundice is caused by a substance called bilirubin, secreted by the liver.

Hepatitis B can be diagnosed by a blood test. There is a vaccine that can prevent HBV infections in about 90 percent of people vaccinated. The vaccine can help if given after exposure, especially if given within the first 48 hours.

In the work setting, the greatest risk comes from puncture wounds, contact with blood or other body fluids when you have cuts or other broken skin, or contact between risky body fluids and the mucous membranes of your eyes, nose, or mouth. It is essential that you report immediately any exposure to high-risk fluids. Remember that the best protection available is to follow standard precautions.

jaundice a yellow coloring of skin and the white portion of the eye caused by the substance bilirubin, which is secreted by the liver

SCABIES

A communicable disease that is prevalent in nursing homes and other kinds of group living is scabies. **Scabies** is a disease caused by mites that burrow under the resident's or staff member's skin. The symptoms include a rash, open sores, and severe itching. Because of the itching, the resident scratches, causing red tracks or lines under the skin. The mites are most often found around fingers, wrists, underarms, and genitals. They are common in any dark, moist area of the body as in the skin folds under the breasts, abdomen, and buttocks. The itching is so severe that the resident not only stays awake at night but may injure the skin by vigorous scratching. Scabies is diagnosed by taking scrapings from the skin where the rash is present. Usually, a **dermatologist** (physician who specializes in diseases of the skin) is consulted to obtain a diagnosis and recommend treatment. Scabies is considered a public health issue, so in most states an outbreak must be reported to the public health department. The department may send a nurse to the facility to make recommendations on the latest effective drugs and methods of stopping the spread of scabies.

scabies a disease caused by mites that burrow under the skin

dermatologist a physician who specializes in diseases of the skin

The mites spread by contact, so it is not unusual for staff to develop scabies also. It is even possible for an infected staff member to take the scabies home to his or her family. There are drugs that are applied as a lotion or ointment. Because of the high incidence and incomplete or ineffective treatments, some mites are resistant to certain drugs. Eliminating the scabies may require treatment and retreatment. It is not enough to treat the resident. Any infected staff members must be treated at the same time. At times, the family or other visitors may require treatment. The mites can live apart from the resident or another "host" for a few days. This means that while the resident is being bathed and treated, all the linens and clothing must be washed. Items that come in close contact with the resident that cannot be washed can be placed in plastic bags for at least 3 days. Treatment for scabies requires a concerted effort by the entire facility.

SECTION 5 The Resident's Unit: Admission and Discharge

OBJECTIVES
What You Will Learn

When you have completed this section, you will be able to:

- List two ways the nursing assistant can help make the resident's unit more homelike

- Compile a list of items you would want to have with you if you were admitted to a long-term facility
- Operate a bed and side rails
- Make an occupied bed

- Participate in a simulated admission procedure
- List four tasks to be accomplished when relocating a resident in a facility

KEY TERMS

discharge
incontinent

occupied bed
prosthesis

transfer
unoccupied bed

THE RESIDENT'S UNIT

The resident's unit includes the room space, furniture, and equipment provided for one person (Figure 2-24). Each unit must be separated with a curtain or screen for privacy.

There are many different room sizes and arrangements, from private rooms to two, three, or more residents to a room. Regardless of the number of residents sharing a room, each needs his or her own "space."

For the majority of residents, the LTC facility is their home. Every effort should be made to create a homelike environment. Although certain items

FIGURE 2-24

The resident's unit.

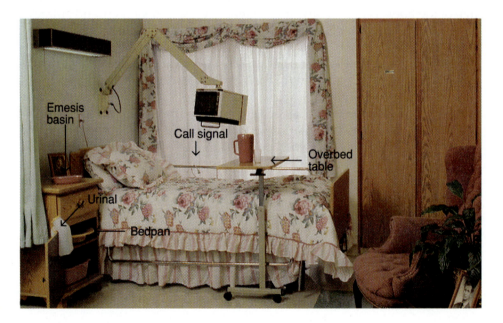

Emesis basin

Call signal

Overbed table

Urinal

Bedpan

are basic, residents are encouraged to bring personal items, including pictures, furniture, and plants. A clock and a calendar will help the resident remain oriented to time and date. When you enter a resident's unit, try to imagine that you are entering their home. Ask permission, particularly if the door is closed or the curtain is drawn. "May I come in?" is a question that shows the residents that you respect their privacy and recognize the unit as their own. You'll notice that when two or three residents share a room they frequently draw imaginary lines to determine which space "belongs" to each. Some will become quite angry if another enters their space.

In most cases, the responsibility for the cleanliness and neatness of the resident's equipment is that of the nursing department. Housekeeping usually is responsible for the cleanliness of the floor, privacy curtains, windows, and the bathrooms, as well as for emptying wastebaskets. You should be aware of your facility's policy on responsibility for the cleanliness of the unit.

There are certain health and safety rules regarding items that may be kept at the resident's bedside. For example, aerosol cans, razor blades, matches, medications, or food that is not in a closed container are items that may not be permitted at the bedside. If you observe any of these items within the resident's unit, report the information to the charge nurse immediately. Be sure you know what items are permitted at the bedside in your facility.

In addition to providing the resident with necessary furnishings and equipment, the unit should be arranged for the safety, comfort, and convenience of the resident.

Convenience is important in helping the resident to be as independent as possible. Many residents can do more for themselves if necessary items are placed within their reach (Figure 2-25). For example, a resident who is paralyzed on one side may need to have the bedside table moved, depending on whatever side is easiest for the resident to use.

Independence is increased for the blind person if necessary items are always kept in the same place. You might even make a chart showing where the items belong. This chart could be kept at the bedside for easy reference by the staff.

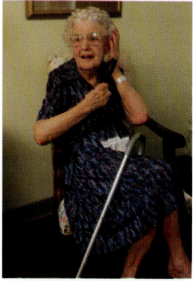

FIGURE 2-25
Promoting independence.

BEDMAKING

Although most residents spend a substantial portion of their time out of bed, the comfort and appearance of the bed is important. The nursing assistant must be able to make a bed that is neat and free of wrinkles. Wrinkles are uncomfortable and can lead to the development of pressure sores (see Chapter 6).

The bed may be made while the resident is in it (called an occupied bed) or when the resident is out of bed (called an **unoccupied bed**). The process is essentially the same, but both procedures will be included here. Review the guidelines for linen handling before you practice bedmaking. Although your facility may use fitted bottom sheets, this procedure includes making mitered corners using a flat bottom sheet.

unoccupied bed   a bed with no one in it

In the LTC facility, you will not be changing the linens completely each day. Although each facility has its own policy, the usual routine is to change the bed completely on the days the resident is bathed or showered (twice weekly) and, of course, when soiled. On a daily basis, you may change only the pillowcase and draw sheet.

Each bed is made with a bottom sheet, top sheet, blanket and/or bedspread, pillow, and pillowcase. Additional bed linens depend on the needs of the resident. For example, a resident who is **incontinent** (has no control over bowel

incontinent   no control over bowel and bladder function

PROCEDURE

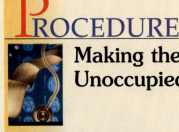

Making the Unoccupied Bed

Preparation

1. Wash your hands.
2. Assemble linens.
3. Place linens on a chair near the bed in the order of use.
4. Adjust the bed to a comfortable working height.

Steps

5. Unfold the bottom sheet and place it lengthwise on the bed. Place the sheet so that the rough edges of the hem will be facing down, away from the resident.
6. Starting at the foot of the bed, open the sheet so that it hangs evenly on each side of the bed. The hem at the foot of the bed is placed so that it is even with the end of the mattress.
7. Raise the mattress and tuck in the sheet at the head of the bed.
8. Miter the corner. Face the head of the bed. With the hand closest to the bed, pick up the edge of the sheet about 12 inches from the edge of the mattress, making a triangle (Figure 2-26). (*Tip:* If you raise the sheet straight up rather than at an angle, you'll form a perfect triangle.)

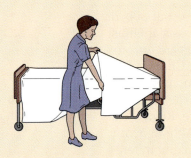

FIGURE 2-26

9. Lay the triangle on the top of the mattress (Figure 2-27).
10. Tuck the hanging portion of the sheet under the mattress.

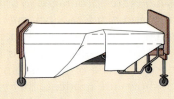

FIGURE 2-27

11. Holding the fold at the edge of the mattress, bring the triangle down and tuck in.
12. Tuck the sheet in all the way to the foot of the bed (Figure 2-28).

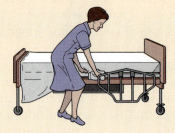

FIGURE 2-28

13. Apply the plastic draw sheet, tuck in (Figure 2-29).

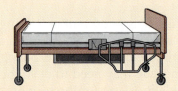

FIGURE 2-29

14. Cover the plastic draw sheet with the cloth draw sheet, tuck in. (Be sure the plastic is completely covered.)
15. Starting at the head of the bed, place the top sheet on the bed with the hem up (leave enough to fold over the edge of the blanket and/or spread).
16. Place the blanket on top of the sheet, unless you are instructed otherwise.
17. Place the spread on top of the blanket.
18. Tuck in the top sheet, blanket, and spread together.
19. Miter the corner but do not tuck in on the side.
20. Move to the opposite side of the bed.
21. Beginning at the head of the bed, tuck in the bottom sheet, pulling tightly as you go.
22. Miter the top corner.
23. Tuck in the plastic draw sheet.
24. Tuck in the cloth draw sheet.
25. Miter the top covers (sheet, blanket, spread). Do not tuck in the sides. *Note:* To prevent pressure on the resident's toes from covers that are too tight, a "toe

pleat" is made. Grasp both sides of the top covers at the mitered corner and gently pull the top covers toward the foot of the bed, making about a 3- to 4-inch fold across the foot of the bed.

26. Fold the hem of the top sheet over the blanket and spread.

27. Put the pillowcase on the pillow:
    - Hold the pillowcase at the center of the end seam.
    - With your hand outside of the case, turn the case back over your hand.
    - Grasp the pillow through the case at the center of one end of the pillow.
    - Bring the case down over the pillow.
    - Fit the corner of the pillow into the seamless corner of the case.
    - Fold the extra material from the side seam under the pillow.

28. Place the pillow on the bed with the open end away from the door.

Ending Steps

29. Adjust the bed to its lowest position.

and/or bladder function) will have a plastic draw sheet (a half-sheet placed from knees to shoulders) covered with a cloth draw sheet and other protective pads or diapers. These additional pads may be cloth or disposable.

A properly made bed will enhance the appearance of the resident's unit. Stand back and look at the bed you've just made. Does it look neat? Is it free of wrinkles? Do the linens hang evenly on either side?

THE OCCUPIED BED

When a resident is unable to be out of bed, it will be necessary to change the linens with the resident in bed. The elements of bedmaking remain the same, with the additional need to protect the privacy, safety, and comfort of the resident.

Making an **occupied bed** frequently is part of giving incontinent care or caring for a resident whose bed is wet or soiled from perspiration, vomiting, or bleeding. You may change all or only part of the linens at this time. A partial bath may be part of the procedure, as well as wiping off the mattress and plastic draw sheet. If the linens of an incontinent resident seem only damp, they should be changed anyway as the odor of urine will be present along with the potential for skin irritation.

occupied bed one with a resident in it

As you practice bedmaking, strive to decrease the number of steps you take as well as the amount of time spent. An efficient nursing assistant can make a bed in 6 minutes!

Make this another opportunity to communicate with the resident. Encourage sharing of past and current events as well as feelings and ideas.

ADMISSION, TRANSFER, AND DISCHARGE

Admission of a resident to an LTC facility is often a time of great stress for both the new resident and the family. The admission process gives the resident and family their first impression of the facility, the staff, and the kind of care given. When the admission is carried out properly and the resident receives a favorable impression, the entire stay is more likely to be a positive one. The importance of this event cannot be overemphasized. If you take time to put yourself in the resident's place, you'll be better able to cope with the resident's feelings and behavior during this stressful experience.

PROCEDURE

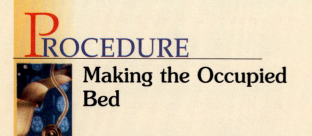

Making the Occupied Bed

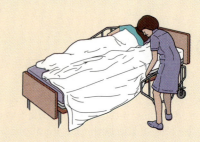

FIGURE 2-31

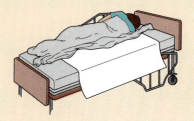

FIGURE 2-32

Preparation

1. Wash your hands.
2. Assemble linens on a chair in order of use.
3. Inform the resident what you are going to do.
4. Provide privacy.
5. Adjust the bed to a comfortable working height with backrest and knee rest flat, if allowed for that resident.
6. Loosen the sheets around the entire bed.

Steps

7. Raise the side rail on the opposite side from where you will be working.
8. Turn the resident to the side toward the raised rail, with the pillow under the head.
9. Roll the cloth draw sheet toward the resident, tucking it against the back (Figure 2-30).

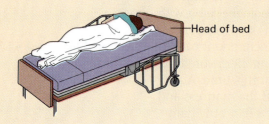

Head of bed

FIGURE 2-30

10. Lay the plastic draw sheet over the resident, after wiping it off, if necessary.
11. Roll the bottom sheet toward the resident and tuck tightly under the back.
12. Unfold the clean bottom sheet and place the center fold in the center of the mattress. Position the sheet as in making the unoccupied bed with the hem even with the foot of the mattress.
13. Tuck in the sheet and miter the top corner. (Figure 2-31)
14. Tuck in the sheet all the way down the bed.
15. Tuck in the plastic draw sheet.
16. Place the clean cloth draw sheet over the plastic draw sheet, tucking in the side closest to you (Figure 2-32).

17. Roll the cloth draw sheet toward the resident. Tuck the sheet under the back (Figure 2-33).

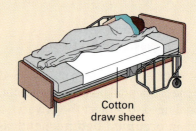

Cotton draw sheet

FIGURE 2-33

18. Raise the side rail on the side where you have been working.
19. Move to the opposite side of the bed.
20. Lower the side rail and roll the resident away from you, over the linens, onto the clean side.
21. Remove the soiled linens and place them at the foot of the bed, between the end of the mattress and the footboard.
22. Pull the clean linens toward you.
23. Tighten the sheets and tuck them in, moving from the head of the bed to the foot (Figure 2-34).
24. Raise the side rail so that you can leave the bedside briefly to dispose of the soiled linens.
25. Change the top sheet by placing it over the soiled sheet so that the resident remains covered. Have the resident hold the clean sheet as you pull the soiled sheet from below. Place at the foot of the bed.

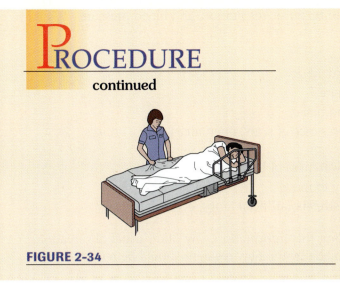

FIGURE 2-34

26. Apply the blanket and/or spread.
27. Tuck in the top covers, mitering the corners.
28. Make the toe pleat.
29. Change the pillowcase.

Ending Steps

30. Position the resident comfortably with the bed in its lowest position.
31. Place the signal cord within reach.
32. Put soiled linens in the appropriate containers.
33. Wash your hands.

One point of view is to look at the losses experienced by the average resident. These may include loss of a home, possessions, pets, a garden, independence and freedom, control over one's life, and privacy. Although facilities make every effort to minimize these losses, to the resident they are highly significant. There indeed is "no place like home." Residents may grieve for the life they once had. Even if they accept the situation, they may never come to like it.

There are some residents who welcome admission to an LTC facility. They may have been lonely, frightened, or unable to meet their own needs. They will enjoy new companionship, good meals, a pleasant environment, and meaningful activities.

Each facility has policies and procedures for the admission of residents. Many procedures are similar regardless of the facility. Find out what the role of the nursing assistant is in the admission process of your facility.

The admission tasks generally include:

- Welcoming the resident
- Gathering information about the resident
- Orienting the resident to new surroundings
- Caring for the resident's personal belongings

WELCOMING THE RESIDENT

To welcome the resident, you should:

- Greet the resident by name
- Introduce yourself
- Explain what you will be doing
- Convey a warm welcome through your facial expression and tone of voice

Gathering information will be accomplished by many health care team members, particularly during the first week. Each will be focusing on a different aspect of the new resident's needs and plans for care.

There is usually an admission form completed by the nursing department. You may be required to fill in all or parts of this form. It usually includes the following information:

- The resident's temperature, pulse, respiration, and blood pressure
- The resident's weight
- The resident's height
- Observation of the resident's:
  —Grooming and hygiene
  —Condition of hair and nails
  —Condition of skin (presence of scars, open areas, sores, bruises, growths, etc.)
  —Level of alertness, awareness of time and place
  —Sight, hearing, ability to move
  —Presence of any **prosthesis** (artificial limbs, eyes, etc.)

prosthesis artificial replacement for a body part such as a limb or eye

In addition to recording this information, any other usual observations, concerns, or complaints made by the new resident should be reported to the charge nurse.

ORIENTATION OF THE RESIDENT

While orienting the new resident to the facility, include any family members who are present. Begin the orientation in the immediate area and gradually include the entire facility. Be sure to emphasize use of the call signal whenever help is needed. Have the new resident practice using the signal once or twice.

A good orientation includes:

- An introduction to facility routines
- A review of facility policies and rules
- An introduction to roommate and staff
- A tour of the facility

It may be necessary to repeat the orientation several times. People who are anxious or frightened do not hear or remember information as well as they normally would.

FIGURE 2-35

Mark items and put them in their proper place.

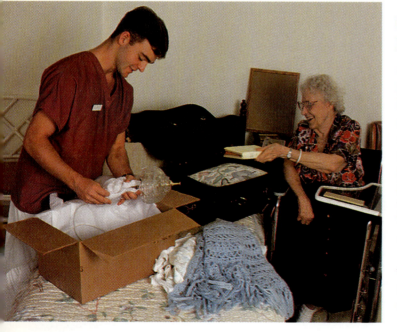

CARE OF PERSONAL BELONGINGS

Care of residents' personal belongings begins at the time of admission. Usually, a personal-effects inventory is made, and all items are listed and made a part of the health record. As a rule, residents should be discouraged from keeping valuable items in the facility. Such items should be placed in the facility safe or sent home with relatives. If the resident insists on keeping valuables, you should notify your charge nurse at once. When listing items brought in with residents, be accurate and complete (Figure 2-35).

Describe items objectively, without placing value on them. For example, if you describe a ring, say, "a gold-colored metal ring with a clear stone," rather than a "gold diamond ring."

In addition to listing items brought into the facility with a resident, the nursing assistant assists in marking items with the resident's name and in putting the items in the proper place. When possible, have residents assist and instruct you where they would like things kept. Allow them to make as many decisions as possible. This helps them feel more "in control" during this time.

Make a special effort during the early admission period to be warm, friendly, and attentive to the new resident. This helps to make the resident's first impression a positive one.

TRANSFERRING THE RESIDENT

The term **transfer** simply means to move from one place to another. You might transfer a resident from a bed to a wheelchair or from one room to another in the same facility or from the LTC facility to an acute-care hospital.

transfer to move from one place to another

There are some general principles to keep in mind when a resident is relocated. Regardless of the reason for the move, the resident should be informed of it as soon as possible. The reason and the destination should be given. Special care must be taken not to lose any of the resident's belongings. A careful check of the entire room and bathroom should be made.

Some residents may become disoriented as a result of a move. Familiar sights are no longer present to remind them of where they are. When moving residents, you may have to remind them frequently of the location of the new room. It may be weeks before they feel at home in their new environment. Because of this, moving residents should be kept to a minimum and done only when absolutely necessary.

Residents and families need to be informed in advance when a room change is planned, to allow them time to adjust to the idea. Helping residents who have formed close relationships with their roommates to remain together and/or introducing them to their new roommates in advance may reduce the anxiety that a room change may cause.

DISCHARGING THE RESIDENT

Residents sometimes may be moved to an acute care hospital. When the resident is expected to return soon, this move is referred to as a transfer. If the resident is gone for a long time or is not going to return at all, the move is called a **discharge.** Facility policy determines how long a resident may be out of the facility before being discharged. Usually, 72 hours is the deadline. At this point the records are closed. If the resident later returns, a new admission is made, and a new medical record is started.

discharge long-time absence or permanent exit from an acute care hospital

If one of your residents is to be transferred, remember that the resident "represents" your facility. The kind of care you give will be judged by the appearance of the resident. Be sure the resident is clean and well groomed and that the hair is combed and nails are trimmed and clean. Send any personal items needed such as dentures, glasses, or hearing aids with the resident. If the resident is to return shortly, personal items may be left in the room. Other times, personal items can be listed, packed, and put into storage. Items sent with the resident should be listed in the chart along with the time and method of transfer, such as by ambulance or by private car.

Residents who leave the facility permanently are considered discharged. They may be discharged to an acute care hospital, to home, or to another level of care, such as a residential care facility. Residents may be discharged only with a physician's order.

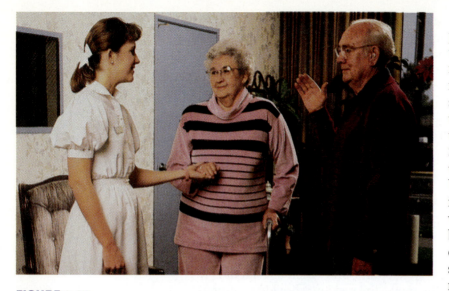

FIGURE 2-36

Discharging the patient: the last impression.

Just as the resident's first impressions are important to the relationship between facility and resident, last impressions are long remembered (Figure 2-36). You should make a special effort to tell the resident good-bye and to extend good wishes for the future. Special care must be taken to see that no belongings are left behind. Usually, there is a personal-effects inventory list of items brought in with the resident. These items must be checked off at the time of discharge and the inventory form signed by the resident or a family member. Check your facility policy to see who is responsible for the various parts of the discharge procedure. The resident should be escorted from the facility by a staff member, who gives assistance with carrying belongings as needed.

SUMMARY

The environment in which you are working and your residents are living needs to be one that is clean, safe, and comfortable. It is also important to prevent injury to residents, staff, and visitors by providing the proper environment, staying alert to potential harm, and taking the right action when there is danger.

Such things as preventing fires, burns, falls, back injury, and transmission of infections require vigilance and skill. You now know what actions to take in the event of a fire (rescue, confine, alert, extinguish) or disaster, how to use protective devices and restraints, and what to do if, despite best efforts, an accident occurs.

You can protect yourself from injury by using proper body mechanics when lifting, moving, or making a bed. Making the bed according to good technique also ensures the resident's comfort and helps reduce risk of pressure ulcers acquired from wrinkles in the sheets. You will be able to protect yourself and others from transmission of infection through handwashing and proper use of protective equipment like gloves, masks, goggles, and gowns.

You have learned about some of the important communicable diseases like AIDs, hepatitis, and tuberculosis. That knowledge can help you recognize and prevent the transmission of these very serious diseases.

Welcoming and making new residents comfortable is a valuable role that you may play. By helping them put their possessions away and by orienting them to the environment, you will reduce some of their fear and anxiety. You'll also help them in transferring to another room, floor, or unit as well as sending them home with a positive impression of both you and the facility where you work.

OBRA HIGHLIGHTS

One of the noteworthy changes brought about through the OBRA legislation on nursing home reform was related to use of restraints. OBRA addresses the need to use restraints carefully and only when proven necessary. The regulations state that the resident has the right to be free from any physical or chemical restraints imposed for purposes of discipline or convenience, and not required to treat the resident's medical symptoms. Other rights relate to the resident's refusing any unwanted treatment, to participate in development of the plan of care, and the right to be in a safe environment. All of these rights are involved when decisions about restraint use are being made.

SELF STUDY

Choose the best answer for each question or statement.

1. Which of the following is **not** a way that the nursing assistant can help prevent falls?
   a. Ensure that wheelchairs and beds are in the locked position during transfers.
   b. Wipe up spills as soon as they occur to prevent slipping.
   c. Keep the bed adjustment gatch (handle) out so it can be reached easily.
   d. Report broken or malfunctioning equipment immediately.

2. When you walk past a resident's room, you notice that a visitor is smoking in the room, which is against facility policy. The visitor has been reminded about smoking policies in the past. What will you do?
   a. Set off the smoke detector, which is wired to the fire alarm.
   b. Insist that the visitor leave the building immediately.
   c. Say nothing since it is a visitor, not the resident, who is smoking.
   d. Report the violation of smoking rules to your supervisor.

3. Which of the following is an example of a postural support?
   a. a seat belt worn while in a wheelchair
   b. a wedge cushion in the seat of a wheelchair
   c. side rails on the bed in the up position
   d. a back brace to hold the resident upright while sitting

4. Mr. Simons has been placed in a restraint according to the doctor's order. How often will you release the restraint?
   a. every 1–2 hours
   b. every 2–3 hours
   c. every 3–4 hours
   d. once during your shift

5. Which of the following actions will you take while Mr. Simons's restraint is off?
   a. Help him change positions.
   b. Help him do range-of-motion exercises.
   c. Allow him to move around without restriction.
   d. all of the above

6. Mrs. Jackson is sometimes unsteady while ambulating, even with her walker. The doctor wants the staff to use alternatives to re-straints. Which of the following would be appropriate action for the nursing assistant to take when caring for Mrs. Jackson?
   a. Use a bedsheet to tie around Mrs. Jackson while she is in her wheelchair.
   b. Place Mrs. Jackson in a wheelchair where she can be easily observed by the staff.
   c. Assign another resident to watch over Mrs. Jackson and call if she tries to get up.
   d. Keep Mrs. Jackson in bed with the side rails up when her family is not available to watch her.

7. You observed Mrs. Jackson slip down in her wheelchair and onto the floor. When you check on her, she does not seem to be hurt. What should you do?
   a. Report it to the charge nurse immediately and assist with completing an incident report.
   b. Assist Mrs. Jackson back into the wheelchair and restrain her so she won't slip again.
   c. Ask another nursing assistant to check Mrs. Jackson too and to help you put her to bed.
   d. Call for a portable x-ray to be done to be sure Mrs. Jackson was not injured when she slipped.

8. Mr. Bernstein uses oxygen continuously. Which of the following would be unsafe for you to do during his care?
   a. Shave him using shaving cream and a disposable razor.
   b. Apply skin lotion to dry areas on his neck and face.
   c. Light a candle to help decrease unpleasant odors.
   d. all of the above

9. You find a fire in Mr. Bernstein's trash can. Which type of fire extinguisher should you use to fight this fire?
   a. Class A   c. Class C
   b. Class B   d. Class D

10. When you use a fire extinguisher to fight a fire, which of the following actions are correct?
   a. Break the safety pin and point the nozzle at the top of the flames.
   b. Pull the handles apart and point the nozzle at the middle of the flames.
   c. Aim the nozzle at the base of the flame and sweep from side to side.
   d. Aim the nozzle beyond the flames and pump the handles together.

11. Which microorganisms occur the most frequently and produce diseases in humans?
   a. viruses and protozoa
   b. viruses and bacteria
   c. bacteria and toxins
   d. bacteria and fungi

12. Which of the following conditions are
needed for bacteria to grow?
   a. dark, dry, cool environment
   b. warm, moist, and light environment
   c. dry, warm, and dark environment
   d. warm, moist, and dark environment

13. Which of these would **not** be considered
medical waste?
   a. used needles and syringes
   b. gowns worn by patients
   c. gloves worn by nursing staff
   d. facial tissues used by patients

14. You are cleaning Ms. Wong's dentures
when another nursing assistant needs your
help immediately with a resident. Which of
these actions should you take?
   a. Leave the room while wearing your
      gloves and go assist him.
   b. Remove your gloves, wash your hands,
      and go to assist him.

   c. Remove one glove and use only the un-
      gloved hand to assist him.
   d. Leave on both gloves, wash your gloved
      hands, and assist him.

15. Which of the following is the most frequent mode of transmitting pathogens in a
health care facility?
   a. by contact transmission
   b. by droplets transmission
   c. by airborne transmission
   d. by reverse transmission

16. When you are bathing Mr. Concho, a new
resident, you notice red lines under his skin
around his fingers and wrists. He is
scratching at the area and has an open sore
on his left wrist. What should you do?
   a. Bathe him well and use an antibacterial
      soap in these areas.
   b. Apply lotion to these areas after the bath
      since his skin must be dry.
   c. Inform your charge nurse immediately
      since he may have scabies.
   d. Put on a mask and gown immediately in
      case he has scabies.

Getting C O N N E C T E D
Multimedia **Extension** Activities

 www.prenhall.com/will-black

Use the above address to access the free, interactive Companion Website created for this textbook. Hear the pronunciation of the key terms in the chapter. Get instant feedback to a variety of chapter-related questions. Link to other interesting sites.

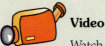 **Video**

Watch the videos *Infection Control, Transmission-Based Precautions,* and *Body Mechanics* from the Care Provider Skills series.

CASE STUDY

Mr. Smith is a 52-year-old man admitted to your facility because he has AIDS in its advanced stages. He is no longer able to care for himself and needs help with all activities of daily living. He is mentally alert and oriented. He has friends who visit frequently.

1. What precautions do you need to take when caring for Mr. Smith?
   a. Always provide care with a buddy so you can watch each other's techniques.
   b. Use standard precautions that you use with all residents.
   c. Use isolation technique when providing direct care.
   d. No precautions are needed since he has no bleeding or open wounds.
2. His friends are coming down the hall with a radio and small television to keep him occupied. You should
   a. inform them that the maintenance man needs to be sure the equipment is electrically safe and add the equipment to the resident's list of personal property
   b. tell them that no personal items are allowed in the room
   c. clean the equipment with alcohol
   d. assist them in finding an extra table and say nothing
3. What do you say about caring for Mr. Smith to your friends and family?
   a. Tell them they have nothing to fear since you are wearing a gown, mask, and gloves.
   b. Tell them you are looking for another job because you don't want to contract AIDS.
   c. Tell them nothing because the resident's diagnosis is confidential.
   d. Tell them nothing, just be sure you change clothes and remove your shoes before coming into the home.

Chapter 3

SPECIAL NEEDS OF THE ELDERLY AND CHRONICALLY ILL

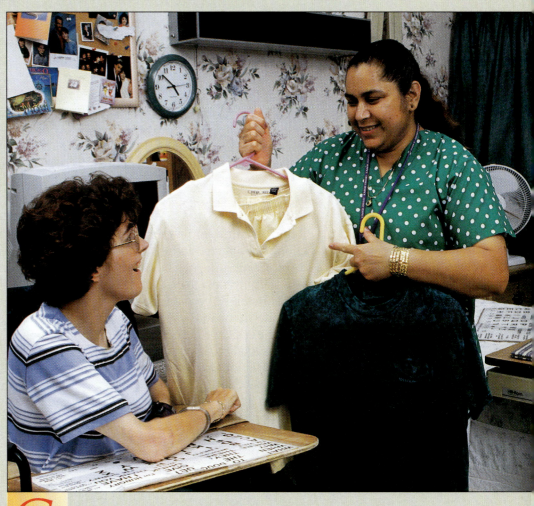

CARING TIP

Show your interest and caring by listening to the resident, by complying with his or her requests, and by giving the resident your full attention whenever you are together.

Andrea O'Connor, EdD, JD, RN
Professor of Nursing
Western Connecticut State University
Danbury, CT

OBJECTIVES
What You Will Learn

When you have completed this section, you will be able to:

- Give three examples of ways the nursing assistant can encourage residents to be more independent

- List three observations you've made that reflect your facility's philosophy of care

KEY TERMS

activities of daily living (ADL)   contracture   quality of life

philosophy   rehabilitation

PHILOSOPHY OF LONG-TERM CARE

philosophy   search for a general understanding of values

The functions, purposes, and types of LTC facilities have been reviewed; however, the "philosophy of care" is something different. The study of **philosophy** is a search for a general understanding of values. It includes the most general beliefs, concepts, and attitudes of an individual or group.

REHABILITATION

rehabilitation   the restoration of the individual to the fullest physical, mental, social, vocational, and economic capacity of which he or she is capable

contracture   shortening of the muscles from inactivity

activities of daily living (ADL)   activities or tasks needed for daily living, such as eating, grooming, dressing, bathing, washing, and toileting

Rehabilitation, or restorative care, is given to each resident. This means that efforts are directed to help each resident become as independent as possible. Rehabilitation includes prevention of complications, retraining in lost skills, and learning new skills. For example, care of a resident who is paralyzed on one side might be planned to prevent **contractures** (shortening of muscles from inactivity) in the affected limbs, to retrain the resident in walking, and to train the resident in the use of a cane.

Included in rehabilitation are all the tasks and skills needed for daily living. These skills are called **activities of daily living (ADL).** ADL include such things as communication, eating, grooming, dressing, bathing, walking, and toileting. The degree to which residents can become independent in ADL depends on both their physical condition and desire to achieve independence. Very often this requires hard work.

The physician, as well as the rest of the health-care team, sets a goal (determines what is possible) and develops a plan for the resident to reach that goal. Most residents can achieve a greater degree of independence when their special needs are addressed in a rehabilitation program (Figure 3-1). As you acquire a rehabilitation philosophy, you will be able to find ways that residents can be more independent. A rehabilitation philosophy includes learning to accept the accomplishment of small, simple goals. Although a total cure may not be possible, you will come to enjoy the rewards from any progress the resident makes. Every resident should be encouraged to do as much as possible independently. Feeling good about oneself is enhanced by being independent. The best way to relearn old skills and to learn new skills is through repetition and practice.

Although the professionals on the health care team are most qualified to teach the resident, the nursing assistant should help encourage the residents, praise their accomplishments, remind them of what has been taught, and report any need for further teaching.

Facilities accept the responsibility to assist the residents in meeting basic human needs. This means care must be provided to meet psychosocial (psychological and emotional) needs as well as physiological (body) needs. Care must be directed to both the mind and the body!

Philosophies, ideas, and goals are worthless unless they become deeds! In other words, a philosophy is of no value unless it is put into practice. You will know what kind of care philosophy your facility has by *what you see!*

The following are just a few examples of what you might see when a facility practices an accepted philosophy of care:

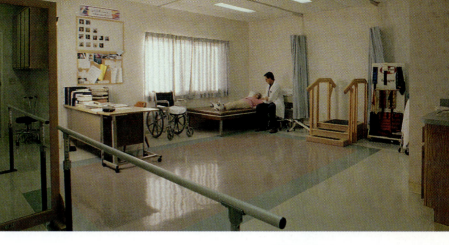

FIGURE 3-1
The rehabilitation unit.

- The facility has a warm, homelike atmosphere.
- Residents are encouraged to make decisions about their care and do as much for themselves as possible.
- Residents take part in social and recreational activities.
- Residents are encouraged and assisted to wear their own clothing and to keep their own belongings.
- Residents are assisted to have good personal hygiene.
- Residents are always treated with respect and dignity.
- Residents are given choices and as much control as possible over their daily care and activities.

PROMOTING INDEPENDENCE

Helping each resident to achieve greater independence is an essential key to improving their **quality of life,** as required under OBRA. Facilities must help each resident "attain their highest practicable functional level." In order to assess and identify resident needs, an assessment tool mandated by federal government is used (the Minimum Data Set, referred to as the MDS). This functional assessment is done upon admission, when significant changes in condition occur, and quarterly in order to plan care that will keep the resident at his or her highest possible functional level.

quality of life a concept that includes all the aspects that make life worth living; best defined by the individual himself

The nursing assistant plays a very important role by reporting changes in functional abilities to the charge nurse promptly so that they can be immediately addressed and helping residents to maintain their abilities by promoting independence. The residents' plan of care should specify which activities of daily living they need assistance with, the goal to be achieved, and the actions or approaches that each team member will use to help residents achieve their goals.

Never risk the safety of the resident by encouraging performance of dangerous tasks like bathing alone or transferring alone unless the interdisciplinary team has determined that it is safe for the resident to do so.

Most residents can perform some activities independently—combing or brushing their hair, holding the bread during a meal, or simply deciding which clothes they would like to wear. It may be difficult to stand by while a resident struggles to perform a task, but remember that function declines without repetition and practice. Encourage and support the resident's efforts toward independence as you carry out daily care. Review the keys to promoting independence (Figure 3-2).

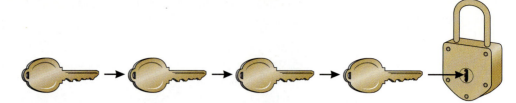

FIGURE 3-2

Keys to promoting independence.

Praise every attempt at independence → Overlook resident's failures → Tell resident you have confidence in his/her ability → Allow resident time to do for him/herself → Independence

SECTION 2 Psychological Aspects of Aging

OBJECTIVES
What You Will Learn

When you have completed this section, you will be able to:

- Define the term **psychosocial**

- List the five basic human needs that Maslow described
- Describe two additional ways by which you can help to meet the residents' need for approval and acceptance, need for recognition and

respect, and need for self-esteem
- List the three developmental tasks of aging
- Complete a questionnaire about aging

KEY TERMS

informed consent
physical needs

psychosocial
security needs
self-fulfillment needs

social needs
status needs

As the number of elderly persons continues to increase, society is becoming more and more aware of the needs and rights of the elderly. The problems of growing old in America are widely publicized. Common myths about aging are being dispelled through education and media programs. It is very important to understand the facts regarding the aging process and to remember that aging is not a disease. In order to measure your own attitudes and knowledge about aging and the aged, complete the "Attitudes about Aging" questionnaire included in your Student Workbook. Most of the nation's elderly are active, productive people who live and function independently. Increasing medical advances and emphasis on living a healthy life and preventing disease are dramatically extending life expectancy.

Aging is an inevitable process and is as yet irreversible. We become old gradually. Most people meet the challenge of aging with imagination and success. America generally is a youth-oriented society. Our culture does not practice the kind of recognition and respect many other societies bestow upon their elderly. In addition, we are an industrial society in which most people have to work outside of their homes, leaving no one at home to provide daily care for the elderly. The long-term care facility very often is the only practical way families can provide for the needs of their elderly loved ones. Contrary to the popular belief that families abandon their elderly in long-term facilities, studies show that most families continue to provide their elderly with loving support. When residents have no families, they often have longtime friends who visit and care for them.

When the elderly become ill and require the care and services of a long-term care facility, many adaptations are necessary. Most important are the psychological and social changes that they experience. Care must be provided to meet their complex **psychosocial** needs.

- Psycho—refers to mental or emotional processes
- Social—refers to interactions and relationships with others

It is not easy to separate mental processes such as behavior and feelings from the social roles and relationships unique to each person. One of the most commonly accepted theories of aging suggests that personalities and their tendency toward certain kinds of behavior are consistent throughout life. A person who is a dynamic leader at age 30 will be a dynamic leader at age 70. When illness and hospitalization disrupt a person's life, role changes occur that make adaptation or adjustment necessary. The nursing assistant can help the resident successfully make these adaptations by understanding human motivation and behavior.

The effort to understand human personality began with Sigmund Freud, an Austrian physician who believed that the human mind has two levels: a conscious and an unconscious. Freud believed that by studying the conscious mind and behavior we would better understand the unconscious mind.

As Freud's theories were examined and expanded, another branch of psychology developed based on the idea that all behavior is learned through a system of rewards and punishments. B. F. Skinner, a scientist, believed that "right" behaviors could be encouraged through a system of rewards and "wrong" behaviors could be eliminated through some types of punishment.

Another branch of psychology, called developmental psychology, was introduced in the 1950s by Erik Erikson, Carl Jung, Abraham Maslow, and others. They supported the idea that emotional well-being, as well as each individual's personality development, depends on the successful completion of a series of developmental tasks at various stages in life. It is believed that successful aging and the completion of these developmental tasks results in increased wisdom.

The developmental tasks to be accomplished for the elderly resident include adjustments and adaptations to the biological, psychological, social, and cultural aspects of aging. These tasks include:

1. An adjustment to the aging process (accepting physical changes and losses). A successful adjustment results in acknowledgment of the realities of aging.
2. Believing that life is important and meaningful; the individual reflects on the meaning of his or her own life.
3. Reviewing life's successes and failures and putting them into perspective as the end of life approaches. Individuals try to determine how valuable their life has been.
4. Accepting that things in the past cannot be changed and a "letting go" of past disappointments and regrets. Individuals focus on the present.
5. An adaptation to the social roles that are appropriate for their own age group.
6. Reconciling moral dilemmas related to personal and social values.

Some of the dilemmas residents and families experience include:

- Role changes related to giving and taking advice and personal freedom
- Changes in living arrangements
- Financial issues

- Legal concerns, transfers of assets: wills, powers of attorney for health care, conservatorship
- Advance directive decisions
- Interpersonal problems with family, friends, others

It is believed that the resident who successfully resolves these developmental tasks will attain a higher level of self-awareness and thus satisfaction with life. Failure to resolve these tasks may inhibit emotional growth and result in emotional instability.

BASIC NEEDS

We all have very basic human needs. Basic needs have been ranked in order of priority by the psychologist Abraham Maslow, who is the author of a classic book in the field of human behavior called *Motivation and Personality.* Maslow identified these basic needs as follows (Figure 3-3):

- Physical needs
- Security needs
- Social needs
- Status needs
- Self-fulfillment needs

physical needs basic human needs for food, water, oxygen, rest, exercise, and sex

security needs basic human needs for physical safety, shelter, and protection

social needs basic human need for approval and acceptance

Physical needs are essential to the survival of each human being. They include the need for food, water, oxygen, rest, exercise, and sex. Even touch is considered necessary for survival. Many studies have been done that show that human beings and animals can become ill or even die when deprived of touch. In your role as a nursing assistant, you will spend a great deal of time assisting residents to meet their physical needs. **Security needs** are concerned with physical safety, feeling protected, and having a job and shelter. You help meet the security needs of residents when you:

- Provide a safe, secure environment.
- Use side rails or postural supports as necessary.
- Help residents feel at home and comfortable in their environment.
- Help them develop trust in those who provide their care by keeping your promises and by speaking well about other staff members.

Next are the **social needs,** the need for approval and acceptance. You help residents meet their social needs when you:

- Praise the resident for accomplishments.
- Encourage the resident to try new things.
- Show acceptance of the individual by respecting his or her individuality.
- Provide care in a kind, considerate manner.
- Provide the essence of human warmth by a gentle touch or a gentle caring voice.
- Show interest in the residents and their family and friends.

FIGURE 3-3

Basic human needs.

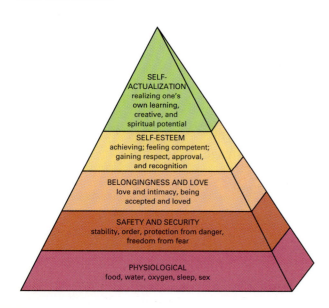

SELF-ACTUALIZATION
realizing one's own learning, creative, and spiritual potential

SELF-ESTEEM
achieving; feeling competent; gaining respect, approval, and recognition

BELONGINGNESS AND LOVE
love and intimacy, being accepted and loved

SAFETY AND SECURITY
stability, order, protection from danger, freedom from fear

PHYSIOLOGICAL
food, water, oxygen, sleep, sex

After social needs are met, the **status needs,** the needs for recognition and respect, become most important. You can help residents meet these status needs when you:

- Address the resident by a proper name and title.
- Listen to residents' concerns and reminiscences.
- Make the resident feel important.
- Protect the residents' privacy needs.
- Ask their opinion and discuss current issues.

The highest level of needs are the **self-fulfillment needs.** These are the needs to achieve as much as possible and to reach the highest potential of development (Figure 3-4). You help the resident meet these self-fulfillment needs when you:

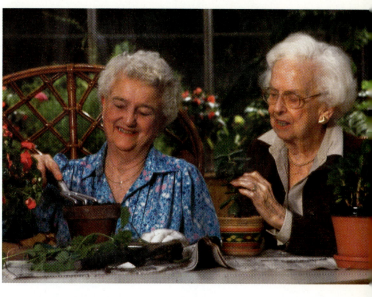

FIGURE 3-4
Help the resident participate in meaningful activities.

status needs basic human needs for recognition and respect

self-fulfillment needs basic human need to reach the highest potential and to accomplish one's life goals

- Share health-care goals with the resident and allow the resident to work toward achieving the goal. Nothing succeeds like success.
- Help the resident to recognize the purpose and direction in his or her life.
- Help the resident to participate in meaningful activities.
- Help the resident recognize the contribution he or she has made throughout a lifetime.
- Assist the resident to look good! Assist with dressing and grooming as needed.
- Allow the resident to direct and control as much of his or her life as possible. Dependency does not foster self-esteem.
- Allow the resident to participate in and approve the plan of care.
- Encourage socialization—the acceptance and approval of friends and family builds self-confidence and self-esteem.

OBRA refers to helping resident's attain the highest quality of life possible; having control of one's life is a major factor. Resident rights are specific:

"The resident has a right to a dignified existence, self-determination and communication with and access to persons and services inside and outside the facility. . . ."

"The resident has the right to make choices about aspects of his/her life in the facility that are significant to the resident. . . ."

"The resident has a right to choose activities, schedules, and health care consistent with his/her interests, assessments, and plans of care. . . ."

We give control to residents when we offer them as many choices as possible. Examples of giving choices include:

- Would you like to shower in the mornings or evenings?
- Would you like to attend the activity exercise program today?
- Would you like to have your family present at the Interdisciplinary Team Conference?

Make offering choices a habit.

INFORMED CONSENT

Another very important resident right is related to informed consent.

> "The resident has the right to be fully informed in advance about care and treatment that may affect the resident's well being. . . ."

This includes prescriptions for new medications or changes in the dosage of routine medications. Residents or their decision makers have the right to know what medications have been prescribed by the physician and what the risks or side effects might be. It is very important when medications are prescribed to control behavior (referred to as psychoactive medications) that residents or their decision makers have a complete understanding of the risks versus the benefits before they consent to their use.

> Residents have "the right to refuse treatment and to refuse to participate in experimental research. . . ."

informed consent permission obtained from a resident to perform or withhold a medical procedure; must be voluntary and in writing

Giving consent is more than saying yes or signing a consent form. Residents and decision makers must give **informed consent.** This means that the resident and/or designated decision maker clearly understands the reasons for the medical treatment, the benefits and risks associated with the treatment, the consequences of not having the treatment, and other possible alternatives. When this kind of accurate information is provided by the physician, the resident or decision maker is able to weigh all the information and give informed consent.

When a resident is not capable of independent decision making, a specific resident right states: "In the case of a resident adjudged incompetent under the laws of a state by a court of competent jurisdiction, the rights of the resident are exercised by the person appointed under state law to act on the resident's behalf. . . ."

Many residents complete legal documents appointing an "agent" to act on their behalf if they are unable to do so; this document is referred to as a Durable Power of Attorney for Health Care in some states and as a Living Will in other states.

State laws differ regarding legal guardians and conservatorship; the important thing for the nursing assistant to understand is that others (often referred to as a surrogate decision maker) may be legally designated to make decisions on behalf of the resident.

PRIVACY

The need for privacy is so important that it requires special mention. Protect privacy of information and privacy of the person as you go about your everyday tasks. Be sure to draw the curtains in the resident's room when performing any kind of personal care. Be aware that the window curtains may also need to be closed. Screen the resident not only from public view but also from view of any roommates who may be present. Never assume that the resident "doesn't mind." Sometimes, when you assist a resident to the toilet, she or he may say "leave the door open, so you'll know when I'm finished." Explain that you can't do that but you'll stay within calling distance. Any time a door is closed or curtains are drawn around a resident's unit, ask permission to enter. Avoid giving personal care in public areas or making public comments like, "You've spilled food all over yourself. Let's go clean you up." That is an invasion of the resident's privacy and right to be treated with dignity.

You will be able to identify many more ways in which to meet the basic human needs of residents. Remember, one of the best ways to recognize and meet their needs is to recognize and understand your own needs. If you treat others as you would like to be treated, you will seldom go wrong.

Perhaps one of the greatest challenges you will face in your role as a nursing assistant will be to develop sensitivity to the needs of others (Figure 3-5). The technical skills are easily taught, but dedication, concern, caring, and wanting to provide the best care possible are traits *you must want to achieve.* A modification of the "Golden Rule" is still the best guide: "Provide care to others as you would have others provide care to you or your loved one."

Aging is inevitable—"unless we can create a world which offers the possibility of aging with grace, honor and meaningfulness, no one can look forward to the future" (Seymour Hallech, *Nursing and the Aged,* McGraw-Hill, 1976).

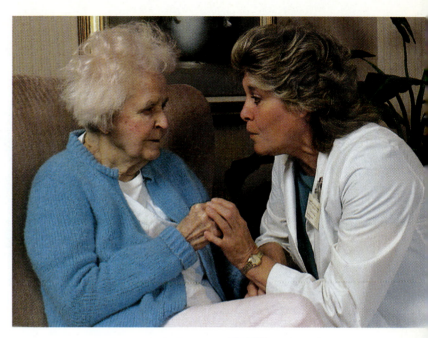

FIGURE 3-5

Developing sensitivity.

SECTION 3 Role Changes

OBJECTIVES
What You Will Learn

When you have completed this section, you will be able to:

- Define the term **role**
- List the roles you play
- Differentiate the characteristics of the sick role from those of the well role
- Give three ways the nursing assistant can minimize role changes experienced by the resident

KEY TERMS

age appropriate

disabled

role

sick role

well role

To understand the feelings, attitudes, and behaviors of the resident in an LTC facility, the nursing assistant must understand the concept of roles and role changes.

A **role** is defined as a part one plays in relationship to others (Figure 3-6). The role we play also affects the way others treat us or respond to us. Roles have specific behavior associated with them. When we are in a particular role, we behave in a particular way.

In a movie or on television, actors are hired to play various roles. Their roles include their lines (the words they speak), their appearance (age, type of clothing), and what they do (behavior). Successful actors are able to perform in many roles during their careers. Even though they personally may be nothing like any of the characters they portray, their skill lies in their ability to convince others that they are.

We, too, play many roles in our everyday lives. Some roles we choose; some are assigned to us. For every role, there are expected behaviors as well as expected ways we are treated. There are roles people associate with age

role   part one plays in relationship to others

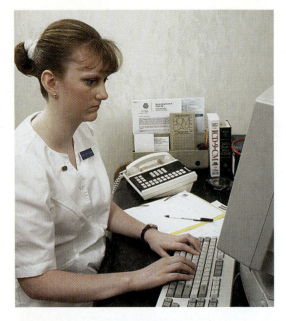

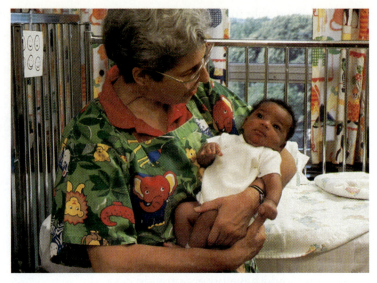

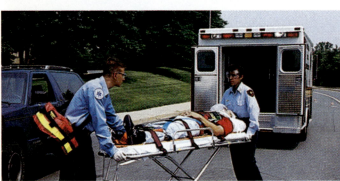

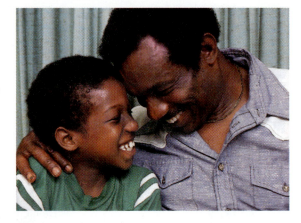

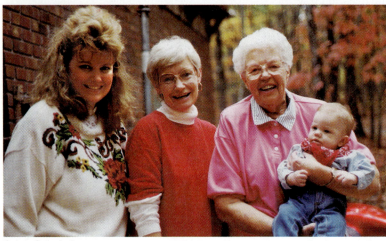

FIGURE 3-6

The varying roles we play.

(2-year-olds are difficult, teenagers are rebellious, older people are cantankerous); roles associated with sex (men are expected to be strong, women are expected to be weak); roles related to social position (the wealthy are snobbish, the poor are humble); and roles associated with professions (lawyers and physicians are intelligent, laborers are not).

As you can see from these examples, the expectations that accompany various roles lead to great conflict at times because each of us wishes to be seen as a unique person. We resent being stereotyped or typecast. Many psychological factors influence how successful an individual is in meeting role expectations as well as how that person adapts to role changes. Nonetheless, to succeed in a given role, certain behaviors must be adopted. Chapter 1 provided the information you need to assume the role of nursing assistant successfully.

Admission to an LTC facility brings about role changes for the resident, regardless of the facility's effort to minimize these changes. Residents frequently grieve over their lost roles and experience difficulty adopting new ones. The resident may have to give up the role of provider and head of the family. It may no longer be possible to be the grandmother who bakes cookies with the children or the grandfather who takes the children to a ball game. Now it is up to the grandchild to visit or take the grandparents on an outing. The reversal of roles presents a difficult adjustment to many residents.

There are other types of roles that influence residents and their behavior. These are the well role, the sick role, and the disabled role.

The **well role** is characterized by independence, responsibility, usefulness, and decision making. The well person is expected to contribute to the well-being of others and is generally regarded as a valuable member of society.

The **sick role** is characterized by dependence, weakness, control by others, lack of responsibility, and uselessness. While the well person gives, the sick person takes.

The **disabled** person suffers from role confusion, being neither sick nor well. Not only is it difficult to know how to behave, but others have difficulty knowing whether to treat the individual as sick or well. Given an opportunity to express their wishes, most disabled people say they prefer to be treated as well. They wish to be as independent as possible, within the limitation of their disability.

Many residents move back and forth between the sick role and the well role. It is important to recognize the role changes that occur and to provide care based on the resident's needs at the time.

Often, people explain a resident's continuing dependency by comparing him or her to a child. An elderly person who may be confused is said to be in his second childhood. This comparison creates a situation where an adult seen as a child is treated like a child and thus continues to behave as a child.

Some residents may behave in childlike ways because of their illness, disability, and dependency. Despite their physical and mental limitations, they are not children and should never be treated like children. Referring to the residents as "kids" or "babies" is never appropriate. By the same token, the manner of dress, grooming, and types of recreational and social activities should be **age appropriate** (appropriate to the chronological age of the person). For example, having adults color in a coloring book with crayons is not age appropriate. Painting a picture or using colored pens to finish a drawing of a farm in the winter would be age appropriate.

Our society often reinforces or rewards illness by paying special attention to those who are ill. We visit the sick and bring them flowers and gifts. We tell the person that we care for them and show our concern. For some, being sick becomes more desirable than being well.

In order to promote well behavior, the facility and its staff must recognize that sickness does have some attractive features and try to make wellness more desirable than sickness. This is accomplished through praising the resident for all efforts at independence, by spending time with the resident, and by showing concern. The family members also need to be involved so that they work with the facility staff by reinforcing or rewarding well behavior and independence.

Perhaps the most difficult role change occurs when residents have to leave their home or normal surroundings to reside in an LTC facility. This role change can be very difficult for some. You can do a great deal to help the resident change roles successfully by the way you provide care.

well role behaviors associated with being well (i.e., independence, increased responsibility, usefulness, control, and decision making)

sick role behavior associated with being sick; dependence, weakness, control by others, decreased responsibility and uselessness

disabled limitation in the ability to function normally

age appropriate appropriate to the chronological age of a person

OBJECTIVES
What You Will Learn

When you have completed this section, you will be able to:

- List four factors influencing individual behavior
- Identify methods of coping with anger that are acceptable for nursing assistants
- Select the most helpful response by the nursing assistant in sample situations

KEY TERMS

culture
environment

feelings or emotions
heredity
interests

standards
values

---

heredity traits we are born with

environment means of providing a safe environment that is as free as possible of pathogenic organisms

culture specimen of body tissue or fluids kept under special laboratory conditions to detect the presence of microorganisms

interests those things we enjoy or care about

feelings or emotions outward expression of mood including happiness, grief, anger, etc.

values what we consider to be most important

standards what is acceptable and unacceptable to us

Performing nursing tasks or skills is quite simple when compared to developing effective interpersonal skills. Although we each have varying abilities to get along with others based on our own personality and life experiences, we can learn to increase our skills in relating to others significantly.

Psychologists and psychiatrists have developed a great body of knowledge about human behavior. Despite many different ideas and philosophies, there are some common principles. Developing skill in interpersonal relations begins with knowing and understanding yourself. Although we are each unique individuals, we are also alike in many ways. We all share the same basic human needs, but we differ in the way we meet those needs.

Our ways of relating to others and our ways of behaving are determined by many factors:

- **Heredity**—traits we are born with
- **Environment**—our surroundings, both physical and social
- **Culture**—habits and customs of our group
- **Interests**—what we enjoy or care about
- **Feelings or emotions**—happiness, grief, anger, jealousy, love
- **Values**—what we consider to be most important
- **Standards**—what is acceptable and unacceptable to us
- Expectations of others—our behavior tends to conform to what others expect of us
- Learning experiences—we learn which behaviors work in certain situations and discard those that don't work
- Stress (such as illness)—affects our behavior

CULTURAL AWARENESS Understanding the effect of cultural differences is necessary to develop successful relationships with residents, family members, and co-workers. Don't assume that everyone is just like you. The best way to learn about other cultures is to ask a person from that culture to describe his or her culture. Be aware that culture affects beliefs and customs about:

- Food
- Clothing
- Relationships

- Religion
- Health practices and health care
- Aging and the old person
- Pain
- Death and dying

Remember that each person is an individual. Avoid the practice of stereotyping (assuming that every person in a group is the same because they are part of a particular group). Learn basic information about the cultural groups that you work with as represented by your co-workers and residents. Use the information to increase your understanding, not to label or judge.

Because all residents are entitled to equally fine care regardless of their behavior, the nursing assistant must develop patience and tolerance through understanding and acceptance. Recognizing that all behavior has meaning, you must study the behavior in an effort to find that meaning (Figure 3-7). The more experience you have with a variety of different people, the greater will be your understanding. The principles of behavior management described in Chapter 16 can be very helpful as you deal with the behavior of any resident.

Acceptance of every resident requires great effort. The key is to focus on the ways the resident is like you, rather than the ways the resident is different from you. Show your interest and caring by listening to the resident, by complying with his or her requests whenever possible, and by giving the resident your full attention whenever you are together.

Some of the behaviors you will be frequently dealing with are:

- Aggressiveness
- Demanding behavior
- Dissatisfied behavior
- Crying
- Self-centeredness
- Being withdrawn or depressed

In health care, the staff must adapt their own behavior in ways that meet the needs of each resident as best they can. Too often the staff will expect the residents to adapt to staff needs, schedules, and routines. The professional health care worker learns how to deal with difficult behaviors without losing control or rejecting the resident.

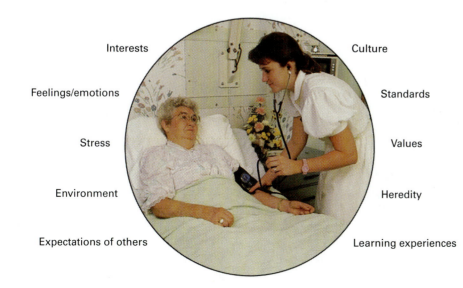

Interests
Feelings/emotions
Stress
Environment
Expectations of others

Culture
Standards
Values
Heredity
Learning experiences

FIGURE 3-7

Factors that determine behavior and ways of relating to others.

There will be times when you experience anger, frustration, or hurt because of a resident's behavior. Coping with your feelings in an acceptable way is essential. Some acceptable ways of coping include:

- Leaving the room (be sure that it is safe to leave; return when you have "cooled off," or send another staff member in)
- Stating your feelings ("I feel very hurt")
- Discussing or venting your feeling to another staff member in private
- Engaging in physical activity (exercise)
- Seeking assistance from your supervisor or social service staff

Unacceptable ways of coping include:

- Yelling
- Threatening
- Striking out
- Slamming doors
- Kicking the furniture
- Drinking or eating excessively when off duty

Determining the reason that a person behaves in a certain way helps us know how best to help (Figure 3-8).

COPING WITH AGGRESSIVE BEHAVIOR

Aggressive behavior can show itself either physically or verbally. As a rule, rational adults do not engage in physical aggression. Usually, the person who strikes out at a staff member is not in control of his or her own behavior due to confusion, mental illness, high fever, or the effects of medication. The individual resident may be frightened by attempts to provide care and can see them as threats of physical harm. This type of behavior can develop if the nursing assistant fails to inform the resident of what he or she is going to do. Imagine a person sleeping soundly at night; the nursing assistant repositions the resident, leaving the light off and saying nothing. Is it any wonder that the resident in the sleeping state might be frightened and fight back? Regardless of the reason for the physical aggression, nursing assistants must protect both the residents and themselves from harm. Usually, it is best simply to back away from the resident rather than try to hold the resident's arms down. If a resident poses a threat to himself or others, seek assistance from your charge nurse immediately. Speak to the resident in a calm, quiet, soothing manner. Give the resident a little time to calm down. Sometimes it is helpful to obtain help from a more experienced staff member or one who knows this particular resident well. Never threaten or attempt to intimidate this resident into cooperating with you. With the right approach, most residents will respond to your requests.

Verbal aggression is a more common event. The key to coping with verbal aggression is to listen without argument or defense and to take action to correct valid complaints. Do not take the attack personally. Your behavior may have nothing to do with the resident's anger.

FIGURE 3-8

Awaken resident gently.

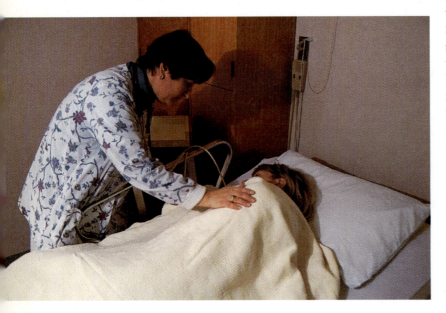

COPING WITH DEMANDING OR DISSATISFIED BEHAVIOR

Many nurses have the most difficulty dealing with the demanding resident who never seems to be satisfied. This person may ring the signal or call light frequently for what seem like unimportant requests. All efforts to please the resident fail. Each action is met with criticism. You might be asked, for instance, to adjust the pillow. Each time the pillow is moved, it is too much or too little, too high or too low. Chances are great that the pillow will end up back where it started. Part of the frustration is that, no matter what you do, it will never be right. It is easy to suffer a loss of confidence and self-esteem if you believe or accept the resident's perception of care provided.

With this type of behavior, the nursing assistant needs to accept the fact that the resident cannot be pleased due to his or her own unique psychological problems. Perhaps because of fears of being alone, excuses are invented to keep the nurse in the room. Sometimes people who suffer from a chronic disease are perceived as demanding because they know more about the condition and their needs than anyone else. After many years of coping with their condition, they develop special ways of doing things that have proved successful. With these residents, it is usually best to do things their way, whenever possible. Imposing your ways and routines on them will only lead to frustration and a poor relationship. Find as many opportunities as you can for the resident to make choices or decisions. Comments like, "Would you like to get out of bed now, or after I finish with Mr. Jones?" or "Would you like to wear the blue pants or the black ones?" are examples of ways you can include the resident in decision making. It is also a good idea to verify with the resident before leaving the room that you have done everything that is needed. Stop by periodically during your shift to see if this individual needs anything. You'll soon find that this person trusts you and will not need to call so often or to invent reasons to keep you in the room.

COPING WITH CRYING AND SELF-CENTEREDNESS

When a resident is crying for any reason, you might feel helpless and uncomfortable. Avoid attempting to stop the resident from crying in order to increase your own comfort. Comments like "Now, now that isn't necessary" or "Let's put a smile on that face" are not helpful. The role of the nursing assistant is to allow the resident to cry, to convey the fact that crying is helpful, and to listen (Figure 3-9). Very often, as you listen the resident will express concern and frustration. Sometimes there are actions you can take to resolve some of the frustration, and other times there may be nothing more to do than to convey a feeling to the resident that you are there and you care. Report to your charge nurse any comments or behavior changes that you feel need to be explored further.

Persons who are ill often become very self-centered. Their world seems to become smaller and smaller as they focus attention on their own needs. This person frequently is demanding of your time and attention. Although it may be tempting to scold

FIGURE 3-9

Listen and allow the resident to cry.

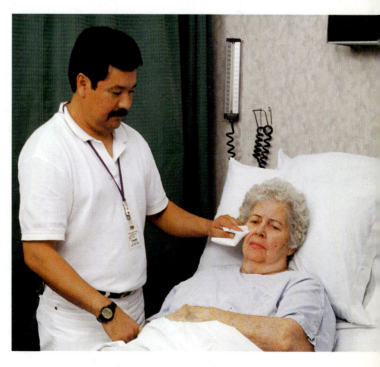

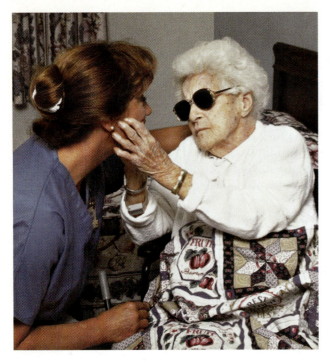

FIGURE 3-10

Show the resident that you care by being there when needed.

the resident or to explain that you have other responsibilities or that there are others who are sicker, resist the temptation. This approach not only increases the anxiety of the resident, but it is also not successful in changing the behavior. Attempting to involve this resident in meaningful activities, particularly those that provide him or her with the opportunity to give to others, will do far more to decrease the self-centered behavior.

Some residents may become depressed and withdraw from contact with family, friends, and staff and give the impression of "lingering sadness."

Depression is the most common emotional disorder for all ages in the United States. The older adult who has retired from the workforce often experiences feelings of uselessness, loneliness, and boredom. When problems of lost physical ability, memory lapses, and the death of many friends and loved ones are added to these feelings, depression results. Usually, the best approach is to be matter of fact. Do not avoid these residents. Spend time with them and give them good care (Figure 3-10). Do not try to "cheer up" the depressed resident. Continue to show affection through your presence, your communication, and your touch. Be sure to report this behavior to your charge nurse.

Developing a positive relationship with your residents can be achieved if these principles are used:

- Recognize your own feelings.
- Put yourself in the resident's place as much as possible.
- Anticipate the resident's needs.
- Explain everything you are doing for the resident.
- Avoid false cheerfulness.
- Listen—allow the resident to express thoughts and feelings.
- Avoid taking the resident's behavior personally.
- Learn to develop tolerance and patience.
- Do things the resident's way whenever possible.
- Give praise for the resident's accomplishments.
- Treat each resident the way you would like to be treated.
- Understand the resident's culture as it affects the resident.

When faced with difficulty relating to a particular resident, remember that you are not alone. Call on the knowledge and experience of the other health-care team members. When you are having a problem, chances are others are having the same problem. A team approach might provide the solution. The decisions made by the team should be entered on the plan of care so that all staff will be consistent in their approach. Many times a team approach can help change behavior in a positive way that proves beneficial to the resident as well as to the staff. Developing good interpersonal relationships with the residents will be your most challenging and rewarding task as a nursing assistant.

SECTION 5 Spiritual Needs

OBJECTIVES
What You Will Learn

When you have completed this section, you will be able to:

- Define the term **spiritual need**
- Choose a religious organization and describe the beliefs regarding illness and death
- Identify those activities that are appropriate to the role of nursing assistant

KEY TERM   spiritual need

RESIDENTS' SPIRITUAL NEEDS

Spiritual needs are difficult to identify and difficult to understand. Spiritual comes from the word *spirit,* which means life or life giving (Figure 3-11). When people have spirit, they are said to be full of life. Spiritual needs might be defined as the need to find meaning in life.

It is easy to see that spiritual needs are very personal and different for everyone. Some find fulfillment in music, art, or nature. Others meet their spiritual needs from within themselves, and still others become part of a group. Groups of people with common beliefs can organize and subscribe to specific religious practices. Some religions have existed since the beginning of human life, while others are young by comparison. It would take volumes to list and describe all the religions present in the world today. Regardless of the way residents meet their spiritual needs, it is never acceptable to criticize or ridicule or to try to impose your own beliefs on the residents.

Most facilities provide some types of religious services for those who wish to participate. Some residents are able to leave the facility to attend services of their choice. Often members of the clergy (ministers, priests, rabbis) visit the resident in the facility.

Spiritual beliefs can affect the resident's life in many ways. For example:

- Diet—various foods may be left out or included in the diet. On special religious occasions, some residents might fast (go without food).
- Clothing—special items of clothing can have religious meaning: for example, the yarmulkes (skullcaps) that Jewish males wear.
- Holidays—special days set aside to remember important events in the history of the religion (Christmas, Hanukkah).
- Customs and rituals—ceremonies or special routines that may be followed.
- Objects or symbols—objects with special meaning (statues, books, photos).
- Death and dying—beliefs about refusing life-sustaining treatment, belief in an afterlife.

Beliefs about illness and death affect the attitudes, feelings, and behavior of

> **spiritual needs** need to finding meaning in life

FIGURE 3-11

Spiritual needs.

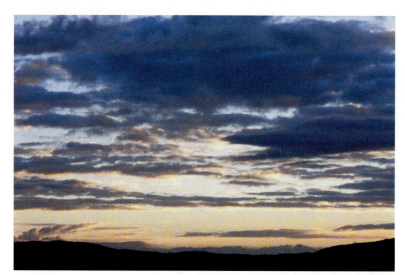

many residents. The resident may choose to endure pain rather than ask for medication because pain is believed to be punishment for previous wrongs or because tolerating pain is considered to be a virtue. Death can also be seen as punishment or as the way to a better existence. Those who believe in a life after death may experience death in a different way than those who do not believe in an afterlife.

As far as spiritual needs are concerned, the role of the nursing assistant is primarily one of accepting and supporting the residents in the expression of their own beliefs. In order to accomplish this, the nursing assistant should:

- Make an effort to learn as much as possible about the resident's beliefs
- Treat any religious objects or items of clothing with respect
- Cooperate cheerfully in preparing the resident to attend religious services, regardless of the day or time of day
- Offer alternatives if foods served are in conflict with religious beliefs
- Listen attentively and respectfully when the resident talks about her or his spiritual beliefs
- Report to the charge nurse when a resident requests to see a member of the clergy
- Provide privacy when clergy visit the resident

SUMMARY

In this chapter, you have learned about the overall goals of care for the long-term care facility. A philosophy of rehabilitation means that efforts are directed toward restoring independence as much as possible and at least by preventing loss of function. The keys to promoting independence include praise and encouragement of residents to do as much as they can for themselves.

One of the keys to your success as a nursing assistant is understanding the needs of all people and how those needs change with aging. By understanding the developmental task of aging, you'll be better able to work with your residents. The processes of adaptation, life review, and reconciliation will be occurring every day as you work with the elderly residents.

The residents will become teachers to you about your own aging process. You'll have the opportunity to care for those who age gracefully and those who do not. The more you learn about your residents, the more you will learn about yourself.

When you know the roles the resident played prior to coming to the facility, it is easier to understand their behavior and feelings. The male resident who likes to "boss you around" might be best understood if you know he was a foreman on a construction crew or a first grade teacher.

Because you will care for and work with people from many different backgrounds, cultures, and beliefs, you need to be able to "get along" with them. The greatest key to understanding is to learn about their culture while remembering that each is an individual.

For reasons of culture, role changes, and the stress of illness and aging, you will care for residents whose behavior is challenging for those around them. This chapter has given you tips for coping with aggressive behavior, demanding and dissatisfied behavior, as well as crying and self-centeredness. Each behavior requires a unique approach that you have learned. Practice these skills with residents and with family and friends.

The final section of this chapter was about the resident as a spiritual being. You have learned that spirituality is a much broader concept than "religious" and is expressed in many diverse ways. The role of the nursing assistant is to accept residents as they are and never to impose your own beliefs on them.

OBRA HIGHLIGHTS

The OBRA regulations place great importance on "quality of life" by devoting a number of specific regulations to it. The regulations state "A facility must care for its residents in a manner and in an environment that promotes maintenance or enhancement of each resident's quality of life." It further states that this includes dignity, individuality, self-determination, and participation. By treating each resident with respect and by assisting with carrying out the resident's choices in grooming, dress, and activity, the nursing assistant is helping to ensure an environment that promotes quality of life.

SELF STUDY

Choose the best answer for each question or statement.

1. When you accept and celebrate the accomplishment of small, simple goals for residents, you are exhibiting
   a. a rehabilitation philosophy
   b. a denial of reality
   c. a philosophy of dependence
   d. a task-oriented behavior

2. How do long-term care facilities assess and identify residents' needs?
   a. by asking the physician what the needs are
   b. by asking the family what the needs are
   c. by using a Minimum Data Set (MDS)
   d. by having the resident perform a set of tasks

3. Mr. Monroe is unable to perform any of his own care, but he is alert and oriented. How can you help promote his independence?
   a. Insist that Mr. Monroe attempt to wash his legs.
   b. Allow Mr. Monroe to decide what clothes he would like to wear.
   c. Perform all of his care as quickly as possible so he won't feel helpless for long.
   d. all of the above

4. Which of the following actions by the nursing assistant can help meet a resident's social needs?
   a. Serve his meal tray promptly while the food is hot.
   b. Keep his side rails up and use postural supports as necessary.
   c. Keep his room clean and neat, with personal items put away.
   d. Praise him for his accomplishments and for trying new things.

5. Which of these is part of informed consent?
   a. understanding the reasons for medical treatment
   b. understanding the benefits and risks of the treatment
   c. understanding the consequences of refusing the treatment
   d. all of the above

6. Mr. Marconi is in the dining room for a meal when he has an episode of incontinence. Which of the following is appropriate for you to say when you escort Mr. Marconi out of the dining room?
   a. "I'll get him cleaned up and be back to help with the meal as soon as I can."
   b. "Come with me, Mr. Marconi. Let's go back to your room for a minute."
   c. "I'm surprised you were incontinent again, Mr. Marconi. I thought you were doing better."
   d. "I'm going to put you in diapers from now on, Mr. Marconi, so we can get through a meal."

7. Most residents who are disabled wish to be considered in which of the following roles?
   a. the sick role
   b. the well role
   c. the dependent role
   d. the child role

8. Julie works in a residential care facility for the developmentally disabled. Which of the following would be appropriate care for Julie to give to these residents?
   a. Calling the residents "her kids."
   b. Putting the female residents' hair in pigtails.
   c. Teaching the residents to make a bowl from clay.
   d. Watching cartoons with the residents.

9. How can the long-term care facility staff make wellness more desirable than sickness for a resident who often assumes the sick role?
   a. Praise the resident for all efforts at independence.
   b. Involve the family members in rewarding well behavior.
   c. Spend time with the resident and show concern.
   d. all of the above

10. Which of the following is a way to show acceptance of a resident?
    a. Focus on the ways the resident is like you, rather then on how he or she is different.
    b. Let the resident talk while you are busy doing other things in the room.
    c. Comply with the resident's requests once in a while, but not very often.
    d. all of the above

11. Mrs. Melvin is a demanding patient who is difficult to please. Which of the following would be appropriate for you to do when caring for Mrs. Melvin?
    a. Ask Mrs. Melvin before you leave the room if you have done everything she needs.
    b. Require Mrs. Melvin to bathe and dress when you are available, not when she wishes to.
    c. Avoid Mrs. Melvin's room once you have done her care so she won't keep asking for things.
    d. Tell Mrs. Melvin you have other residents who need your help more than she does.

12. Ms. Jefferson demands a great deal of your time and attention. She cries often and exhibits self-centered behavior. Which of the following would be appropriate for you to do when caring for Ms. Jefferson?
    a. Tell Ms. Jefferson about other residents who are sicker than she is but don't demand as much attention.
    b. Tell Ms. Jefferson that you do not have time to sit and listen to her cry, but that you'll come back later.
    c. Encourage Ms. Jefferson to participate in a project knitting slippers for children who have cancer.
    d. Tell Ms. Jefferson not to cry and to count her blessings instead of feeling sorry for herself.

13. Ms. Jefferson continues to cry and complain that no one cares about what happens to her. You are feeling very frustrated with her. Which of the following actions should you take?
    a. Leave the room and get a different staff member to check on Ms. Jefferson.
    b. Tell Ms. Jefferson you have heard enough for today, and now it is time to get dressed.

c. Take a break and discuss Ms. Jefferson's behavior with others in the break room.
    d. Tell Ms. Jefferson that if she doesn't quit crying and complaining, no one will take care of her.

14. Mr. Goldstein is sometimes confused and becomes aggressive at times. When you prepare to assist him back to bed, he becomes combative. He yells, "Get away from me, get out of here you dirty pig!" Which of the following actions should you take?
    a. Hold his arms down and call for assistance to get him back to bed.
    b. Yell back at Mr. Goldstein, telling him that you are a nursing assistant here to help him.
    c. Speak to Mr. Goldstein in a calm, soothing manner, giving him some time to calm down.
    d. Tell Mr. Goldstein to calm down right now or he will have to sleep in the chair tonight.

15. Mrs. Evans is a resident who is depressed over several losses in her life. Which of the following is appropriate for you to do when you are caring for Mrs. Evans?
    a. Avoid Mrs. Evans's room unless you must go in there, since she is such a downer.
    b. Point out what a beautiful day it is today and the good things in Mrs. Evans's life.
    c. Encourage Mrs. Evans to at least try to cheer up while you are with her.
    d. Accept Mrs. Evans depression by showing affection through touch and talking.

16. Which of the following can be affected by a resident's spiritual beliefs?
    a. diet
    b. clothing
    c. death and dying
    d. all of the above

Getting C O N N E C T E D
Multimedia Extension Activities

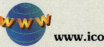 **www.icon** *www.prenhall.com/will-black*

Use the above address to access the free, interactive Companion Website created for this textbook. Hear the pronunciation of the key terms in the chapter. Get instant feedback to a variety of chapter-related questions. Link to other interesting sites.

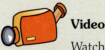 **Video**

Watch the *"Honoring Cultural Diversity"* section of the *Focus on Professionalism* video.

CASE STUDY

Mr. Black is a 42-year-old man injured in an accident. He is divorced and lives alone, so there is no one to care for him at home. He is in the facility for rehabilitation following his treatment in the acute hospital. Both legs were broken, and the physical therapist is beginning to get him out of bed. He seems angry and frustrated. No matter what you do for him, it never seems to please him.

1. Mr. Black's behavior is probably related to
   a. the fact that he doesn't like you
   b. the fact that you are new at your job and are not yet competent
   c. the fact that he is adjusting to a role change brought on by his loss of independence
   d. the fact that he is just a nasty person
2. You and your fellow nursing assistants decide to come up with an approach to caring for him. The best plan would be to
   a. give him choices about all aspects of his care
   b. ask the charge nurse to have a talk with him about how he is behaving
   c. assign a more experienced CNA
   d. ignore his bad attitude and take charge of his care
3. When a younger resident like Mr. Black is in a long-term facility, which of his needs might be more difficult to meet?
   a. his physical needs
   b. his social needs
   c. his security and safety needs
   d. his entertainment needs
4. You enter his room one morning and find that he is crying. Your action is to
   a. tell him to look around the facility and see how many residents are worse off than he is
   b. call the nurse immediately so she can given him medication to treat his depression
   c. distract him by talking to him about your plans for the weekend
   d. listen and stand by quietly

BASIC NURSING CARE

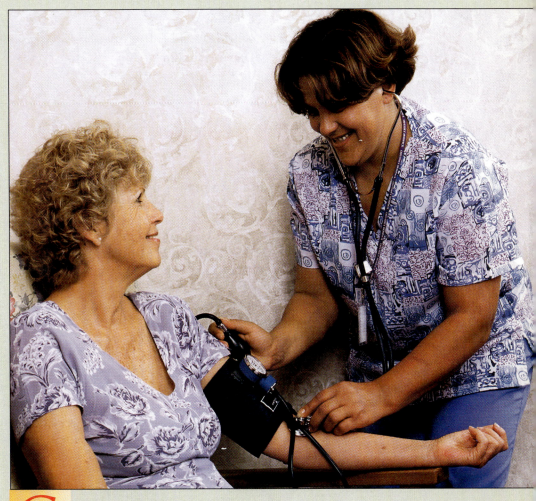

CARING TIP

Accuracy in taking vital signs allows for

accuracy in giving care.

Patricia Edwards, RN, BA
Director of Education
Royal Park Care Center
Spokane, WA

OBJECTIVES
What You Will Learn

When you have completed this section, you will be able to:

• Review the health care plan of 10 residents in your facility and list the different health care disciplines involved

• Explain how the nursing assistant can contribute to the development of the plan of care

• List four ways the health care plan can help you as you provide daily care

KEY TERMS

continuity
health care plan

individualized health care plan
MDS coordinator
minimum data set (MDS)

resident-assessment protocols
(RAPs)

CHARACTERISTICS OF THE HEALTH CARE PLAN

health care plan written guidelines for providing care

individualized health care plan plan of care tailored to reflect the individuality of each resident

Minimum Data Set (MDS) a written, standardized assessment of all residents living in a skilled nursing facility

MDS coordinator title of the registered nurse responsible for completion of the resident assessment or MDS

Resident Assessment Protocols (RAPs) in-depth focused assessments on specific aspects of care such as risk for falls or tube feeding

The **health care plan** is similar to an architect's blueprint—it gives members of the health care team the written guidelines for providing care. A building is never successfully completed without a plan. Similarly, good resident care cannot be provided without a plan!

An **individualized health care plan** is a legal requirement for all residents of a health care facility. Just as we are all different, with our own problems and needs, each resident must be viewed as a unique individual, and a plan of care must be tailored to reflect the individuality of each resident. You can test whether a care plan is individualized by reading the plan and seeing if you can identify the resident without referring to name or room number. Good health care plans are sketches of the residents and their problems and needs. An individualized care plan is tailor-made to reflect the unique needs of a single resident.

To develop an individualized health care plan, all members of the health care team must learn as much as possible about the resident. The team observes the resident, interviews the resident and family members, and reviews the medical record. The form used is called the **Minimum Data Set (MDS).** This form is required to be used at all nursing homes across the country. Usually there is a Registered Nurse appointed as the **MDS coordinator.** The coordinator gathers information about the resident over a two-week period. You may be asked for information to contribute to the assessment. The nurse will want to know things like how much help the resident needs to bathe, dress, groom, transfer, walk, and go to the toilet. The nurse needs to determine the care needed, the resident's strengths, and the risks the resident has. The answers on the assessment may trigger a more in-depth review of the patient. These in-depth assessments are called **Resident Assessment Protocols (RAPs).** The team will determine what actions need to be taken to prevent the resident from losing function, falling, or otherwise harming himself or herself as well as risk of developing a pressure ulcer.

CULTURAL AWARENESS Other considerations in developing the health care plan are determining from the resident and family any individual or cultural needs and preferences about food, activities, dress, or other practices. It is important to include in writing any cultural or individual "do's and don'ts."

Residents and families are encouraged to participate in the development of the plan and resident's must approve their plan of care. As you review the health care plans of residents in your facility, identify the entries made by other members of the health care team.

It is important to include the resident and family members in the development of the health care plan whenever possible. It's surprising to see how positively residents respond when they are involved in planning their own care. Residents generally are more motivated to achieve goals when they have taken part in the goal-setting process.

There may be health care professionals from outside the facility involved in the management and planning of the resident's care. The resident may be enrolled in a managed care or health maintenance organization or in a hospice program. In this case, the other organization may have the primary responsibility to plan the care, though the facility staff must follow the plan in providing care. In these cases, the facility has agreed to provide the care under the direction of the outside professionals.

As a nursing assistant, you are in the best position to gather important information about the residents' needs and problems. You can contribute to the development of the care plan by:

- Making factual observations
- Reporting and recording those observations accurately

USING THE HEALTH CARE PLAN

Too often, the health care plan is developed carefully but not used appropriately. It is of no value if the caregivers do not follow the plan! If actions or approaches listed are not effective, they must be changed. When the health care plan is well developed and used appropriately, it is *the single most important tool* in providing high-quality care to residents (Figure 4-1).

Without a plan, residents generally get the same care. What is right for one resident may not be right for another. When an individualized plan of care is not used, psychosocial needs are almost never met.

There are a number of ways the health care plan can help you as you provide daily care.

- *It provides specific instructions regarding care to be given:* for example, "keep head of bed elevated at all times; report any complaints of burning, frequency, or pain on urination."
- *It provides necessary information needed prior to giving care:* for example, "hard of hearing—face resident and speak slowly; unsteady when ambulating—ambulate with assistance only."
- *It provides all caregivers with the same guidelines:* **Continuity** means doing the same things in the same way—when everyone works together to achieve the same goal, positive results are more likely to occur. Residents feel more secure and comfortable when there is continuity of care.

  continuity doing the same things in the same way

- *It provides the nursing assistant with essential data or facts necessary for organizing and planning work:* You will be able to determine what special assignments or tasks must be performed, such as Clinitests, intake and output (I&O), scheduling of special appointments or tests. You will also be better prepared to set your priorities in giving care when you have all the data available.

Resident Care Plan Form

Diagnosis: CVA with paralysis on the left side

Admit date: 9/1/00   **DOB** 5/13/17   **Sex/Age** 87
Recap date: ____   **Religion:** Protestant

☒ Dentures ____
☐ Hearing Aid ____
☒ Glasses ____

Allergies: Penicillin   **Alerts:** DNR

Evaluations

Date	Dept.	Signature
		Sample

Initial identification

Initials	Signature/Title

Long Term Goal: Return of independence in ADLS

Discharge Plan Statement: Return home independent in ADLS

Prob. # 1   Problem: L-side paralysis

Goal: Able to ambulate with walker
Target Date: 3\01

Date	Approach/Plan	Disc	Init	DC
9/8	Dress for PT appoint by 830/Am		CNA	
9/8	To wear tennis shoes To PT daily		CNA	
	Record progress in Ambulation		RNA	

Prob. # 2   Problem: Risk for falls due to paralysis & weakness

Goal: Will be free of falls
Target Date: 2/1/00

Date	Approach/Plan	Disc	Init	DC
9/3	Respond promptly to call light		All	
9/3	Therapy 5 x wk for Strength & balance		PT	
9/3	Supervise all activities to assure safety			
9/3	Remind to ask for assistance when getting out of bed or walking		All	

Last Name: Jones	First Name: Martha	Med. Rec. #: 1234	Physician: Dr Good	Page # 1

JWA-117A 5/91   **RESIDENT CARE PLAN**

FIGURE 4-1

Resident care plan.

Remember: The health care plan is your most important resource in providing care. Each LTC facility will have specific policies and procedures related to the health care plans. Be sure you understand how to use them in your facility.

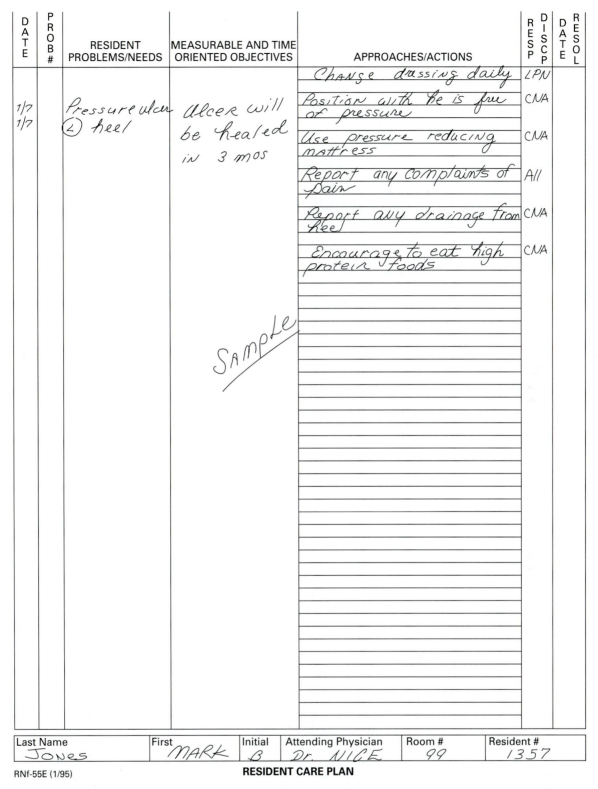

DATE	PROB #	RESIDENT PROBLEMS/NEEDS	MEASURABLE AND TIME ORIENTED OBJECTIVES	APPROACHES/ACTIONS	RESP DISCP	DATE	RESOL
1/7 1/7	②	Pressure ulcer heel	Ulcer will be healed in 3 mos	Change dressing daily	LPN		
				Position with he is free of pressure	CNA		
				Use pressure reducing mattress	CNA		
				Report any complaints of pain	All		
				Report any drainage from heel	CNA		
				Encourage to eat high protein foods	CNA		

Sample

Last Name	First	Initial	Attending Physician	Room #	Resident #
JONES	MARK	B	Dr. NICE	99	1357

RNf-55E (1/95)

RESIDENT CARE PLAN

FIGURE 4-1

(Continued)

OBJECTIVES
What You Will Learn

When you have completed this section, you will be able to:

- List the four steps involved in organizing time
- Define the term **planning**
- Place four tasks in the sequence in which they should be completed
- Write a sample plan for completing your assignment for one day

---

KEY TERMS

implement

planning
procrastination

rounds
setting priorities

When you are doing your job as a nursing assistant, you will soon realize that there is not enough time to do everything you would like to do. In fact, lack of time is a common complaint of most people. Unfortunately, there is only so much time—60 minutes in an hour, 24 hours in a day. Since you cannot control time, you must learn to control or manage yourself.

ORGANIZING

Organizing or managing yourself in order to complete your assignments is a four-step process that includes:

- Gathering information
- Planning
- Carrying out the plan
- Revising the plan

Your job description provides the foundation of information on which you base your organization. Begin with obtaining your assignment from your charge nurse. You'll be told which residents you'll be caring for and given specific task assignments. These tasks may vary from taking vital signs to cleaning the utility room. Most facilities use a written assignment form. Some are designed to show all the assignments for the unit, while others are individualized to each nursing assistant. You may complete the form yourself or it could be written in advance for you. Review the sample to see the kinds of information you would need to plan and organize your work.

Check the health care plan or nursing care Kardex to find out the specific needs of each resident. Determine if any residents have timed schedules that must be followed, such as testing urine before meals or keeping an appointment inside or outside the facility. You must also find out any planned events that affect the facility as a whole. Check the activity calendar for resident activities. Find out if there are employee classes or meetings scheduled.

rounds, making   going to each resident to determine briefly whether they have any immediate needs

Gathering information includes making **rounds** of your assigned residents. Making rounds means going to each resident to determine briefly whether they have any immediate needs.

PLANNING

planning   devising a way of getting a job done

Once all the information is gathered, it is time to plan (Figure 4-2). **Planning** is devising a way of getting the job done. It includes thinking about the information you have gathered and writing down your plan. The written plan may simply be a "things to do" list or notes that list the names of the residents to whom you're assigned and specific tasks to be done. Planning involves:

- What you are going to do
- How you are going to do it
- When you are going to do it

SETTING PRIORITIES

Setting priorities is part of planning. It refers to looking at all things that need to be done and putting them in order of what should be done first, second, and so on. You must decide who needs your attention first as well as which tasks must be done and which can, if necessary, wait until later (Figure 4-3). Priorities tend to change from moment to moment, so there are no set rules. Your common sense will help you decide which jobs are most important. The charge nurse will help you set priorities.

There are some principles that will guide you in your planning:

- Protecting the welfare and safety of the resident is always a high priority. This includes, for example, staying with the resident in the shower, rescuing a resident who is falling, or carrying out emergency procedures in case of choking.
- Carrying out specific orders from the physician.
- Helping those who are most dependent. Needs of residents always take priority over cleaning duties.

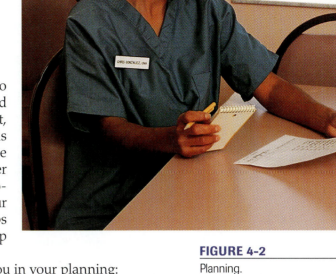

FIGURE 4-2

Planning.

setting priorities looking at things that need to be done and putting them in the order of importance

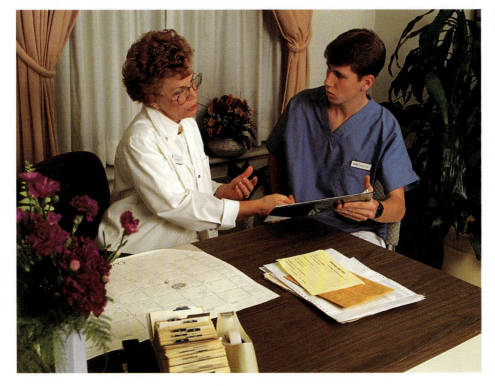

FIGURE 4-3

Set priorities.

implement to carry out or accomplish a given plan

procrastination putting off doing something until some other time

Once your plan is developed, it is time to **implement** or carry out the plan. Learning to think through each task in advance will save you both time and energy. One of the biggest wasters of time is procrastination. **Procrastination** is putting off doing something until some other time. People most often put off tasks that they find unpleasant. Successful managers of time do not procrastinate. In fact, they usually do unpleasant tasks first so they are free to enjoy more pleasant ones.

Performing a task usually consists of three steps—preparation, action, and completion. Preparation involves gathering needed equipment. This will save you much time and energy. Action is the actual doing of the procedure or task. Remember to follow principles of good body mechanics and infection control. In giving direct care to a resident, you can be more efficient if you describe out loud what you will be doing in a step-by-step manner. Not only will the resident know what to expect, but you will also do a better, more efficient job.

One of the most effective ways you can make your job easier is to allow for and to encourage self-care. At first, it may take more time for residents to feed, dress, or groom themselves. Many of your residents may be very slow. If you find yourself becoming impatient, leave the room briefly or do some other tasks in the room. Don't just stand and watch. Once they have learned, they benefit by feeling better, and you benefit by having less work to do.

To complete a task, there is usually "cleanup" to do. You must return equipment to the proper place and dispose of waste materials properly.

Throughout the day's work, you might have to revise your plan. If you are getting behind or are unable to complete a particular task, ask your charge nurse for help. Be sure to ask as soon as possible so that the job can be completed. Don't wait until the shift is over to say, "By the way, I didn't have time to. . . ."

Just as you can ask for help from your co-workers, be ready to help them when they ask. Be particularly sensitive to the needs of new employees. In addition to showing a friendly and welcoming attitude, take time to help. You'll benefit in the long run by having a stronger and more capable co-worker and team member. At the end of your shift of duty, take time to make rounds one last time to be sure that your residents' needs have been taken care of and that your assigned tasks have been done. Then you will be able to leave work with the knowledge and good feeling of a job well done.

SECTION 3 Observation and Charting

OBJECTIVES
What You Will Learn

When you have completed this section, you will be able to:

- Define the term **observation** and explain why it is an important responsibility of the nursing assistant

- Differentiate between statements that are fact and those that express an opinion
- List three basic principles of making entries into the resident's health record

- Identify proper charting principles
- Match abbreviations and symbols with their definitions

KEY TERMS

objective observations

observation

subjective observations

ELEMENTS OF OBSERVATION

One responsibility of the nursing assistant is to observe, report, and record changes in the resident's condition and her or his response or lack of response to care and treatment provided. Because you, the nursing assistant, provide *more direct care* than anyone else on the health care team, you are the most valuable resource available for observation of the resident!

Observation is recognizing and noticing a fact or occurrence. It means taking note of or paying attention to what is happening around you. Developing your ability to make accurate observations will take time and practice. You must be alert to obvious visible changes as well as to subtle changes in a resident's physical condition, mental attitude, or behavior patterns. Observation is not merely looking—it is planned, careful, and focused. *Observation involves using all the senses.*

In order to recognize changes, you must have "stored information" as to what is normal for a particular resident. If you make a habit of quickly observing the "head-to-toe" condition of each resident as you provide care, you will be prepared to recognize any changes.

It is very important to learn to make **objective observations.** Objective observations are facts you notice that are not distorted by your personal feelings. In other words, objective means free from bias or judgment. Entries in the health record must be fact, not judgments or impressions.

Subjective observations are individual judgments based on personal feelings. Although it is not appropriate for you to make subjective statements, you may record subjective information when you quote or describe a resident's statement of how he or she feels.

Examples of objective and subjective observations are:

Objective	**Subjective**
The dress is red.	The dress is pretty.
The resident weighs 80 pounds.	The resident is thin.
The resident wanders from the facility twice a day.	The resident is confused.
The resident refused a shower today.	The resident is uncooperative.
The resident was crying after her daughter visited.	The resident was depressed by the daughter's visit.

observation recognizing and noticing a fact or occurrence

objective observations facts observed and not distorted by personal feelings

subjective observations individual judgments based on personal feeings

CHARTING

In addition to making accurate observations, you must write them in the resident's health record (Figure 4-4). The amount of charting you will do, as well as the kinds of information you record, will vary from state to state and from one facility to another. *Usually, you will record:*

- Care and treatment provided to each resident
- Their response or lack of response to care and treatment provided
- The safety measures you use in providing care that protect the resident

FIGURE 4-4
Charting.

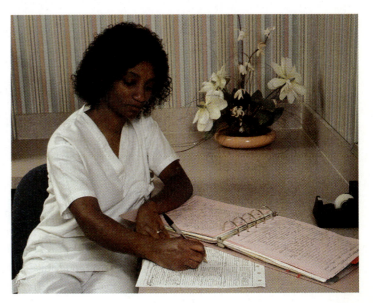

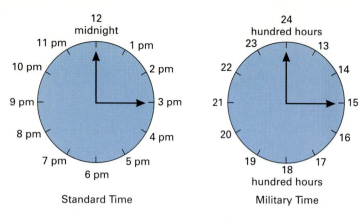

FIGURE 4-5

Standard time; military time.

• What you do with the resident's personal belongings or property
• Any events that occur that involve the resident

Your charting should reflect the fact that you are carrying out the actions specified on the health care plan and indicate the resident's progress toward achieving the established goals. Review the care plan as you give care and as you record the care given.

The resident's health record is most commonly called the medical record or chart. The chart is a permanent legal record. The physician uses it to direct the care to be given, to record observations and progress, and to check what care has been given.

The physician will also gather information from entries made by other health team members to use in further diagnosis and treatment. The nursing staff uses the chart as a resource on how to provide care (based on the physician's orders) and also records all observations, progress, or lack of progress. The chart should contain an accurate picture of the resident, the care provided, and the resident's response to the care. The information and observations contained in the chart assist other health team members in planning the care to be given. Although you'll be learning new terminology and abbreviations, remember that clear communication is most important. If you don't know or aren't sure of the medical term, just use simple descriptive words.

Accuracy of charting includes recording the date and time of your observations. Some facilities use a 24-hour "clock," often called *military time,* instead of the standard 12-hour clock with A.M. and P.M. To use the 24-hour clock, the hours from midnight to noon are called "_____ hundred hours," written as "0100" (1:00 A.M.). After noon (twelve hundred hours) add the time on the 12-hour clock to 12 to obtain the military time. For example, if the time is 3 P.M., military time would be 12 + 3 or 1500 hours. Use the conversion clock to help you (Figure 4-5).

PRINCIPLES OF CHARTING

There are certain principles of charting that you should follow:

• All entries must be made in *ink* and should be printed or written so they are *legible.*
• All entries must be *signed* with your first initial and full last name along with your title.
• All entries must be in *chronological order* (in the sequence of occurrence) and must contain *date* and *time* in order to determine when entries are made.
• All entries must be *factual* because the chart is a legal document.
• The chart must be *complete*—it must contain all information regarding the resident.
• All entries should be *brief* and *exact.*
• The chart is a *confidential* record. Each resident is guaranteed the right to confidential treatment of his or her medical records.
• The chart is the *property of the facility* and should not be removed from the premises.

- There should be no empty spaces left on a line when charting. Draw a line through the center of an empty space. This prevents anyone charting in a space signed by someone else.
- When an error is made while charting, no erasures, whiteouts, or any type of obliteration of any entry may be made. If an incorrect entry is made, a single line should be drawn through the entry and a notation made (Figure 4-6).
- Use the present tense on all entries and use only approved abbreviations. Ditto marks are not acceptable.
- Make sure that any new forms added to the chart are properly identified with the resident's name, room number, and physician's name.

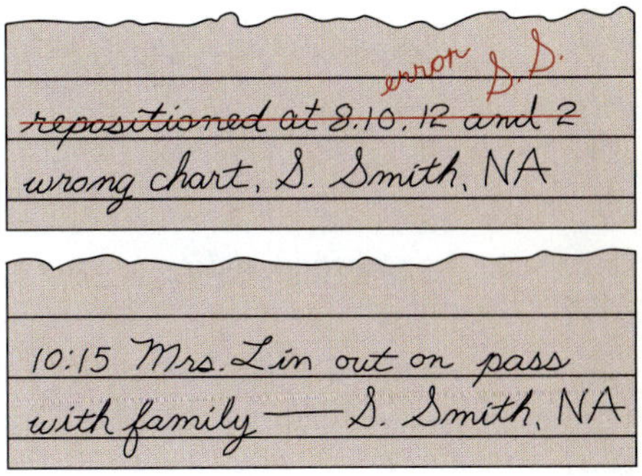

The following charting tips should be helpful as you make entries into the resident's health record.

As you continue to improve your skills in observation, you will find yourself relying on more of your senses to note unusual signs and symptoms. Being a good observer and putting your observations into clear, concise language takes skill and practice.

FIGURE 4-6

Correcting an error on the chart.

```
                              error  S. S.
repositioned at 8.10.12 and 2
wrong chart, S. Smith, NA
```

```
10:15  Mrs. Lin out on pass
with family ——— S. Smith, NA
```

CHARTING

Describe what you see:

- The activity of the resident, including activities of daily living (dressing, bathing, feeding, personal hygiene, ambulation, continence, etc.)

  Describe what *kind* of assistance is required (total, minimal) and describe what the resident is able to do.

  Describe how the resident tolerates the activities—(fatigued, short of breath, without difficulty, etc.)

  Describe the resident's reaction to performing activities of daily living, by recording the resident's nonverbal reactions (looks of disgust, shaking fist, uninterested look, etc.).

- The resident's appetite or lack of appetite

  Describe what percentage of the food was eaten. If less than 50 percent, list and report what was eaten.

  On diabetic residents, list any food items not eaten, and report.

  Describe unusual food habits, likes/dislikes (always eats fruit and dessert, never eats meat, always eating food from other trays, etc.).

- The resident's body position: how the resident appears while in bed, up in chair, ambulating

  Describe contractures or other limitations of movement, posture, gait; special assistive devices (cane, walker, etc.).

- The resident's skin condition: any changes from normal; always refer to the location, size, and special characteristics of any abnormal skin condition

  Describe unusual dryness, discolored areas, breaks in the skin, drainage, scratches, bruises.

- The presence of any abnormal discharge or drainage from any part of the body or present in excretions of the body

  Describe the substance, the amount, the color, the odor, and the consistency.

Guidelines

Describe what you hear:

- The way the resident talks

Describe any difficulties in speaking, special patterns of speech (repetitive words, mumbling, slurred speech, etc.).

Describe any differences in how the resident talks to different people (staff, family, friends, etc.).

- What the resident says: ordinary conversations need not be described, but any unusual comments or conversations should be recorded and reported

State exactly what the resident has said that is unusual. Clarify with residents any statements made to obtain additional information and to avoid misunderstandings or "snap" judgments. If the resident complains of pain, ask and record:

- How and when it occurs
- Where it is
- What kind of pain
- How long it lasts

- Unusual sounds or noises made by the resident

Describe any unusual coughing, wheezing, gurgling, sounds in throat, and so on.

Describe what you smell:

- Note changes in the normal odors of the resident's body; poor personal hygiene can lead to disease and infection

Describe unusual odors (fruity, ammonialike, foul, sour, etc.).

- Bad mouth odor can indicate an infection in the mouth
- Drainage from wounds is usually foul-smelling when present

Describe what you touch:

- Use your hands to examine the resident; note reactions of the resident to touch

Describe any abnormal areas (smooth, enlarged, swollen, tender, thin, flat, distended, etc.).

Notice and describe changes you feel in skin temperature (cold, clammy, hot, dry, etc.). Describe the resident's reactions to touch (painful, no sensation).

Record what the resident tells you:

- If the resident has any complaints or concerns, state in the resident's words what the concerns are. Be sure to report and write down any complaints of pain or discomfort. Also write down that you reported to the charge nurse.

COMMONLY USED ABBREVIATIONS

If you look at a typical medical dictionary, you will see that the medical profession has developed a language of its own. This section introduces you to common abbreviations used in long-term care facilities so that you can accurately record data in the resident's health record. Study the following abbreviations and definitions until you can use them comfortably.

Related to Time

a.c.	before meals	a.m.	morning
p.c.	after meals	p.m.	afternoon or evening
q.d.	every day	h.s.	hour of sleep (bedtime)
b.i.d.	two times a day	n.o.c.	night
t.i.d.	three times a day	stat	immediately
q.i.d.	four times a day	P.R.N.	as necessary
q.o.d.	every other day	D/C	discontinue or stop
q.h.	every hour	$\bar{c}$	with
min.	minute	$\bar{s}$	without

Related to Diagnostic Terms and Body Parts

abd.	abdomen	nephro	kidney
ax	axilla	O.D.	right eye
Ca	cancer or carcinoma	O.S.	left eye
CHF	congestive heart failure	O.U.	both eyes
CVA	cerebral vacular accident (stroke)	osteo	bone
DX	diagnosis	psych	related to psychology
Fx	fracture	pneumo	lung
gastric	stomach	resp	respirations
G.I.	gastrointestinal	Rt	right
G.U.	genitourinary	R.B.C.	red blood cell
H.O.H.	hard of hearing	staph	staphylococcus
Lt	left	S.O.B.	short of breath
M.I.	mycocardial infarction (heart attack)	W.B.C.	white blood cell
N/V	nausea/vomiting		

Related to Measurements

amt.	amount	ht	height
approx.	approximately	kg	kilogram
C	centigrade or Celsius	lb	pound
cc	cubic centimeters	L	liter
dr	dram	min	minim
F	Fahrenheit	mg	milligram
g	gram	no	number
gr	grain	oz	ounce
gtt	drop	ss	one-half

Related to Measurements

tbsp	tablespoon	wt	weight
tsp	teaspoon	I, II, III, IV	one, two, three, four

Related to Treatment

B/p	blood pressure	Sub-Q	subcutaneous (injection just into the superficial layers of skin)
cap	capsule	PT	physical therapy
cath	catheter or catheterization	R	rectal
C/S	culture and sensitivity (laboratory procedure)	ROM	range of motion
drsg.	dressing	Rx	prescription
EEG	electroencephalogram (brain wave tracing)	S/A	sugar/acetone (test of urine)
EKG or ECG	electrocardiogram (tracing of heart function)	supp	suppository
		SSE	soap suds enema
Foley	type of urinary catheter	tab	tablet
H_2O	water	TPR	temperature, pulse, respiration
H_2O_2	hydrogen peroxide	TWE	tap water enema
O_2	oxygen	U/A	urinalysis (laboratory procedure)
IM	intramuscular (injection into the muscle)	UNG	ointment
IV	intravenous (injection within the vein)	V/S	vital signs (temperature, pulse, respiration, blood pressure)

Related to Resident Orders/Activity

ADL	activities of daily living	C/O	complains of
ad lib	as desired	Dr.	doctor
amb	ambulate	pt	patient
assist	assistance	I&O	intake and output
BM	bowel movement	NPO	nothing by mouth
BR	bathroom	PCP	patient care plan
BRP	bathroom privileges	W/C	wheelchair

Each facility has a particular form or type of charting to be completed by the nurse assistant. The goals, however, are the same: to provide a record of care and treatment given and to record resident response to the care and to record changes in condition and unusual observations and events. In addition to observing and recording changes in the resident's condition, the nursing assistant must report to the charge nurse:

- Accident with or without injury
- Change in:
  Appearance   Appetite
  Behavior   Elimination
  Function

- Presence of unusual odors
- Reddened or broken skin
- Complaints of pain or nausea
- Presence of swelling
- Presence of drainage
- Any bleeding
- Any tubes that are dislodged

SECTION 4 Weight and Vital Signs

OBJECTIVES
What You Will Learn

When you have completed this section, you will be able to:

- List the necessary criteria for obtaining accurate weights
- Weigh a resident on a standing scale
- Weigh a resident using a mechanical lift
- Weigh a resident on a bed scale
- Measure a resident's height using a tape measure
- Distinguish between conditions that increase body temperature from those that decrease body temperature

- Identify temperature readings that should be reported to the charge nurse immediately
- Read sample thermometers accurately
- Measure an oral, rectal, and axillary temperature using a glass thermometer
- Measure an oral, rectal, and axillary temperature using a battery-operated electronic thermometer
- Identify four sites on the body where the pulse can be measured
- Distinguish between those conditions that increase the pulse from those that decrease the pulse

- Measure the resident's pulse accurately
- Identify different types of respirations
- Measure a resident's respirations accurately
- Identify which reading represents the systolic blood pressure and the diastolic blood pressure
- Identify those conditions that cause the blood pressure to increase and those that cause it to decrease
- Measure a resident's blood pressure accurately

KEY TERMS

abdominal respirations
apical pulse
axillary
blood pressure
bulb (thermometer)
calibrated
Celsius or centigrade
Cheyne–Stokes respiration
diastolic pressure

Farenheit
force of the beat (pulse)
hypertension
hypotension
irregular respiration
labored respirations
oral
perpendicular
pulse
radial pulse

rate (pulse)
rectal
respiration
rhythm (pulse)
shallow respiration
sphygmomanometer
stem (thermometer)
stertorous respirations
stethoscope
systolic pressure

WEIGHING THE RESIDENT

As part of the admission procedure, and on a periodic basis thereafter, residents are weighed. Many facilities weigh residents monthly or more often according to the physician's orders.

Weight loss is considered to be a sign of poor-quality care. The loss may be beyond the control of the facility as when it is due to the medical condition of the resident. A loss of weight may mean that the resident needs more help to eat, that the food is not good, or that the resident is sad or even depressed. Emphasis in the facility is placed on finding out the reason for the loss and making an effort to stop or reverse it. The weight taken at the time of admission gives the physician a standard to compare with future weights. *Weight measurements must be accurate to be useful!*

There are many types of scales used to weigh residents in long-term care facilities. They include the bathroom scale like the one you have at home, the standing scale, scales attached to hydraulic lifts, wheelchair scales, and bed scales (Figure 4-7).

You need to learn how to use the scales in your facility safely and correctly. Scales used in your facility might measure the resident's weight according to the U.S. customary scale (pounds and ounces) or the metric scale (kilograms and grams). There are 2.2 pounds in each kilogram. If you wish to change kilograms into pounds, multiply the number of kilograms by 2.2. You may have to read the numbers on the scale, or it may have a digital readout that prints the numbers.

There are some basic guidelines you should follow when weighing residents.

- Residents should always be weighed each time at the same time of day. (Weight varies during different periods of the day, so when weights are compared, they need to be taken as close as possible to the same time of day.)
- Residents should be weighed each time wearing the *same* type or amount of clothing.
- Residents should be weighed using the *same* scale each time.

As with any procedure, the safety of the resident is most important. Be sure the equipment is in proper working order and that you know how to use it. If you need help or instructions, ask. Never risk injuring the resident!

FIGURE 4-7

Types of scales: (a) standing scale, (b) scale with mechanical lift, (c) wheel chair scale.

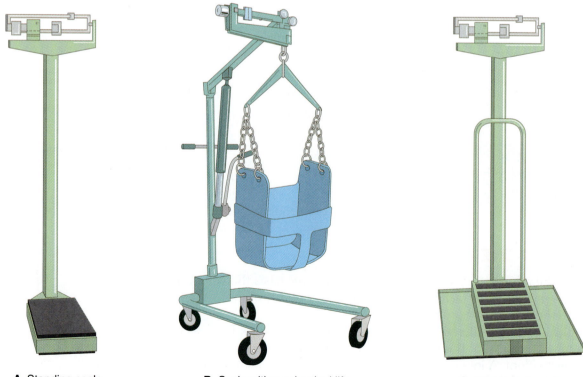

A Standing scale   **B** Scale with mechanical lift   **C** Wheelchair scale

The most commonly used scales are the standing balance scale, the scale with a hydraulic lift, and the bed scale.

Residents who are unable to stand can be weighed using a chair scale, a modification of the standing balance scale that is operated in the same fashion. Allowance is made for the weight of the chair and platform by subtracting a certain amount from the weight or by having the scale adjusted to allow for the extra weight. Follow the procedures established in your facility for the specific equipment used.

Another method of weighing a resident who is unable to stand is with a mechanical lift with a scale attached. Mechanical lifts operate using a hydraulic pump to raise and lower the resident. There are different types of lifts. Since one of the most commonly used lifts was made by the Hoyer Company, the mechanical lift may be called the Hoyer lift.

Although mechanical lifts are designed to allow one person to lift the resident, it is a good idea to use two people whenever possible. The lift may seem frightening to the resident, so explain the procedure carefully and reassure the resident that the procedure is safe.

Remember, the resident's weight measurement must be accurate. This information is vital in the diagnosis and treatment prescribed by the physician. If you have any questions as to the accuracy of the weight obtained, ask your charge nurse to verify the weight with you. You can test the accuracy of the scales by weighing yourself and comparing the results to your known weight.

VITAL SIGNS

Vital signs are measurements used to evaluate a resident's condition. The vital signs include body temperature, pulse rate, and respiration rate. Although not strictly considered a vital sign, blood pressure is also included. In some settings, the rating of pain intensity is called "the fifth vital sign" because it is so important to the well-being of the resident (Figure 4-8).

BODY TEMPERATURE

Body temperature is measured by a clinical thermometer, and it represents a balance between the heat produced by the body and the heat lost by the body.

FIGURE 4-8

Vital signs.

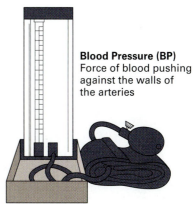

Blood Pressure (BP)
Force of blood pushing against the walls of the arteries

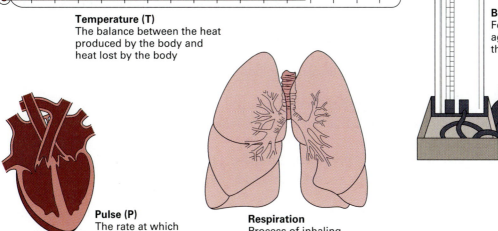

Temperature (T)
The balance between the heat produced by the body and heat lost by the body

Pulse (P)
The rate at which the heart is beating

Respiration
Process of inhaling and exhaling

PROCEDURE

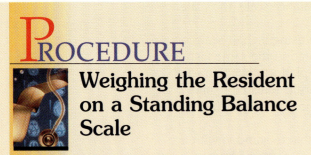

Weighing the Resident on a Standing Balance Scale

Preparation

1. Prior to weighing the resident, obtain the previous weight from the chart. If this is an admission, ask the resident what his or her normal weight is. This provides a standard for comparison.
2. Explain to the resident what you are going to do.

Steps

3. Take the resident to the scale (scales will remain accurate longer if they are moved as little as possible).
4. Level the scales if necessary. Some have a level bar with a bubble that is centered when the scale is level. Balance the scale. (With both weights at zero, the balance beam should be balanced in the center. If not, use the balance adjustment to bring the scale to balance.) (Figure 4-9)

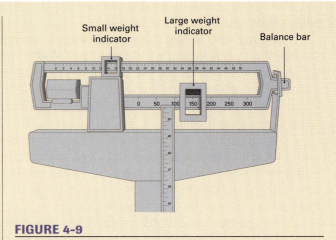

FIGURE 4-9

5. Assist the resident to stand on the scale with hands at the sides. Be sure the resident is balanced and centered on the scale. If the resident is unable to stand alone safely, another type of scale should be used.
6. Adjust the weights until the scale is in balance.
7. Write down the weight immediately.

Ending Steps

8. Assist the resident to return to the room.
9. Record the weight in the proper place and report any weight losses or gains to the charge nurse.

Fahrenheit (F) measurement of temperature in which 32 degrees is the freezing point and 212 degrees is the boiling point for water

Celsius or centigrade (C) measurement of temperature in which 0 degrees is the freezing point and 100 degrees is the boiling point for water

The normal adult temperature is measured in degrees **Fahrenheit (F)** or degrees **Celsius** or **centigrade (C).** The normal adult body temperature taken orally is 98.6°F or 37°C.

Factors that *increase* the body temperature include:

- Infection
- Shivering
- Physical activity and exercise
- Warmer external environment (hot weather, warm blankets or clothing, hot bath)
- Dehydration (lack of enough fluid in the body)

Factors that *decrease* the body temperature include:

- Shock (decreased circulation)
- Colder external environment (cold weather, cold shower, alcohol sponge bath)
- Age (older people tend to have a lower "normal" body temperature)
- Drugs such as aspirin or acetaminophen

Regulation of temperature is one of the many ways the body protects itself. The temperature increases to fight infection and decreases to save strength and energy.

PROCEDURE

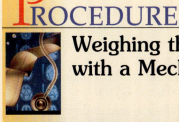

Weighing the Resident with a Mechanical Lift

Preparation

1. Assemble your equipment at the bedside:
   - Lift
   - Sling
   - Clean sheet
2. Explain to the resident what you are going to do.
3. Provide privacy.
4. Roll the resident on one side and place half the sling between the shoulders and the knees. Roll the resident to the opposite side and pull the other half of the sheet and sling under (Figure 4-10a).
5. Wheel the lift into place over the resident with the base beneath the bed.
6. Attach the sling using the chains and hooks provided. *Note:* The open part of the hook should be *away* from the resident (Figure 4-10b).

Steps

7. Using the hand crank or pump handle, raise the resident until the buttocks are clear of the bed. Make sure that the resident is aligned in the sling and is securely suspended.

8. Swing the feet and legs over the edge of the bed. If the bed is low enough and the lift goes high enough for the resident to be clear of the bed, weigh the resident while still over the bed.
9. If not, move the lift back from the bed so that no part of the resident's body is in contact with the bed (Figure 4-10c).
10. Adjust the weights until the scale is balanced. Follow the balancing directions for the scale in use. Read and record the weight shown immediately (Figure 4-10d).
11. Return the resident to a position over the bed.
12. Slowly release the knob and lower the resident onto the bed.
13. Remove the sheet and sling from beneath the resident.

Ending Steps

14. Position the resident comfortably with call signal within reach.
15. Return equipment to proper place.
16. Report any weight losses or gains to the charge nurse.

FIGURE 4-10

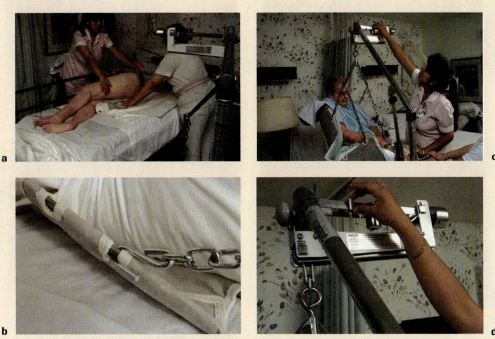

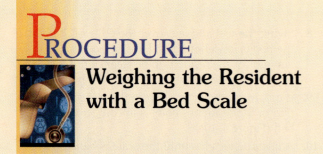

PROCEDURE

Weighing the Resident with a Bed Scale

Preparation

1. Assemble your equipment at the bedside.
   - Scale
   - Clean sheet
2. Explain to the resident what you are going to do.
3. Provide privacy.

Steps

4. Roll the resident toward one side and place the clean sheet beneath the resident (Figure 4-11a). (Use a folded sheet to allow you to use it as a lift sheet.) Roll the resident to the opposite side and pull the other half of the sheet under.
5. Place the bed scale next to the bed or, if possible, roll the scale so that the platform is over the bed.

6. Lock the wheels of the scale.
7. Using two people, either
   a. Roll the resident onto the weighing platform, or
   b. Use the lifting sheet to lift the resident onto the platform (Figure 4-11b)
8. Release the brake and move the resident and scale away from the bed (Figure 4-11c).
9. When using a digital scale, read and record the weight provided. If weights are used, add until the scale is balanced. Record the weight immediately (Figure 4-11d).
10. Return the resident to the bed by rolling or lifting him or her from the scale onto the bed.
11. Remove the sheet from under the resident.

Ending Steps

12. Position the resident comfortably.
13. Place the call signal within reach.
14. Return the equipment to the proper place. Disinfect pads on bed scale unless sheets were used. (Sheets must be changed.)
15. Wash your hands.

FIGURE 4-11

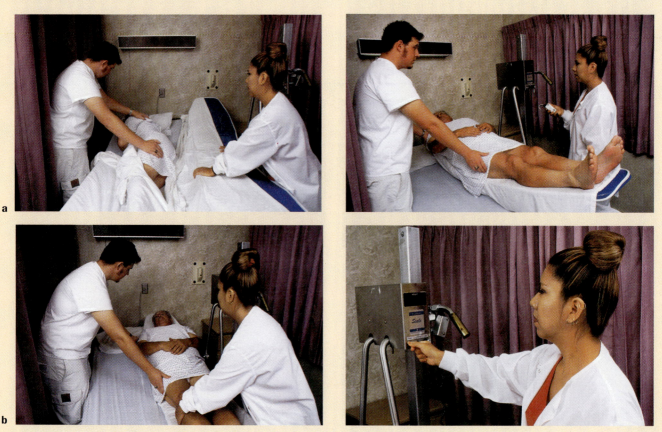

a

b

c

d

MEASURING HEIGHT

In order to determine the appropriate or ideal weight for an individual resident, it is necessary to know the resident's height. You may be asked to measure height by using either the height measurement device on the standing scale or by using a tape measure.

Height is measured in feet, inches, or centimeters. When using a tape measure, make sure the bed is in a flat position; then position the resident in the supine (back lying) position, with the body extended. Place a mark on the sheet at the top of the head and at the bottom of the feet; then measure the distance between the marks. An alternative for a resident who cannot "straighten out" due to contractures is to extend one arm so that it is **perpendicular** (at a right angle) to the body. Measure from the center of the neck to the tip of the longest finger, multiply the result by 2 and subtract 2 inches. The final number will be the resident's height.

TYPES OF THERMOMETERS AND INDICATIONS FOR USE

We measure body temperature with a clinical thermometer. There are glass thermometers (Figure 4-12), battery-operated electronic thermometers, and chemically treated paper or plastic single-use thermometers. Recently, an ear (aural) thermometer has been developed (Figure 4-13). This is another type of electronic thermometer. The ear probe is inserted gently into the outer ear to measure the temperature of the eardrum. The probe is covered with a disposable sheath, which is replaced with each use. The device converts and displays the temperature as equal to either the oral or rectal method. Be sure to indicate whether it is oral or rectal when you write the temperature reading.

Glass thermometers are filled with mercury, a silver liquid that expands with heat. The thermometer is **calibrated** (marked) in degrees and fractions of degrees (Figure 4-14). There are thermometers with Fahrenheit scales and thermometers with centigrade scales (Figure 4-15).

perpendicular   at a right angle

calibrated   marked with graduations, as on a thermometer or graduate

TYPES OF MEASUREMENT

The Fahrenheit thermometer has been most commonly used in the United States. The numbers start at 94°F and go up to 110°F (Figure 4-16). The long lines represent 1 degree, the short lines represent two-tenths of a degree. There is usually an arrow at 98.6°F, which is the "normal" body temperature reading.

The centigrade thermometer begins with 34°C and ends at 43°C (Figure 4-17). Each long line represents 1 degree; each short line represents one-tenth of a degree.

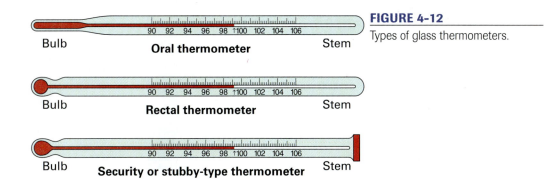

Oral thermometer

Rectal thermometer

Security or stubby-type thermometer

FIGURE 4-12
Types of glass thermometers.

bulb (thermometer) portion of the thermometer that is placed in direct contact with the resident's body

stem (thermometer) long narrow portion of a thermometer, opposite from the bulb

oral in the mouth

rectal in the rectum

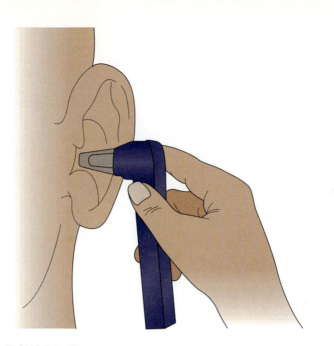

FIGURE 4-13

Tympanic membrane sensor measures body temperature. A probe is inserted into the ear canal.

The parts of a thermometer consist of the **bulb,** which is the portion placed in direct contact with the resident's body, and the **stem,** which is the opposite end of the thermometer.

Temperature is measured orally (by mouth), axillary (under the armpit), or rectally (inserted through the anus into the rectum). These sites are chosen because each has a rich supply of blood close to the surface that will produce an accurate temperature reading.

METHODS OF MEASUREMENT

The decision as to how a temperature should be measured will depend on several factors. In some instances, the physician will specify which method to use. Other factors are related to the condition of the resident. For example, you would never measure an **oral** (in the mouth) temperature on an unconscious or very confused resident who might accidentally bite down on the thermometer. Generally, a **rectal** (in the rectum) temperature is ordered when the resident:

FIGURE 4-14

Temperature conversion.

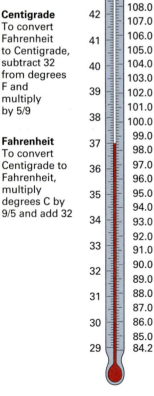

Temperature Conversion

Centigrade
To convert Fahrenheit to Centigrade, subtract 32 from degrees F and multiply by 5/9

Fahrenheit
To convert Centigrade to Fahrenheit, multiply degrees C by 9/5 and add 32

FIGURE 4-15

The two major scales used for measuring temperature in the United States.

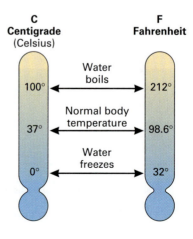

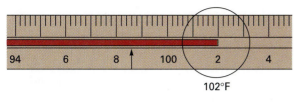

100.2°F

102°F

FIGURE 4-16

Fahrenheit thermometer.

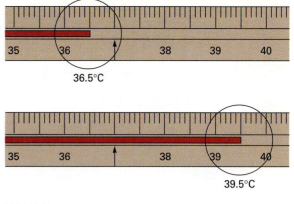

36.5°C

39.5°C

FIGURE 4-17

Centigrade thermometer.

- Has a history of seizures
- Is under 8 years old
- Cannot keep his or her mouth closed around the thermometer
- Is unable to breathe through the nose

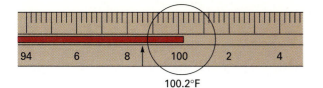

PROCEDURE

Reading a Fahrenheit Thermometer

Preparation

1. With your thumb and first two fingers, hold the thermometer at the stem.
2. Hold the thermometer at eye level. Turn the thermometer back and forth between your fingers until you can clearly see the column of mercury.
3. Notice the scale of calibrations. Each long line stands for 1 degree.
4. There are four short lines between each of the long lines. Each short line stands for two-tenths (or 0.2) of a degree.
5. Between the long lines that represent 98 and 99, look for a longer line with an arrow directly beneath it. This arrow points to "normal" oral body temperature (98.6).

Step

6. Look at the end of the mercury. Notice the line where the mercury ends. If it is one of the short lines, notice the previously long line toward the bulb end. The temperature reading is the degree marked by that long line plus two-, four-, six-, or eight-tenths of a degree. If the mercury ends on the second short line after 99, the temperature is 99.4°F. If the mercury ends between two lines, use the closer line (Figure 4-18).

Ending Step

7. Write down the temperature reading right away. The temperature reading may be written 99.4°F or 99[4]. If the temperature is taken rectally, write 99.4 R. If the temperature is taken in the axilla, write 99.4 A. If not marked R or A, the temperature is assumed to be an oral reading.

FIGURE 4-18

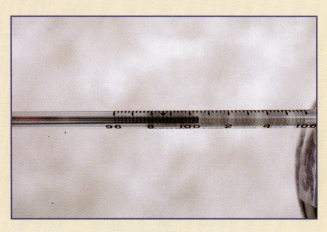

PROCEDURE

Measuring an Oral Temperature

Preparation

1. Assemble your equipment:
   - Oral thermometer
   - Pen or pencil and paper
   - Tissue or paper towel
   - Disposable plastic shield

2. Wash your hands.
3. Identify the resident.
4. Tell the resident that you are going to measure the temperature.
5. Ask if the resident has recently had hot or cold fluids or has been smoking. If yes, wait 20 minutes before taking an oral temperature.
6. If the thermometer has been soaking in a solution, rinse it with cool tap water and dry with paper towel or tissue.

7. Shake the mercury down, if necessary.

Steps

8. Gently put the bulb end in the resident's mouth under the tongue. The mouth and the lips should stay closed (Figure 4-19a and 19b).
9. For the most accurate reading, leave the thermometer in the resident's mouth for 8 minutes.
10. Take the thermometer out. Hold the stem end and wipe the thermometer with the tissue from the stem toward the bulb.
11. Read the thermometer (Figure 4-19c).
12. Record the temperature. Report any abnormal reading immediately to your charge nurse.
13. Shake the mercury down. Replace the thermometer in its container or return it to the proper area for cleaning.

Ending Steps

14. Make the resident comfortable.
15. Wash your hands.

FIGURE 4-19

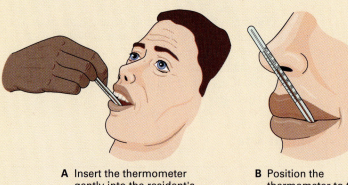

A Insert the thermometer gently into the resident's mouth under the tongue.

B Position the thermometer to the side of the mouth.

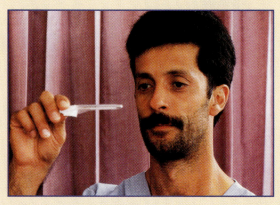

C Read the thermometer.

PROCEDURE

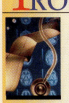

Measuring Rectal Temperature

Preparation

1. Assemble your equipment:
   - Rectal thermometer
   - Tissue or paper towel
   - Lubricating jelly
   - Disposable gloves
   - Pencil or pen and paper

2. Wash your hands.
3. Identify the resident.
4. Provide privacy.
5. Tell the resident that you are going to measure the temperature by rectum.

Steps

6. Place the bed in a flat position, if possible.
7. Inspect the bulb of the thermometer carefully for cracks or chipped places (Figure 4-20a). A broken thermometer could seriously injure the resident. **Never** use a chipped, cracked, or broken thermometer.
8. Shake the thermometer down, if necessary.
9. Put a small amount of lubricating jelly on a piece of tissue. Then lubricate the bulb of the thermometer with the lubricated tissue. This makes insertion easier and also makes it more comfortable for the resident (Figure 4-20b).

10. Assist the resident to turn to one side. Turn back the covers just enough so that you can see the buttocks. Avoid overexposing.
11. Put on your gloves.
12. Raise the upper buttock until you can see the anus (the opening of the rectum) and gently insert the bulb 1 inch through the anus into the rectum.
13. Hold the thermometer in place for 3 minutes. Never leave a resident with a rectal thermometer in the rectum (Figure 4-20c).
14. Remove the thermometer. Holding the stem, wipe it with a tissue from stem to bulb to remove any particles of feces.
15. Read the thermometer.

Ending Steps

16. Remove your gloves.
17. Record the temperature. Note that this is a rectal temperature by writing an R after the figure. Report any abnormal readings immediately to your charge nurse.
18. Return the thermometer to the appropriate area for cleaning.
19. Wash your hands.
20. Make the resident comfortable.
21. Place the call signal within reach.

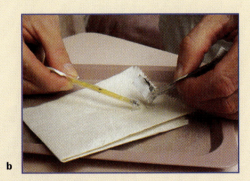

b

FIGURE 4-20

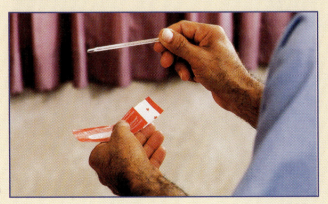

a

c

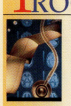

PROCEDURE

Measuring Axillary Temperature

Preparation

1. Assemble your equipment:

   • Oral thermometer
   • Tissue or paper towel
   • Pen or pencil and paper

2. Wash your hands.
3. Identify the resident.
4. Tell the resident that you have to measure the temperature.
5. Provide privacy.

Steps

6. If the thermometer is kept in a solution, rinse the thermometer with cool tap water and dry it with tissue.
7. Shake down the mercury if necessary.

8. Remove the resident's arm from the sleeve of the gown. If the axillary region is moist with perspiration, dry it with a towel.
9. Place the bulb of the thermometer in the center of the armpit (axilla). The thermometer then should be held upright by the arm.
10. Put the resident's arm across the chest or abdomen (Figure 4–21).
11. If the resident is unconscious or too weak to help, you will have to hold the thermometer in place.
12. Leave the thermometer in place for 10 minutes. Stay with the resident.
13. Remove the thermometer. Wipe it off with tissue from the stem to the bulb.
14. Read the thermometer.
15. Record the temperature. Note that this is an axillary temperature by writing an A after the figure.

Ending Steps

16. Report any abnormal readings immediately to your charge nurse.
17. Replace the thermometer in its container or return it to the proper area for cleaning.
18. Put the resident's arm back in the sleeve of the gown.
19. Make the resident comfortable.

FIGURE 4-21

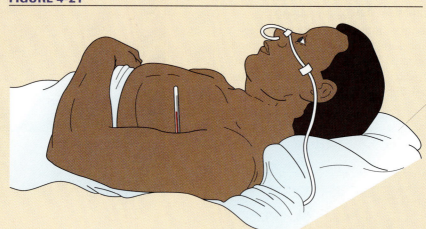

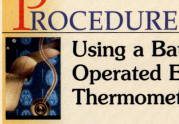

PROCEDURE

Using a Battery-Operated Electronic Thermometer

FIGURE 4-22

Preparation

1. Assemble your equipment:
   - Battery-operated electronic thermometer
   - Plastic disposable probe cover
   - Appropriate attachment for type of temperature (oral, rectal, axillary)
   - Pen or pencil and paper
   - Gloves for rectal temperature

2. Wash your hands.
3. Identify the resident.
4. Tell the resident that you are going to measure the temperature.
5. Provide privacy.

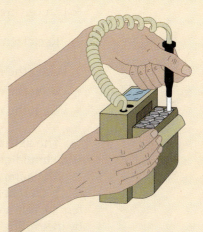

A Insert the probe into a probe cover.

Steps

6. Remove the probe from its stored position and insert it into the probe cover (Figure 4–22a).
7. Insert the covered probe into the appropriate opening (mouth, rectum, or axilla). If taking the temperature rectally, lubricate the probe cover with a water-soluble lubricant.
8. Hold the probe in place.
9. Wait for the buzzer or beep to signal that the temperature reading is complete.
10. Remove the probe and discard the probe cover without touching it (Figure 4–22b).

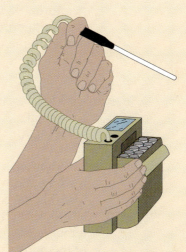

B After measuring the temperature, press to eject the probe cover.

Ending Steps

11. Return the probe to its stored position (Figure 4–22c).
12. Record the temperature.
13. Make the resident comfortable.
14. Wash your hands.
15. Report any abnormal reading to the charge nurse.

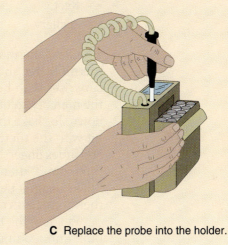

C Replace the probe into the holder.

- Is restless, unconscious, or confused
- Has coughing or sneezing spells
- Is receiving warm or cold applications to the face or neck

Rectal temperature should *not* be measured under the following conditions:

- When the resident has any sign of hemorrhoids or rectal bleeding
- When the resident is very combative
- When the resident has diarrhea

The **axillary** (in the armpit) method of measurement is the least reliable and should only be used if the oral and rectal methods would be unsafe.

The aural (ear) thermometer is a good alternative to both the oral and rectal thermometer. It is safe and comfortable for the resident. Aural thermometers are also accurate and easy to use. The sensor measures the body temperature by measuring the temperature of the tympanic membrane (eardrum).

Thermometers vary according to how the temperature is to be measured. One type is used for oral and axillary, another is used for measuring rectal temperature.

The "normal" reading varies with the method of measurement and the type of thermometer used.

	Fahrenheit	Centigrade
Oral	98.6	37.0
Rectal	99.6	37.5
Axillary	97.6	36.4

Memorize these normal readings so that you can recognize an abnormal reading and report it promptly. There are small variations in body temperature that are considered normal. For example, the body temperature is generally lower in the morning and increases in the afternoon. However, when the temperature reaches any of the following readings, it should be considered out of the normal range and reported immediately.

Oral	100°F or 37.6°C
Rectal	101°F or 38.0°C
Axillary	99°F or 37.2°C

Glass thermometers are very fragile and must be handled with care. The thermometer should be checked for cracks before each use. Although mercury rises with heat, it does not constrict with cold. This means that to move the mercury column down after it has risen, the thermometer must be shaken down. To shake the thermometer down, stand away from objects that you might hit with the thermometer. Grasp the stem end securely between your thumb and index finger. Using a snapping motion of your wrist, shake the thermometer three times, then check to see how far the mercury column has gone down. Shake again if necessary. It should be below the 94°F or 34°C mark before the thermometer is ready for use.

Reading the thermometer consists of locating the end of the mercury column and reading or calculating the number of degrees represented (Figure 4-23). Write down the information immediately. Don't try to remember it. Accuracy is essential! Practice reading as many thermometers as possible and have your charge nurse verify your readings to ensure that you have learned to read a thermometer correctly.

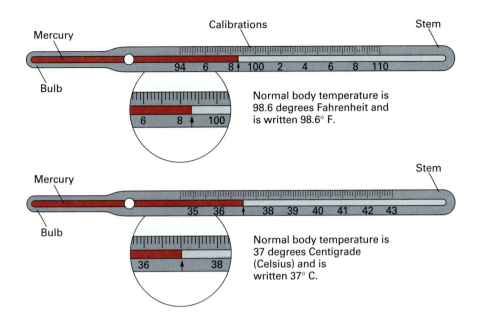

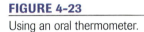

FIGURE 4-23

Using an oral thermometer.

Remember that you will always use a rectal thermometer for taking rectal temperatures. Note that the rectal thermometer has a small round bulb on one end. This bulb prevents the thermometer from injuring the sensitive lining of the resident's rectum.

If the battery-operated electronic thermometer is used in your facility, follow the general principles of measuring temperature along with the manufacturer's instructions.

CHARACTERISTICS OF THE PULSE

Each time the heart beats, it pumps a certain amount of blood into the arteries. This causes the arteries to expand (get bigger). Between heartbeats, the arteries contract, returning to their normal size. The heart pumps the blood in a steady rhythm. The rhythmic expansion and contraction of the arteries, which can be measured to show how fast the heart is beating, is called the **pulse** (Figure 4-24).

Measuring the pulse is a simple method of determining how the circulatory system is functioning. The pulse measures how fast the heart is beating. The pulse can be felt at certain places on the body. The normal pulse can be felt easily by your fingertips. If circulation is decreased, the pulse can be weak or absent.

One of the easiest places to feel the pulse is at the wrist (Figure 4-25). This is called a **radial pulse** because you are feeling the radial artery. When measuring the pulse, you must accurately note the following.

- **Rate**—the number of pulse beats per minute
- **Rhythm**—the regularity of the pulse beats
- **Force of the beat**—weak or bounding

Each person has a "normal" rate somewhere within the normal range. The nursing assistant must report any significant changes in pulse rate, rhythm, or force. If the resident's rate is below 60 or above 90 beats per minute, report

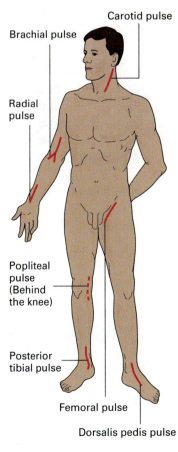

FIGURE 4-24

Places where the pulse may be taken.

pulse   the rhythmic expansion and contraction of the arteries, which can be measured to show how fast the heart is beating

radial pulse   pulse felt at the inner aspect of the wrist (radial artery)

rate pulse   the number of pulse beats per minute

rhythm pulse   the regularity of the pulse beats

force of the beat pulse strength or power described as weak or bounding

apical pulse   heartbeat measured at the apex of the heart

this to your charge nurse immediately. Remember, the pulse rate will increase with physical activity, stress, emotional disturbances, fever, and some illnesses. Make sure that you measure the routine pulse when the resident is at rest.

Normal Pulse Rates (per Minute) for Different Age Groups	
Childhood years	80–115
Adult years	72–80
Later years	60–70

APICAL PULSE

The pulse rate should be the same as the heart rate. However, in some residents, the heartbeats are not strong enough to be felt along the arteries. This can be due to some forms of heart disease. For these residents, an apical pulse would be taken with a stethoscope (Figure 4-26).

An **apical pulse** is a measurement of the heartbeats at the apex of the heart, located just under the left breast (Figure 4-27).

You will be using a stethoscope to listen to the apical pulse. The **stethoscope** is an instrument used to listen to various sounds in the body, such as

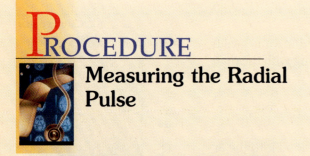

PROCEDURE

Measuring the Radial Pulse

Preparation

1. Assemble your equipment:
   - Watch with a second hand
   - Pen or pencil and paper
2. Wash your hands.
3. Identify the resident.
4. Tell the resident that you are going to measure the pulse.

Steps

5. Her hand and arm should be well supported and resting comfortably.
6. Find the pulse by placing the tips of your middle three fingers on the palm side of the resident's wrist, in a line with the thumb, directly next to the bone. Press lightly until you feel the beat. If you press too hard, you may stop the flow of blood and the pulse. Never use your thumb. It has its own

pulse and you might count your own pulse instead of the resident's. When you have found the pulse, note the rhythm. Is the beat steady or irregular? Note the force of the beat. Is it strong or weak?

7. Note the position of the second hand on your watch. Count the pulse beats until the second hand comes back to the same position.
   - Method A: Count the pulse beats for 1 full minute and report the full minute count. Always do this if the resident has an irregular beat.
   - Method B: Count for 30 seconds, until the second hand is opposite from the position when you started. Then multiply the number of beats by 2. This is the number you record. For example, if you count 35 for 30 seconds, the count for 1 full minute would be 70.

8. Record the pulse count.

Ending Steps

9. Make the resident comfortable.
10. Wash your hands.
11. Report to your charge nurse:
    - If the pulse rate was under 60 or over 90 beats per minute
    - If the rhythm was irregular
    - If the force was weak or bounding
    - If there was a change in rate, rhythm, or force from previous measurements

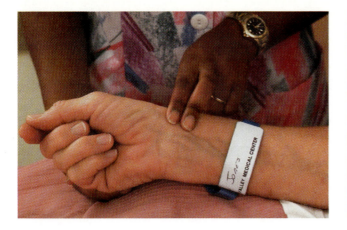

FIGURE 4-25
Radial pulse.

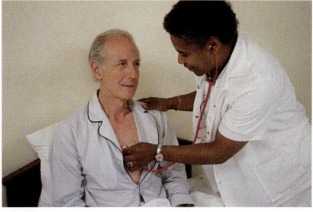

FIGURE 4-26
Taking an apical pulse with a stethoscope.

the heartbeat or breathing sounds. The stethoscope is a tube that picks up sound when it is placed against a part of the body. One end is either bell-shaped (called a bell), or it is round and flat (called a diaphragm) (Figure 4-28). The other end of the tube is split into two parts. These parts have tips on the ends and fit into the listener's ears.

MEASURING RESPIRATIONS

Respiration is the process of inhaling and exhaling (Figure 4-29). One respiration includes breathing in once and breathing out once. When a person breathes out, the chest contracts (gets smaller). When you count respirations, you watch the resident's chest rise and fall or feel the chest rise and fall with your hand.

When a person knows that respiration is being counted, he or she may not breathe naturally. What you want to count is the natural breathing rate. Normally, adults breathe at a rate of 16 to 20 times a minute. Children breathe more rapidly. The elderly breathe more slowly. Exercise, digestion, emotional stress, disease, drugs, stimulants, heat, and cold can all affect the number of times per minute that a person breathes.

While you are counting the resident's respirations, it is important to observe and make note of anything about the breathing that appears to be abnormal. Different types of abnormal respiration include:

- **Labored**—the resident struggles or works hard to breathe and may make gurgling, rattling, or wheezing sounds.
- **Stertorous**—the resident makes abnormal noises like snoring when breathing.
- **Abdominal**—breathing using mostly the abdominal muscles.
- **Shallow**—breathing with only the upper part of the lungs.
- **Irregular**—the depth of breathing changes and the rate of the rise and fall of the chest is not steady.
- **Cheyne–Stokes**—irregular breathing. At first the breathing is slow and shallow, then respiration becomes

stethoscope instrument that picks up sound when placed against part of the body

respiration process of inhaling and exhaling

labored respirations difficult breathing that may include gurgling, rattling, or wheezing sounds

stertorous respirations abnormal noises like snoring when breathing

FIGURE 4-27
Position of heart in the chest.

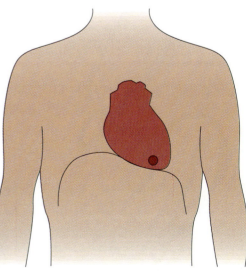

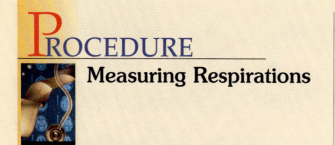

PROCEDURE

Measuring Respirations

5. Hold the resident's wrist as if you were measuring the pulse. Count the respirations immediately after counting the pulse rate.
6. One rise and one fall of the chest counts as one respiration.
7. If you cannot clearly see the chest rise and fall, hold the resident's arms across the chest and feel the chest rise.
8. Count the respirations for one full minute.
9. Write down the figure.

Ending Steps

10. Make the resident comfortable.
11. Wash your hands.
12. Report any unusual observations to your charge nurse immediately.

Preparation

1. Assemble your equipment:
   - Watch with a second hand
   - Pen or pencil and paper
2. Wash your hands.
3. Identify the resident.
4. Provide privacy.

---

abdominal respirations
breathing using mostly the abdominal muscles

shallow respiration
breathing with only the upper part of the lungs

faster and deeper until it reaches a kind of peak. It then slows and becomes shallow again. Breathing may stop completely for 10 seconds and begin the same pattern again.

Temperature, pulse, and respiration (TPR) are usually measured at the same time as one procedure. Careful, accurate recording of this information is very important. The procedures for measuring the vital signs must be practiced many times for you to be able to carry them out skillfully and accurately (Figure 4-30).

FIGURE 4-28

Stethoscopes.

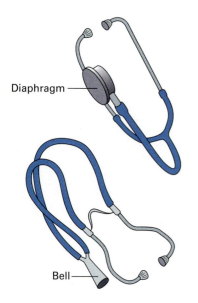

Diaphragm

Bell

FIGURE 4-29

The patient must be unaware that you are counting respirations.

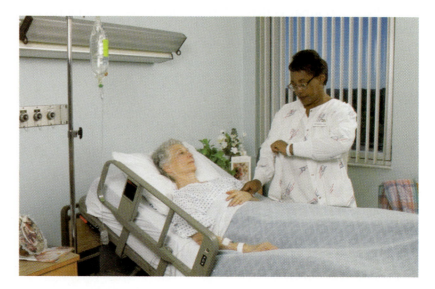

BLOOD PRESSURE

Blood pressure is the force of the blood pushing against the walls of the blood vessels. When you measure a resident's blood pressure, you are measuring the force of the blood flowing through the arteries.

There is always a certain amount of pressure in the arteries. This is because the heart, by pumping, is constantly forcing blood to circulate. The amount of pressure in the arteries depends on two things:

- The rate of the heartbeat
- How easily the blood flows through the blood vessels

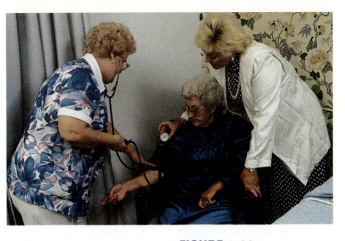

FIGURE 4-30

Learning basic skills.

The heart contracts as it pumps blood into the arteries. When the heart is contracting, the pressure is highest. This pressure is called **systolic pressure.** As the heart relaxes between each contraction, the pressure goes down. When the heart is most relaxed, the pressure is lowest. This pressure is called the **diastolic pressure.** When you measure a resident's blood pressure, you are measuring the systolic and diastolic pressures.

In healthy adults, the normal systolic blood pressure range is between 100 and 140 millimeters (mm) of mercury (Hg). The normal diastolic pressure is between 60 and 90 millimeters (mm) of mercury (Hg). The way to write these figures is: 120/80. The systolic pressure is always the first or top number.

When a resident's blood pressure is higher than the normal range for his or her age and condition, it is referred to as **hypertension** or high blood pressure. When a resident's blood pressure is lower than the normal range, it is referred to as **hypotension** or low blood pressure.

The elderly tend to have higher blood pressure due to a loss of elasticity of the arteries. There are many residents with hypertension in LTC facilities. The blood pressure will normally increase with physical activity, stress, emotional disturbances, fever, and some illnesses. It will decrease when the resident is sleeping or at rest or if the resident is in shock (a condition related to the circulatory system). Certain medications also increase or decrease blood pressure. All individuals have a "normal" range of blood pressure for their age and physical health. Any significant changes in blood pressure should be reported to the charge nurse immediately.

The position of the resident will also change the measurement. Generally, the blood pressure increases when the resident is lying flat, and it decreases when the resident is in a sitting or standing position. You should try to measure the blood pressure each time with the resident in the same position (usually sitting if tolerated).

INSTRUMENTS FOR MEASURING BLOOD PRESSURE

When you measure blood pressure, you will be using a stethoscope and an instrument called a sphygmomanometer. **Sphygmomanometer** is a combination of three Greek words:

- *Sphygmo,* meaning pulse
- *Mano,* meaning pressure
- *Meter,* meaning measure

irregular respiration   a change in the depth of breathing and an unsteady rate of rise and fall of the chest

Cheyne–Stokes respiration   a kind of breathing that can be observed when a resident is near death. The breathing is slow and shallow at first, followed by faster and deeper breathing, which reaches a peak, then stops completely. The pattern then repeats until breathing stops completely

blood pressure   measurable force of the blood against the walls of a blood vessel

systolic pressure   pressure created when the heart is contracting; highest pressure

diastolic pressure   pressure when the heart is relaxed (the lowest pressure)

hypertension   high blood pressure

hypotension   low blood pressure

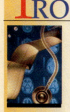

PROCEDURE

Measuring Blood Pressure

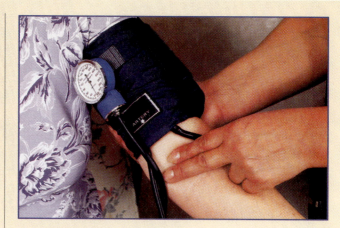

FIGURE 4-31b

Preparation

1. Assemble your equipment:
   - Sphygmomanometer
   - Stethoscope
   - Antiseptic pad
   - Pen or pencil and paper
2. Wash your hands.
3. Identify the resident.
4. Tell the resident that you are going to measure the blood pressure.
5. Wipe the earplugs of the stethoscope with antiseptic pads.

Steps

6. Have the resident resting quietly, either lying down or sitting in a chair.
7. If you are using the mercury type, the measuring scale should be at eye level.
8. The resident's arm should be bare up to the shoulder.
9. The resident's arm from the elbow down should be resting fully extended on the bed or on the arm of a chair.
10. Unroll the cuff and loosen the valve on the bulb. Then squeeze the compression bag to deflate it completely.

11. Wrap the cuff snugly and smoothly around the resident's arm about 1 inch above the elbow with the arrows on the cuff pointing toward the brachial pulse. Do not wrap it so tightly that the resident is uncomfortable from the pressure (Figure 4-31a).
12. Be sure the manometer is in position so that you can read the numbers easily.
13. Put the earplugs of the stethoscope into your ears.
14. With your fingertips, find the brachial pulse at the inner side of the arm above the elbow (Figure 4-31b). Place the diaphragm or bell of the stethoscope there. It should be held firmly against the skin, but should not touch the cuff (Figure 4-31c).
15. Tighten the thumbscrew of the valve to close it. Turn it clockwise. Be careful not to turn it too tightly or you will have trouble opening it.
16. Hold the stethoscope in place. Inflate the cuff so that the dial points to 170 (200 on an older person) and you no longer hear the pulse.

FIGURE 4-31c

FIGURE 4-31a

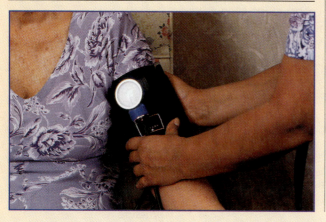

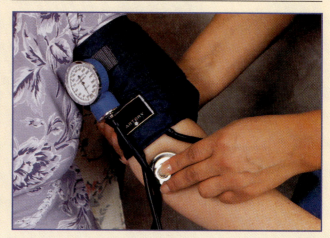

PROCEDURE

continued

17. Open the valve counterclockwise. This allows the air to escape. Let it out *slowly* until the sound of the pulse comes back. A few seconds must go by without any pulse sounds. If you do hear pulse sounds immediately, completely deflate the cuff and wait a few seconds. Then inflate the cuff to a higher calibration, above 200. Again, loosen the thumbscrew slowly to let out the air. Listen for a repeated pulse sound. At the same time, watch the indicator (Figure 4-31d).

18. Note the calibration the pointer (or the mercury) passes as you hear the first sound. This point indicates the systolic pressure. Remember it.

19. Continue releasing air from the cuff. When the sounds change to a softer and faster thud or disap-pear, note the calibration. This is the diastolic pressure. Remember it.

20. Deflate the cuff completely. Remove it from the resident's arm.

21. Record your reading.

Ending Steps

22. After using the blood pressure cuff, roll it up over the manometer and place it in the proper storage area.

23. Wipe the earplugs of the stethoscope with an antiseptic wipe. Put the stethoscope back in its proper place (Figure 4-31e).

24. Make the resident comfortable.

25. Wash your hands.

26. Report anything unusual to your charge nurse.

FIGURE 4-31d

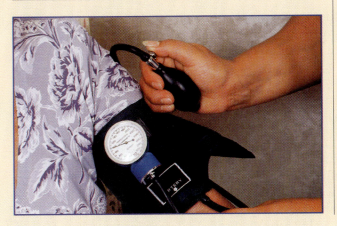

FIGURE 4-31e

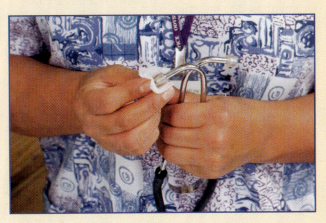

This instrument, however, is usually called a *blood pressure cuff.* The four main parts of this instrument are the manometer, valve, cuff, and bulb.

Three kinds of manometers are used for taking blood pressure. One is called the mercury type (Figure 4-32). Another is called the aneroid (dial) type (Figure 4-33). The third type is an electronic manometer with a digital display. All three use an inflatable cloth-cover rubber bag or cuff. The cuff is wrapped around the resident's arm. The electronic device inflates and deflates the cuff automatically, while the mercury and the aneroid type have a rubber bulb for pumping air into the cuff. The procedure for measuring blood pressure is the same, except for reading the measurement. The electronic type has a simple-to-read digital display. When you use the mercury type, you will be watching the level of a column of mercury on a measuring scale. When you use the dial or aneroid type, you will be watching a pointer on a dial.

FIGURE 4-32

Mercury sphygmomanometer.

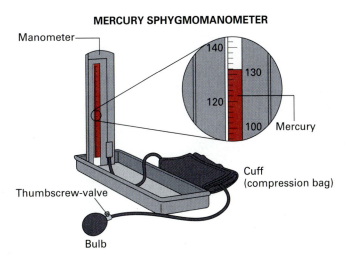

MERCURY SPHYGMOMANOMETER

Manometer

Thumbscrew-valve

Bulb

140
130
120
100 — Mercury

Cuff (compression bag)

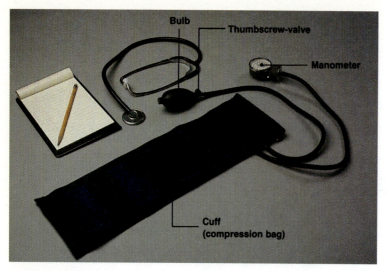

FIGURE 4-33

Aneroid sphygmomanometer.

sphygmomanometer instrument used to measure blood pressure; can be either aneroid (measurer watches a calibrated dial) or mercury type (measurer watches a column of mercury)

When you measure a resident's blood pressure, you are doing two things at the same time. You are listening to the brachial pulse as it sounds in the brachial artery in the resident's arm. You also are watching an indicator (either a column of mercury or a dial) in order to take a reading.

Accurately measuring blood pressure requires a lot of practice. Blood pressure can vary each time it is taken and in each arm. If you need to repeat the measurement, allow the resident several minutes to rest. Do not inflate and deflate the cuff several times in a row because the results will be inaccurate. The cuff that wraps around the resident's arm must fit properly in order to obtain an accurate result. For this reason, there are cuffs made in small (pediatric) sizes as well as extra-large sizes. For residents who are so thin that the cuff slides up and down on the arm, request a small cuff. If the resident is so heavy that the cuff just barely meets, ask for a large cuff.

Usually, blood pressure is measured in the left arm in order to have consistent readings. Do not measure blood pressure in an arm with an IV, an AV shunt (dialysis patient), a cast, or any kind of wound or sore.

SUMMARY

In this chapter, you have learned how a long-term care facility determines what the resident needs and develops a written plan to meet those needs. The health care plan is written in language that is probably new to you. It includes abbreviations as well as new terms. Throughout your training, you will be learning new words to add to those in this chapter. Your role as an observer of the resident's behavior, of physical and functional changes, is very important to assuring high-quality care. You have also learned what to look for and what to report and record in the chart.

New skills that you will be practicing daily in your role as a nursing assistant include weighing residents using several different types of scales as well as measuring and recording vital signs. You've learned the importance of the vital signs and what causes changes in the vital signs. Measuring blood pressure is a skill that needs regular practice to ensure your competency and accuracy. A number of studies have shown that even physicians make errors in measuring the blood pressure.

OBRA HIGHLIGHTS

The OBRA regulations place great importance on the resident's weight. The regulations tell us that one way to determine if the resident's nutritional status is maintained is to monitor the resident's weight loss and gain. The nursing assistant is responsible for following the correct procedures needed to provide accurate weights. Inaccurate weights would lead to false conclusions about the resident's nutritional and general health status.

SELF STUDY

Choose the best answer for each question or statement.

1. When a care plan is truly individualized, you could read it and be able to
   a. identify the resident without looking at the room number or name
   b. identify a few obvious needs of the resident, but not all of his or her needs
   c. explain to family members the reason for all the resident's medications
   d. identify which nursing unit the patient is on without seeing the name

2. Mr. Martinez is a new resident to your facility. The MDS coordinator asks you for information about how much assistance he needs with specific activities of daily living. What is the reason for this?
   a. The MDS coordinator does not have time to observe these things herself, so she asks you.
   b. The MDS coordinator will use the information to develop the resident's health care plan.
   c. The physician wants a report of how the resident is doing in the facility.
   d. The information will be shared with the family to determine if placement is appropriate.

3. Which of the following is true of the health care plan for a long-term care resident?
   a. The plan gives general suggestions about how to handle the resident while giving care.
   b. The plan is an outline of the steps needed to complete specific tasks, such as giving a shower.
   c. The plan provides all caregivers with the same guidelines for care, establishing continuity of care.
   d. The plan is not important for planning your work; the assignment sheet and bath schedule are all you need.

4. Which of the following actions should you take to gather information to organize your work day?
   a. Check for any time schedules that must be followed to complete care.
   b. Make rounds on each of your assigned residents.
   c. Check for any events planned for residents or staff during the day.
   d. all of the above

5. How do you set priorities in resident care?
   a. Determine what care should be done first and what care can, if necessary, wait until later.
   b. Determine how long you can take breaks and still complete your work before the end of your shift.
   c. Decide who you can get to help you with your assigned residents so your work won't take as long.
   d. Decide what tasks you would rather do first and what tasks you would rather do later.

6. What should you do if you get behind or are unable to complete your work during your shift?
   a. Tell your charge nurse at the end of the shift what you didn't get done.
   b. Ask your charge nurse for help as soon as you get behind.
   c. Ask another nursing assistant to do part of your assignment for you.
   d. Say nothing about what you did not get done and try to do better tomorrow.

7. Which of the following is an example of an objective observation?
   a. The resident refused breakfast.
   b. The resident does not cooperate.
   c. The resident is depressed and won't eat.
   d. The resident thinks her family is neglecting her.

8. Which of the following would be inappropriate for the nursing assistant to chart?
   a. Resident was given a shower and stated, "That felt good."
   b. Resident is resting in bed with side rails up.
   c. Resident's doctor does not seem to care about his ulcer.
   d. Resident attended activities and church service.

9. When you document the care you gave for a resident, you make an error. How should you correct the error?
   a. Erase the error, then write the correct information.
   b. Use whiteout over the error, then write the correct information.
   c. Draw a line through the error, and make a notation of the error.
   d. Skip one line to indicate an error, then begin the notation again.

10. Which of the following would be an example of inappropriate charting?
    a. Foul odor is noted from resident's mouth.
    b. Resident slurs words as he speaks.
    c. Large, hard, reddened area is noted on left ankle.
    d. Resident complains of pain to get attention.

11. Your assignment sheet states: "Mr. Smith is H.O.H. with a Lt CVA. He is to be up in w/c t.i.d." Which of the following translations is correct?
    a. Mr. Smith is hard of hearing in his left ear, has congestive heart failure, and is to have white blood cell count three times a day.
    b. Mr. Smith is hard of hearing, has had a stroke on his left side, and is to be up in the wheelchair three times a day.
    c. Mr. Smith is hard of hearing in his left ear, has had a heart attack, and is to be weighed in a chair scale once each day.
    d. Mr. Smith is hard of hearing, has had a stroke on his left side, and is to be up in the wheelchair for as long as he desires each day.

12. Mr. Smith is to be weighed today. He has lost 6 pounds since admission. Which of the following is true about measuring Mr. Smith's weight?
    a. It must be done accurately to be useful.
    b. It must be done at the same time of day as his previous weights.
    c. He must wear the same type or amount of clothing as he did for previous weights.
    d. all of the above

13. Which of the following observations about Mr. Smith should you report to your charge nurse?
    a. His ankles are slightly swollen after his bath.
    b. He complains of being cold at the beginning of his bath.
    c. He does not want to wear his usual sweatsuit today.
    d. His gastrostomy tube is in place, without redness around it.

14. Mrs. Marconi's temperature is elevated. When you read the Fahrenheit thermometer, the mercury stops two short marks past the long line indicating 101 degrees. What is Mrs. Marconi's temperature reading?
    a. 101.2 degrees
    b. 101.4 degrees
    c. 102 degrees
    d. 103 degrees

15. When you take Mrs. Marconi's apical pulse, you find it is 10 beats faster than her radial pulse. What is the reason for this?
    a. You heard other sounds in the stethoscope and accidentally counted them as heartbeats.
    b. Some of her heartbeats are not strong enough to be felt in the radial artery.
    c. You must have miscounted her radial pulse, because the two pulses are always the same.
    d. The apical heart rate is like the systolic blood pressure and will always be highest.

16. When you take Mrs. Marconi's blood pressure, you have difficulty hearing it. You need to repeat the blood pressure. What should you do?
    a. Immediately reinflate the cuff to repeat the blood pressure.
    b. Take the blood pressure in her leg instead of her arm.
    c. Allow her to rest a few minutes, then repeat the blood pressure.
    d. Have her get in bed, then repeat the blood pressure while she is lying down.

Getting C O N N E C T E D
Multimedia **Extension** Activities

www.prenhall.com/will-black

Use the above address to access the free, interactive Companion Website created for this textbook. Hear the pronunciation of the key terms in the chapter. Get instant feedback to a variety of chapter-related questions. Link to other interesting sites.

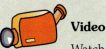
Video

Watch the video *Measuring Vital Signs* from the Care Provider Skills series. Watch the *Age-Specific Competencies* video from the Care Provider Skills series.

CASE STUDY

You are caring for Mrs. Garcia, a 90-year-old who has just been admitted with a hip fracture. She has been living with her daughter, son-in-law, and three grandchildren until she fell while walking her dog. You find out that her English is limited. She came here from Mexico when in her twenties and was married. Her two children were born here. Her religion is Roman Catholic.

1. You notice that Mrs. Garcia is wearing a ribbon around her neck with some sort of picture hanging from it. It is time for her shower. You
   a. take it off and put it in the laundry with her gown
   b. ask her if she wants to wear it or remove it for her shower
   c. take it off and put it in the bedside table
   d. ask her to tell you what it is and whether she would like to remove it for her shower
2. You notice when removing her dinner tray that she hasn't eaten much. You ask her:
   a. "Are there other foods that your prefer?"
   b. "I bet you'd like some beans and tortillas."
   c. "Why don't I call your daughter? She can get you to eat."
   d. "Don't you want to get better? You'd better eat!"
3. Discuss with your fellow nursing assistants or students your answers and explain why you chose the answer you did.
4. Mrs. Garcia complains to you that her roommate won't stop talking to her. She has beads in her hand and explains she is praying the rosary. You should
   a. Ignore it; they must learn to live together.
   b. Tell her roommate to leave her alone.
   c. Inform the nurse so she can discuss it with the other staff and add it to the health care plan.
   d. Pull the curtain around her bed and hope the roommate gets the hint.

Chapter 5

ANATOMY, PHYSIOLOGY, CANCER, AND SENSES

CARING TIP

You care for special people—not diseases

or problems. Each one is a unique individual.

Joan M. Scribner, RN, BSN
Affiliate Faculty
Penn Valley Community College
Kansas City, Missouri

KEY TERMS

anatomical position
anatomy
cell
cell membrane
chromosomes
cytoplasm
homeostasis
inferior
metabolism
nucleus
physiology
protoplasm
superior
tissue

BASIC PHYSICAL NEEDS

All people have basic human needs that must be met to survive. These needs are divided into two categories:

- Basic psychosocial needs (mind)
- Basic physiological needs (body)

The psychosocial needs have been studied in Chapter 3. In the chapters dealing with the body systems, you will study the physiological needs. In addition to the sections on basic human physiology, systems, and the senses in this and following chapters, also study the color illustrations of these topics presented in each chapter.

- Need for air (oxygen)
- Need for food and fluids
- Need for activity and rest
- Need for protection (shelter)
- Need for elimination of body wastes

During your study of normal body structure and function, you will see how chronic illness, disease, injury, and age-related problems interfere with the resident's ability to meet these basic physical needs.

ANATOMY AND PHYSIOLOGY

As you provide residents with care, you will need to understand the *anatomy* (basic structure) and *physiology* (function) of the body. This knowledge will help you understand why certain kinds of nursing care are necessary.

- **Anatomy** is the study of body parts, how the body is made, and what it is made of.
- **Physiology** is the study of how the body functions and how all the body parts work independently and together.

In the study of anatomy, all terms of reference are made in relation to the **anatomical position** (Figure 5-1). When in the anatomical position, the per-

anatomy study of body parts, how the body is made, and what it is made of

physiology study of how the body functions, how all the body parts work independently and collectively

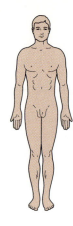

FIGURE 5-1

Anatomical position.

anatomical position
term of reference used when a person is standing facing you, with palms out and feet together

superior   toward the head

inferior   toward the feet

homeostasis   the body's attempt to keep its internal environment stable and in balance

son is standing straight facing you, with palms out and feet together. When you look at a person in the anatomical position, the left side is always on your right side—like looking into a mirror.

Many of the terms used to describe body parts and their relationships are familiar words, but they assume different meanings when used in anatomical description (Figures 5-2 and 5-3). For example, **superior** means toward the head and **inferior** means toward the feet. These terms may also be used to describe the position of an organ in the body. For example, the shoulder is superior to the elbow.

HOMEOSTASIS

The human body is a complex structure. This section provides you with only a basic introduction to the study of anatomy and physiology. A very important concept in the field of physiology is homeostasis. **Homeostasis** is the body's attempt to keep its internal environment stable or in balance.

Examples of the body's ability to maintain homeostasis are:

- The body temperature stays very constant.
- The blood pressure stays within specific limits.
- The chemistry of the blood stays within certain normal limits.

Only when illness, disease, injury, or emotional disturbances occur does this balance of our inner environment change. The body then has a great ability to adapt to overcome these problems.

FIGURE 5-2

Terms that describe where body parts are located.

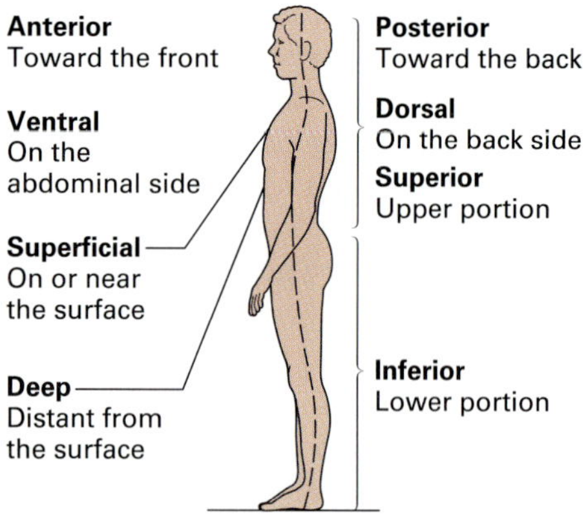

Anterior
Toward the front

Ventral
On the abdominal side

Superficial
On or near the surface

Deep
Distant from the surface

Posterior
Toward the back

Dorsal
On the back side

Superior
Upper portion

Inferior
Lower portion

FIGURE 5-3

Terms that describe anatomical postures.

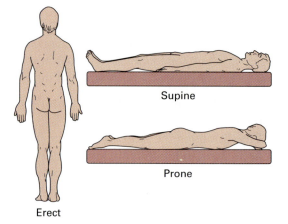

Supine

Prone

Erect

THE CELL

The **cell** is the fundamental building block of all living organisms (Figure 5-4). Cells are so small they can be seen only through a microscope. The human body is made up of about 100 trillion cells. There are many different kinds of cells and each has a special function. Living cells have many things in common. Cells:

- Come from preexisting cells
- Use food for energy
- Use oxygen to break down food
- Use water to transport various substances
- Grow and repair themselves
- Reproduce themselves
- Die

Cells are made of **protoplasm,** the basic substance of life. The cell consists of three main parts:

- **Nucleus**—directs the activities of the cell, like a command center. The nucleus directs the growth of the cell and cell division. Cells also contain **chromosomes,** threadlike structures that carry the genetic material.
- **Cytoplasm**—the protoplasm *outside* the nucleus. It contains structures that have specialized functions in performing the work of the cell (work center of the cell).
- **Cell membrane**—the rim or edge of the cell. It keeps the protoplasm in but allows certain other materials to pass in and out of the cell.

All living cells carry out complex processes that use oxygen and give off carbon dioxide. These processes are called **metabolism,** or the work of the cell.

Cells are constantly dying; therefore, they must reproduce themselves. Cells reproduce by dividing. Cell division simply means that the cell splits into two parts, each exactly like the other. Then these two parts divide again and again.

Currently, there is a great deal of research involving the cell and its environment. Because the cell is considered the building block of all living matter, scientists are constantly searching for new knowledge that can lead to cures for diseases such as cancer, muscular dystrophy, and leukemia.

TISSUE

Cells usually do not work alone but are organized together into tissue. **Tissue** is a group of the same type of cells functioning in the same way. The types of body tissue are grouped into five distinct categories (Figure 5-5):

- Epithelial
- Connective
- Nervous
- Blood and lymph
- Muscular

Tissues do not work alone, they combine to form organs (Figure 5-6). An organ is a body part where two or more tissues work together to perform a particular function. Examples of important organs and their location within the body are shown in Figures 5-7 and 5-8.

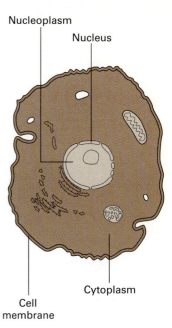

FIGURE 5-4

Structure of the cell.

cell the fundamental building block of all living organisms

protoplasm essential living matter of all animal and plant cells

nucleus part of the cell that directs growth of the cell and cell division

chromosomes threadlike structures that carry genetic material

cytoplasm material surrounding the nucleus of a cell

cell membrane rim or edge of the cell

metabolism complex processes of the living cells in which oxygen is used and carbon dioxide is given off (called the work of the cell)

tissue group of the same type of cells functioning in the same way

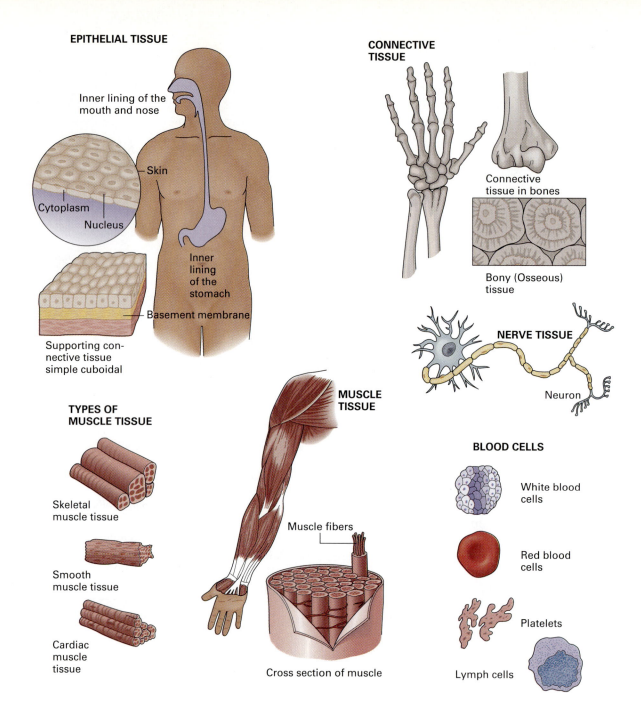

EPITHELIAL TISSUE

Inner lining of the mouth and nose

Skin

Cytoplasm

Nucleus

Inner lining of the stomach

Basement membrane

Supporting connective tissue simple cuboidal

CONNECTIVE TISSUE

Connective tissue in bones

Bony (Osseous) tissue

NERVE TISSUE

Neuron

TYPES OF MUSCLE TISSUE

Skeletal muscle tissue

Smooth muscle tissue

Cardiac muscle tissue

MUSCLE TISSUE

Muscle fibers

Cross section of muscle

BLOOD CELLS

White blood cells

Red blood cells

Platelets

Lymph cells

FIGURE 5-5

Types of body tissues.

SYSTEMS

Organs do not function independently either. They work together with other organs to perform a specific function, thereby creating a body system. A system consists of a group of organs that perform the same function (Figure 5-9). The systems of the body are:

- Integumentary
- Digestive
- Skeletal
- Respiratory

- Muscular
- Circulatory
- Nervous

- Endocrine
- Urinary
- Reproductive

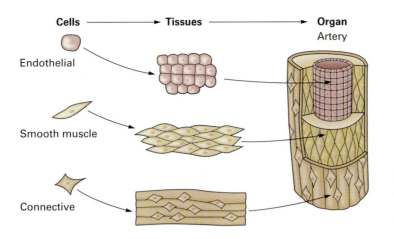

Cells ———→ Tissues ———————→ Organ
Artery

Endothelial

Smooth muscle

Connective

FIGURE 5-6

Cells combine to form tissues, and tissues combine to form organs.

When all the body systems are working normally, a person is *physically well*. As you review each body system, you will study:

- The normal anatomy and physiology of each system
- The common abnormalities associated with each system
- Age- and disuse-related changes associated with each system
- The related nursing measures and skills associated with each body system

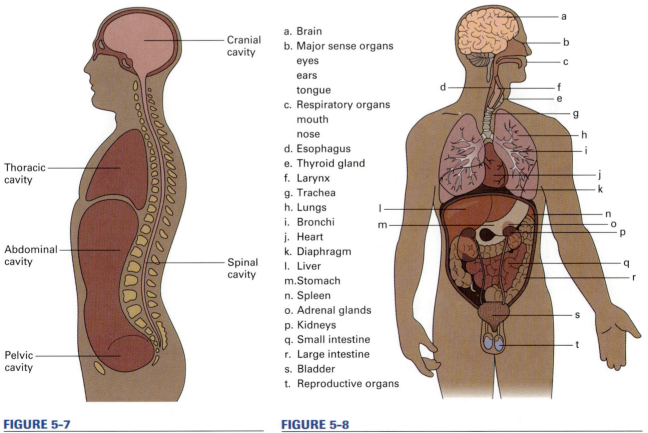

Cranial cavity

Thoracic cavity

Abdominal cavity

Spinal cavity

Pelvic cavity

a. Brain
b. Major sense organs
   eyes
   ears
   tongue
c. Respiratory organs
   mouth
   nose
d. Esophagus
e. Thyroid gland
f. Larynx
g. Trachea
h. Lungs
i. Bronchi
j. Heart
k. Diaphragm
l. Liver
m. Stomach
n. Spleen
o. Adrenal glands
p. Kidneys
q. Small intestine
r. Large intestine
s. Bladder
t. Reproductive organs

FIGURE 5-7

Body cavities.

FIGURE 5-8

Location of important organs.

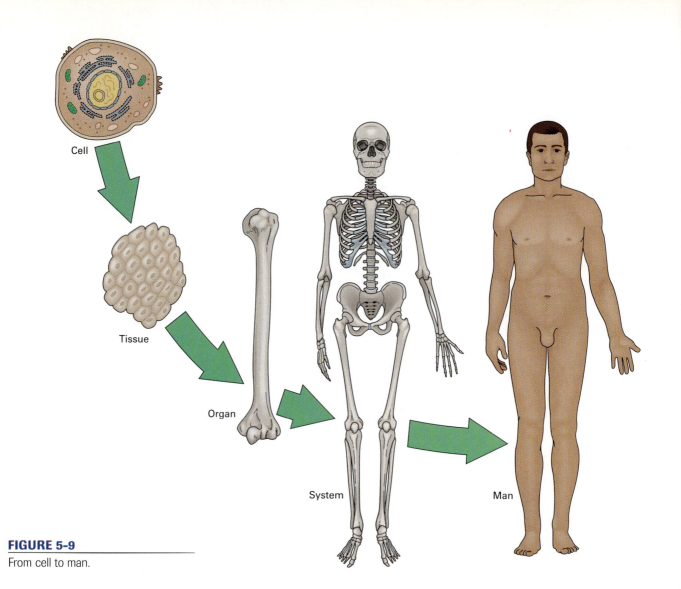

FIGURE 5-9

From cell to man.

Cell

Tissue

Organ

System

Man

SECTION 2 Cancer

OBJECTIVES
What You Will Learn

When you have completed this section, you will be able to:

- Describe the basic mechanisms of cancer
- List cancer's seven warning signals
- Describe the three most common types of cancer and treatment

KEY TERMS

cancer
carcinogens
carcinoma
chemotherapy
control

cure
intramuscularly
intravenously
metastasize
orally

palliation
radiation therapy
rehabilitation
sarcoma
surgery

Cancer is often considered a disease of modern humanity caused by chemical irritants, pollution, and radiation. However, some of the earliest writings refer to the Greek work *kapklvoo,* which means "crab," spreading its pincers throughout the body to choke off life.

Cancer is a form of cellular disorder in which the normal mechanisms of the cell that control the rate of growth, cell division, and movement are disturbed. If you think of the cell as a tiny computer, when cancer invades the cell's normal mechanisms that control rate of growth, cell division and movement are destroyed (Figure 5-10). The American Cancer Society describes cancer as "a group of diseases caused by the runaway growth of useless cells that crowd out tissues needed for essential body functions . . . such as digestion, circulation, motion, excretion, etc."

Research has identified approximately 100 viruses and over 1,000 substances capable of producing cancer in animals when concentrations of these substances are high. There continue to be many advances made in the prevention, diagnosis, treatment, and rehabilitation of cancer victims, yet no "miracle cure" has been discovered.

Cancer cells can originate in any body tissue and grow to invade other tissues, or cancer can **metastasize** (spread) to other parts of the body through blood and lymphatic vessels, where the cancer cells continue to grow to form additional tumors. Tumors that form and are not cancerous are called *benign.* Cancerous tumors are called *malignant.* There are over 250 different kinds of cancer that can occur in different sites in the body (Figure 5-11). The two main types of cancer are:

- **Carcinoma**—found most often in skin and the lining of hollow organs and passageways
- **Sarcoma**—found most often in bone, muscle, cartilage, and lymph systems

Cancer is the second leading cause of death behind heart disease in the United States. Of the 250 million Americans now living, approximately 75 million will develop cancer. Cancer will strike about three of four families.

In 1937, when the National Cancer Institute was founded, only 20 percent of those diagnosed were cured. By 1950 the cure rate had increased to 33 percent. Currently, the cure rate is about 60 percent. Almost two of every three diagnosed will be saved—a more positive outlook than ever before. As the population is aging, the number of people diagnosed is increasing. For 1999, the American Cancer Society predicted 1,221,800 new cases of cancer. Each year, about 563,100 are expected to die from cancer—more than 1,500 per day. One

cancer   form of cellular disorder in which the normal mechanisms of the cell (that control rate of growth, cell division, and movement) are disrupted

metastasize   spread to other parts of the body

carcinoma   a form of cancer found most often in the skin and the lining of hollow organisms and passageways

sarcoma   a form of cancer found most often in bone, muscle, cartilage, and lymph systems

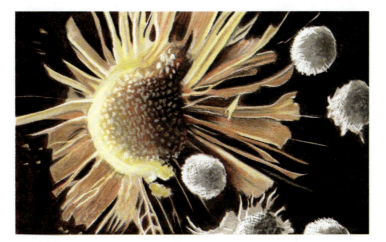

FIGURE 5-10

Cancer cell surrounded by killer T cells. Unregulated cells that avoid detection by T cells cause cancer.

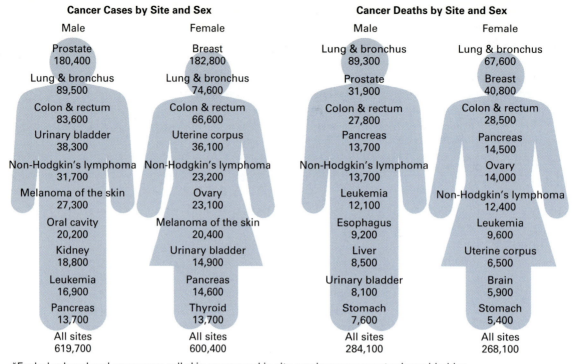

Cancer Cases by Site and Sex

Male	Female
Prostate 180,400	Breast 182,800
Lung & bronchus 89,500	Lung & bronchus 74,600
Colon & rectum 83,600	Colon & rectum 66,600
Urinary bladder 38,300	Uterine corpus 36,100
Non-Hodgkin's lymphoma 31,700	Non-Hodgkin's lymphoma 23,200
Melanoma of the skin 27,300	Ovary 23,100
Oral cavity 20,200	Melanoma of the skin 20,400
Kidney 18,800	Urinary bladder 14,900
Leukemia 16,900	Pancreas 14,600
Pancreas 13,700	Thyroid 13,700
All sites 619,700	All sites 600,400

Cancer Deaths by Site and Sex

Male	Female
Lung & bronchus 89,300	Lung & bronchus 67,600
Prostate 31,900	Breast 40,800
Colon & rectum 27,800	Colon & rectum 28,500
Pancreas 13,700	Pancreas 14,500
Non-Hodgkin's lymphoma 13,700	Ovary 14,000
Leukemia 12,100	Non-Hodgkin's lymphoma 12,400
Esophagus 9,200	Leukemia 9,600
Liver 8,500	Uterine corpus 6,500
Urinary bladder 8,100	Brain 5,900
Stomach 7,600	Stomach 5,400
All sites 284,100	All sites 268,100

*Excludes basal and squamous cell skin cancer and in situ carcinomas except urinary bladder.

© 2000, American Cancer Society, Inc., Surveillance Research

FIGURE 5-11

Leading sites of cancer incidence and death—2000 estimates*.

of four deaths in the United States is from cancer. It is estimated that 160,000 to 170,000 of those cancer patients could have been cured if treated earlier. Early detection and prompt treatment increase the possibility of both control and cure. Annual checkups that include examination of the mouth, breast, rectum, cervix, prostate, and skin are essential to early cancer detection. When people neglect regular physical examinations and wait until symptoms occur, valuable treatment time is lost.

carcinogens substances known to cause cancer

Research has helped to identify **carcinogens** (substances known to cause cancer) (Figure 5-12). Education and control are directed toward either removing carcinogens from the environment or reducing exposure to them; for example, it is well known that overexposure to the sun increases the risk of skin cancer and that cigarette smoking and alcohol consumption increase the risk for a number of different types of cancer. In fact, smokers are 10 times more likely to die of lung cancer than nonsmokers!

Cancer is frequently referred to as a disease of old age—*50 percent of all cancer cases occur after the age of 65.* It is the second leading cause of death in the elderly. Because cancer is so common among the elderly, it is very impor-

Cancer's Seven Warning Signals

- Change in bowel or bladder habits
- A sore that does not heal
- Unusual bleeding or discharge
- Thickening or lump in breast or elsewhere
- Indigestion or difficulty swallowing
- Obvious changes in a wart or a mole
- Nagging cough or hoarseness

tant for all members of the health care team to be aware of cancer's seven warning signals. Being alert and recognizing a problem can make the difference between life and death.

Report any observations of the above to your charge nurse immediately.

Diet is now considered a *suspected* risk factor. Studies suggest that diets high in fat as well as obesity increase the risk of developing cancer.

The American Institute for Cancer Research lists the following dietary guidelines to lower cancer risk:

- Reduce the intake of dietary fat—saturated and unsaturated—from the current average of approximately 40 percent to a level of 30 percent of total calories.
- Increase the consumption of fruits, vegetables, and whole-grain cereals.
- Consume salt-cured, smoked, and charcoal-broiled foods in moderation only.
- Drink alcoholic beverages in moderation only.
- Stop smoking.

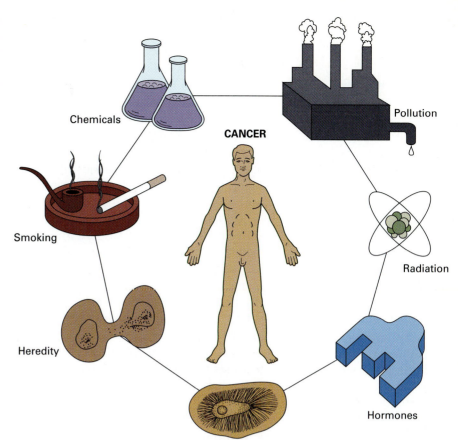

FIGURE 5-12
Possible causes of cancer.

The diagnosis of cancer evokes many negative emotions, including shock, denial, anxiety, and fear. Fear of the unknown, fear of pain, and fear of dying are some of the most commonly expressed concerns. The diagnosis of cancer has a tremendous impact on all aspects of a resident's life as well as on those family members and friends who are in regular contact. There are many agencies that can provide support to residents and families during this difficult period.

The Cancer Information Service (CIS) is a toll-free telephone inquiry network funded by the National Cancer Institute, Bethesda, Maryland 20205. It is affiliated with state divisions of the American Cancer Society. It is an important resource available to everyone. Specially trained volunteers and professionals are available to answer questions. Call (800) 638-6694. Each state has local numbers that can be obtained from the national center.

Once cancer is diagnosed, treatment is generally directed toward:

- **Cure**—to correct or remove a problem
- **Control**—to stop or limit growth
- **Palliation**—to relieve symptoms
- **Rehabilitation**—to restore or return function

Cure is most often achieved by **surgery** that removes the cancerous tissue by means of an operation. The use of radiation and chemotherapy are the second and third most commonly used forms of treatment.

cure   correction or removal of a problem

control   to stop or limit growth

palliation   to relieve symptoms

rehabilitation   the restoration of the individual to the fullest physical, mental, social, vocational, and economic capacity of which he or she is capable

surgery   a process of removing or cutting out tissue from the body

radiation therapy use of high-energy rays to stop cancer cells from growing and multiplying

In the LTC facility, you will see residents who have already experienced one or more of the above treatments and, in some cases, are currently receiving either radiation therapy or chemotherapy on an outpatient basis through an acute care hospital or oncology center (treatment center for cancer patients).

Radiation therapy is the use of high-energy rays to stop cancer cells from growing and multiplying. Radiation destroys the ability of *all* cells, both cancerous and normal, to grow and reproduce. Radiation therapy may be either external or internal. In external therapy, the most common type of treatment, a machine beams high-energy rays toward the cancer site. The treatment itself is painless, but unpleasant side effects frequently result. With internal radiation therapy, a very small amount of radioactive material is placed inside the body and left for a short time period. This type of therapy is carried out in the acute care hospital.

Radiation is sometimes used alone to destroy cancer and sometimes used with chemotherapy and surgery. Radiation is an aggressive form of cancer treatment and will often affect normal tissues, causing side effects. The side effects vary according to the extent of the cancer, the amount of radiation given, the part of the body being treated, and the individual resident's response. There are a number of nursing measures to help the resident receiving radiation therapy to tolerate the treatments better. Review these nursing measures carefully in the next section.

chemotherapy use of drugs or medications to treat disease

Chemotherapy refers to the use of drugs or medications to treat disease. It comes from combining the two words *chemical* and *treatment.* Chemotherapy may be given:

orally taken by mouth

intramuscularly injection into muscle

intravenously injection into the vein

- **Orally** (taken by mouth)
- **Intramuscularly** (injection into muscle)
- **Intravenously** (injection into the vein)

These medications enter the bloodstream and are distributed to all parts of the body. The medication acts to interfere with the duplication and growth of the rapidly multiplying cancer cells. Unfortunately, anticancer drugs also affect normal cells, especially those that normally divide rapidly, like those of the bone marrow and gastrointestinal tract. However, these normal cells have the ability to regenerate and usually repair themselves.

Anticancer drugs produce side effects in some but not all people. Each drug may react differently in different people. Generally, chemotherapy drugs affect:

- Gastrointestinal tract
- Mouth
- Bone marrow
- Hair
- Skin
- Reproductive system (ovaries and testes)
- Urinary tract
- Emotional state

There are a number of nursing measures to help reduce the side effects of chemotherapy, which will be explained in the next section. After finishing a treatment program of either surgery, radiation, chemotherapy, or some combination of these, the patient waits and hopes for control or cure. Many are optimistic and are able to move positively toward any necessary rehabilitation and a return to normal life. Others face recurrence of the disease accompanied by emotional trauma and disappointment. Even those who have experienced cure or control live with the fear that the disease will recur. One patient stated, "It's like living on top of a powder keg, a time bomb. You don't know when it's going to go off and destroy you!"

For those residents or patients whose cancer has reached an uncontrollable state, the goals of treatment change from cure and control to palliation.

Palliative measures are used to reduce pain and discomfort. Pain control and symptom management are the primary focus of care.

Treatment must not only be directed toward destroying cancerous cells; it must also take into consideration the emotional and psychosocial needs of each resident. Family members and friends must be assisted and given support to help them deal with the shock, fear, anxiety, frustration, and role changes they face when a loved one has cancer. The trauma to a family can be tremendous and the responsibilities overwhelming.

Section 3 Care of the Resident with Cancer

OBJECTIVES
What You Will Learn

When you have completed this section, you will be able to:

- List four common side effects associated with radiation and chemotherapy

- List two specific nursing measures that can help reduce side effects or complications

- Describe ways you would like others to provide you with emotional support if you were a cancer victim

KEY TERMS

alopecia

apathy

CANCER TREATMENT

Cancer treatment can extend over weeks and months. Some residents continue to take chemotherapy or hormones for years to prevent recurrence of the cancer. The treatments have side effects that are sometimes more unpleasant than the symptoms caused by the cancer. The following guidelines will help you provide better nursing care to the resident receiving radiation or chemotherapy:

- *Fatigue*—Residents easily become tired because the body uses a good deal of its energy to fight the cancer and to rebuild injured cells. Allow residents time for rest and recognize their limitations. Help them understand why they feel so tired.

- *Loss of appetite leading to malnutrition*—Nausea and vomiting are frequently associated with chemotherapy. Loss of appetite is common. It is especially important for residents to maintain good nutrition because the body needs wholesome food to restore its strength and to rebuild and repair injured cells.

  The following tips can help the resident maintain good nutrition:
  —Provide food whenever they feel hungry, even if it is not mealtime.
  —Encourage smaller meals more frequently, offering fluids 1 hour before meals rather than with meals.
  —Have nutritious snacks available: cottage cheese, juice, milk. Discourage sweets and fatty foods.
  —Create a pleasant mealtime atmosphere to make it a positive experience.
  —If odor of hot foods increases nausea, provide cold substitutions.
  Encourage the resident to chew food well so that it is easily digested. Instruct the resident not to lie down flat for 2 hours after eating. Food is

digested easier if the resident is not supine and if activities are limited. Notify the charge nurse so that medications prescribed to reduce nausea and vomiting can be given promptly.

- *Skin effects*—Sometimes the skin may begin to look reddened or irritated or even burned during radiation therapy. A variety of rashes and itching can develop during chemotherapy:

  —Keep skin clean.

  —Avoid any type of irritation, pressure, or injury to the skin.

  —Avoid use of scented or perfumed lotions or powders.

  —Report rashes, irritation, or broken areas to the charge nurse immediately.

- *Mouth effects*—Some anticancer drugs can cause the mouth and throat to be dry and sore. Radiation therapy to the head and neck can cause difficulty swallowing and chewing. The following tips should increase the patient's comfort:

  —Cut food into small pieces or if necessary mechanically alter the diet so that it is tolerated by the resident.

  —Discourage rough or coarse foods.

  —Encourage plenty of fluids.

  —Keep the mouth very clean, using a soft brush.

  —Avoid use of commercial mouth washes that contain alcohol and are drying to the mucous membranes of the mouth.

- *Hair effects*—The hair follicles of the scalp, beard, eyebrows, eyelashes, armpits, and pubic areas are very sensitive to some of the anticancer drugs and radiation therapy, resulting in loss of scalp and body hair. This side effect is called **alopecia.**

  alopecia loss of scalp and body hair

  This is particularly disturbing because it changes the body image of the resident. Once treatments are finished, the hair generally grows back, but in the meantime help the resident to select some form of head covering, such as a wig, scarf, turban, or hat. Some residents prefer to cut their hair or shave their hair rather than watch it fall out in clumps every day. Some friends and family members have been known to shave their heads too in a gesture of love and support.

- *Emotional effects*—Having cancer and receiving treatments is a very stressful experience. The side effects of therapy can be very distressing, and many residents have difficulty accepting them. They find it hard to believe they are "getting better" when they feel so ill. Some emotional changes are directly related to the drug therapy—feelings of depression, fear, anger, and even **apathy** (not caring) are common.

  apathy lack of feeling or interest in things

There are other side effects that should be observed for and reported at once:

- Fever
- Sudden weight loss or gain
- Bleeding or hemorrhage
- Changes in vital signs
- Intense or severe pain
- Changes in behavior
- Severe constipation or diarrhea

One of the most important aspects of providing care is to be sensitive to the emotional needs of the cancer resident and the family and friends (Figure

5-13). You must allow them to express their feelings and fears. It is not appropriate to give false cheer and try to lift the resident's spirits; this merely keeps the residents from being able to express what they really feel. Listening, sharing, being yourself is the best you can offer. There is no "right thing" to say or do in most cases. Just being there and conveying to the resident "I care" may be enough.

There are always ways to find hope during difficult times. Even if the future is uncertain, there may be remissions or periods of control. There can still be good days, special times, and shared experiences.

The cancer resident needs to stay as involved as possible with responsibilities, diversions, and activities. It seems that cancer patients who have things to do live longer. Help your residents engage in useful and meaningful activities.

Caring for the resident who has cancer requires an understanding of the nature of the disease and its side effects and, most important, an understanding of the unique individual who is experiencing the disease. There are a number of excellent references and resource groups that will assist you in expanding your knowledge and understanding.

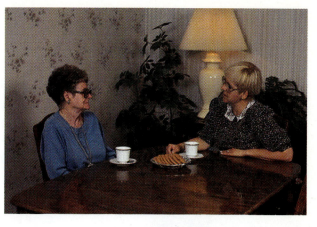

FIGURE 5-13
Being sensitive to the emotional needs of the cancer resident.

Section 4 The Senses

OBJECTIVES
What You Will Learn

When you have completed this section, you will be able to:

- Match three types of visual disturbance with their descriptions
- Identify age-related changes in the sense of taste
- Describe how loss of sensation of temperature and pain can pose a hazard to the safety of the resident

KEY TERMS

cataract
glaucoma

olfaction
presbyopia
sensory neurons

stimuli
tympanic membrane

SENSORY SYSTEM

The sensory system (Figure 5-14) consists of:

- Eyes
- Ears
- Nose
- Tongue
- Skin

The functions of the sensory system are:

- Vision
- Hearing
- Balance
- Smell
- Taste
- Touch

Through the actions of specialized cells called **sensory neurons,** a person is made aware of changes in the outside environment. These changes are re-

sensory neurons specialized type of nerve cell

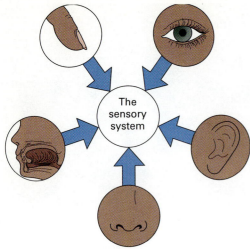

stimuli action or agent that causes a response in an organ or organism

ferred to as **stimuli** (an action or agent that causes a response in an organ or organism).

- Eyes respond to visual stimuli (what you see).
- Ears respond to sound stimuli (what you hear).
- Membranes lining the nose respond to smells.
- Taste buds located chiefly on the tongue respond to bitter, sweet, sour, and salty tastes.
- Skin responds to touch, pressure, heat, cold, and pain.

THE EYE

The eye is similar to a camera. It has a lens, a shutter, and an adjustable opening, as well as light-sensitive film (Figure 5-15). The parts of the eye are as follows:

- *Sclera*—white of the eye
- *Vitreous humor*—transparent liquid that fills the eyeball
- *Aqueous humor*—fluid produced in the eye; fills space between cornea and lens
- *Cornea*—clear plasticlike covering

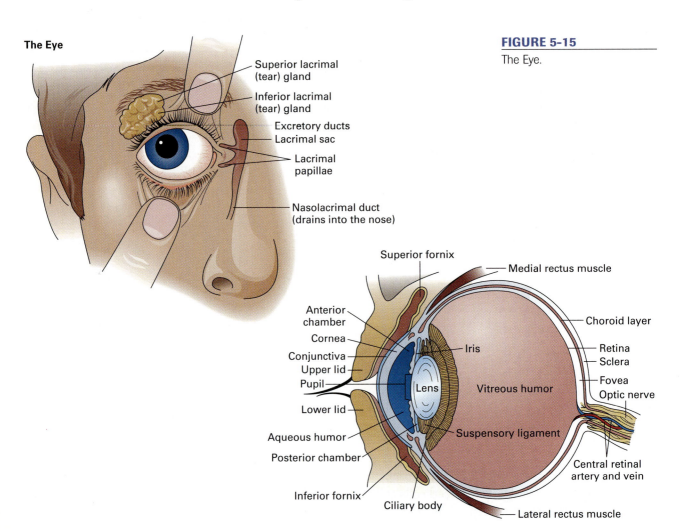

- *Iris*—circle of color
- *Pupil*—the opening in the center of the iris through which light enters
- *Lens*—directly behind the pupil, focuses the image upon the retina
- *Retina*—back part of the eye; receives image and sends impulses to the optic nerve
- *Optic nerve*—receives impulses from the rods and cones in the retina and transmits them to the brain

AGE-RELATED CHANGES AND ABNORMALITIES OF THE EYE

As a person ages, various changes occur and diseases of the eye are common. Generally, there is a decrease in peripheral (side) vision and vision at night. The eye also adjusts more slowly to changes in both light and distance.

Some conditions of the eye include:

- **Presbyopia**—lens of eye loses its ability to focus clearly due to loss of elasticity of the lens. The individual with presbyopia must hold small print at arm's length in order to read. Frequently, eyeglasses will improve vision. If an individual has difficulty seeing at a distance, bifocals (glasses with two different lenses) might be needed.

- **Cataract**—the lens undergoes changes that decreases its transparency. The lens becomes more and more opaque (cloudy) to the point of complete blindness. The only cure for a cataract is surgery. Many recent advances in surgical techniques make this a relatively safe and simple procedure. A person with cataracts may describe his or her vision "like looking through glasses covered with Vaseline." The individual usually experiences sensitivity to bright light and glare.

- **Glaucoma**—occurs when pressure within the eye increases. This pressure can increase to dangerous levels leading to blindness from pressure on the optic nerve. The resident may complain of pain over the eye at night, indicating the pressure is increasing. Glaucoma is usually treated with eye drops. If this therapy fails, a small hole is made surgically to reduce pressure. Glaucoma may be acute, with sudden severe symptoms, or chronic, with slowly developing symptoms. The person may describe "halos" around lights and decreased peripheral and central vision. Such things as physical strain and emotional stress tend to increase the pressure within the eye and to increase the damage done by the pressure.

Loss of vision can affect the resident physically, socially, and emotionally. Simple tasks may become much more difficult. Grooming and hygiene may decline. A woman may apply excessive makeup because she is unable to see the softer or subtle colors. Residents may not see stains on their clothing or may mismatch colors. Activities that the resident enjoyed, such as reading or watching television, may be more difficult or impossible. Residents also need twice as much light to see as they did when in their twenties. Loss of vision increases the risk for falls and accidents leading to bruises, skin tears, and even fractures.

THE EAR

The ear is a special sense organ associated with hearing and equilibrium (balance). The ear has three main parts (Figure 5-16).

presbyopia condition in which the lens of the eye loses its ability to focus clearly due to loss of elasticity

cataract condition in which the lens becomes cloudy to the point of complete blindness

glaucoma increased pressure within the eye that can lead to blindness due to pressure on the optic nerve

The Ear

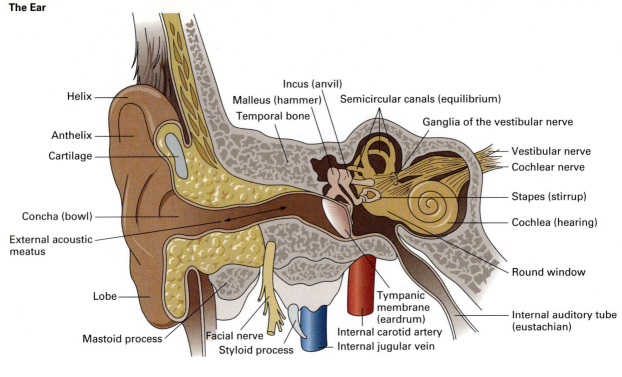

FIGURE 5-16

The ear.

- *Outer ear*—leads to the small sound opening of the middle ear. The small membrane that separates the outer and middle ear is the eardrum.
- *Middle ear*—contains three small bones that serve as a bridge to the inner ear. The middle ear also contains the eustachian tube arising from an area of the throat.
- *Inner ear*—contains canals that hold fluid necessary for maintaining equilibrium or balance. Also within the inner ear are tiny hairlike nerve cells that receive sound and send signals to the brain.

tympanic membrane
thin membrane inside the ear that vibrates when struck by sound waves; the eardrum

Sound waves enter the outer ear and strike the **tympanic membrane** (eardrum), causing it to vibrate. The vibration of the membrane causes the tiny bones of the middle ear to move, carrying the sound to the inner ear. Through a complex process, sound stimuli are transmitted to nerves that transport the signal to the brain.

AGE-RELATED CHANGES AND ABNORMALITIES

Disturbances of any part of the hearing mechanism can lead to partial or complete deafness. Most elderly people experience some hearing loss as a result of the aging process. Ninety percent of the elderly have some hearing loss. A progressive hearing loss of high-pitched sounds is most common. The hearing loss may be compared to a radio that is not quite tuned correctly. There is distortion of sound that is not improved by turning up the volume. Severe loss of hearing can seriously interfere with a person's ability to interact and communicate with others. This loss of socialization can contribute to increased confusion, disruptive behavior, and withdrawal. You have an important nursing responsibility to assist hard-of-hearing residents in all aspects of communication.

SMELL, TASTE, TOUCH

Olfaction or the sense of smell is associated with the special lining of the upper part of the nose. Of all the senses, the sense of smell is the least understood. You can detect, by smell, various substances and can even tell the difference between substances. How this occurs is not known. The sense of smell is often affected when infection of the nasal sinuses occurs. The sense of smell decreases during the aging processes.

Generally, the sense of taste is associated with the tongue. The tongue allows us to tell the difference between sweet, sour, bitter, and salty tastes (Figure 5-17). The taste buds are special sensory nerve cells. There is an important relationship between the sense of taste and the sense of smell. The elderly resident will also experience a decrease in the sense of taste. The taste for sweet and salty seem to decrease first. Residents have a tendency to oversalt their food and prefer to eat very sweet foods. The loss of taste contributes to a loss of appetite, a common problem of residents in LTC facilities.

The skin has special sensory nerve cells that transmit messages to and from the brain allowing us to recognize pressure, heat, cold, pain, and pleasure. The same sensory nerve cells allow us to identify and tell the difference between objects as they are touched.

Frequently, chronically ill or elderly residents will have decreased awareness of touch. They lose the ability to perceive heat and cold as well as pain and pressure. This places them at risk for burns due to water that is too hot and for pressure sores because they may not feel the discomfort that reminds them to change positions. They can also ignore treatment of minor cuts and scrapes because they are not aware that an injury has occurred. The nursing assistant can protect the resident from harm by checking the temperature of bath water carefully and by inspecting the resident's skin at least daily to observe for signs of injury or pressure.

One sensory experience that does not change with age is that of pain. There is a myth that says that the elderly do not feel pain in the same way others do. There is no evidence to support that myth. In fact, research has shown that pain in the elderly is undertreated and that elderly living in nursing homes receive the poorest pain management.

CULTURAL AWARENESS Pain and how it is expressed is an individual matter that is influenced by gender, age, culture, and even by religious beliefs. Although all persons experience pain, they may behave in many different ways. For example, in Asian cultures it is common to be "stoic." People who are stoic do not express their emotions outwardly, especially pain. They act as if they are not in pain at all. In other cultures, it is common to be vocal about pain. The person may moan, cry, or even yell. Because of the difference in how people show their pain, the only way to know how much pain a person is experiencing is to ask him. Pain is becoming an important political issue as the public views relief of pain as a right. In some states, there are initiatives that make the relief of pain their mission. Medical boards and boards of registered nursing have issued position papers making the relief of pain a professional requirement. The fact is that the knowledge and methods exist today that can keep most people comfortable without sacrificing alertness. In California, the legislature passed a law that referred to pain as "the fifth vital sign." Health care professionals in all settings are to make relief of pain a priority. All patients/residents are to be asked about pain just as their temperature, pulse, respirations, and blood pressure are measured on a routine basis.

Pain is defined as "an unpleasant sensory experience associated with actual or potential tissue damage." A more useful definition is "Pain is whatever

olfaction   sense of smell

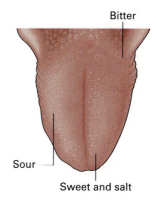

FIGURE 5-17

The tongue.

the experiencing person says it is, existing whenever he says it does." This definition points out that the experience of pain is entirely subjective. We have learned how to talk about pain and how to describe it, but there is no objective measurement. Because of that, the philosophy of care is to believe the resident. Only persons in pain know where their pain is, how much pain they are experiencing, and what their pain feels like.

Pain is part of the body's natural defenses. Experiencing pain tells you that something is wrong. It is often an early symptom of illness, disease, or injury. Usually, if it hurts to perform a certain activity or to move in a certain way, we stop. Sometimes, serious injury is prevented because pain keeps us from going further. Pain often is the reason the medical care is sought. This may make the difference in early diagnosis of serious illness.

The existence of pain that does not go away or pain that is not being treated well has a great impact on quality of life. One model of quality of life says that quality of life has physical, social, spiritual, and emotional aspects. Pain affects the person physically because most people reduce their activity in order to reduce the pain. By limiting movement, the person may become less and less able to function. If the pain is severe, the person may remain at home or may even stay in bed. Staying in bed leads to muscle weakness and loss of strength, risk for pneumonia, pressure ulcers, and stiff and immovable joints. Socially, people in pain may withdraw and lose interest in others. They become more and more focused on themselves and their pain. They may be unable to attend to the needs of others. It is difficult for others to spend time in the presence of a person in pain because they feel helpless and uncomfortable. It is easier to avoid contact. Emotionally, when people have endured pain without relief, they may become discouraged and depressed. People have been known to commit suicide in an effort to end their pain. Spiritually, they may lose their faith in a higher power or faith in the future. They may question their previously held beliefs in a kind and good God. Some may believe they are being punished for their sins or wrongdoing.

SECTION 5 Problems Related to the Sensory System

OBJECTIVES
What You Will Learn

When you have completed this section, you will be able to:

- List four ways the nursing assistant can help prevent sensory deprivation

- Indicate by the "clock" the location of foods on a tray
- Give four nursing approaches that are appropriate when caring for blind residents

- Identify correct statements describing care of the hard-of-hearing resident
- Describe the role of the nursing assistant when the resident is experiencing pain

KEY TERMS

hearing aid

otologist
pain

sensory deprivation
unconscious

SENSORY DEPRIVATION

Under normal circumstances, human beings receive constant stimulation from the world around them. We see, hear, smell, taste, and touch during all of our waking hours. The need for stimulation is as basic as the need for water and food.

Some people experience a loss or lack of stimulation from the environment called **sensory deprivation.** Stories of the isolation of war prisoners or use of brainwashing techniques tell of the effects on the body and mind of sensory deprivation. The person deprived of sensory stimulation experiences tension, anxiety, and an inability to concentrate. Confusion, hostility, and aggression are common. Some individuals withdraw and become depressed.

sensory deprivation loss or lack of stimulation from the environment

One does not have to be in prison to experience deprivation. The same phenomenon can occur in people living in LTC facilities. When a person is blind, she is deprived of visual stimulation. When she is deaf, she is deprived of auditory stimulation. The unconscious resident receives little stimulation other than the touch involved when care is given. Even those who are confused or difficult to get along with can experience sensory deprivation when the staff avoids contact with them.

Good nursing care is designed to provide stimulation of all of the senses (Figure 5-18). Some examples of ways to stimulate the senses are:

- *Sight*—television, movies, pictures on the wall, plants, flowers, mobiles above the bed, bulletin boards with greeting cards, magazines, books, newspapers, outdoor activities, pets (Figure 5-19)
- *Hearing*—radio, television, records and tapes, conversation, outdoor activities, pets
- *Smell*—flowers in the room, using colognes, aftershaves, providing personal cleanliness, the smell of coffee brewing or food cooking, the smell of popcorn (Figure 5-20)
- *Taste*—offering a variety of foods on the menu, serving foods at the proper temperature, offering different kinds of liquids
- *Touch*—gentle touching when care is given, a warm bubble bath, hugs, pats on the shoulders, holding a hand, arts and crafts, touching flowers, animals, or children (Figure 5-21)

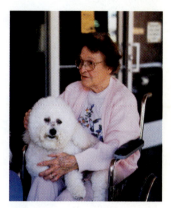

FIGURE 5-18
Stimulate all the senses.

Even the **unconscious** resident, one who is unaware of the surrounding environment, must be provided with sensory stimulation. Because we do not know what is understood by the unconscious person, that person must be treated as if he could understand everything.

unconscious unaware of the surrounding environment

When giving care to these residents, always introduce yourself and explain what you are going to do. If you are working with another staff member, avoid chatting with one another and excluding the resident. Nothing should be said in the presence of the resident that you would not want him or her to hear.

VISUAL IMPAIRMENT

Visual problems are a great threat to the safety and independence of the resident in an LTC facility. About 80 percent of the residents have some type of visual problem. These approaches will help to provide care:

- Identify yourself to the resident, "It's Mary, Mrs. Jones, your nursing assistant."
- Describe what you are doing, "I'm going to roll your bed up for breakfast now."
- Keep the resident's glasses clean.
- Relocate possessions or furnishings only if necessary and tell the resident where you are placing them.

FIGURE 5-19
Sight.

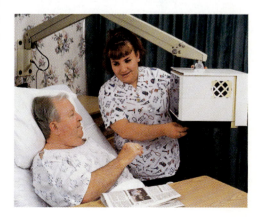

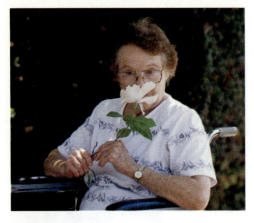

FIGURE 5-20

Smell.

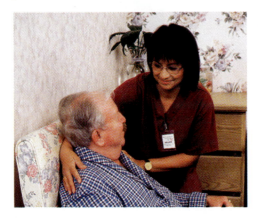

FIGURE 5-21

Touch.

FIGURE 5-22

Use the clock as a reference.

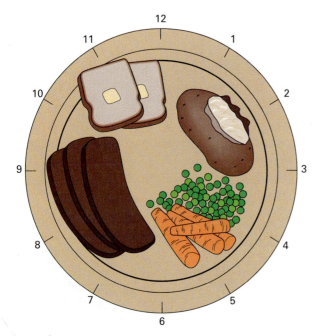

- Describe events occurring or the surroundings in a way that creates a word picture.
- Watch for safety hazards.

All staff members need to help prevent the blind or visually impaired resident from withdrawing and becoming increasingly dependent. Being able to feed oneself is an important activity for every resident, and loss of vision need not change this. When serving the visually impaired resident, describe the various items on the tray by location. One technique often used with the blind is to use a clock as a reference point in describing the location of foods on a plate (Figure 5-22). You may also wish to remove very hot items such as coffee, tea, or soup to be served separately. Sometimes a plate with a lip-guard will assist residents in feeding themselves. Overlook any spills or sloppiness. Give lots of praise for success.

If the blind resident must be fed, be sure to describe the food on the plate as well as the content of each bite. Tell the resident the temperature of the food, too. Determine if the resident prefers to eat all of one food before going on to another or a bite or two of each food. Allow the resident to make as many choices as possible to help him or her feel less dependent, more in control.

When assisting blind residents to ambulate, have them take your arm rather than you taking their arm. Describe where you are going, mentioning obstacles along the way. Most facilities have rooms and bathrooms marked with raised numbers or symbols. Show the resident how to locate these numbers. When staff consistently explain locations of items inside and outside of the room, most residents will be able to function more independently.

Be sure to assist the blind resident with grooming and hygiene. The loss of vision need not make the resident less attractive in appearance. It is up to you to be the eyes of the resident and be sure that her or his appearance is neat, clean, and appropriate.

In a fire or disaster, the blind resident will require your assistance to leave the building. A list of the blind residents is kept at the nursing station, and some type of sign is placed at the bedside. You should be aware of those residents who have visual impairments; but remember, even though many can have the same disability, each is a unique individual with different ways of coping.

HEARING LOSS

Communicating with the hard-of-hearing or deaf resident will be more effective if you follow these guidelines:

- Always face the person when speaking (this provides visual cues and increases understanding).
- Do not cover your mouth with your hand.
- Touch the person to gain his or her attention.
- Speak slowly and clearly, but do not pronounce words unnaturally (avoid overarticulating or mumbling).

- If you are not understood, find new words to say the same thing rather than repeating the same words at a higher volume.
- Use gestures and body movements to help get your point across.
- Avoid talking while chewing gum or smoking.
- Do not shout. Since the resident hears distorted sounds, making them louder does not make them easier to understand.
- Speak slowly.
- Write hard-to-understand messages on paper or a "magic slate."

There is a tendency to avoid contact with residents who have communication problems because of the difficulty and frustration in communicating. It is very important to make every effort to establish contact. It may take patience, time, and understanding on your part to accomplish good communication with the resident who has a hearing loss, but it is necessary to prevent isolation, withdrawal, and deprivation.

Some types of hearing loss can be improved through use of a **hearing aid** (Figure 5-23). Only an **otologist,** a specialist in hearing, makes this determination. Hearing aids are mechanical devices used to make certain sounds louder. They do not make sound clearer.

When a resident has a hearing aid, you will be responsible to help care for and properly use this expensive device. There are many different devices. Some are very small and are contained entirely within the ear, while others may be part of a pair of eyeglasses. Regardless of the type, remember to:

- Protect the hearing aid from damage. Keep it in a safe place when not in use. Do not drop it or expose it to water.
- Turn off the aid when not in use. Report the need for batteries to the charge nurse.
- Observe for wax buildup and sores in the ears, and report any you see to the charge nurse.
- Keep the earmold clean.
- When talking with the resident, keep background noise to a minimum. It may be helpful to turn off the radio or television or close windows and doors.
- Follow the same principles or guidelines for communicating as you do in communicating with the hard-of-hearing resident.

Residents with hearing aids experience a great deal of distortion of sound in large, noisy groups, and they may avoid such situations or turn off the aid during those times. The resident with a hearing loss must be identified, just as the blind person is. In the event of fire or disaster, the deaf resident will need special assistance to leave the building safely. There is usually a list of hard-of-hearing residents at the nursing station. The resident's room or bed may also be identified with a sign or symbol.

CARE OF THE RESIDENT WITH PAIN

The nursing assistant can play a valuable role when a resident has **pain.** It is important to re-

hearing aid   a mechanical device used to make certain sounds louder

otologist   a specialist in hearing

pain   an unpleasant sensory experience caused by actual or potential tissue damage

FIGURE 5-23

Hearing aid.

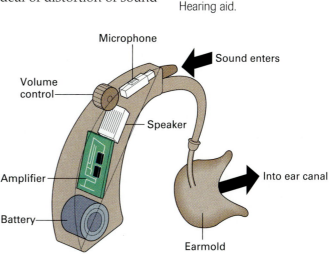

Microphone

Sound enters

Volume control

Speaker

Amplifier

Into ear canal

Battery

Earmold

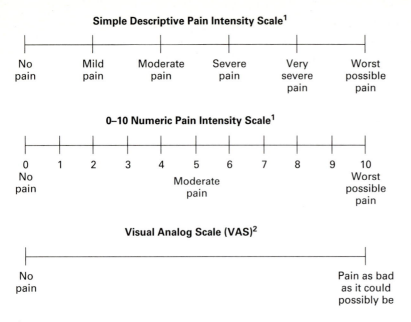

Simple Descriptive Pain Intensity Scale[1]

| No pain | Mild pain | Moderate pain | Severe pain | Very severe pain | Worst possible pain |

0–10 Numeric Pain Intensity Scale[1]

| 0 No pain | 1 | 2 | 3 | 4 | 5 Moderate pain | 6 | 7 | 8 | 9 | 10 Worst possible pain |

Visual Analog Scale (VAS)[2]

No pain ←———————————————————→ Pain as bad as it could possibly be

[1]If used as a graphic rating scale, a 10-cm baseline is recommended.
[2]A 10-cm baseline is recommended for VAS scales.

FIGURE 5-24

Pain Rating Scales.
Source: U.S. Dept. of Health and Human Services, Agency for Health Care Policy and Research, #94-0593. March, 1994.

port and record the pain so that an effort can be made to find the cause. Once the cause is found, treating the cause of the pain may eliminate the pain. For example, a bladder infection may cause pain upon urination, or voiding. Curing the infection with an antibiotic medication will eliminate the pain. When reporting and recoding pain, it is helpful to use the right language. Residents who are able to communicate may be asked to give a rating of their pain (Figure 5-24). On a scale of 0 to 10, with 0 being no pain and 10 being the worst pain you can imagine, how would you rate your pain right now? They also are asked to tell where the pain is and to describe how it feels. Words like *dull, aching, stabbing, piercing, electrical, throbbing,* and *cramping* can help the physician and the nurse identify the type of pain so they can decide how best to treat it. When a resident cannot communicate due to a stroke, dementia, or other conditions, your observations can help recognize pain so that it can be treated. Some residents may cry, moan, or yell when in pain. Some may only make a face or withdraw from touch. You may notice when moving residents that they "stiffen" or "tense up." This may be a sign that they are in pain. Common sense comes into play when observing a resident who can't tell you they hurt; that is, if it hurts in someone who can say it hurts, then it hurts in everyone. Good pain management means that you treat the pain if your good judgment tells you it is probably present. Put yourself in the place of a resident who can't communicate and imagine what it would be like to suffer without any hope that your pain would be treated. Sometimes, the cause of pain cannot be cured and the pain becomes chronic. The word *chronic* refers to how long the pain lasts, not how severe it is. Those with chronic pain can be given medication to control their pain. Sometimes, over-the-counter drugs given on a regular basis are enough to keep the resident comfortable. Remember, pain is the fifth vital sign, so ask about pain—don't wait for the resident to complain. Because you spend so much time with each resident, you will learn to recognize when they are hurting. Be sure to take it seriously and tell the charge nurse.

SUMMARY In this chapter, you have learned the basic ways the body is made and how it works. Knowing what is normal makes it easier to understand the abnormal. The care given to residents is designed to meet the needs created because of their illness or their functional limitations. The more you understand the consequences when the body isn't working as it should, the better grasp you will have of what care should be given.

This chapter has focused on what happens when the sensory system isn't working or when it is impaired. You learned how to care for those who have limited vision and hearing. You learned about pain and the importance of recognizing it and treating it. It should be clear to you now how important you are to the care of the residents. You can make a great difference in the quality of care and quality of life for the residents you care for.

Cancer is primarily a disease of the elderly. The longer one lives, the greater the chance of having cancer. Many of your residents will have cancer or will have had it in the past. You now know what their needs are and how you can give them the best care. Hopefully, by learning risk factors and warning signs, you can take actions to improve your own health.

OBRA HIGHLIGHTS

The OBRA regulations, in addressing quality of care in a nursing facility, emphasize the need to provide all the care and services to help the resident reach or keep the highest level of physical, mental, and psychosocial well-being. One aspect of reaching or keeping the level of well-being is to continue to be as independent as possible in all activities of daily living. One condition that may affect the ability to care for oneself is pain. The regulations address the need for pain relief and control as a way to help residents keep their independence in activities of daily living. The regulations also mention the importance of maintaining both vision and hearing abilities. The facility is responsible for helping the resident obtain and use any assistive devices like eyeglasses or hearing aids. Your responsibility as a nursing assistant is to observe the resident's problems and needs related to pain, vision, and hearing; to report to the proper staff member; and to care for residents and for their assistive devices as you have learned in this chapter.

Choose the best answer for each question or statement.

1. Mr. Johnson is resting in the anatomical position. Which of the following is true about his left side?
   a. As you face him, his left side is on your right side, just like looking into a mirror.
   b. As you face him, his left side is on your left side, so you won't be confused.
   c. As you face him, his left side is against the bed and his right side is up.
   d. As you face him, his left side is up and his right side is against the bed.

2. Which of the following is an example of the body's ability to maintain homeostasis?
   a. The body temperature varies widely with the environmental temperature.
   b. The blood pressure varies widely depending on the body's position.
   c. The blood chemistry stays within certain normal limits.
   d. The body becomes overwhelmed by illness or disease.

3. When a cell uses oxygen and gives off carbon dioxide while carrying out complex processes, this is called
   a. cytoplasm
   b. metabolism
   c. homeostasis
   d. protoplasm

4. Which of the following is not a category of body tissue?
   a. nervous
   b. muscular
   c. blood and lymph
   d. bones

5. Which of the following would be considered an organ?
   a. big toe
   b. right arm
   c. heart
   d. skull

6. When organs work together with other organs, they form which of the following?
   a. a system
   b. a type of tissue
   c. a body
   d. any of the above

7. Which of the following is located inferior to the knee?
   a. ankle
   b. hip
   c. elbow
   d. waist

8. The three main parts of the cell are the
   a. heart, cytoplasm, and nucleus
   b. cytoplasm, cell membrane, and nucleus
   c. cell membrane, protoplasm, and brain
   d. chromosomes, cell membrane, and brain

9. The lungs are located in which body cavity?
   a. cranial cavity
   b. abdominal cavity
   c. thoracic cavity
   d. pelvic cavity

10. Which of the following is *not* a body system?
    a. digestive
    b. skeletal
    c. circulatory
    d. brain

11. The lens of the eye is normally clear. If it becomes cloudy and less transparent, which of the following eye conditions results?
    a. glaucoma
    b. presbyopia
    c. retinal detachment
    d. cataract

12. When pressure within the eye is higher than normal, which of the following eye conditions results?
    a. glaucoma
    b. presbyopia
    c. retinal detachment
    d. cataract

13. Which of the following is considered the "fifth vital sign"?
    a. vision
    b. hearing
    c. pain
    d. touch

Chapter Review

14. Mrs. Joseph is complaining of arm pain. Which of the following would you report to your charge nurse?
    a. "She rates her left arm pain as a 7 on a 1 to 10 scale."
    b. "She says her arm hurts."
    c. "She says her arm hurts but she was using it during her shower."
    d. "She says her arm hurts. It's probably because she went to physical therapy."

15. Which of the following is *not* a way to prevent sensory deprivation?
    a. hanging pictures and mobiles in the room
    b. offering different kinds of foods and liquids

    c. holding the resident's hand
    d. keeping silent while caring for an unconscious resident

16. When you communicate with a resident who is hard of hearing, which of the following actions should you take?
    a. Speak loudly and carefully, saying each syllable of the word slowly.
    b. If you are not understood, find new words to say the same thing.
    c. If you are not understood, repeat the same words at a higher volume.
    d. Shout when you need to be heard over background noises.

Getting C O N N E C T E D
Multimedia Extension Activities

 www.prenhall.com/will-black

Use the above address to access the free, interactive Companion Website created for this textbook. Hear the pronunciation of the key terms in the chapter. Get instant feedback to a variety of chapter-related questions. Link to other interesting sites.

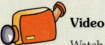 **Video**

Watch the "Anatomy" section of the video *Body Mechanics* from the Care Provider Skills series.

CASE STUDY

Miss Jackson is 74 years old. She is living in the facility since she never married and had no other family. She has had some strokes that left her paralyzed on her left side. She is able to communicate. She remembers the names of the staff, although at times she doesn't know the date. A year ago she had treatment for breast cancer that included removing the lump (tumor) and radiation.

1. You notice that she has what looks like a sunburn on her breast. She says it doesn't hurt. You should
   a. ignore it since there is no pain
   b. notify the charge nurse, it may be a radiation burn
   c. wash the area with soap and water and apply her favorite perfumed lotion
   d. take her to the patio to get some sun on the area

2. She complains of pain in her back. Your best course of action is to
   a. encourage her to attend exercise class to get the "kinks out"
   b. ask her "on a scale of 0 to 10, how bad does it hurt?" Report results to the charge nurse
   c. ignore it—pain at her age is normal
   d. write a note in the chart that her cancer has metastasized to the bone of her spine

3. When providing personal care to Miss Jackson, it is very important to
   a. be gentle in how you lift, move, and position her
   b. scrub the skin thoroughly, particularly around the site of her breast cancer
   c. distract her from her pain by telling her about your family life
   d. treat her just like you treat everyone else

4. Miss Jackson begins spending more and more time in bed. When you touch her, she groans, but when you ask her if she has pain, she says "no." The best action for you is to
   a. take her at her word—she may just be depressed
   b. tell her if she will get up, you will bring her some ice cream after lunch
   c. pay no attention—it is not part of the responsibility of the nursing assistant
   d. discuss the behavior—she appears to be in pain even though she isn't admitting it—with the charge nurse

Chapter 6

THE INTEGUMENTARY SYSTEM

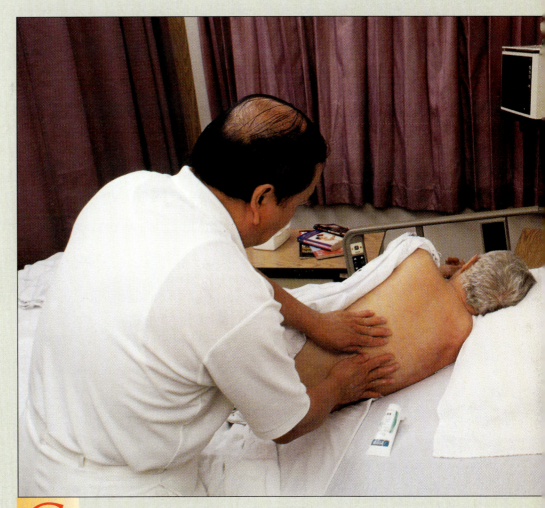

CARING TIP

Bathing is about more than cleaning the skin—it is a time for talking, sharing, observing, and enjoying.

Dr. Anne Woodtli
Professor of Nursing
University of Arizona
Tucson, Arizona

OBJECTIVES
What You Will Learn

When you complete this section, you will be able to:

- List four functions of the integumentary system
- Relate changes in skin condition to possible causes
- Explain how the skin helps to regulate body temperature

KEY TERMS

appendages	dermis	eschar
cyanosis	epidermis	follicles
	erythema	podiatrist

THE SKIN

The integumentary system is composed of:

- Skin
- Hair
- Nails
- Sweat and oil glands

The functions of the integumentary system are to:

- Protect the body
- Improve one's appearance
- Eliminate wastes through the sweat glands
- Regulate body temperature
- Produce vitamin D when exposed to sunlight

The skin, which is the largest organ, covers the entire body and has two layers (Figure 6-1):

epidermis   outer layer of the skin

dermis   second layer of skin

- **Epidermis**—the outer layer of skin (the skin you see)
- **Dermis**—the second layer of skin, which is made up of new cells that replace discarded cells from the epidermis

The epidermis or outer layer of skin is very thin on most parts of the body, with the exception of the palms of the hands and the soles of the feet. Because these areas get the most "wear and tear," the cells there die and rub off constantly, producing dead flaking skin. Within the dermis or second layer of skin, new cells grow to replace the dead ones.

Under the dermis is a fatty tissue. When more food is taken in than is needed, fat is manufactured. Fat is the way the body stores energy until it is needed. Because there are few blood vessels in fatty tissue, the fat acts as insulation for the body, keeping warmth in and cold out. Fat also adds protection or padding to the body.

Because of the skin's protective function, it must be kept clean, dry, and properly lubricated. Moisture on the skin picks up dust and particles from the air, which creates an environment where bacteria can grow. Moisture also causes chafing, excoriation, rashes, and lesions, leading to skin breakdown and infection. Injuries to the skin destroy its protective nature and provide openings for disease-producing organisms to enter the body.

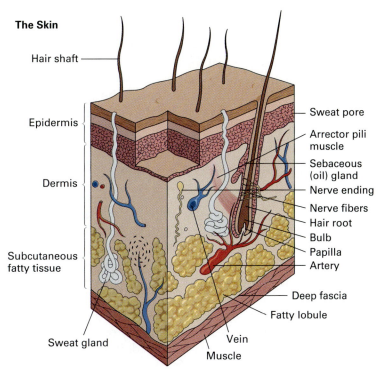

The Skin

Hair shaft

Epidermis

Dermis

Subcutaneous
fatty tissue

Sweat gland

Sweat pore

Arrector pili
muscle

Sebaceous
(oil) gland

Nerve ending

Nerve fibers

Hair root

Bulb

Papilla

Artery

Deep fascia

Fatty lobule

Vein

Muscle

FIGURE 6-1

The skin.

Oil glands in the skin keep it lubricated, soft, and flexible, and they also supply the hair **follicles** (roots) with oil. The skin has a role in the production of vitamin D when exposed to sunlight. Vitamin D produces calcium and plays a role in potassium metabolism.

The skin helps to eliminate certain body wastes. Perspiration is released from the body through sweat glands, which are distributed over the entire skin surface. Water and salts are excreted through the sweat glands.

Body temperature is controlled by the skin. The skin helps reduce body temperature when blood vessels near the surface of the skin dilate (become larger). This brings more body heat to the skin surface. There, the heat is lost through exposure to the cooler air. Even more important, the evaporation of perspiration carries heat away from the skin.

When the body needs to increase its temperature in order to stay warm, perspiration stops. Blood vessels near the surface contract (become smaller). This decreases the heat brought to the surface of the skin, and the skin temperature falls. When we feel too cold, we begin to shiver. This creates warmth due to muscle activity.

The *homeostatic* or balance mechanism is important in keeping body temperature the same most of the time. Only when illness or injury occurs does the body temperature exceed its normal limits.

The hair and nails are **appendages** or attachments of the skin. Fingernails and toenails grow from nailbeds. Some illnesses, diseases, drugs, and injuries affect the growth and condition of hair and nails.

CULTURAL AWARENESS There are many differences in the skin based on race, ethnicity, lifestyle, and age. Some of the differences are in the shade or color of the skin, while others are in the texture. The best way to observe for injury such as bruising, swelling, "redness," or other signs is to compare one area of the body with another. For example, black skin may simply appear darker than the surrounding skin or the skin on the opposite side of the body. If you are unsure of what you are seeing, ask the

follicles roots of the hair

appendages attachments of the skin

resident or other staff members to confirm your observations. Because of the different textures of skin, some residents may have special products that they prefer to use on their skin. Ask them and make every effort to follow their requests. Some cultures—Cambodian, Vietnamese, and some Chinese, for example—practice a healing method knowns as "coining" or "coin rubbing." Coining may leave red and blue marks on the skin that would make you suspect abuse. Be sure you are aware of the cultural practices before you jump to conclusions.

AGE-RELATED CHANGES

Age-related changes in the integumentary system can be seen easily. The skin loses elasticity and becomes dry, wrinkled, thin, and easily damaged. The skin becomes so thin that it almost feels like tissue paper. This fragile skin tears and scrapes easily, which can lead to infection. Because of this, the nursing assistant must be very gentle when lifting, moving, positioning, and bathing elderly residents. Remember to use a transfer belt in order to decrease the risk of injury.

There may be brown spots on the skin, particularly on the hands and arms. The hair usually becomes sparse and gray or white. Fingernails and toenails thicken and become abnormally shaped. It is frequently necessary to have a **podiatrist** (foot specialist) care for the toenails of the elderly. Just as you observe the skin for changes, it is also important to observe and report changes in the fingernails and toenails that may indicate a problem (complaints of pain, redness, drainage, or swelling).

Some women experience growth of hair on the face, especially around the mouth and chin. These residents may require special personal care for the removal of facial hair.

Most elderly residents experience loss of the fat under the skin. They lose the comfort from the padding provided by the fat and may become uncomfortable sitting or lying on hard surfaces. Because of the loss of insulation, they often complain of feeling cold even when the room temperature seems fine or even warm to others. For this reason, you must take special care to keep elderly residents warmly dressed or well-covered when giving nursing care.

The protective function of the skin is *very important* in the prevention of disease and infection. Therefore, some of your responsibilities as a nursing assistant are to:

- Keep the resident's skin clean and dry.
- Protect the residents from injury to the skin.
- Report *any* changes in skin condition or color to your charge nurse immediately:
  —Redness of the skin **(erythema)** can mean increased body temperature, prolonged pressure, infection, or injury.
  —A blue or gray color **(cyanosis)** can mean decreased circulation, a life-threatening problem.
  —A black or "scablike" skin area can mean **eschar,** disguising a more serious skin problem underneath. A scab does not necessarily mean a wound is healing well.
  —A very pale or white color can mean circulatory problems related to shock.

Accurate observation and reporting of the resident's skin color and condition are of life and death importance!

podiatrist   a physician who specializes in treating the feet

erythema   redness of the skin

cyanosis   blue or gray color of the skin, lips, and nailbeds, indicating lack of oxygen

eschar   a slough produced after an injury (often called a scab)

SECTION 2 Pressure Ulcers

OBJECTIVES
What You Will Learn

When you have completed this section, you will be able to:

- List the three causes of pressure ulcers

- Identify the sites on the body where pressure ulcers are most likely to occur
- Select those conditions that increase the risk of developing a pressure ulcer

- List five ways the nursing assistant can prevent pressure ulcers from occurring
- Describe correct usage of two pressure ulcer prevention devices

KEY TERMS
anemia

debridement
hydrated

pressure ulcers
shearing

EFFECTS OF IMMOBILITY ON THE SKIN

Immobility can cause serious changes in the skin. The most important is development of **pressure ulcers,** often called decubitus ulcers or bed sores. Pressure on an area of skin prevents the flow of blood, resulting in tissue that dies from lack of oxygen and other necessary nutrients. The dead tissue comes off, leaving an open, painful sore that provides a way for microorganisms to enter the body, causing infection.

The areas most likely to break down are those parts of the body where little fat exists between the skin and the bone. Examples are the back of the head, rim of the ears, shoulder blades, spine (especially the coccyx or tailbone), shoulders, elbows, hips, knees, ankles, heels, and toes (Figure 6-2).

The residents most likely to develop pressure sores are those who are unable or unwilling to move.

Residents may be unable to move because of:

- *Paralysis*—due to stroke, spinal injury, or disease
- *Weakness*—may be very frail, ill, or anemic
- *Coma*—illness or injury resulting in unconsciousness

Residents may be unwilling to move because of:

- *Pain*—it hurts to move, as with arthritis
- *Depression*—may have "given up"
- *Disorientation*—not aware of the consequences of remaining in one position

pressure ulcers an inflammation, sore, or ulcer in the skin over a bony prominence caused by shearing or pressure

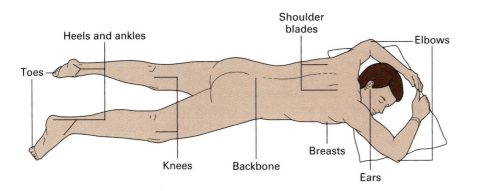

FIGURE 6-2
Pressure points.

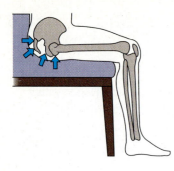

FIGURE 6-3

Pressure from the ischial bones and sacrum with the resident in the sitting position.

shearing   force that occurs when skin moves one way while bone and tissue under the skin move another way

anemia   insufficient supply of red blood cells

Residents who spend a lot of time sitting may also experience skin breakdown in the center of the buttocks due to pressure from the ischial bones and sacrum (Figure 6-3). Those who remain on their abdomen (prone) for long periods of time often develop pressure ulcers on their cheeks, ears, ribs, collarbones, breasts, genitalia, knees, and toes.

Although *intense* pressure can cause death of tissue after only 90 minutes, it usually takes 6 to 8 hours to occur.

Skin breakdown can also be caused by a force called **shearing.** Shearing takes place when the skin moves one way while the bone and tissue under the skin move another way (Figure 6-4). This pinches the tiny blood vessels and cuts off the supply of oxygen and other nutrients, leading to tissue death. An example of shearing force can be seen when a resident slides down in bed or a wheelchair. The nursing assistant can cause shearing by pulling a sheet from under the resident. If the sheet is wet, the damage increases. This is why the resident should be *rolled* from side to side to remove linens from underneath or assisted to stand if in a wheelchair. The fragile skin of the elderly is highly susceptible to shearing.

In addition to pressure and shearing, moisture is the greatest contributor to skin breakdown. Moisture on the skin from saliva, perspiration, urine, or feces reacts chemically with the skin, leading to redness, irritation, and damage.

RISK FACTORS FOR SKIN BREAKDOWN

Some residents have a higher risk of developing a pressure ulcer than others. In addition to those unable or unwilling to move, high-risk residents include those who are underweight or overweight and those with **anemia** (usually not enough red blood cells), diabetes, or poor circulation. Also at risk are residents in casts, braces, or splints. It is important for you to be able to recognize which residents are most likely to experience skin breakdown. Then you can take extra precautions to prevent breakdown.

Now that you know why a pressure ulcer develops, let's examine what happens if nothing is done to prevent or treat it. You've probably heard the expression "an ounce of prevention is worth a pound of cure." In no case is this saying more true than with pressure ulcers. Once an ulcer is allowed to develop, it is very difficult to heal. It is also painful to the resident and requires a great deal of nursing time and energy to heal.

FIGURE 6-4

Shearing of blood vessels due to opposing forces.

STAGES OF DEVELOPMENT FOR PRESSURE ULCERS

Pressure ulcers develop in stages or steps (Figure 6-5). First, the skin becomes reddened (or in the case of the dark-skinned resident becomes darker). This redness does not immediately disappear when pressure is relieved. To understand the first-stage development of a pressure sore, hold a clear drinking glass tightly in your hand. Notice that your fingers become pale, showing that the supply of blood has been cut off. Let go and note how quickly the blood returns to the area. This is the redness seen when there has been pressure on a particular area. You can see another example simply by crossing your knees for a few minutes and then uncrossing them. Observe the skin. You'll see that it is red from the pressure. In both examples, the skin quickly returns to normal. When a resident is developing a pressure sore, the area remains red even after pressure is relieved.

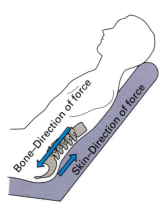

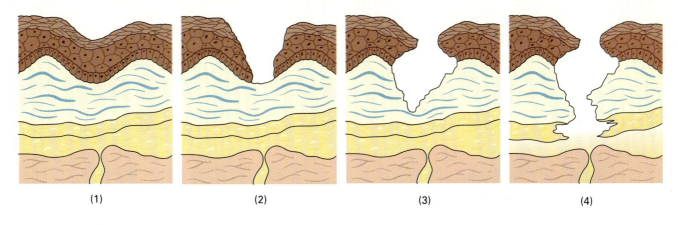

FIGURE 6-5

Stages of pressure ulcer development.

(1)   (2)   (3)   (4)

The reddened area is tender and warm to touch. If nothing is done at this point, the next stage will be development of a blister. The blister then breaks open, leaving an ulcer that may grow in width and depth. Some might even progress through the tissue and muscle to the bone!

Infection is often recognized when foul-smelling drainage is present and the area is reddened and warm. In its most advanced stages, the sore can be covered with eschar. Eschar prevents healing and must be removed with surgical instruments or medication. This process is called **debridement.**

Remember, regardless of the special preventive devices used, *there is no substitute for position changes and avoidance of prolonged pressure!*

debridement removal of dead or unhealthy tissue

PREVENTING PRESSURE ULCERS

Other measures to prevent development of pressure ulcers include keeping the skin clean and dry, providing lotion and gentle massage, and protecting the skin from scratching, rubbing, or other trauma. Gentle massage helps to increase circulation to the area and is an important preventive measure. The bed should be free of wrinkles or objects that could cause irritation. Clothing, shoes, braces, and splints must fit properly so there is no injury or pressure. The resident's nails should also be kept short and smooth to prevent scratching. Carrying out these measures, together with being sure that the resident is adequately nourished and **hydrated** (receives enough liquids), is necessary to prevent the development of pressure sores.

hydrated having enough fluid

Frequent changes of position as well as the use of proper positioning techniques are essential! A dependent resident's position should be changed at least every 2 hours. Residents who are very frail or seriously ill may need to be positioned even more often.

You will use certain devices to help decrease pressure and reduce friction or rubbing. Review Table 6-1 and study the various devices available as well as the purpose of each. Regardless of the devices used, the resident continues to require frequent position changes. Never assume that because special beds or mattresses are in use that you need not reposition the resident.

All measures used to prevent pressure ulcers must be documented or recorded in the resident's health record. There is a saying in health care that "if it isn't documented, it wasn't done." Take credit for your efforts by recording them.

TABLE 6-1 Pressure Sore Prevention Devices

DEVICE	PURPOSE	PRECAUTIONS FOR USE
Fiber-filled mattress overlay 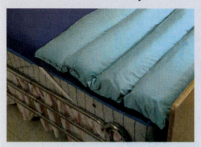	Provides cushioning and a light redistribution of pressure as well as some circulation of air beneath resident.	Not as effective for incontinent patients unless a very thin plastic sleeve covering is used to protect the mattress. The mattress will retain a urine odor unless protected. It is most effective when used with *only one* loosely applied sheet between the resident and the mattress.
Water mattress	Redistributes the body weight during any movement. Conforms to body shape and weight.	Do not puncture. Must not be over- or underfilled.
Air mattress 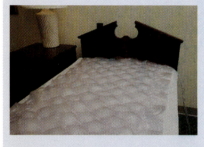	Redistributes pressure on a timed automatic basis.	Be careful not to puncture. Be sure that motor and mattress are working correctly. Use only one loosely applied sheet between the resident and the mattress.
Sheepskin pad 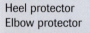	Reduces friction or rubbing against sheets.	*Does not* eliminate pressure.
Heel protector Elbow protector 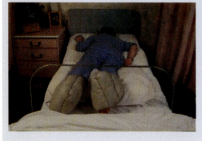	Cushions against trauma. Decreases friction on rubbing against bedclothes.	Must be removed for daily washing of feet/elbows and inspection of skin. Creates warm moist environment favoring growth of bacteria.

TABLE 6-1 Pressure Sore Prevention Devices (continued)

DEVICE	PURPOSE	PRECAUTIONS FOR USE
Foot elevator	Reduces pressure on heels.	Must be properly applied. Check skin for rubbing.
Wheelchair cushion (solid)	Conforms to body when sitting. Provides comfort.	Place properly in chair. Cover with cloth.
Foot cradle (tentlike device attached to the lower third of the bed)	Keeps bed coverings off legs and feet.	Be sure the bed covering is off legs. Residents may feel cold, requiring pajamas, etc., to provide additional warmth.
Air fluidized therapy	Relieves pressure through continuous motion. Resident "floats."	Produces heat in the room; resident needs additional fluids to prevent dehydration. Must use wedges to elevate head.

SECTION 3 Care of the Skin

OBJECTIVES
What You Will Learn

When you have completed this section, you will be able to:

- List three goals of good skin care
- Give four reasons for bathing residents
- Recognize appropriate guidelines for bathing residents
- Give a complete bed bath
- Give a back rub
- Give perineal care
- Give a tub bath
- Give a shower

KEY TERMS

partial bath

perineal

GOALS OF SKIN CARE

Nursing care of the skin is designed to:

- Provide cleanliness
- Prevent injury
- Promote circulation

Cleanliness is maintained by bathing. There are several important reasons for bathing the resident. Bathing removes dirt from the resident's body. It also eliminates body odors and cools and refreshes the resident. A bath stimulates circulation and helps prevent pressure ulcers. Bathing requires movement of certain parts of the body: the resident's legs and arms are lifted, and the head and torso are turned. This activity exercises muscles that might otherwise remain unused. At bath time, the nursing assistant has the opportunity to observe the resident for any unusual body changes, such as skin rashes, pressure ulcers, or reddened areas. Bath time is also an excellent time to communicate with the resident. All measures used to prevent pressure ulcers must be documented or recorded in the resident's health record.

A resident may be bathed in one of four ways, depending on his condition. He may be given a complete bed bath, a partial bath, a tub bath, or a shower. Some areas of the body require a daily bathing to remain clean. These areas include the face, hands, underarms, groin, and areas where body folds and creases exist. When a resident perspires greatly (due to fever) or has lost control of bowel and bladder function, bathing is required more often. This type of bathing is called a **partial bath.**

partial bath bathing of only those areas of the body that require daily bathing to remain clean

The frequency for giving a total bath will vary with the individual resident. The elderly resident usually receives a complete bath at least twice a week. More frequent bathing is likely to cause further drying of the skin. Younger and more active residents may be bathed more often.

perineal in the female, the area between the vagina and the anus; in the male, the area between the scrotum and the anus

When the term *partial bath* is used in an LTC facility, it refers to bathing only part of the body. A partial bath usually includes face, underarms, hands, and perineal area. The **perineal** area in the female is the area between the vagina and the anus. In the male, the perineal area is between the scrotum and the anus. Partial baths are usually given on the days between showers or tub baths and if a resident is very ill or incontinent. When the resident is incontinent, you will always give perineal care.

Record in the chart the type of bath, shower, or skin care given. Include the response of the resident, degree of independence, and any observations you have made.

Although you have learned many tasks that make up care of the resident's skin, it is important not to treat the person as an object and perform these tasks in a mechanical, routine way. Each resident is unique, and the performance of nursing care activities provides an opportunity to establish meaningful contact with the residents. Such care also allows you to experience the rewards that come from helping others.

It is very important to prevent injuries to the resident's skin when you provide care. The smallest bump or scrape may result in severe bruising or skin tears because the skin of the elderly resident is often very fragile. Ways to prevent injuries to the skin include:

- Taking time to protect limbs when transferring and repositioning
- Padding side rails or wheelchair parts
- Transporting carefully in wheelchair to avoid dragging feet and/or bumping arms against door frames, etc.
- Using long-sleeved clothes
- Keeping shoes and socks on
- Using assistance or mechanical lifts to avoid dragging across bed or wheelchair

When skin tears occur, they are often difficult to heal and frequently become a site for infection. Any bruising or skin tear should be reported to the charge nurse immediately.

BATHING A RESIDENT

- Always protect the welfare and safety of the resident. Take all safety precautions to prevent slips and falls (Figure 6-6). *Never* leave a resident unattended in the bath tub or shower!

- Use good body mechanics to protect yourself as well as the resident.

- Rinse the resident carefully. Soap has a drying effect and can cause itching and skin rashes if not rinsed off completely.

- Make bath time a pleasant experience for the resident by:
  —Protecting the privacy of the resident
  —Avoiding exposure or chilling
  —Using comfortably warm water and changing it whenever it becomes soapy, dirty, or cold
  —Talking with the resident so that bath time becomes a social experience

- Always encourage the resident to do as much of the bath as possible.

- Be alert and carefully observe the condition of the resident's skin as you are giving a bath. Report any redness, rashes, broken skin, tender places, or complaints of pain to your charge nurse immediately.

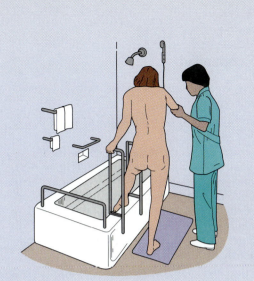

FIGURE 6-6

- If you must transport the resident through the halls for a bath or shower, be sure that she is adequately covered to protect her privacy and to keep her warm. It is a good idea to dress and undress the resident in the shower room.

PROCEDURE

Giving a Complete Bed Bath

Beginning Steps

1. Assemble your equipment on the overbed table:
   - Soap and soap dish
   - Washcloth
   - Wash basin
   - Towels
   - Gloves, if indicated
   - Talcum powder or cornstarch (optional)
   - Clean gown or clothing
   - Bath blanket, if available
   - Orange stick for nail care, if used by your facility
   - Lotion
   - Comb or hairbrush
   - Clean bed linen, stacked on the chair in order of use, if the bed is to be made following the bed bath

2. Wash your hands.
3. Identify the resident.
4. Tell the resident what you are going to do.
5. Provide privacy.

Steps

6. Offer the bedpan or urinal (see Chapter 10).
7. Take the bedspread and regular blanket off the bed.
8. Fold them loosely over the back of the chair, leaving the resident covered with the top sheet or bath blanket, if available.
9. Lower the headrest and kneerest of the bed, if permitted. The resident should be as flat as is comfortable for him and as is permitted.
10. Raise the bed to a comfortable working height with the side rail up on the side opposite from where you are working.
11. Assist the resident to move closer to you so you can work easily without straining your back.

12. Remove the gown, but keep the resident covered to avoid chilling.

13. Fill the wash basin two-thirds full of water at 105° to 110°F (43°C).

14. Put a towel across the resident's chest (Figure 6-7) and make a mitt with the washcloth (Figure 6-8). This prevents flopping edges from dropping across the skin. Wash the eyes from the nose to the outside of the face. Ask if the resident wants soap used on his or her face. Wash the face. Be careful not to get soap in the eyes. Rinse, and dry by patting gently with the bath towel.

15. Place the towel lengthwise under the arm farthest from you. Support the arm with the palm of your hand under the elbow. Then wash the shoulder, axilla (armpit), and arm. Use long, firm, circular strokes. Rinse and dry the area well.

16. Place the basin of water on the towel on the bed. Put the resident's hand into the water. Wash, rinse, and dry the hand well. Place it under the sheet.

17. Wash, rinse, and dry the arm, hand, axilla, and shoulder closest to you in the same way.

18. Clean the fingernails with an orange stick, if used by your facility (Figure 6-9).

19. Fold the sheet down to the resident's abdomen. Wash and rinse the resident's ears, neck, and chest. Take note of the condition of the skin under the female resident's breasts. Dry the area thoroughly.

20. Cover the entire chest with the towel. Fold the sheet down to the pubic area.

21. Wash the resident's abdomen. Be sure to wash the umbilicus (navel) and any creases of the skin. Dry the abdomen. Then pull the sheet up over the abdomen and chest and remove the towel.

22. Empty the dirty water. Rinse the basin and fill it with clean water at 105–110°F (40.5–43°C).

23. Fold the sheet back from the resident's leg farthest from you.

24. Bend the knee, and wash, rinse, and dry the leg and foot. Hold the heel for more support when flexing the knee. If the resident can easily bend the knee, put the wash basin on the towel. Then put the foot directly into the basin to wash it (Figure 6-10).

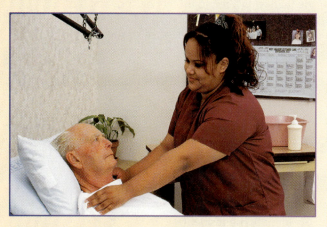

FIGURE 6-7
Put a towel across the chest.

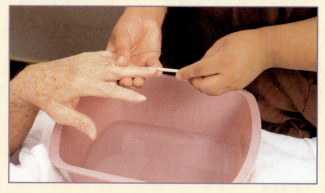

FIGURE 6-9
Cleaning the fingernails with an orangewood stick.

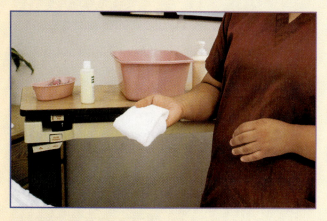

FIGURE 6-8
Make a mitt with the washcloth.

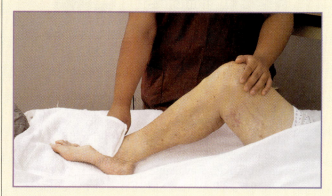

FIGURE 6-10
Bend the knee and wash, rinse, and dry the leg and foot.

PROCEDURE

continued

25. Observe the toenails and the skin between the toes for general appearance and condition. Look especially for redness and cracking. Remove the basin. Dry the leg and foot and between the toes. Cover the leg and foot with the sheet and remove the towel.

26. Repeat the entire procedure for the leg and foot closest to you. Empty the basin, rinse and refill it with clean water at 105–110°F (40.5–43°C).

27. Assist the resident to turn to one side with his or her back toward you.

28. Put the towel lengthwise on the bottom sheet near the resident's back. Wash, rinse, and dry the back, buttocks, and back of the neck behind the ears with long, firm, circular strokes.

29. Look for reddened areas, dry the resident's back, remove the towel, and assist the resident to turn over.

30. Offer the resident a soapy washcloth to wash the genital area (Figure 6-11). Offer a clean wet washcloth to rinse with, and a dry towel for drying. If the resident is unable to do this, you must wash the resident's genital area. Allow for privacy at all times. Put on your gloves when washing the genital area.

> **Ending Steps**

31. Give the resident a back rub.

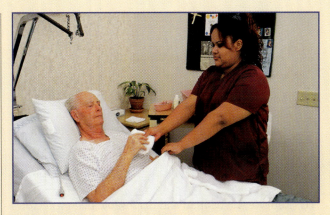

FIGURE 6-11
Offer the resident a soapy washcloth.

32. Follow the procedures for dressing the resident (see Chapter 6) and transferring to a wheelchair (see Chapter 8) if indicated. If the resident is to remain in bed, put a clean gown on the resident.

33. Comb the hair if the resident is unable.

34. Change the linens and make the bed.

35. Clean your equipment and put it in its proper place. Discard disposable equipment.

36. Wipe off the overbed table. Discard soiled linen in the dirty linen container.

37. Make the resident comfortable.

38. Place the signal cord within reach.

39. Wash your hands.

40. Report and record your observation of anything unusual.

PROCEDURE

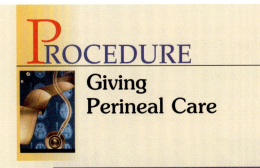

Giving Perineal Care

> **Beginning Steps**

1. Assemble your equipment:
   - Disposable bed protector
   - Bedpan
   - Basin of warm water (or special perineal washing solution)
   - Soap
   - Washcloth
   - Towels
   - Gloves

2. Wash your hands.
3. Provide privacy.
4. Explain to the resident what you are going to do.

> **Steps**

5. Obtain a basin of warm water, or special peri-wash solution used in the facility.

6. Place the disposable bed protector under the buttocks.

7. Assist the resident onto the bedpan.

8. Put on your gloves.

9. Using a disposable paper cup or peri-wash squeeze bottle, pour warm solution over the perineal area. Spread the labia in the female and wash from front to back. In the uncircumcised male, retract the foreskin and clean thoroughly, rinse thoroughly and dry.

PROCEDURE

continued

10. If the resident is soiled with urine and feces, use soap and warm water to wash thoroughly. Change water in basin as necessary. Rinse and dry thoroughly. Remember, bacteria normally found in the bowel will cause urinary tract infections—take every precaution to ensure that residents are properly cleaned.
11. Remove the bedpan and disposable bed protector.
12. Cover the resident.

13. Empty, rinse, and clean equipment and return to appropriate storage area.
14. Discard disposable equipment.
15. Remove your gloves.
16. Wash your hands.
17. Assist the resident with handwashing.
18. Reposition and make the resident comfortable, and replace the call signal cord.
19. Wash your hands.
20. Report and record care given and any unusual observations.

Guidelines

GIVING A BACK RUB

Rubbing a resident's back is refreshing; it relaxes muscles and stimulates circulation. Because of pressure caused by the bedclothes and the lack of movement to stimulate circulation, the skin of a bedridden resident needs special care.

Back rubs are usually given right after the bath. They are also given:

- As part of bedtime care
- When changing the position of a dependent resident
- For restless residents who need relaxing
- On doctor's orders

Proceed to rub the back as follows (Figure 6-12a–c):

- Warm the lotion by placing it in a basin of warm water or by pouring a small amount into your hand and using friction to warm it.
- Apply the lotion to the entire back with the palms of your hands. Use long, firm strokes from the buttocks to the shoulders and back of the neck.

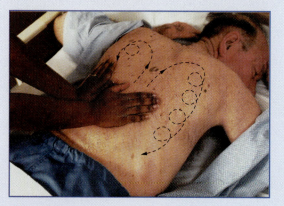

FIGURE 6-12b

- Exert firm pressure as you stroke upward from the buttocks toward the shoulders. Use gentle pressure as you stroke downward from shoulders to buttocks.
- Use circular motion on each bony area.
- Continue rubbing for 1½ to 3 minutes.

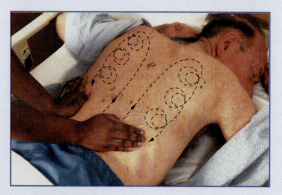

FIGURE 6-12a

Giving a back rub.

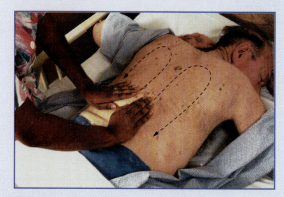

FIGURE 6-12c

PROCEDURE

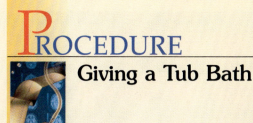

Giving a Tub Bath

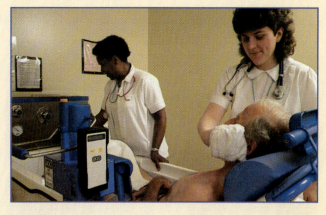

FIGURE 6-13

Giving a tub bath.

Beginning Steps

1. Assemble your equipment on a chair near the bathtub:
   - Towels
   - Washcloth
   - Bath thermometer, if available
   - Chair (place this near the bathtub)
   - Clean clothing
   - Disinfectant solution

2. Wash your hands.
3. Identify the resident.
4. Tell the resident what you are going to do.

Steps

5. Take the resident to the tub room, being sure that he or she is covered to avoid chilling.
6. Wash the tub with disinfectant solution.
7. Fill the tub half full of water at 105°F (40.5°C). Test the temperature with a bath thermometer.
8. Place one towel on the floor where the resident will step out of the tub to prevent slipping.
9. Allow the resident to test the water temperature for comfort.
10. Assist the resident to undress and get into the tub. Get additional assistance if necessary.
11. Let the resident stay in the tub according to your instructions (usually about 15 minutes).

12. Assist the resident with washing as needed (Figure 6-13).
13. Never leave the resident alone in the tub.
14. Put a towel across the chair.
15. Assist the resident out of the tub and onto the towel-covered chair.
16. Dry the resident well by patting gently with a towel.

Ending Steps

17. Assist with dressing.
18. Take the resident back to his or her room.
19. Make the resident comfortable.
20. Return to the tub room. Clean the tub with disinfectant solution.
21. Remove all used linen and put it in the dirty linen container.
22. Wash your hands.
23. Record in the chart:
    - That you have given the resident a tub bath
    - Your observations of anything unusual

PROCEDURE

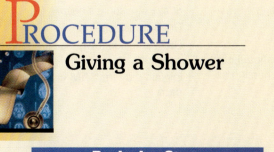

Giving a Shower

Beginning Steps

1. Assemble your equipment on a chair near the shower:
   - Towels
   - Soap
   - Washcloth
   - Clean clothing

2. Wash your hands.
3. Identify the resident.
4. Tell the resident what you are going to do.
5. Provide privacy.
6. Be sure the resident is properly covered (Figure 6-14).

Steps

7. Turn on the shower and adjust the water temperature to the resident's comfort.
8. Assist the resident into the shower.
9. Give the resident soap and washcloth so he or she can wash as much as possible. Assist as necessary.

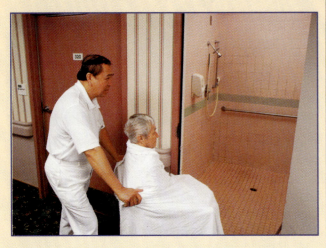

FIGURE 6-14

Be sure the resident is properly covered.

10. Turn off the water and assist the resident out of the shower.
11. Dry the resident well by patting gently with the towel.

Ending Steps

12. Assist with dressing.
13. Take the resident back to his or her room (Figure 6-15).

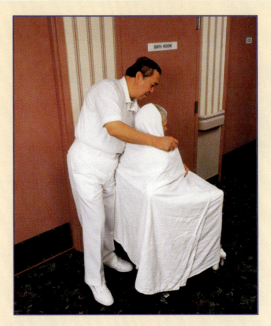

FIGURE 6-15

Take the resident back to his or her room.

14. Return to the shower room. Remove all used linen and put it in the dirty linen container.
15. Put your equipment back in its proper place.
16. Wash your hands.
17. Record in the chart:
    • That you have helped the resident with a shower
    • Your observations of anything unusual

SECTION 4 PERSONAL CARE AND GROOMING

OBJECTIVES
What You Will Learn

When you have completed this section, you will be able to:

• List the procedures included in personal grooming
• List three conditions that increase the need for oral hygiene

• Brush the teeth of a dependent resident
• Care for dentures
• Indicate which residents should not be given nail care by the nursing assistant
• Trim fingernails or toenails
• Care for the hair

• Shave a resident's beard
• Dress a resident in bed
• Dress a resident who is paralyzed on one side
• Explain the terms **AM care** and **PM care**

KEY TERMS

AM care   oral hygiene   PM care

PERSONAL GROOMING

Personal grooming includes oral hygiene, care of nails, care of hair, shaving, makeup, and dressing. Personal grooming is particularly important to the resident's feelings of self-worth and well-being. The dignity of all human beings is directly related to their grooming. No matter what the personal grooming activity, encourage as much resident involvement as possible. Even if the participation is limited simply to making decisions, the resident must be included in the process.

Residents should be encouraged to use deodorant, perfume, and cosmetics just as they did prior to admission. If you need to apply makeup for the resident, make every effort to obtain a pleasing result. Some residents with poor vision might apply too much makeup and will need your help to determine the right amount.

ASSISTIVE DEVICES

Greater independence can sometimes be achieved through use of assistive devices. Assistive devices are tools designed to help the resident perform tasks that would otherwise be impossible. Use of any assistive devices requires training the resident, along with consistent encouragement from the staff. At first it may take the resident more time to use the device than if you performed the task, but remember the independence and self-esteem that come with it are very important to the resident. A good nursing assistant will not perform tasks for residents that they are capable of doing for themselves. A good nursing assistant will be patient and assist each resident toward independent functioning. Some of the devices available for grooming and dressing are shown in Figure 6-16.

As you give care to residents, remember that there are many assistive devices available. Do not hesitate to suggest to the charge nurse that they be used when appropriate. The services of an occupational therapist may be indicated to recommend special devices and to train the resident in their use.

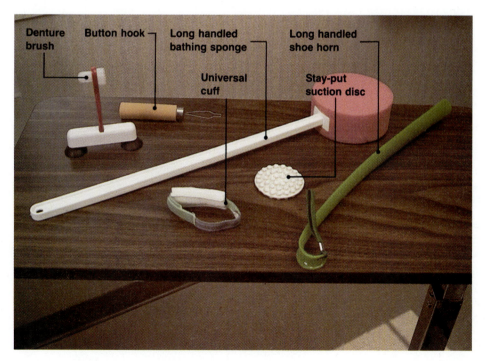

FIGURE 6-16

Some grooming and dressing devices.

ORAL HYGIENE

Oral hygiene is part of the daily care of every resident and includes care of the mouth, teeth, gums, and tongue. The purpose of oral hygiene is to keep the mouth, teeth, gums, and tongue healthy. A mouth in poor condition can be uncomfortable and can cause loss of appetite as well as decreased fluid intake. Poor nutrition and dehydration contribute to lowered resistance of the mouth, tongue, teeth, and gums to infection. When mouth care is poor, tartar, plaque, and food collect around the teeth, leading to irritation, tooth decay, gum disease, and loss of teeth. Other parts of the body are often affected by infection and disease of the mouth.

Residents who are disabled or elderly may be unable to provide their own mouth care. They can fail to recognize the importance of oral hygiene, forget to perform it, or be physically unable to do so. Having a clean, fresh mouth is part of the dignity to which each resident is entitled.

PROCEDURE

Cleaning Dentures (False Teeth)

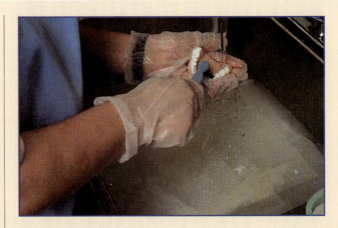

FIGURE 6-17
Hold the dentures in the palm of your hand.

Beginning Steps

1. Assemble your equipment on the bedside table:
   - Tissues
   - Mouthwash
   - Denture cup
   - Toothbrush or denture brush
   - Towel
   - Denture toothpaste or baking soda
   - Gloves

2. Wash your hands.
3. Identify the resident.
4. Tell the resident what you are going to do.
5. Provide privacy.
6. Spread the towel across the resident's chest to protect the gown and the top sheets.
7. Put on your gloves.

Steps

8. Ask the resident to remove the dentures. Assist residents who cannot remove their own dentures by pushing gently to break the suction.
9. Take the dentures to the sink in the denture cup. Hold the dentures securely in the basin.
10. Line the sink with a paper towel or fill the sink with water to guard against breaking the dentures if you drop them.
11. Apply toothpaste or denture cleanser. With the dentures in the palm of your hand, brush them until they are clean (Figure 6-17).
12. Rinse them thoroughly under cool running water.
13. Fill the clean denture cup with cool water and place the dentures in the cup.
14. Help the resident rinse with the mouthwash and water solution.
15. Have the resident replace the dentures.
16. Leave the labeled denture cup with the clean solution where the resident can reach it easily.

Ending Steps

17. Clean all equipment and put it in the proper place. Discard disposable equipment in the proper container.
18. Remove and discard your gloves.
19. Wash your hands.
20. Record and report any unusual observations.

PROCEDURE

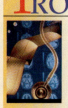

Giving Special Mouth Care to the Unconscious Resident

Beginning Steps

1. Assemble your equipment:
   - Towel
   - Emesis basin
   - Mouth care kit of commercially prepared swabs. Or if such kit is not available:
     - —Tongue depressor
     - —Applicators or gauze sponges
     - —Lubricant such as glycerine, or a substance used by your facility, or a solution of lemon juice and glycerine
   - Gloves

2. Wash your hands.
3. Identify the resident.
4. Tell the resident what you are going to do. Even though a resident seems to be unconscious, he or she still may be able to hear you.
5. Provide privacy.

Steps

6. Stand at the side of the bed with the resident facing you.
7. Put a towel on the pillow under the resident's head and partly under the face.
8. Put the emesis basin on the towel under the resident's chin.

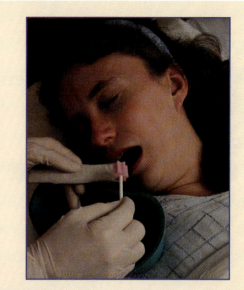

FIGURE 6-18

Hold the tongue with a tongue depressor.

9. Put on your gloves.
10. Press on the cheeks and hold the tongue in place with a tongue depressor (Figure 6-18).
11. Open the commercial package of swabs and wipe the resident's entire mouth, roof, tongue, and inside the cheeks and lips.
12. If a disposable swab is not available, use applicators moistened with diluted mouthwash.

Ending Steps

13. Clean your equipment and put it back in the proper place. Discard disposable equipment in the proper container.
14. Remove your gloves.
15. Make the resident comfortable.
16. Wash your hands.
17. Report and record any unusual observations.

Some nursing assistants find giving mouth and denture care an unpleasant task. It is so important that you must learn to overcome your own feelings and put the needs of the resident first. The more you practice this skill, the less unpleasant it will become.

In addition to performing mouth and denture care, the nursing assistant should observe and report signs of disease or injury of the mouth, tongue, teeth, and gums. Report such things as:

- Sores in the mouth
- Bleeding
- Dry, coated tongue
- Loose or broken teeth
- Bad mouth odor

These problems must be reported immediately and recorded in the health record.

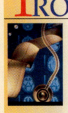

PROCEDURE

Assisting the Resident with Oral Hygiene

Beginning Steps

1. Assemble your equipment on the overbed table:
   - Mouthwash
   - Fresh water
   - Disposable cup
   - Straw
   - Toothbrush
   - Toothpaste
   - Emesis basin
   - Face towel

2. Wash your hands.
3. Identify the resident.
4. Tell the resident what you are going to do.
5. Provide privacy.

Steps

6. Spread the towel across the resident's chest to protect the gown and top sheet. (If possible, assist the resident into the bathroom.) (Figure 6-19)
7. Dilute the mouthwash with four parts of water to one part of mouthwash. (Full-strength mouthwash may be harmful to delicate gums.)
8. Let the resident take a mouthful of the mixture and rinse the mouth.
9. Hold the emesis basin under the chin so that the resident can spit out the mouthwash solution.
10. Put toothpaste on the wet toothbrush (Figure 6-20). Encourage the resident to brush his or her own teeth if possible (Figure 6-21). Assist as necessary.
11. Help the resident rinse out the toothpaste using the fresh water.

Ending Steps

12. Make the resident comfortable.
13. Clean and put your equipment in its proper place. Discard disposable equipment.
14. Wash your hands.
15. Record that you have assisted the resident with oral hygiene.

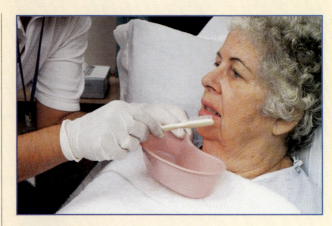

FIGURE 6-19

Spread the towel across the resident's chest.

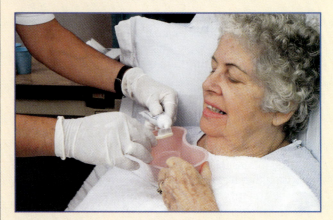

FIGURE 6-20

Put toothpaste on the wet toothbrush.

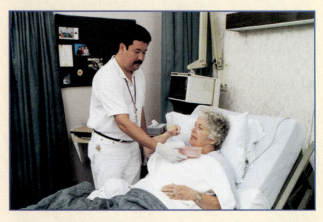

FIGURE 6-21

Encourage the resident to brush his or her own teeth.

Every resident should receive oral hygiene twice daily. Certain residents require more frequent care. They are residents who are:

- Unconscious
- Receiving oxygen
- Unable to take fluids by mouth
- Breathing through the mouth
- Feverish

Brushing the teeth is the most important aspect of mouth care! Although you also may refresh and lubricate the mouth with mouthwash, swabs, and sponge-type devices, there is no adequate substitute for brushing the teeth and gums.

Ideally, a soft-bristle, junior-size brush is used for the resident. This allows you to do a good job without injuring the mouth and gums.

Dental hygienists have recommended that the teeth of long-term residents be brushed using the following principles:

- Wear gloves.
- Use a *dry* brush first to stimulate gums.
- Hold the brush at a 45-degree angle to the teeth.
- Use a circular motion.
- Massage the area where the teeth and gums meet.
- Brush the upper teeth first since brushing the lower teeth produces excessive saliva.
- Brush outer surface, inner surface, then chewing surface.
- After about 1½ minutes, repeat this process using toothpaste.

If a resident is able to brush his own teeth, he should be encouraged to do so. Your role would be to provide the necessary equipment and supplies and to assist as needed. Use the following procedure when assisting a resident with oral hygiene.

CARE OF NAILS AND HAIR

As a nursing assistant in an LTC facility, you will assist residents with nail care and care of the hair (Figure 6-22). As with the skin, cleanliness is very important. The hair and fingernails are a critical part of personal grooming and will have an effect on how the residents feel about themselves. Cleanliness and good grooming contribute to the dignity and self-esteem of every resident.

The fingernails and toenails must be kept short, clean, and free of rough edges. This prevents damage to the skin and provides a pleasant appearance. With the inactive or elderly resident, the nails may become thick, brittle, and difficult to trim. For this reason, you will find it easier if the nails are trimmed after soaking in warm water. Trimming the nails weekly also makes the job easier. If the nails are long, they are more likely to split when being trimmed. Usually, clippers are used rather than scissors. Take care not to injure the skin while trimming.

Certain residents will have their nails trimmed only by the licensed nurse or podiatrist. These are residents who have diabetes or poor circulation and heal slowly if injured. Follow the policies and procedures established in your facility regarding trimming the resident's nails. If you are to trim nails, follow the procedure above.

Daily care of the resident's hair consists of combing, brushing, and arranging. Any resident who is able to should be encouraged and assisted to care for her own hair. Your role may be

FIGURE 6-22

Assisting resident with nail care.

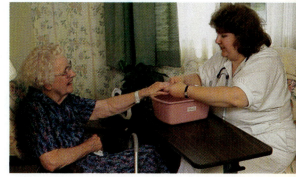

PROCEDURE

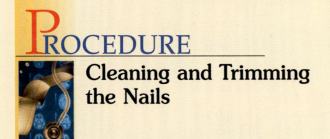

Cleaning and Trimming the Nails

Beginning Steps

1. Assemble your equipment:
   - Nail clippers
   - Emery board or file
   - Orange stick, if available
   - Basin of warm water
   - Towel
   - Lotion

2. Wash your hands.
3. Explain to the resident what you are going to do.

Steps

4. Protect the bed with a towel.
5. Place the hands or feet in warm water and wash.
6. Clean the nails using the orangewood stick.
7. Dry the hands or feet.
8. Trim the nails using the clippers.
9. File rough edges using an emery board or nail file.
10. Apply lotion and gently massage the hands or feet.
11. Repeat steps 6 to 10 on the feet or hands.

Ending Steps

12. Return the equipment to its proper place.
13. Wash your hands.
14. Record and report your actions and any unusual observations in the chart.
15. Report any injury immediately.

simply to take the resident with the proper equipment to the bathroom to perform her own hair care. Some residents, due to blindness, paralysis, weakness, or disorientation, may need to have their hair care done entirely by you.

The goals for choosing a particular style should include simplicity and neatness, but most important are the preference and dignity of the individual. Most facilities have a professional hairdresser who visits on a regular basis. When an age-appropriate or dignified hairstyle cannot be achieved, the resident may need an appointment with the hairdresser. It is always necessary to obtain permission of the family and the resident before making the appointment.

SHAVING THE RESIDENT

A regular morning activity for most men is shaving. This is a *daily* activity, not every other day. If the resident is able to shave himself, encourage him and only provide help if necessary.

Guidelines

SHAMPOOING THE RESIDENT'S HAIR

Shampooing hair is part of the routine care of the resident. Some residents will have a regular appointment with a hairdresser or may even go out to a beauty salon for shampooing. Do not shampoo the hair as part of the shower if the resident has a regularly scheduled beauty salon appointment.

Most often you will shampoo the hair as part of the shower. Younger residents may be shampooed daily, while the elderly may receive a shampoo once a week. Check with your facility for the policy on frequency of shampoos.

Regardless of the method used, the procedure should be done in such a way that the:

- Hair is thoroughly cleansed
- Resident is not chilled
- Soap is rinsed completely
- Eyes are not irritated by the shampoo

Residents who are unable to sit in a shower or shampoo chair may have their hair shampooed by placing them on a wheeled stretcher set over the sink, shower, or tub.

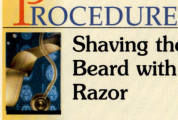

PROCEDURE

Shaving the Resident's Beard with a Safety Razor

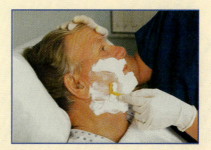

FIGURE 6-23
Use short, firm strokes.

Beginning Steps

1. Assemble your equipment on the bedside table:
   - Basin of water at 115°F (46.1°C)
   - Shaving cream
   - Safety razor
   - Face towel
   - Washcloth
   - Mirror
   - Tissues
   - Aftershave lotion, if available
   - Gloves

2. Wash your hands.
3. Identify the resident.
4. Tell the resident that you are going to shave his beard.

Steps

5. Adjust the light so that it shines on the resident's face.
6. Raise the head of the bed, if allowed.
7. Spread the face towel under the resident's chin. If he has dentures, be sure they are in his mouth.
8. Put on your gloves.
9. Pat some warm water or use a damp washcloth on the resident's face to soften his beard.
10. Apply shaving soap generously to the face.
11. With the fingers of one hand, hold the skin taut (tight) as you shave in the direction that the hair grows. Start under the sideburns and work downward over the cheeks. Continue carefully over the chin. Work upward on the neck under the chin. Use short, firm strokes (Figure 6-23).
12. Rinse the razor often.
13. Areas under the nose and around the lips are sensitive. Take special care in these areas.
14. If you nick the resident's skin, report this to your charge nurse.
15. Wash off the remaining soap when you have finished.
16. Apply aftershave lotion if the resident prefers.

Ending Steps

17. Clean your equipment and put it in its proper place. Discard disposable equipment.
18. Remove your gloves.
19. Make the resident comfortable.
20. Wash your hands.

Shaving can be done with an electric razor or a safety razor. If the resident has his own electric razor, it should be used to shave him. Electric razors are *never* used if the resident is receiving oxygen or if oxygen is being given to any other person in the room because this presents a fire hazard.

DRESSING THE RESIDENT

In most LTC facilities, residents are encouraged to wear street clothing rather than hospital gowns or pajamas, robes, and slippers. As a nursing assistant you will not only help the resident to dress but also to select clothing that is neat, clean, in good repair, and appropriate for the environment and weather.

Types of clothing that are particularly useful are jogging suits (they are warm and loose fitting, without buttons, snaps, or zippers), brunch coats (loose-fitting dresses that snap down the front), or specially made clothing for those who spend time in wheelchairs or in bed. Most of this type of clothing uses Velcro fasteners and opens in the back. These items can be obtained from some of the major department stores as well as specialty companies.

PROCEDURE

Dressing and Undressing the Totally Dependent Resident

Note: It is usually easier to dress the dependent resident completely in bed before transferring the resident to a chair. Generally, the resident sleeps in a hospital gown at night.

Beginning Steps

1. Wash your hands.
2. Identify the resident.
3. Explain what you are going to do.
4. Assist the resident to select clothing.
5. Provide privacy.
6. Fold back the bed covers.

Steps

7. Turn the resident to the supine (face up) position.
8. Untie the gown.
9. Remove the gown by pulling the sleeves down and over the arms.
10. Lay the gown across the resident to provide covering.
11. With all the buttons, fasteners, or zippers open, apply the clothing as follows:

    To apply pants or slacks: Gather the pant leg for the leg farthest from you. Reach through the leg to grasp the resident's ankle. Pull the pant leg over your hand and the resident's leg. Repeat for the leg nearest you (Figure 6-24). Pull the pants up as high as possible. If the resident is able, have him or her raise the buttocks as you pull the pants up to the waist. If the resident is unable to raise the buttocks, roll the resident on the side away from you as you pull up the other side. Fasten as indicated.

    Shirt or dress that opens down the front: Reach inside the sleeve farthest from you and grasp the resi-

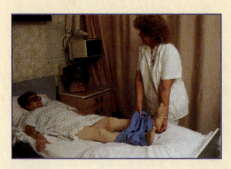

FIGURE 6-24

Pull the pant leg over your hand and the resident's leg.

dent's wrist. Slide the sleeve over your hand and the resident's arm. Roll the resident toward you and tuck the remainder of the item under the resident. Roll the resident away from you and pull the item free. Reach through the sleeve and grasp the resident's wrist. Pull the sleeve over your hand and the resident's wrist. Secure the fasteners.

Pullover-type shirt or dress: Place both the resident's hands, one at a time in the sleeves. Pull the item as high on the arms as possible. Grasp the neck opening and slide over the head (Figure 6-25). Either assist the resident to sit and pull the item down, or roll the resident from side to side, pulling the clothing down as you go.

Ending Steps

12. Apply socks or stockings and shoes.
13. Wash your hands.

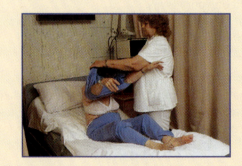

FIGURE 6-25

Grasp the neck opening and slide over the head.

Offering the resident the opportunity to choose his or her own clothing is one way of encouraging the resident to participate in his or her own care and to make decisions. It also allows the resident a measure of control that is important to most individuals. When offering a choice of clothing, select two or three appropriate items and ask the resident, "Which one do you want to wear today?" Elderly residents tend to require warmer clothing due to decreased circulation. Take this need into consideration as you assist with dressing.

For residents who have a problem that results in their constantly disrobing (taking their clothes off), jump suits can be very helpful as a deterrent. For those who don't remain covered when in bed or who are exposed when up in a chair, try pants or pajama bottoms to protect privacy and dignity.

The dressing procedure varies with the abilities and limitations of each resident. You may need to combine parts of the above procedures on dressing, depending on the needs of the residents. Remember to allow residents to do as much for themselves as possible.

You may have times when you are dressing residents who have either tubes (feeding tubes or catheters) or intravenous (in the veins) catheters. Use caution so that you do not place any tension on the tube that might dislodge or displace it. Treat the IV and the tubing as a part of the person. Some facilities will provide gowns that snap on over the arm and shoulder to make it easier to dress the resident. If you have no special clothing, be careful in both clothing selection and application. If there is an IV in an arm, use short-sleeved clothing. The nurse needs to be able to observe the site where the needle or catheter enters the vein. Loose-fitting clothing will be easier to apply than tight-fitting clothing. You will be learning more about the purposes and types of tubes and catheters in Chapters 9, 10, and 18.

Undressing a helpless resident is simply the reverse of the dressing procedure.

Dressing a resident with one paralyzed side, a cast, an IV, or other impairment requires that you remember one thing. *Always dress the affected side first and undress it last.* It is also important that residents be dressed with proper underclothing in keeping with their personal preferences.

Most of the basic skills you have learned in this section are carried out on a daily basis and make up some of the facility routines or daily procedures performed for each resident.

These activities are often referred to as *AM care* or *PM care* because of the time of day they are carried out.

AM care includes:

- Providing an opportunity to go to the bathroom (see Chapter 10)
- Washing the resident's face and hands
- Providing oral hygiene
- Preparing the resident for breakfast (see Chapter 9)

PM or **HS** (hour of sleep) **care** includes:

- Providing an opportunity to go to the bathroom
- Washing face and hands
- Providing a bedtime snack or nourishment
- Providing oral hygiene
- Dressing in sleeping attire
- Giving a back rub

Most facilities have specific procedures for both AM and PM care that can include other activities.

AM care   assisting the resident with toileting needs, washing face and hands, providing oral hygiene, and preparing the resident for breakfast

PM care   assisting the resident with toileting needs, washing face and hands, giving bedtime nourishment, providing oral hygiene, dressing for bed, and giving a back rub

OBJECTIVES
What You Will Learn

When you have completed this section, you will be able to:

- Describe the effect of heat and cold on blood vessels
- List appropriate temperatures for different types of heat application
- List four safety precautions to be followed when using heat or cold

KEY TERMS   dry application   moist application

APPLYING HEAT AND COLD

You may be given the job of applying heat or cold to a resident's body. To carry out this task safely requires an understanding of how both heat and cold work (Figure 6-26) and the safety precautions that must be followed. Each facility has policies that include the kinds of applications used and the personnel who may apply them. Some facilities permit only licensed nurses to apply heat and cold.

Heat is used to speed up the healing process, to decrease swelling, or to relieve pain. When heat is applied to the skin, the blood vessels dilate (open). This causes more blood with oxygen and nutrients to reach the injured area.

FIGURE 6-26

Principles of warm and cold application.

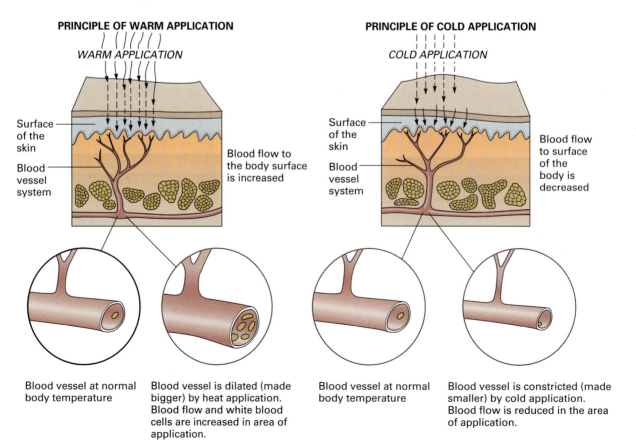

PRINCIPLE OF WARM APPLICATION

WARM APPLICATION

Surface of the skin

Blood vessel system

Blood flow to the body surface is increased

Blood vessel at normal body temperature

Blood vessel is dilated (made bigger) by heat application. Blood flow and white blood cells are increased in area of application.

PRINCIPLE OF COLD APPLICATION

COLD APPLICATION

Surface of the skin

Blood vessel system

Blood flow to surface of the body is decreased

Blood vessel at normal body temperature

Blood vessel is constricted (made smaller) by cold application. Blood flow is reduced in the area of application.

Fluids that may be causing swelling and pain are absorbed and carried away as the blood circulates. The warmth also relaxes the muscles, decreasing pain due to tension.

Cold is used to prevent swelling, control bleeding, relieve pain, or lower body temperature. When cold is applied, the blood vessels contract (narrow), reducing the flow of blood to the area. The physician will order the kind of heat or cold to be applied, the frequency of application, and the length of treatment. Moist or dry applications may be ordered.

Moist applications include:

- Soak (warm or cold)
- Compress (warm or cold)
- Tub
- Alcohol sponge bath
- Sitz bath
- Cool wet packs

Dry applications include:

- Ice pack and ice collar
- Warm water bottle
- Heat lamp
- Aquamatic K-pad

A **moist application** is one in which water touches the skin. A **dry application** is one in which no water touches the skin. Compresses and soaks are both moist applications. They can be either warm or cold. A compress is a

moist application application in which water touches the skin

dry application application in which no water touches the skin

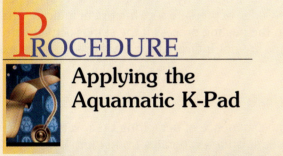

PROCEDURE

Applying the Aquamatic K-Pad

Beginning Steps

1. Assemble your equipment:
   - Aquamatic K-pad and control unit
   - Cover for pad

2. Inspect the K-pad for leaks, and make sure the cord and plug are in good condition.
3. Wash your hands.
4. Identify the resident.
5. Explain to the resident what you are going to do.
6. Provide privacy.

Steps

7. Plug the cord into an electrical outlet.
8. Place the pad in the cover. *Do not use pins!* (Figure 6-27)
9. Place the pump on the bedside table. Arrange the tubing at the level of the pad. Do not allow the tubing to hang below the level of the bed.

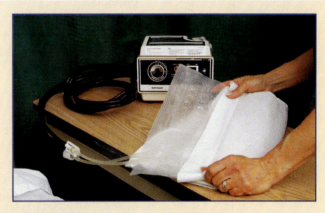

FIGURE 6-27

Place the pad in the cover.

10. Gently apply the covered pad to the proper body area.
11. Check the skin under the pad every hour.

Ending Steps

12. When the treatment is finished, return the equipment to its proper place.
13. Make the resident comfortable.
14. Wash your hands.
15. Record in the chart:
    - The time the K-pad was applied
    - The length of treatment
    - The area of application
    - Your observations of anything unusual

localized application. A soak can be either localized or generalized. In applying a compress, a cloth is dipped into water, wrung out, and applied to a specific area. To apply a soak, you immerse the body or body part completely in water. Warm water bottles, ice caps, and Aquamatic K-pads are considered dry applications because they have a dry surface. Water is used only inside the equipment and never touches the skin. Dry applications are sometimes used to keep moist applications at the correct temperature.

Although some facilities still use warm water bottles to apply dry heat, most have discontinued the practice for several reasons:

- The elderly and chronically ill often have decreased perception of the temperature and pain, increasing the risk of burns.
- The weight of the bottle can create additional pressure on an already injured or damaged area.
- It is difficult to keep the bottle in position.
- It is difficult to control the temperature of the water.

Electric heating pads are equally dangerous to older residents. Sometimes families bring in heating pads in an attempt to be helpful. Refer them to the charge nurse, who can explain the dangers to the resident. Most facilities have policies excluding the use of electric heating pads.

Use of a heat lamp also contains great risk of burning the resident. This procedure is being used much less frequently than in the past. A heat lamp can provide soothing and drying to skin irritated from moisture as a result of perspiration or urine. Current knowledge of pressure sore treatment indicates that use of a heat lamp slows down the healing process if the skin is actually broken. In other words, heat lamps are not indicated for any pressure sores except perhaps stage 1.

THE ALCOHOL SPONGE BATH

You can probably remember the experience of perspiring on a warm summer day. You often feel cooler as the moisture evaporates from your skin. As perspiration evaporates into the air, it carries heat away with it and this cools the body. An alcohol sponge bath cools in the same way. Alcohol is applied to the resident's body because it will evaporate from the skin much faster than water. The purpose of the alcohol sponge bath is to lower the body temperature.

Either heat or cold applications can damage the skin if not observed frequently and carefully. Since the elderly and chronically ill residents have fragile skin and a decreased ability to feel pain and temperature, they are at risk for burns.

Guidelines

GIVING THE ALCOHOL SPONGE BATH

- Alcohol sponge baths are *never* given without doctor's orders.
- Never apply alcohol to the resident's face.
- If the resident starts to shiver, stop the treatment. Call the charge nurse. If the shivering cannot be controlled, the alcohol sponge bath will do no good because the shivering causes increased cell and muscle activity. This produces more heat and causes the body temperature to rise.
- Follow your facility's step-by-step procedures for giving the bath.

- Follow the instructions of the charge nurse.
- Check the application often to keep it at the right temperature throughout the treatment. Suggested times for checking different kinds of applications are:
  —Soaks and intermittent compresses: every 5 minutes
  —Heat lamps: every 5 minutes
  —Continuous compresses: every 30 minutes
  —Ice bags: at least every hour
- Keep the resident comfortable. Make sure that the resident is comfortably positioned during the application of heat or cold (Figure 6-28).
- If the resident begins to shiver during cold applications, stop the treatment, cover the resident with a blanket, and report to your charge nurse for further instructions.
- For a warm application, always use a bath thermometer to test the temperature of the water. Temperatures for different kinds of heat application are:
  —Warm soak 100°F (37.8°C)
  —Warm compress 115° (46.1°C)
  —Tub bath 105°F (40.5°C)
- For cold applications, use cubed ice if available. Crushed ice will melt too quickly. Also, it may stick to the cloth and be too cold for the resi-

dent's skin. Keep the application cold by adding ice as necessary.
- Always dry the bags after checking for leaks.
- Always apply the ice cap with the metal or plastic stopper away from the resident's body. The stopper should never touch the resident's skin. It will burn the resident. Remember, ice can also burn the skin.
- Never put an ice cap directly on the skin. Always cover it with a cloth (Figure 6-29).
- Never put an ice bag on top of the painful area. The weight will probably increase the pain.
- Check the resident's skin. Watch for too much redness. Look for darker discolorations that might mean the resident is being burned. Listen to any complaints. If you think a resident is being burned, remove the heat application immediately and report to your charge nurse at once!
- Check the resident's skin where cold is being applied. If the area appears to be blanched or bluish, tell the charge nurse at once!
- When you have finished the moist application, dry the resident's skin thoroughly and gently, using a patting motion. Do not rub the resident's skin.

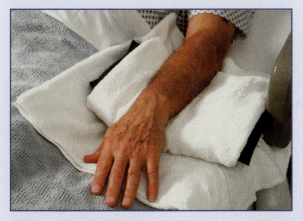

FIGURE 6-28
Check the application often.

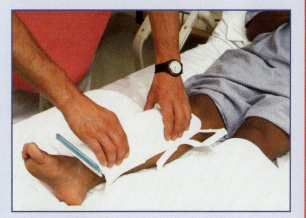

FIGURE 6-29
Never put ice directly on skin.

SUMMARY

SUMMARY This chapter has given you the knowledge and information needed to provide your residents with excellent personal care. Many elderly come to live in a nursing home because they are unable to provide their own personal care. Being clean and well groomed is important to each resident's quality of life and feeling of well-being. The quality of care of the facility is evaluated based on the grooming, hygiene, and personal care you provide.

The Health Care Financing Administration, which has jurisdiction of nursing homes, has developed some "Quality Indicators" that they use to evaluate nursing homes on their annual surveys. The most serious conditions are called sentinel events. If even one sentinel event occurs, it will be investigated. One example is the development of pressure ulcers, stages 1 through 4. You have learned in this chapter how important your role is in preventing the development of pressure ulcers. You learned the importance of bathing and good skin care. You know about the need for frequent changes of position and how to use pressure-reducing devices. Remember also that your observation, reporting, and documentation about any changes in the skin are essential to good resident care.

The skin of elderly residents is fragile and easily injured. One important aspect of your care is to proceed slowly and gently. Be careful to avoid bumping the resident's body on the wheelchair, doorway, or bed rails. Watch for tight-fitting clothing or objects in the bed that might cause pressure or injury.

OBRA HIGHLIGHTS

The OBRA regulations are very specific when it comes to the development of pressure ulcers or pressure sores. In fact, the regulations state that a person who enters the facility without pressure sores must not develop them unless the medical condition of the resident made them impossible to prevent. Development of pressure sores is considered an indication of poor-quality care. If pressure sores do develop, the facility must provide care and treatment to heal and to prevent development of additional pressure sores. Preventive measures include turning and proper positioning, application of pressure reducing or relief devices, providing good skin care, clean and dry bed linens, and maintaining adequate nutrition and hydration.

SELF STUDY

Choose the best answer for each question or statement.

1. Why do elderly residents often complain of feeling cold?
   a. because they have thinner blood than younger people
   b. because they have lost insulating fat from under the skin
   c. because they have decreased heat sensors in their skin
   d. because they are not accustomed to using fans and air conditioners

2. If a resident's skin takes on a blue or gray color, it can mean that the resident
   a. has a serious problem due to decreased circulation
   b. is taking certain medications that discolor the skin
   c. is about to go into shock
   d. has a fever or infection

3. Which of the following residents would be **least** likely to develop a pressure ulcer?
   a. a resident with arthritis who experiences pain when changing positions
   b. a resident with heart disease who ambulates with a walker
   c. a resident with paralysis who cannot turn himself
   d. a resident who is depressed and remains in one position in bed

4. Which of the following actions by a nursing assistant could cause shearing?
   a. pulling a wet sheet from underneath a resident
   b. rolling a resident from side to side to remove a sheet
   c. assisting a resident to stand to remove a wet sheet from beneath him
   d. using a turn sheet to turn a resident from one side to the other

5. Which of the following is true of a pressure ulcer?
   a. It is not painful but is difficult to heal.
   b. It is painful but heals quickly with the correct treatment.
   c. It is painful and is very difficult to heal.
   d. It is not painful and will heal quickly with treatment.

6. Mrs. Washington is a new resident and is at risk for developing pressure ulcers. Which of the following care should you provide for her?
   a. Change her position at least every 2 hours.
   b. Change her position at least every 3 hours.
   c. Change her position at least every 4 hours.
   d. Apply lotion and powder to pressure areas every hour.

7. You are asked to give Mrs. Washington a partial bath. Which of the following will you do when you bathe her?
   a. Have her wash all her body that she can reach, then you wash the rest.
   b. Wash her face, underarms, hands, and perineal area.
   c. Wash her face and hands only to prevent drying the skin.
   d. Limit the bath to whatever the resident feels like washing.

8. Mrs. Washington has very fragile skin. Which of the following should you do to prevent injuries to her skin?
   a. Dress her in long-sleeved clothes.
   b. Pad her side rails and wheelchair arms.
   c. Keep her from dragging her feet in the wheelchair.
   d. All of these actions will prevent skin injuries.

9. Mrs. Washington's arm accidentally was scraped when you pushed her wheelchair through the doorway. What should you do?
   a. Cover the scrape with ointment and a bandage immediately.
   b. If the scrap isn't bleeding, just cover it with her clothing.
   c. Report the incident to your charge nurse immediately.
   d. Wash the scrape with soap and water, but there is no need to report it.

10. What is the purpose of an assistive device?
    a. to help the resident perform tasks that would otherwise be impossible
    b. to keep the resident from having to bend or stretch to perform a task
    c. to help the resident walk without falling
    d. to save the resident and the staff time and effort

11. How should you provide oral care to an unconscious resident?
    a. Use a toothbrush and very little toothpaste without rinsing.
    b. Use swabs to wipe inside the mouth and cheeks and clean the tongue and lips.
    c. Use mouthwash to moisten a toothbrush, then brush all teeth.
    d. Use mouthwash in a small syringe to rinse the mouth and tongue.

12. Mr. Morganstein has very poor circulation to his feet. Nursing assistants are not allowed to trim his toenails because
    a. he will heal slowly if his feet are injured
    b. his nails will not grow due to poor circulation
    c. poor circulation causes contagious fungus on his nails
    d. poor circulation causes his nails to be very thick

13. How often should male residents be shaved?
    a. daily
    b. every other day
    c. twice a week
    d. weekly

14. Mr. Morganstein's roommate is receiving oxygen through a mask. How will you shave Mr. Morganstein?

    a. Take him into the hall and shave him with a safety razor.
    b. Shave him with an electric razor in his room.
    c. Shave him with a safety razor in his room.
    d. Take him into the hall and shave him with an electric razor.

15. Ms. Chavez has an IV in her right arm. Which of the following actions will you take when you dress her?
    a. Dress her right arm first using a short-sleeved top.
    b. Dress her left arm first using a short-sleeved top.
    c. Dress her right arm first using a long-sleeved top.
    d. Dress her left arm first using a long-sleeved top.

16. What happens when heat is applied to the skin?
    a. The blood vessels narrow and reduce the blood to the area.
    b. The blood vessels in the area open to bring more oxygen to the area.
    c. The heat paralyzes the nerve endings so that pain is not felt.
    d. The blood vessles open, which controls bleeding in the area.

Getting C O N N E C T E D
Multimedia Extension Activities

 www.prenhall.com/will-black

Use the above address to access the free, interactive Companion Website created for this textbook. Hear the pronunciation of the key terms in the chapter. Get instant feedback to a variety of chapter-related questions. Link to other interesting sites.

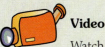 **Video**

Watch the videos *The Bed Bath* and *Personal Care* from the Care Provider Skills series.

CASE STUDY

Harold Green is a 43-year-old African American man who was paralyzed following a car accident. He is unable to walk and uses a wheelchair to get around. He can't move his legs or feel anything below the waist. Although he wants to do everything for himself, he needs some help with bathing and dressing.

1. You return from 2 days off and notice he is wearing the same clothes he was wearing before you left. You offer to help him bathe and change clothes and explain to him that
    a. he will look much nicer if he puts on clean clothes
    b. his roommate will complain if he doesn't smell good
    c. keeping his skin clean will help prevent skin breakdown with pressure ulcers
    d. you'll get in trouble with the charge nurse if you don't give him a bath
2. When you remove his shoes and socks, you notice that his heels feel warm to the touch. His skin looks darker than the rest of his foot. Your action is:
    a. Notify the charge nurse, he might have the beginning of a pressure ulcer.
    b. Tell him not to wear his shoes for a few days.
    c. Massage his heels with lotion.
    d. Ignore it since he can't feel any pain.
3. When you walk by the activity room in the morning, Mr. Green is sitting in his wheelchair working on building a birdhouse. You notice that he is sitting in the same place when you leave at 3:00 P.M. You approach him and remind him that
    a. he will get bored if he works on the birdhouse for long hours
    b. he is at risk for pressure ulcers because he is sitting in the same position for hours without relief
    c. it is important to stay out of bed as much as possible
    d. he missed the movie in the day room
4. Your co-worker says that you have nothing to do for Mr. Green since he is so independent. Your reply is
    a. "That is true but the rest of my residents require a lot of care."
    b. "I do almost everything for him even when he can do it for himself."
    c. "I tell him jokes and keep his spirits up."
    d. "I make sure that I observe his skin every day from head to toe, remind him to reposition himself, use care to prevent injury to his skin, and urge him to eat and drink to maintain his nutrition and hydration."

Chapter 7

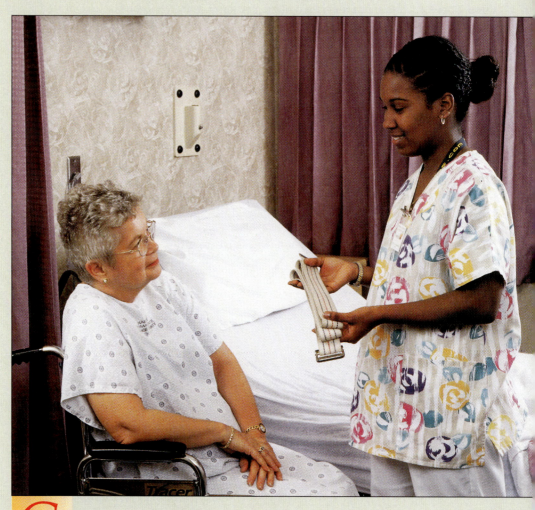

CARING TIP

A successful transfer is one in which both the resident and the caregiver are safe.

Patricia Edwards, RN, BA
Director of Education
Royal Park Care Center
Spokane, Washington

SECTION 1 Anatomy and Physiology

OBJECTIVES
What You Will Learn

When you have completed this section, you will be able to:

- List four functions of the skeletal system
- Identify examples of the different types of bones

- Define the terms **ligament, tendon, bursa,** and **cartilage**
- Identify two age-related changes that affect the skeletal system

KEY TERMS

bursa	joints	rheumatoid arthritis
bursitis	kyphosis	scoliosis
cartilage	ligament	sprain
cranium	osteoarthritis	tendon
dislocation	osteocytes	vertebrae
	osteoporosis	

THE SKELETAL SYSTEM

The skeletal system (Figure 7-1) is composed of:

- Bones
- Joints

The skeletal system functions are to:

- Protect
- Support
- Provide leverage
- Store vital minerals
- Produce blood cells

The human skeleton is made up of 206 bones. The bones act as a framework for the body, giving it structure and support. The bones are passive organs of motion—they do not move by themselves. They must be moved by the muscles of the body, which are stimulated to move by nerve impulses. Most muscles attach to bones, providing the leverage necessary for body movement.

BONES

The bones surround our vital organs and provide protection:

- **Cranium** (bones of the head)—protect the brain (Figure 7-2)
- **Vertebrae** (bones of the spine)—protect the spinal cord (Figure 7-3)
- *Bones* of the rib cage—protect the heart and lungs

Bones are composed of living cells called **osteocytes,** which store vital minerals like calcium, phosphorus, magnesium, and sodium that are essential for other body functions. Bones are not dead, they are the site of many body activities. Red blood cells are produced in the marrow of certain bones.

There are several types of bones (Figure 7-4), each of which has a different function. The skeletal system interacts with the muscular system, the nervous system, and the circulatory system to achieve movement of the body. Movement occurs at the joints. Bones of the hands and feet are shown in Figure 7-5.

cranium bones of the head

vertebrae bones of the spine

osteocytes living cells of the bone

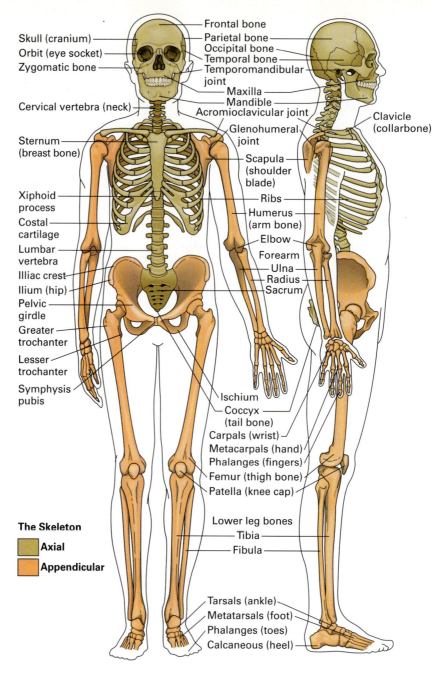

The Skeleton
- Axial
- Appendicular

JOINTS

joint any connection between bones

ligament tough, white, fibrous cord that connect bone to bone

tendon elastic cordlike structures that connect muscles to bone

Joints are areas where one bone connects with one or more other bones. Joints are necessary as levers in all motion. Joints are classified by their type of motion (Figure 7-6). Joints are made up of different structures (Figure 7-7):

- **Ligament**—tough, white, fibrous cord that connects bone to bone.
- **Tendon**—an elastic cordlike structure that connects muscle to bone.
- **Bursa**—small fluid-filled sac that allows one bone to move easily over another. The fluid prevents friction so that the ends of the bones do not wear out. Bursas are located throughout the body, but the most important are in the shoulder, elbow, knee, and hip.
- **Cartilage**—a tough gristlelike substance that forms a pad at the end of or between bones, which acts as a cushion. Cartilage looks like white elastic.

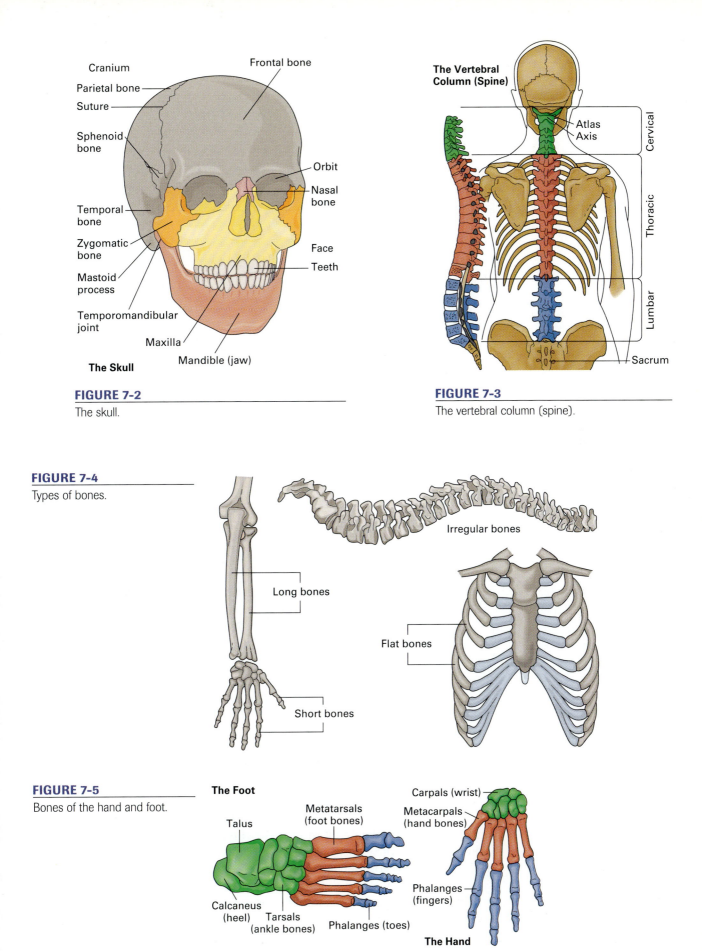

Cranium
Parietal bone
Suture
Sphenoid bone
Temporal bone
Zygomatic bone
Mastoid process
Temporomandibular joint
Maxilla

Frontal bone
Orbit
Nasal bone
Face
Teeth
Mandible (jaw)

The Skull

FIGURE 7-2
The skull.

The Vertebral Column (Spine)
Atlas
Axis
Cervical
Thoracic
Lumbar
Sacrum

FIGURE 7-3
The vertebral column (spine).

FIGURE 7-4
Types of bones.

Irregular bones
Long bones
Flat bones
Short bones

FIGURE 7-5
Bones of the hand and foot.

The Foot
Talus
Metatarsals (foot bones)
Calcaneus (heel)
Tarsals (ankle bones)
Phalanges (toes)

Carpals (wrist)
Metacarpals (hand bones)
Phalanges (fingers)
The Hand

Section 1 The Long-Term Care Facility   **197**

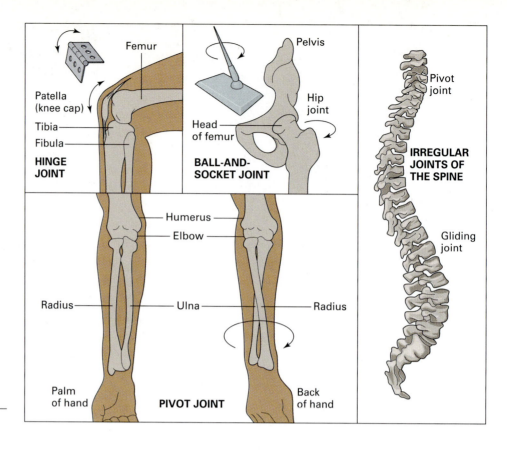

FIGURE 7-6

Movable joints.

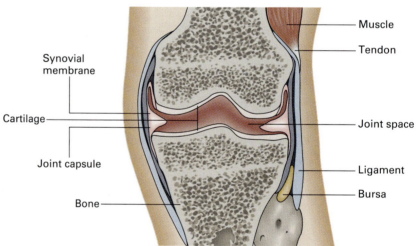

FIGURE 7-7

Normal joint.

ABNORMALITIES OF THE SKELETAL SYSTEM

bursa small fluid-filled sac that allows one bone to move easily over another bone

cartilage tough gristle-like substance that forms a pad at the end of or between bones

Abnormalities of the skeletal system include skeletal or postural deformities. Due to aging or chronic illness, scoliosis and kyphosis can occur. **Scoliosis** refers to an S-shaped curving of the spine. **Kyphosis** is a hunchback or forward curving of the spine. Both of these conditions affect the body's balance and distribution of weight. Ambulation is usually affected, resulting in the resident's need to compensate or adjust his gait.

Osteoarthritis is the deterioration and abrasion of joint cartilage, with formation of new bone at the joint surfaces. Osteoarthritis affects many joints, but usually the weight-bearing ones—knee, hips, vertebrae, and fingers. Symptoms include aching, stiffness, and limited motion. Osteoarthritis does not cause inflammation, deformity, or crippling, as does **rheumatoid arthritis.**

Rheumatoid arthritis affects people of all ages. The joints become extremely painful, stiff, swollen, red, and warm to the touch. The joints become gradually more deformed and often function is completely lost (Figure 7-8). The pain experienced is severe, even at rest. Application of heat and gentle massage and medications may provide some relief.

Common injuries of the skeletal system include:

- **Fracture**—breaking or cracking a bone (injury, cancer of the bone, and osteoporosis are common causes).
- **Dislocation**—disruption of the normal alignment of bones where they form a joint.
- **Sprain**—stretched or torn ligaments or tendons that support a joint.
- **Bursitis**—inflammation of the fluid-filled sac, causing pain on movement.

Broken bones mend solidly, but the process is gradual. Bone cells grow and reproduce slowly. The blood supply to bone tissue is poor compared to other tissues of the body. This decreased circulation makes bone more susceptible to infection. Once infection is present in bone, it is very difficult to clear up.

AGE- AND DISUSE-RELATED CHANGES

Both aging and disuse have profound effects on the skeletal system. There is a loss of bone mass and a shortening of the vertebral column. Some people lose as much as 2 inches in height. If an individual is unable to bear weight (stand), the long bones of the body lose calcium, which is eliminated by the kidneys. This same loss of calcium has been reported when astronauts are in a weightless or zero-gravity state. With the loss of calcium, the bones become porous and chalklike. The resulting condition is known as **osteoporosis.** The bone is weakened and breaks easily. Sometimes a slight fall or stumble can result in a fracture. Fractures of the hip (the neck of the femur) are life-threatening to the elderly. Confinement to bed while the fracture heals means the resident has a greater risk of developing other complications related to immobility.

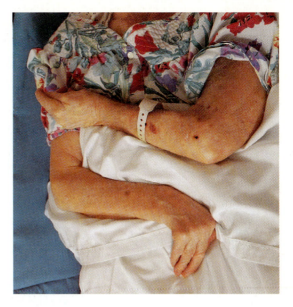

FIGURE 7-8
The resident with arthritis.

scoliosis   S-shaped curving of the spine

kyphosis   hunchback or forward curving of the spine

osteoarthritis   disease characterized by deterioration of joint cartilage and formation of new bone at joint surfaces

rheumatoid arthritis   disease characterized by painful, stiff, swollen red joints that eventually become deformed.

SECTION 2   The Resident with a Fracture

OBJECTIVES
What You Will Learn

When you have completed this section, you will be able to:

- Define the term **fracture**
- List the three goals of fracture treatment
- Match common problems of the resident with a cast to their related causes

---

KEY TERMS

abducted
countertraction

fracture
immobilized
prosthesis

reduction
rehabilitation
traction

FRACTURES

dislocation   disruption of the normal alignment of bones where they form a joint

sprain   stretched or torn ligaments or tendons

bursitis   inflammation of the fluid-filled sacs between bones, causing pain on movement

osteoporosis   disease characterized by porous or chalklike bones that fracture very easily

fracture   breaking or cracking of a bone

The term **fracture** refers to a break in a bone (Figure 7-9). A fracture usually results from some type of trauma, but in the elderly or residents with certain types of disease, it can occur spontaneously. Frequently, hip fractures in the elderly are spontaneous. Instead of falling and fracturing the hip, the spontaneous fracture of the hip causes the person to fall. Regardless of the cause of the fracture, the symptoms are similar:

- Loss of strength and movement
- Bruising and swelling
- Pain and tenderness over the fracture site
- Deformity or misalignment

If any of these symptoms are observed, report and document them immediately.

Any time a resident in your facility sustains a fall or other trauma, the resident should be evaluated by a licensed nurse *before being moved.* The licensed nurse will observe for the signs and symptoms mentioned above. One sign of a fractured hip is misalignment—usually external rotation of the hip (Figure 7-10).

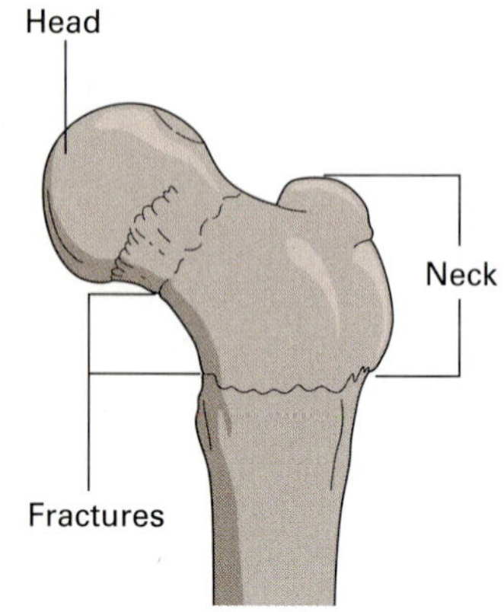

FRACTURE TREATMENT: REDUCTION, IMMOBILIZATION, REHABILITATION

Whatever the cause of the fracture, the goals of treatment are the same:

- Reduction
- Immobilization
- Rehabilitation

Reduction means setting the bone in a proper position so that it heals correctly. The reduction may be closed (by movement or traction) or open (surgical procedure). Reduction is done by a physician.

Once the fracture is reduced, it must be **immobilized** (unable to move) to allow healing to take place. Immobilization is also done by the physician in several basic ways (Figure 7-11):

- External (casts, splints, traction)
- Internal (pin and plaster; nails, plates, screws)

FIGURE 7-9

Fractures of the femur.

Head

Neck

Fractures

FIGURE 7-10

External (outward) rotation of the hip.

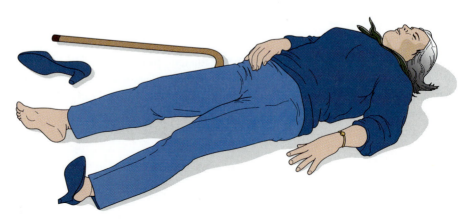

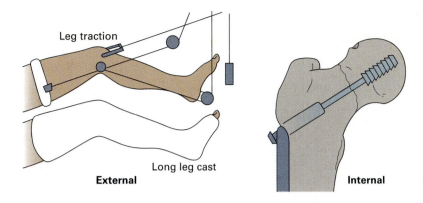

Leg traction

Long leg cast

External

Internal

FIGURE 7-11

Ways to immobilize.

PREVENTING COMPLICATIONS

Whether the immobilization requires casts, traction, or internal fixation, good nursing care is required to protect the fracture and prevent complications. Complications can be prevented by correctly positioning and repositioning, providing the proper exercise, and giving fluids and foods in sufficient quantities to promote healing.

Positioning requires special knowledge and skill. Positioning guidelines for each resident with a fracture should be written in detail on the health-care plan. *Do not reposition* a resident with a fracture until you have received instructions from the licensed nurse. The positions vary with each resident, fracture location, and method used to immobilize. Failure to follow positioning guidelines could result in displacement of the fracture.

Often a special foam wedge or pillow is ordered by the physician to maintain proper alignment of the fractured hip. This device is called an abductor pillow or an abduction wedge because it keeps the leg **abducted** (away from the center of the body) and prevents strain on the fracture site or the hip **prosthesis** (artificial joint).

The placement of the abduction device is the responsibility of the physical therapist or licensed nurse. Report any displacement of the device to the charge nurse immediately. Provide good skin care and report any signs of skin irritation or pressure to the charge nurse.

Some common precautions for the resident who has had a hip fracture include (Figure 7-12):

- Do not cross the legs
- Do not rotate (turn) the affected leg outward
- Do not bring the affected leg past the midline of the body
- Do not raise the knee on the affected side higher than the hip
- Do not allow the resident to bend forward from the waist more than 90 degrees

reduction setting a bone in proper position for healing

immobilized unable to move

abducted to move an arm or leg away from the center of the body

prosthesis artificial replacement for a body part such as a limb or eye

FIGURE 7-12

Hip fracture precautions.

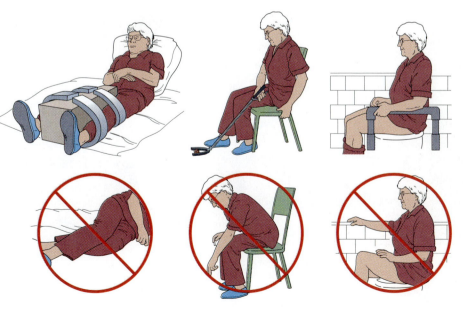

OBSERVATION OF A RESIDENT WITH A CAST

If you observe:	It is caused by:	You should then:
A. Staining of the cast	Bleeding or drainage from a sore under the cast	Circle and date the stained area. (Figure 7-13A) Notify charge nurse.
B. Resident unable to move fingers or toes or complains of numbness, tingling or pain	Pressure on the nerves from a cast that is too tight or positioned improperly	Check for swelling. (Figure 7-13B) Reposition the limb. Check for signs of decreased circulation. Notify charge nurse.
C. Skin cool below the cast	Pressure that decreases circulation	Check for pressure. (Figure 7-13C) Notify charge nurse immediately.
D. Swelling of fingers and toes	New injury or decreased circulation	Support the cast. (Figure 7-13D) Notify charge nurse immediately.
E. Cast becomes soiled or stained around upper leg or perineal area	Urine or feces	Wipe with damp cloth. Do not soak with water. Protect from future soiling by placing plastic wrap around the edges. Plastic wrap can be washed or changed when necessary. (Figure 7-13E)
F. Slow return of nailbeds to pink after pressing ("blanching")	Decreased circulation from pressure of cast	Notify charge nurse immediately.
G. Foul or musty odor from cast	Infection under the cast	Notify charge nurse.
H. Complaints of itching from resident	Dry flaky skin under cast or loose plaster	Wash as far as possible with a damp cloth. Use a bulb syringe to blow air under the cast. Discourage resident from scratching with a sharp object.
I. Cast has sharp or rough edges	Cast breaking down around edges	Petal the cast. Cut 1-inch pieces of 1-inch-wide adhesive tape. Place the tape over the edge, half on the inside and half on the outside. This procedure is carried out by a licensed nurse.

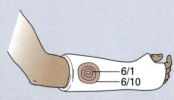

A. Circle the stained area

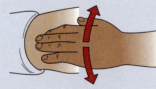

B. Check the skin

FIGURE 7-13

Observation of a resident with a cast.

C. Check for pressure

D. Support the cast

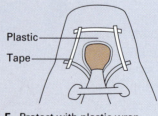

Plastic

Tape

E. Protect with plastic wrap

THE RESIDENT WITH A CAST

The nursing assistant provides valuable information through daily observations of the resident with a cast. During your routine nursing care, notice the condition of the resident and the condition of the cast itself. Report any changes promptly.

On those occasions when traction is used to promote and maintain alignment of broken bones or other conditions (back or neck pain), good body alignment is essential. **Traction** means the exertion of pull by means of weights and pulleys. **Countertraction** (exertion of pull in the opposite direction) must be present to maintain body alignment. Although the nursing assistant never adjusts or changes the equipment used, you must observe and report to your charge nurse.

When caring for the resident in traction, be sure to ask yourself:

- Are ropes frayed?
- Are weights hanging freely?
- Is the rope on the pulley?
- Is the resident positioned properly in the bed?
- Is the splint positioned correctly?
- Does the resident complain of pain?

Because a resident is less active when in a cast or traction, the risk of pressure ulcers is increased. In addition to checking the cast or traction, check the skin on the rest of the resident's body as part of your routine care. Be alert for signs of pressure!

The third goal of care for the resident with a fracture is **rehabilitation,** restoring normal function. Restoring normal function begins by preventing complications of the fracture. When enough time has passed, a program of exercise and mobility is begun. The physician directs the program through the physical therapist. This program is meaningless if poor nursing care has allowed the resident to develop pressure sores or contractures.

CULTURAL AWARENESS Although much of the American culture places high value on their independence and returning those sick and injured to their previous level of function, other cultures differ. For example, in the Japanese culture, which is known for respecting elders, family members step in and do for the injured elder. The Japanese elder often expects to be cared for by others rather than maintain or regain independence. This resident may not appear motivated, or staff who are unaware of the cultural differences may perceive the resident as lazy, uncooperative, or demanding. Remember, not all cultures value independence. The challenge will be to motivate the resident in other ways. Find out what the individual resident does value and attempt to use the information to motivate. For example, if the resident values appearance, he or she might be motivated by the unsightly appearance of contractures of the joints.

During the entire time of recovery from a fracture, the nursing staff must have a positive, hopeful attitude that the resident will regain maximum independence. Attitudes are contagious! The mental attitude of the resident can speed up or slow down the recovery process.

traction exertion of "pull" by means of weights

countertraction exertion of pull in the opposite direction of traction

rehabilitation the restoration of the individual to the fullest physical, mental, social, vocational, and economic capacity of which he or she is capable

OBJECTIVES
What You Will Learn

When you have completed this section, you will be able to:

• Describe four tips for teamwork

• Move a resident by using a lift sheet
• Move residents up in bed with their help
• Turn a resident onto the side away from you or toward you

• Turn a resident by using the log-rolling technique
• Identify proper lifting and moving techniques

KEY TERM   Log rolling

LIFTING AND MOVING THE RESIDENT

Nursing assistants are required to lift and move residents many times a day. In order to protect yourself from injury, you need to observe the following principles:

1. Use any mechanical devices available to help you. They may seem time consuming, but a back injury may cause a lifetime of pain and suffering. These devices include mechanical lifts, transfer boards, sliding boards, and so on.
2. Always get help. It is safer for both you and the resident.
3. When appropriate, use a transfer belt on the resident to provide a "handle."
4. As a last resort, use a back support. These supports are controversial since they may make you think you can lift more weight that is safe for you. Also, if not properly used (tightened for lifting and released when no lifting), the muscles of the back may actually weaken from lack of use.

You'll need to use the principles of body mechanics learned in Chapter 2 to protect yourself and the resident from injury.

Every time a resident needs to be moved, you must ask yourself, "Can I do it alone or do I need help?" When in doubt, ask for help. It is also important to gain the cooperation and assistance of those residents who are able to help themselves. Remember, it is good for residents to do as much as they can for themselves.

WORKING AS A TEAM

Regardless of the specific task, whenever two or more people are needed, there are some tips that will help you work better as a team.

• Before asking for help, be sure you are ready. Do as much of the task as possible. For example, have the resident "ready." If you are going to move the resident up in bed, have the bed in the proper position. You'll find that being considerate of your co-workers this way will assure their willingness to help you.
• Decide who is in charge. Usually, it is the person assigned to that resident, but it could also be the most experienced person. Regardless of who it will be, the decision must be made in advance.

PROCEDURE

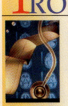

Moving the Resident by Using a Lift Sheet

Beginning Steps

1. Explain to the resident what you are going to do.
2. Provide privacy.
3. Remove the pillow from under the resident's head.
4. Stabilize the bed by locking the wheels. (Figure 7-14)
5. Raise the bed to a comfortable working height, if possible.

Steps

6. With one nursing assistant on each side of the bed, roll the lift sheet as close as possible to the resident's body. (Figure 7-15)
7. Stand straight with feet about 12 inches apart. Your body should be turned slightly toward the head of the bed, with your feet pointed in the direction of the move (toward the head of the bed). If moving side to side, your toes point toward the side of the bed.
8. Grasp the rolled sheet with your hands at the resident's shoulder and at the hip. (Figure 7-16)

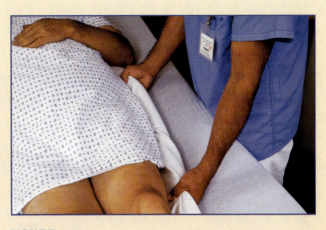

FIGURE 7-15
Roll the lift sheet as close as possible to the resident's body.

9. Count "one, two, three."
10. Keeping your back straight and knees bent, slide the resident toward the head of the bed (or toward the side of the bed) as you shift your weight from one foot to the other.

Ending Steps

11. Replace the pillow.
12. Position the resident comfortably.
13. Lower the bed to the lowest position.
14. Place the call signal within reach.
15. Wash your hands.

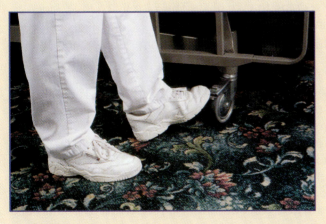

FIGURE 7-14
Stabilize the bed by locking the wheels.

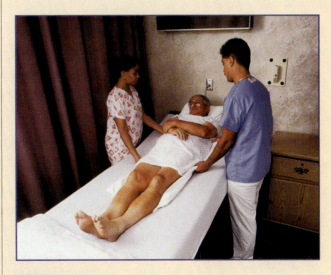

FIGURE 7-16
Grasp the rolled sheet with your hands at the resident's shoulder and hip.

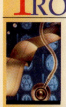

PROCEDURE

Assisting the Resident to Move Up in Bed

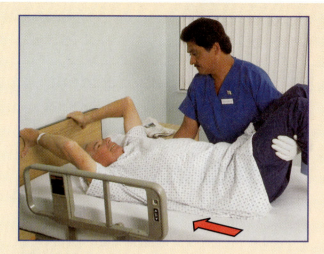

FIGURE 7-17
Slide the resident toward the head of the bed.

Beginning Steps

1. Wash your hands.
2. Tell the resident what you are going to do.
3. Provide privacy.
4. Raise the bed to a comfortable working height. Lower the headrest.
5. Stabilize the bed.

Steps

6. Stand next to the bed with your feet about 12 inches apart. The foot closer to the head of the bed should be pointed in that direction.
7. Place one hand under the resident's shoulder and one under the buttocks.
8. Ask the resident to bend the knees and brace the feet firmly against the mattress. If not using a trapeze, the resident may either reach up and grasp the headboard or place the hands on the mattress about hip level with the elbows bent.
9. On the signal "one, two, three," have the resident push toward the head of the bed with hands and feet against the mattress as you slide the resident toward the head, with your back straight and knees bent. (Figure 7-17)

Ending Steps

10. Replace the pillow.
11. Position the resident comfortably.
12. Lower the bed to its lowest position.
13. Place the call signal within reach.
14. Wash your hands.

- Review out loud what is going to take place. This also helps the resident know what is happening.
- Coordinate your activities by counting out loud. For example, "one, two, three, lift."

Some residents are best moved with a "lift" or "turn" sheet. This is simply a sheet (folded for extra strength) placed under the resident from shoulders to knees. The turn sheet prevents friction between the resident's skin and the bed, and it lessens the effort required of the nursing assistant. You may use the lift sheet to move the resident toward the head of the bed or to one side of the bed. The procedure is essentially the same, except for the direction of the move.

Whenever residents are able to help, encourage them to do so. Not only do they feel better about themselves, but they also receive exercise and build strength. Some residents can utilize an overhead trapeze to help them lift, turn, and move about in bed. If you feel that one of your residents has the strength and coordination to use a trapeze, suggest it to your charge nurse so that a physician's order can be obtained.

With or without a trapeze, the procedure for moving residents up in bed with their help is essentially the same.

In addition to moving the resident toward the head of the bed, you will also move the resident from one side of the bed to the other. This may be

PROCEDURE

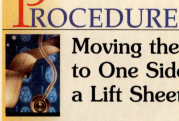

Moving the Resident to One Side Without a Lift Sheet

Beginning Steps

1. Wash your hands.
2. Tell the resident what you are going to do.
3. Provide privacy.
4. Raise the bed to a comfortable working position.
5. Lower the headrest.
6. Lower the side rail on the side where you will be working (you will be moving the resident toward you).

Steps

7. With your hand under the knees and ankles, move the resident's feet and legs toward you. (Figure 7-18)

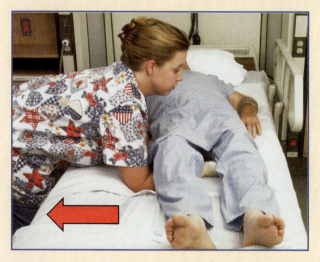

FIGURE 7-18

8. Place your forearms under the small of the back and the buttocks and slide the resident toward you (Figure 7-19). (Remember to keep your back straight and knees bent.)
9. Place your hands under the resident's shoulders and slide the resident toward you.

Ending Steps

10. Replace the pillow.
11. Place the call signal within reach.
12. Adjust the height of the bed and headrest.
13. Wash your hands.

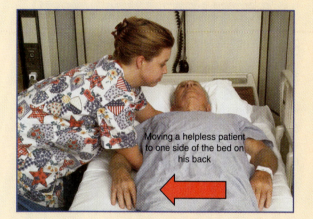

Moving a helpless patient to one side of the bed on his back

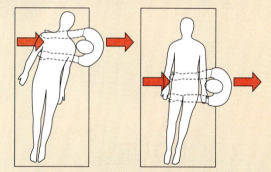

As a safety measure, this procedure must be done before turning a patient onto his side. It insures that the patient, when turned, is located in the center of the mattress.

FIGURE 7-19

done by one or two people and with or without a turn sheet. The principles of safety for resident and staff members are most important. Not only must we guard against falls and back injury, but also against injury to the resident's skin.

Usually, a person is moved to one side of the bed in order to be turned and repositioned. This ensures that when turned the resident will be positioned safely in the center of the bed.

Although turning a resident away from you requires less effort, there may be times when you will turn the resident toward you. This usually occurs when you are assisting a doctor or nurse with an examination or treatment.

PROCEDURE

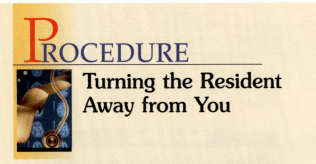

Turning the Resident Away from You

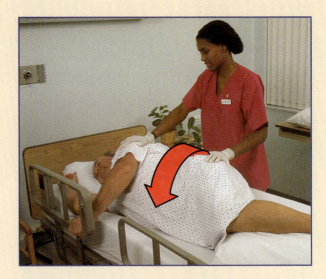

FIGURE 7-20

Move your hand from knee to hip to shoulder to complete the turn.

Beginning Steps

1. See steps 1 to 9, "Moving the Resident to One Side Without a Lift Sheet."

Steps

2. If possible, flex (bend) the resident's knee of the leg nearest you.
3. If the knee cannot be bent, cross the near leg over the far leg.
4. Place one hand on the knee and one on the hip.
5. Push down on the knee and over on the hip to roll the resident over.
6. Move your hand from the knee to the hip and from the hip to the shoulder to complete the turn. (Figure 7-20)
7. Position in either the semisupine or semiprone position.

Ending Steps

8. Replace the head pillow.
9. Place the call signal within reach.
10. Lower the bed.
11. Wash your hands.

PROCEDURE

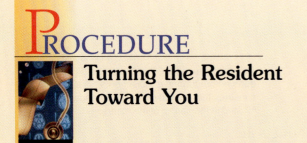

Turning the Resident Toward You

Beginning Steps

1. Wash your hands.
2. Tell the resident what you are going to do.
3. Provide privacy.
4. Stabilize the bed.
5. Raise the bed to a comfortable working height.
6. Lower the backrest and footrest, if this is allowed.
7. Raise the side rail on the far side of the bed.

8. Loosen the top sheets without exposing the resident.

Steps

9. When you are turning the resident toward you, cross the leg furthest from you over the leg closest to you. (Figure 7-21)

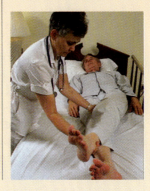

FIGURE 7-21

Cross the leg.

PROCEDURE
continued

10. Cross the resident's arms over the chest.
11. Reach across the resident and put one hand behind the shoulder. (Figure 7-22)
12. Place your other hand behind the hip and gently roll the resident toward you. (Figure 7-23)

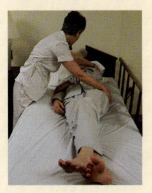

FIGURE 7-22
Place one hand behind the shoulder.

Ending Steps

13. Replace the head pillow.
14. Place the resident in a comfortable position.
15. Check to make sure the call signal is within easy reach of the resident.
16. Lower the bed to its lowest horizontal position.
17. Wash your hands.

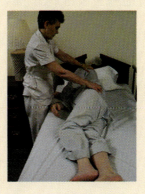

FIGURE 7-23
Roll the resident toward you.

PROCEDURE
Turning the Resident by Using the Log-Rolling Technique

Beginning Steps

1. Wash your hands.
2. Identify the resident.
3. Tell the resident what you are going to do.
4. Provide privacy.
5. Stabilize the bed.
6. Raise the bed to a comfortable working height.
7. Raise the side rail on the far side of the bed.

Steps

8. Request help.
9. Remove the pillow from under the resident's head, if allowed.
10. Use a lift sheet. Roll the sheet up as close as possible to the resident's body.

11. Keep your knees bent and your back straight as you lift the resident to one side of the bed. Remember to count "one, two, three" to coordinate your movements.
12. Using the turn sheet, roll the resident onto one side like a log, turning the body as a whole unit, without bending the joints. Turn gently. You may need one person to support the leg during the turn. (Figure 7-24)

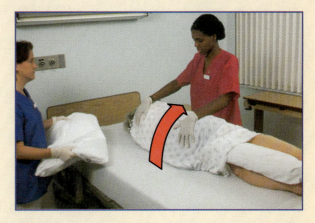

FIGURE 7-24
Roll the resident like a log.

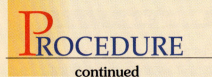
Ending Steps

13. Replace the pillow under the resident's head, if allowed.
14. Use pillows against the resident's back to keep the body in proper alignment. (Figure 7-25)
15. Remake the top of the bed.
16. Make the resident comfortable. Lower the bed to its lowest horizontal position.
17. Place the call cord within reach.
18. Wash your hands.

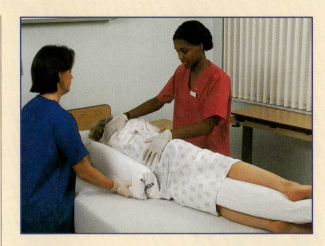

FIGURE 7-25
Use pillows against the back.

log rolling a technique of turning a patient

There are residents who must be moved and turned without disturbing the alignment of the body. Rather than being moved in sections, they must be moved as one unit. This technique of turning is called **log-rolling.** Residents who must be log-rolled are usually those who have had recent back or hip surgery. Your charge nurse will tell you which residents must be log-rolled. This information will be on the health-care plan and may be posted at the bedside. Log-rolling should be done with at least two people and a turn or lift sheet.

Always remember to use good body mechanics when lifting and moving residents. Be alert for safety hazards to protect yourself as well as the resident!

SECTION 4 Transfer Techniques

OBJECTIVES
What You Will Learn

When you have completed this section, you will be able to:

- Transfer a resident using the pivot technique
- Transfer a dependent resident
- List four principles related to transfer technique
- Distinguish proper from improper transfer techniques

KEY TERMS

hemiplegic

transfer belt

transferring

TRANSFERRING THE RESIDENT

transferring to move from one place to another

The need to move a resident from bed to wheelchair or wheelchair to toilet occurs many times each day. This process is called **transferring.** Many techniques are used to transfer a resident depending on the strength and ability of both the nursing assistant and the resident. This is a time when safety must be uppermost in your mind. Good body mechanics are a must! Review the section on body mechanics before you proceed with learning transfer techniques.

In keeping with the philosophy of rehabilitation, the resident should be encouraged to do as much as possible. Each step of the procedure must be explained to the resident to ensure cooperation in completing a smooth transfer.

You will learn to pivot transfer a person who is paralyzed on one side of the body (**hemiplegic**) or one who has general weakness and to transfer a person who is completely unable to assist you. Transfer technique must be demonstrated and practiced many times before skill is developed.

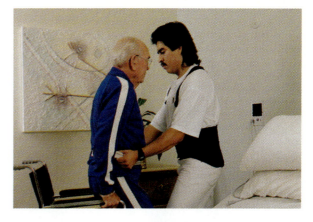

FIGURE 7-26
Using a transfer belt.

TRANSFER BELT

Use of a **transfer belt** is one technique that protects both the resident and you from injury. The belt is placed around the waist of the resident to provide the nursing assistant with a "handle" to hold during transfer (Figure 7-26). This allows good control of the transfer as well as eliminating injury to the resident's skin. Many facilities issue each nursing assistant a transfer belt. For convenience, the nursing assistant wears the belt around his or her own waist so that it will be readily available when needed.

Transferring a resident on or off a toilet or from a wheelchair to bed incorporates the same techniques as those just described. Remember the principles and apply them.

hemiplegic   paralyzed on one side of the body

transfer belt   belt placed around the resident's waist to provide a "handle" to hold during transfer

PROCEDURE

Pivot Transfer of the Hemiplegic Resident

Beginning Steps

1. Wash your hands.
2. Bring necessary equipment to the bedside:
   - Wheelchair
   - Transfer belt
   - Cushion
   - Lap robe or blanket
3. Tell the resident what you are going to do.

Steps

4. Prepare the resident (dress appropriately), including shoes with nonskid soles.
5. Position the wheelchair on the resident's nonparalyzed side so that you can move the resident toward the stronger side. Do not refer to the resident's "good" or "bad" side.

6. Place the chair at a 45-degree angle to the bed with the brakes on the chair in the locked position. Place the pedals up and out of the way. If possible, remove the armrest on the side next to the bed.
7. Stabilize the bed.
8. Place the bed in the lowest position, if possible.
9. Assist the resident to a sitting position with feet "dangling" over the edge of the bed.
10. Place the transfer belt around the resident's waist. (Figure 7-27)

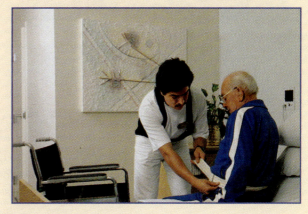

FIGURE 7-27
Place the transfer belt around the waist.

PROCEDURE

continued

11. Allow the resident to gain balance by sitting for a few minutes on the edge of the bed.

12. Stand in front of the resident with your hands gripping the transfer belt, one on either side of the resident's waist. Never allow residents to place their arms around your neck. This could lead to a serious injury, and you would lose control of the transfer.

13. Position yourself so that the resident's paralyzed leg is between your knees, keeping your base of support about 18 inches.

14. Assist the resident to stand while you support the paralyzed leg with your knees. (Figure 7-28)

15. Instruct the resident to reach with the nonparalyzed hand and grasp the farthest armrest of the wheelchair.

16. Assist the resident to pivot (turn) toward the nonparalyzed leg by pivoting your own body. Do not twist. Turn your body as a unit. (Figure 7-29)

17. Gently lower the resident into the chair by bending your knees and keeping your back straight. (Figure 7-30)

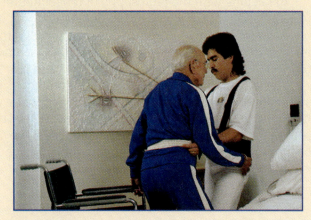

FIGURE 7-29

Assist the resident to pivot.

Ending Steps

18. Remove the transfer belt.

19. Position the paralyzed arm and leg properly on the armrest and footrest. The resident may now use the footrest on his or her strong side to allow him to guide the chair by pushing against the floor.

20. Apply a safety belt or soft-tie protective device if ordered by the doctor and if necessary for resident safety.

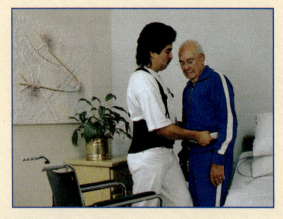

FIGURE 7-28

Assist the resident to stand.

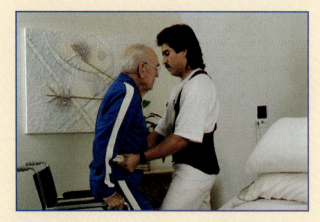

FIGURE 7-30

Lower the resident into the chair.

- Plan and organize what you're going to do before you begin.
- Encourage the resident to do as much as possible.
- Remember, safety first for both the resident and yourself.
- Use your transfer belt.
- Use good body mechanics.

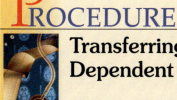

PROCEDURE

Transferring the Dependent Resident

Beginning Steps

1. Wash your hands.
2. Take the necessary equipment to the bedside.
3. Explain to the resident what you are going to do.
4. Provide privacy.
5. Dress the resident appropriately. *Note:* Do not seek help until you have done everything possible in advance. This allows the helper to spend a minimal amount of time, helping only when necessary.

Steps

6. Position the wheelchair next to the bed at a 45-degree angle facing the foot of the bed. Remove the near armrest if possible. Lock the brakes. (Figure 7-31)
7. Obtain the help of one or two persons, depending on the resident's weight and ability to cooperate.
8. Place the taller nursing assistant at the head of the bed and the shorter at the level of the resident's knees.
9. Assist the resident to sit up in bed with legs remaining on the bed. Apply the transfer belt around the resident's waist.

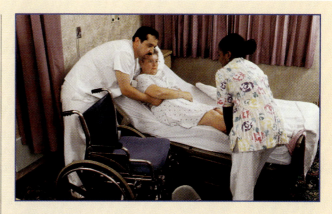

FIGURE 7-32

One grasps the belt, the other reaches under the legs.

10. Have the person at the head reach around the resident and grasp the belt on either side of the resident's waist. The person at the foot reaches under the resident's knees and thighs. (Figure 7-32)
11. Count "one, two, three," and move the resident to the edge of the bed.
12. Reestablish your base of support. Count "one, two, three" again and carefully lift the resident into the chair.

Ending Steps

13. Remove the transfer belt. (Figure 7-33)
14. Position the resident properly with feet on the pedals and hips well back in the chair. Apply a seat belt or soft-tie protective device if needed and ordered by the doctor.

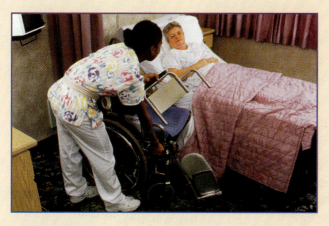

FIGURE 7-31

Remove the armrest and lock the brakes.

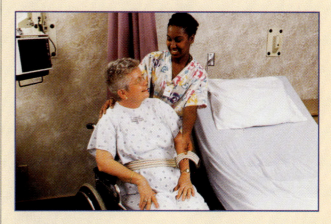

FIGURE 7-33

Remove the transfer belt.

SUMMARY

SUMMARY This chapter contained some difficult and complex skills. The skills are used many times each day and involve great risk to both the resident and the nursing assistant. There is risk of back injury and of sprained wrists, arms, and shoulders for the nursing assistant. For the resident, there is danger of scratching, bruising, skin tears, and even falling. Work at perfecting the skills of lifting, moving, and transferring your residents in a safe and efficient way. Remember to use mechanical lifts if at all possible. Once you get used to them, it becomes easier and your back will thank you. If you are uncertain or believe that you have not mastered the skills, ask for help. Your instructor, the facility educator, and the physical therapist are good resources.

All residents must be told what you are going to do in a step-by-step manner as you are lifting and moving them. Probably the most important difference in caring for the elderly is that everything should be done *slowly*. Think about how you can slow your pace as you lift, move, and transfer the resident.

OBRA HIGHLIGHTS

According to the regulations, "A resident's abilities in activities of daily living do not diminish unless circumstances of the individual's clinical condition demonstrate that diminution was unavoidable. This includes the resident's ability to bathe, dress, and groom; transfer and ambulate; toilet; eat; and use speech, language, or other functional communication systems."

SELF STUDY

Choose the best answer for each question or statement.

1. Which of the following structures make up the skeletal system?
   a. bones and muscles
   b. bones and joints
   c. bones and teeth
   d. cranium and vertebrae

2. A resident fell and tore a ligament in his knee. The damaged structure serves what purpose?
   a. connects bone to bone
   b. connects muscle to bone
   c. pads the ends of the bones
   d. prevents friction on the ends of bones

3. Mr. Melvin has osteoarthritis in his knees and hips. Which of the following is true of osteoarthritis?
   a. It affects people of all ages, especially young adults.
   b. It causes deformity of joints and crippling.
   c. It is caused by deterioration and abrasion of cartilage in the joints.
   d. It causes joints to become stiff, red, and swollen.

4. A condition of the bones that causes them to become chalklike and break easily is called
   a. osteoarthritis
   b. rheumatoid arthritis
   c. osteobursitis
   d. osteoporosis

5. Which of the following are symptoms of a fracture?
   a. bruising and swelling in the affected area
   b. pain and tenderness over the site
   c. deformity or misalignment of the area
   d. all of these are fracture symptoms

6. Mrs. Micah has a fractured hip. She has just returned to the long-term care facility from the hospital where she had surgery to repair the hip fracture. Which of the following actions will you take when you care for Mrs. Micah?
   a. Keep an abduction wedge between her legs at all times.

b. Exercise her affected leg vigorously, bending her knee and hip past 90 degrees.
   c. Cross her legs before you get her out of bed to keep the hip stable.
   d. all of the above

7. Mr. Stevens has a fractured left wrist. He has a cast on his left lower arm and hand. You notice a dark reddish-brown stain on the underneath side of the cast. Which of the following actions should you take?
   a. Wash the cast with soap and water to remove the stain, and notify the charge nurse.
   b. Circle and date the stained area; then notify the charge nurse.
   c. Check for pressure of the cast against the arm in the stained area.
   d. Blow air under the cast with a bulb syringe in the area of the stain.

8. Mr. Stevens complains of itching under his cast. Which of the following should you do to help relieve the itching?
   a. Cut pieces of tape and cover the edge of the cast with petals so the edges of the cast don't cause further itching.
   b. Give him a straightened wire hanger to use to scratch underneath the cast.
   c. Sprinkle a generous amount of powder down the cast to absorb moisture that causes itching.
   d. Wash under the cast with a damp cloth, then blow air under the cast with a bulb syringe.

9. Mrs. Jefferson is in a long leg cast. Because she is less active than usual, which of the following observations would you make?
   a. Look for areas that could form pressure ulcers.
   b. Ask her the date, time, and who the president is.
   c. Look for ways to attach traction to the cast in case it is needed.
   d. Look for a rash on her toes or upper body.

10. Which of the following actions should you take when you move or lift a resident?
    a. Do not use mechanical devices such as lifts unless absolutely necessary.
    b. Avoid asking others for help unless the resident is much too heavy for you to lift alone.
    c. Use a transfer belt on the resident when appropriate.
    d. Use a back support only if you have previously injured your back.

11. Which of the following actions should you take when you work as a team to lift or move a resident?
    a. Do as much of the task as possible before asking for help.
    b. Decide who is in charge of the procedure.
    c. Count out loud so you coordinate your movements.
    d. Use all of these actions to work as a team.

12. Mr. Mathis has had back surgery and must be turned by log rolling. How will you turn him?
    a. Turn his body in sections: first the feet, then the trunk, then the head.
    b. Turn his body in sections: first the head, then the trunk, then the feet.
    c. Turn his body as one unit using a turn sheet and two other people.
    d. Turn his body as one unit using a mechanical lift or other device.

13. How does a transfer belt help protect you and the resident from injury?
    a. The belt is placed around the resident's waist and serves as a handle for you to hold during transfers.
    b. The belt is placed around your waist to give you support and give the resident a handle to hold during transfers.
    c. The belt is placed under the resident's armpits and is used to lift the resident to a standing position.
    d. The belt is placed around the resident's hips and is used to lift the hips without causing strain on your back.

14. When you transfer a patient, which of the following guidelines should you follow?
    a. Get help, then plan how you will complete the transfer.
    b. Instruct the resident to relax and let the staff do the moving.
    c. Use good body mechanics and a transfer belt.
    d. All of these guidelines should be followed during transfers.

15. The tough, gristle-like substance that pads the ends of bones is called
    a. a tendon
    b. cartilage
    c. bursa
    d. a joint

16. When the bones of a joint are no longer aligned correctly, which of the following conditions exist?
    a. osteoarthritis
    b. fracture
    c. dislocation
    d. sprain

Getting C O N N E C T E D
Multimedia Extension Activities

www.prenhall.com/will-black

Use the above address to access the free, interactive Companion Website created for this textbook. Hear the pronunciation of the key terms in the chapter. Get instant feedback to a variety of chapter-related questions. Link to other interesting sites.

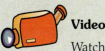

Video

Watch the video *Transfer and Ambulation* from the Care Provider Skills series.

CASE STUDY

Mrs. Jones is a 55-year-old woman admitted to the facility for rehabilitation following a serious automobile accident. She has a fracture of her left arm and of her left femur, tibia, and fibula. She weighs about 280 pounds. You are assigned to care for her the day after she arrives.

1. She complains to you of pain in her left arm, which is in a cast. You notice a dark stain around the elbow. You should
   a. ignore it because it must be old
   b. notify the charge nurse immediately so she can mark the cast and notify the doctor
   c. mark the darkened area by drawing a circle and dating and timing it
   d. tell the resident that she should get used to a little pain

2. When you review your assignment, you are pleased that you don't have to get her out of bed until the therapist authorizes it. Your care should be directed toward
   a. avoiding disturbing her
   b. preventing the harmful effects of immobility including contractures
   c. protecting yourself from injury
   d. being an active listener

3. The therapist needs your help to get her out of bed for her therapy appointment. Your preparation should include all of the following *except*
   a. informing her that you will be helping to get her out of bed
   b. placing the wheelchair on her right side
   c. placing the wheelchair on her left side
   d. obtaining additional help for her transfer

4. Because she has been in bed for over a week since her accident, plans to get her up should include
   a. taking her temperature
   b. raising the head of the bed so she adjusts to being upright
   c. getting her up quickly so it will be less painful
   d. being sure her family is present to watch

Chapter 8

THE MUSCULAR SYSTEM

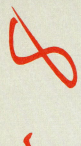

CARING TIP

Safety is the primary concern while walking a resident.

Becki Ross, RN
Health Occupations Instructor
Puxico, Missouri

SECTION 1 Anatomy and Physiology

KEY TERMS

ankylosed
atrophy
cardiac muscle tissue

contracture
edema
ligaments
muscular dystrophy

paralysis
smooth muscle tissue
striated muscle tissue
tendons

THE MUSCULAR SYSTEM

The muscular system is composed of:

- Muscles
- Tendons
- Ligaments

Muscles are made of three different kinds of tissue (Figure 8-1). **Striated muscle tissue,** also called the *voluntary muscles,* resembles a group of ropes held together tightly. This type of tissue makes up all the muscles that you can move consciously.

Smooth muscle tissue is also called the *involuntary muscles.* These muscles work on their own and include the muscles that push food and water through the gastrointestinal tract. Smooth muscle allows actions such as dilation and contraction of the pupil of the eye and blood vessels.

Cardiac muscle tissue controls the heartbeat. It is involuntary and contracts and relaxes about 72 times per minute in the average adult, creating the pulse.

Tendons are elastic cordlike structures that connect muscles to bone. **Ligaments** are tough, white, fibrous cords that connect bone to bone.

The muscular system functions to provide the body with:

- Movement
- Heat
- Posture
- Protection

striated muscle tissue
type of voluntary muscle tissue

smooth muscle tissue
involuntary muscle tissue

cardiac muscle tissue
type of muscle in the heart that controls the heartbeat

tendons elastic cordlike structures that connect muscles to bone

ligaments tough, white, fibrous cords that connect bone to bone

FIGURE 8-1

Types of muscle tissue.

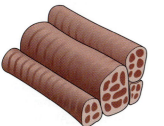

Striated muscle tissue

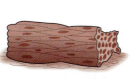

Smooth muscle tissue

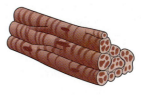

Cardiac muscle tissue

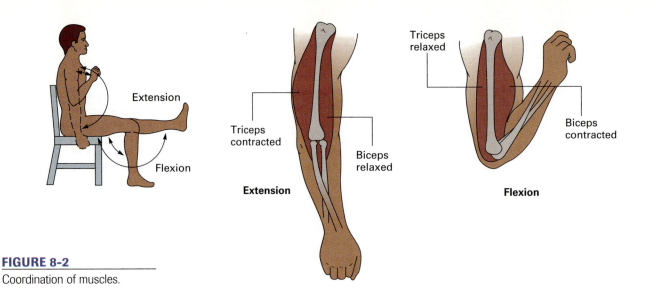

FIGURE 8-2
Coordination of muscles.

The muscular system makes all motion possible inside and outside the body. Muscles are able to provide movement because they are attached to movable parts of the body. The attachments are usually to bones that function as levers in movement. However, attachment may also be to soft tissue, other muscles, connective tissue, and even to skin.

Muscles seldom move independently. Most movement is a result of the co-ordinated action of several muscles (Figure 8-2). Flex your arm by bringing it toward you. The large muscle, the biceps, on the anterior portion of your upper arm contracts (tightens) while the large muscle on the posterior portion of your upper arm, the triceps, relaxes. When you extend or straighten your arm, the opposite occurs—the triceps contracts and the biceps relaxes.

There is a complex system of chemical reactions that allows muscles to con-tract and relax, producing movement. The end result of this process is the pro-duction of energy (heat). The muscles not only move the body, but they also produce heat. This heat production is increased during physical activity or exercise.

Muscles have an abundant blood supply that delivers oxygen and nutri-ents to the muscle cells. This rich blood supply makes the muscle tissue more resistant to infection than all other body tissues. The muscles provide support to the bones of the skeleton and give posture to the body.

MUSCULAR SYSTEM ABNORMALITIES

paralysis loss of volun-tary movement

Paralysis means loss of voluntary movement. Paralysis of a body part can occur as a result of injury or illness. Damage to the brain or spinal cord makes it im-possible to transmit the necessary signals that tell the muscles to act or react, so voluntary movement is lost.

muscular dystrophy a group of related muscle dis-eases that are progressively crippling due to weakness and atrophy of muscles

Muscular dystrophy is a group of related muscle diseases that are pro-gressively crippling due to weakness and atrophy of muscles. It affects the muscles themselves. This disease is different from multiple sclerosis, where the muscles become useless due to damage to the nerves that control them. Muscular dystrophy affects almost a quarter of a million Americans. These people frequently require ongoing nursing care in LTC facilities. At this time, all the causes of muscular dystrophy are not known, and there is no specific cure.

EFFECTS OF AGING AND DISUSE ON THE MUSCULAR SYSTEM

Older persons usually lose some muscle strength and muscle bulk. When people remain physically active, these changes do not occur, or they occur more slowly. Since the body is designed to function most efficiently when movement is present, immobility (the limitation of movement) through disuse results in many changes. Most of these changes are serious and tend to be permanent.

Atrophy occurs when muscle mass decreases in size (also called wasting of muscle). When muscles are not used for any reason (paralysis, limb in a cast or brace, pain, lack of motivation to move, etc.), atrophy occurs.

atrophy decreasing of muscle mass; wasting of muscle tissue

Contracture is a permanent shortening of the muscle. When a muscle is not used, it becomes "fixed" or very resistant to stretching. Contractures occur most often in well-developed muscles, usually the muscles that allow flexion or bending of the joints. They commonly occur in the hands, fingers, elbows, hips, and knees. Contractures can lead to permanent disability or loss of function. If untreated, the joints themselves become **ankylosed** or "frozen."

contracture shortening of the muscles from inactivity

Contractures are painful and unsightly. Even though a resident may never walk or perform activities of daily living independently, you should not allow contractures to develop. The resident has a right to be free of the deformity and pain that results from inadequate care. Contractures contribute to skin breakdown because of a change in the distribution of body weight. Residents with contractures are more difficult to move, position, bathe, and dress.

ankylosed condition in which joints become very stiff, unmovable, and frozen

Contractures occur as a result of improper support and positioning of joints affected by arthritis, injury, inadequate movement, and exercise. **Edema** (swelling) of tissue or a joint for any reason contributes to the development of contractures. The fluid that produces edema becomes like glue and limits movement of the swollen joint. Residents who are dependent on others are especially prone to developing contractures. Special range-of-motion exercises must be given to residents as a preventive measure. Learning how to perform these exercises is an important part of your training.

edema swelling of joints, tissue, or organs

SECTION 2 Nursing Care Related to the Muscular System

OBJECTIVES
What You Will Learn

When you have completed this section, you will be able to:

- Correctly perform range of motion for a dependent resident
- List four observations to be made, reported, and recorded while performing range of motion

- List the steps depicting readiness for ambulation
- Ambulate a resident using the step-by-step procedure
- List the safety precautions for ambulation devices
- List four reasons why dependent residents must be repositioned frequently

- Properly position a dependent resident in a wheelchair
- Correctly position a dependent resident in the:
  a. Supine position
  b. Semisupine
  c. Prone position
  d. Semiprone position

KEY TERMS

abduction	bridging	passive	spasticity
active	dorsiflexion	plantar flexion	supination
adduction	extension	pronation	trochanter roll
alignment	flexion	radial deviation	ulnar deviation
ambulation	gait belt	range of motion	
	hyperextension	rotation	

ambulation   walking or moving about in an upright position

range of motion   extent to which a joint can be moved before causing pain

passive   done for the patient by the nursing assistant

active   done by the resident independently

adduction   to move an arm or leg toward the center of the body

abduction   to move an arm or leg away from the center of the body

extension   to straighten an arm or leg

hyperextension   to move beyond the normal extension

flexion   to bend a joint (elbow, wrist, knee)

plantar flexion   extending the ankle (toward the sole of the foot)

dorsiflexion   to flex the ankle (away from the sole of the foot)

rotation   to move a joint in a circular motion around its axis

pronation   turning palms down

supination   to turn palms up

radial deviation   toward the thumb side of the hand

ulnar deviation   away from the thumb side of the hand

RANGE-OF-MOTION EXERCISES

Nursing care of dependent residents is aimed at the prevention or reduction of the effects of disuse on the body through:

- Range-of-motion exercises
- Assisting with **ambulation** (walking)
- Positioning residents properly

   Range of motion means that each joint is put through its normal range of activity. The exercises may be either **passive** (done for the resident by the nursing assistant) or **active** (done by the resident independently).
   Regardless of whether the exercises are active or passive, there are several guidelines to be followed:

- Exercise in an organized, systematic way.
- Never exercise a swollen, reddened joint.
- Be gentle—never exercise beyond the point of pain.
- Support the limb at the joint as it is exercised.
- Put each joint through each movement three times.
- Be particularly careful with exercise of the head and neck since many residents experience pain.

TYPES OF MOVEMENT

The following terms are used to describe the many types of motion that are included in range-of-motion exercises:

- **Adduction**—to move an arm or leg toward the center of the body
- **Abduction**—to move an arm or leg away from the center of the body
- **Extension**—to straighten an arm or leg
- **Hyperextension**—beyond the normal extension
- **Flexion**—to bend a joint (elbow, wrist, knee)
- **Plantar flexion**—to extend the ankle (toward the sole of the foot)
- **Dorsiflexion**—to flex the ankle (away from the sole of the foot)
- **Rotation**—to move a joint in a circular motion around its axis
  —Internal rotation—to turn in toward center
  —External rotation—to turn out away from center
- **Pronation**—to turn palms down
- **Supination**—to turn palms up
- **Radial deviation**—toward the thumb side of the hand
- **Ulnar deviation**—away from the thumb side of the hand

   As you read through the procedure, put your own joints through their range of motion by closely following the illustrations.
   The time spent in performing range-of-motion exercises gives the nursing assistant the chance to observe for special problems and communicate with the resident. You should note and report:

- Swollen joints
- Reddened skin over a joint
- Complaints of pain on movement
- Painful joints
- Weakness

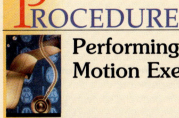

Performing Range-of-Motion Exercises

Beginning Steps

1. Wash your hands.
2. Identify the resident.
3. Explain to the resident what you are going to do.
4. Pull the curtain around the bed for privacy.

Steps

5. Place the resident in a supine position with knees extended and arms at the side.
6. Lower the side rail on the near side of the bed.
7. Exercise the neck.

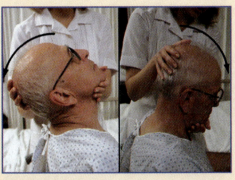

FIGURE 8-3

Head Flexion and Extension: With body straight, gently move head down, up, and backward, then straighten neck again.

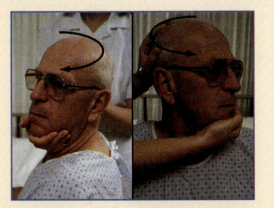

FIGURE 8-4

Right/Left Rotation: With head and body straight, gently rotate head to the right. Come back to the starting position, then rotate head to the left.

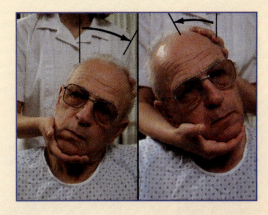

FIGURE 8-5

Right/Left Lateral Flexion: With body and head straight, move head gently toward the right shoulder. Come back to the starting position, then move head toward the left shoulder. Use the weight of the head to help move it.

8. Hold the extremity to be exercised at the joint (i.e., knee, wrist, elbow).
9. Exercise each shoulder.

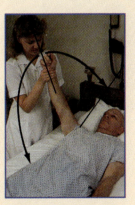

FIGURE 8-6

Shoulder Flexion: With elbow straight, raise arm over head, then lower, *keeping arm in front of you.*

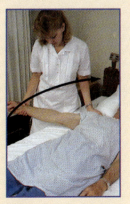

FIGURE 8-7

Shoulder Abduction and Adduction: With elbow straight, raise arm over head, then lower, *keeping arm out to the side.*

PROCEDURE

continued

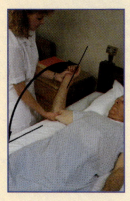

FIGURE 8-8

Shoulder Internal and External Rotation: Bring arm out to the side. Do not bring elbow out to shoulder level. Turn arm back and forth so forearm points down toward feet, then up toward head. With arm alongside body and elbow bent at 90°, turn arm so forearm points across stomach, then out to the side.

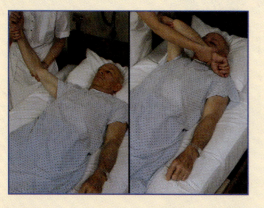

FIGURE 8-9

Shoulder Horizontal Abduction and Adduction: *Keeping arm at shoulder level*, reach across chest past opposite shoulder, then reach out to the side.

10. Exercise each elbow, wrist, and forearm.

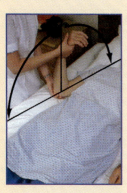

FIGURE 8-10

Elbow Flexion and Extension: With arm alongside body, bend elbow to touch shoulder, then straighten elbow out again.

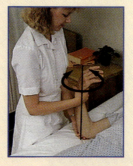

FIGURE 8-11

Forearm Pronation and Supination: With arm alongside the body and elbow bent to 90°, turn forearm so palm faces first toward head, then toward feet.

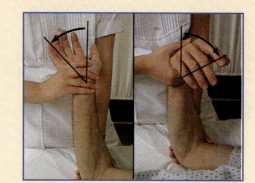
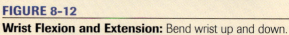

FIGURE 8-12

Wrist Flexion and Extension: Bend wrist up and down.

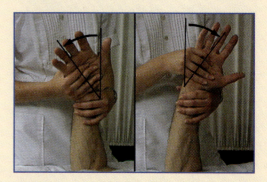

FIGURE 8-13

Ulnar and Radial Deviation: Bend wrist from side to side.

11. Exercise each finger.

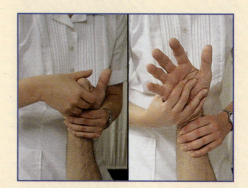

FIGURE 8-14

Finger Flexion and Extension: Make a fist, then straighten fingers out together.

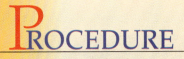
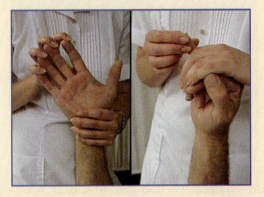

FIGURE 8-15
Individual Finger Flexion and Extension: Move each joint individually. Touch tip of each finger to its base, then straighten each finger in turn.

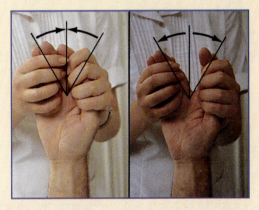

FIGURE 8-16
Finger Adduction and Abduction: With fingers straight, squeeze fingers together, then spread them apart.

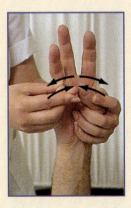

FIGURE 8-17
Finger/Thumb Opposition: Touch thumb to the tip of each finger to make a circle. Open hand fully between touching each finger.

12. Exercise the hip.

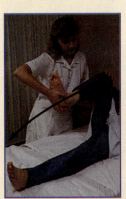

FIGURE 8-18
Hip/Knee Flexion and Extension: Bend knee and bring it up toward chest, keeping foot off bed. Lower leg to bed, straightening knee as it goes down.

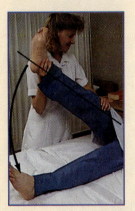

FIGURE 8-19
Straight Leg Raising: Keeping the knee straight, raise leg up off the bed. Return slowly to the bed, keeping the knee straight.

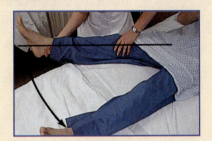

FIGURE 8-20
Hip Abduction and Adduction: With leg flat on bed and knee kept pointing to ceiling, slide leg out to the side. Then slide it back to touch across the other leg.

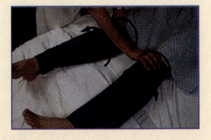

FIGURE 8-21
Hip Internal and External Rotation: With legs flat on bed and feet apart, turn both legs so knees face outward. Then turn them in so knees face each other.

PROCEDURE
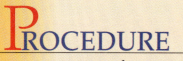
continued

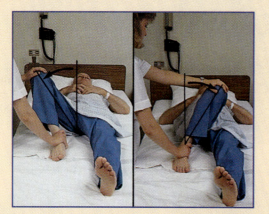

FIGURE 8-22

Hip Internal and External Rotation (Variation): With one knee bent and foot flat on bed, turn leg so knee moves out to the side, then inward across the other leg. Do each leg separately.

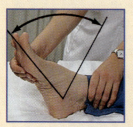

FIGURE 8-23

Ankle Dorsiflexion and Plantar Flexion: Bend ankles up, down, and from side to side.

13. Exercise the toes.

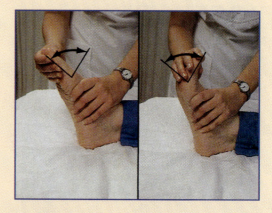

FIGURE 8-24

Toe Flexion and Extension: Bend and straighten each toe.

Ending Steps

14. Make the resident comfortable.
15. Be sure the signal cord is within easy reach.
16. Raise the side rails.
17. Wash your hands.
18. Record in the chart that you have completed range-of-motion exercises with the resident and how the exercises were tolerated. Also record and report your observations of anything unusual.

ENCOURAGING ACTIVE RANGE OF MOTION

Those residents who are able should be encouraged and instructed in active range of motion. Active exercise has the additional benefit of increasing muscle strength as well as maintaining range of joint movement.

Many residents will enjoy the increased responsibility and independence that comes from performing their own exercises. Some see it as an activity that occupies time and interest during the day. Some residents may get "carried away" and exercise too much. Tell the resident to go through each motion three times and to exercise each extremity two or three times a day.

Even when residents do their own range-of-motion exercises, the nursing assistant needs to verify that the exercises are being done and to record that fact in the chart. Ask the residents to show you how they exercise and remind them during the day to exercise. Compliment their efforts: "You're doing a great job, Mr. Green. I can see the improvement in just one week."

CULTURAL AWARENESS When it comes to taking action to prevent complications from inactivity, there are cultural variations. Some cultures such as Hispanic and African American are said to be present-time oriented. Other cultures are past oriented, and Anglo Americans are more future oriented. Those who are present-time oriented may not see the value of range-of-motion exercises to prevent contractures because they don't have a problem in the present. They may choose to avoid the discomfort of the exercises over preventing a possible future problem. When a resident does not respond to the instructions, it is important to ask why. You may have to find another reason to motivate other than explaining future complications.

As strength and movement in joints increase, self-care activities will begin to substitute for exercises in providing range of joint motion. Encourage self-care such as brushing hair and assisting with bathing and dressing.

Residents confined to wheelchairs may quickly develop hip and knee contractures. In addition to range-of-motion exercises, they need to stand frequently during the day and be positioned with hips and legs extended when in bed.

AMBULATION

Another skill that the nursing assistant will use to promote proper body functioning, exercise, and activity is assisting residents to ambulate. Ambulation means walking or moving about in an upright position.

Frequently, residents who need help with ambulation are weak or unsteady on their feet, or they experience dizziness. These residents are more likely to slip or fall. In order to protect yourself and the resident from injury, you will need to understand and use good body mechanics. Review the principles of body mechanics in Chapter 2. Ambulation has positive effects on body systems:

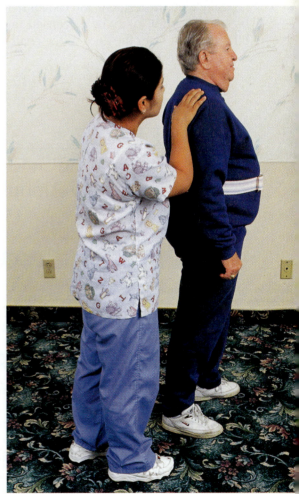

FIGURE 8-25

Use the gait belt to assure control if the resident falls.

- Circulation is stimulated.
- Muscles are strengthened.
- Pressure on certain body parts is relieved.
- Joints are extended and moved.
- Weight is borne on the large bones.
- The urinary and digestive systems work more efficiently.
- Independence is increased, leading to a more positive self-image.

Most residents want to be able to ambulate. The physician, along with input from the physical therapist and nurse, will determine the resident's readiness to ambulate and prescribe how and under what conditions the resident will ambulate. To be ready to ambulate, the resident needs strength and balance. There is a natural progression of abilities needed. The resident must first be able to come from a sitting position to a standing position. Then the resident must have balance while standing, and the legs must be strong enough to support the weight of the body. Last, the resident must be able to move forward one step at a time, requiring balance, strength, and coordination.

The first time a resident ambulates after a period of illness is very important in building confidence and increasing motivation. The first ambulation is often performed or supervised by a physical therapist, a specially trained rehabilitation aide, or a restorative nursing assistant (Figure 8-25). Safety is essential! It is wise to use two people to reassure the resident that there is no danger.

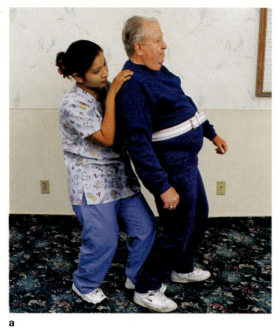

a

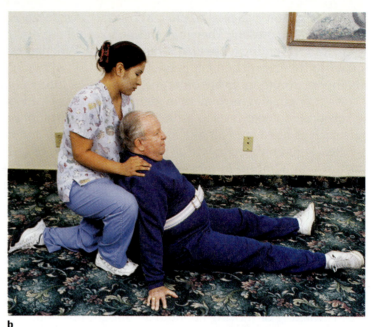

b

FIGURE 8-26

(a) Bring the resident close to your body and ease him or her to the floor; (b) support the resident and call for help.

Sometimes a resident can fall due to leg collapse or loss of balance. When this happens, gently ease the resident to the floor (Figure 8-26), being careful to protect yourself by using good body mechanics (bending your legs instead of your back).

Stay with the resident and call for help. Before moving, the resident should be examined for injury by a licensed nurse. You will need additional help to lift a resident from the floor to the chair or bed.

PROCEDURE

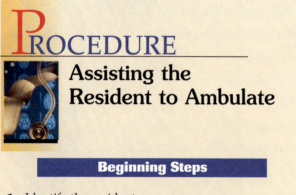

Assisting the Resident to Ambulate

Beginning Steps

1. Identify the resident.
2. Explain what you are going to do, as well as what is expected of the resident.

Steps

3. Assist the resident to a sitting position and allow the resident time to gain balance.
4. Assist in dressing and putting on appropriate shoes (firm support with rubber heels are best).
5. Assist to stand. You may either stand directly in front or to one side.

6. Again, give the resident time to gain balance.
7. Remind the resident to stand up straight, with the chin parallel to the floor.
8. The first step is taken with the affected foot or leg with the weight borne by the unaffected or stronger side.
9. As you walk, observe the resident for signs of fatigue, such as difficulty breathing, sweating, dizziness, and rapid heart rate. Allow the resident to rest if these signs occur.
10. Be on the alert for hazards such as untied shoes, objects on the floor, and wet spots.

Ending Steps

11. Return the resident to bed or a chair.
12. Record in the chart the distance ambulated and the response of the resident. You may estimate distance by number of feet or number of steps. You may also describe from one place to another, such as "ambulated from the bed to the bathroom door" or indicate the time spent, "ambulated in hallway for 10 minutes."

AMBULATION DEVICES

Sometimes a **gait belt** is used for ambulation. This belt (made of leather or nylon webbing) is placed around the resident's waist (Figure 8-27). The nursing assistant stands behind the resident with one hand holding onto the belt. The belt allows residents better control over their center of gravity.

As residents progress in their ability to ambulate, they may graduate from needing the assistance of another person to use of an ambulation device. Ambulation devices include braces, canes, crutches, and walkers (Table 8-1). Although a wheelchair is not a true ambulation device, it is included here since it provides mobility for about 35 percent of LTC facility residents. Also, some residents use a wheelchair somewhat like a walker. They stand behind it, pushing the wheelchair for balance and support.

POSITIONING DEPENDENT RESIDENTS

Positioning dependent residents properly is a very important nursing function. Improper positioning leads to serious complications, such as:

- Skin breakdown from prolonged pressure
- Development of contractures due to improper support
- Decreased circulation from lack of movement
- Pneumonia—secretions collect in the lungs when position is not changed
- Discomfort and pain
- Edema in limbs that are in dependent positions

The dependent or inactive resident must be repositioned at least every 2 hours. Many residents need position changes even more frequently. The healthy person changes positions as often as 30 to 50 times during an 8-hour period of sleep. This movement prevents prolonged pressure in any one area. Prolonged pressure causes decreased circulation and eventual skin breakdown. The dependent resident must trust those who provide care to assume this responsibility. The dependent resident must have position changes made on a 24-hour basis while in bed or when up in a wheelchair.

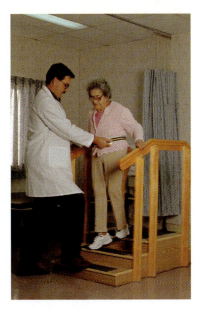

FIGURE 8-27
Using the gait belt.

gait belt a belt placed around a patient's waist that allows better control over the center of gravity

POSITIONING THE RESIDENT IN A WHEELCHAIR

Residents need positioning in wheelchairs for the same reasons they need repositioning when in bed—to reduce pressure, to promote increased circulation, and to increase comfort. Most facilities place cushions in wheelchairs to help reduce pressure on the buttocks.

Once the resident is placed in the wheelchair, check alignment:

- Position the resident's hips well back in the chair.
- Make sure that the feet are resting on the foot rests or on the floor.
- The trunk of the body should be balanced.
- Be sure that male patients are not sitting on the genitalia.

- If necessary, place pillows at the resident's side to prevent sliding over to one side of the chair.
- Place arms on armrests or on a pillow placed across the lap.

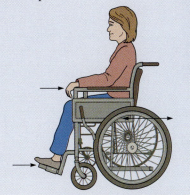

Guidelines

TABLE 8-1: **Ambulation Devices**

DEVICES	PURPOSE	USERS	SAFEGUARDS
Back brace Short leg brace	To promote or limit movement of a body part	Residents with a weak or unstable back, knee, ankle, etc.	Observe the skin under brace for irritation or injury. Report needed repairs such as missing or loose screws. Note if device fits properly.
Conventional cane "Quad cane"	To provide balance and confidence or to decrease weight borne by one foot or leg	Residents who have strength but lack balance or confidence in their activity; used on the opposite side of affected part	Rubber tip(s) must be checked for wear. Report changes in resident that would indicate that cane is no longer appropriate. Inspect rubber tip(s) for wear. Should not be used if resident is weak, unsteady, or unable to maintain balance.
Conventional crutches Canadian crutches	To decrease weight borne by one or both feet and legs; to provide stability	Lower extremity amputees; resident who is normally ambulatory but has suffered a sprain or fracture; someone with lower extremity paralysis or weakness	
Wheeled walker	To provide stability and support	Residents with poor backward/forward balance (Parkinson's disease); resident with general weakness (arthritis)	Be sure wheels turn properly. Check brakes.
Pick-up walker	To provide stability	Resident with weakness or balance problems; frequently, those recovering from a hip fracture	Inspect rubber tip(s) for wear. Report increased weakness.
Standard wheelchair Battery-powered wheelchair	To provide mobility for nonambulatory resident	Residents unable to stand due to weakness, paralysis, amputations, contractures, serious illness; residents unable to propel their own chair; generally used with younger, disabled people	Inspect brakes for proper function. Report needed repairs on torn upholstery.

Maintaining proper body alignment is a fundamental principle of all positioning. **Alignment** means to put in a straight line (Figure 8-28). We look better, feel better, and our bodies function more efficiently when in good alignment.

Caution: Most dependent residents cannot tolerate sitting in a wheelchair for prolonged periods. These residents should be repositioned every 1 to 2 hours while in the wheelchair, and they should never be up in a wheelchair for more than 3 hours without being returned to bed for a rest period. If possible, the resident should be helped to stand for a minute or two at least hourly when up in a wheelchair. Those who are able should shift their position by using the arms of the chair to lift themselves up briefly and adjust their position.

If the resident slips down in the wheelchair, reposition as follows:

• Lock the wheels of the wheelchair.
• Cross the resident's arms over the waist.
• Stand behind the resident, grasp wrists, and simply stand up straight. This moves the resident up in the wheelchair easily.

Whenever you reposition a resident, make sure that you consider nasogastric tubes, catheters, urinary drainage tubing, special dressings, and braces. Always turn and position the resident carefully to avoid dislodging or pulling on tubes, and always make sure that tubing is not obstructed or kinked.

There are special devices used to assist with positioning residents properly. Some of these are presented in Table 8-2.

POSITIONING THE RESIDENT IN BED

Four basic positions are used for most residents:

• Supine
• Semisupine
• Semiprone
• Prone

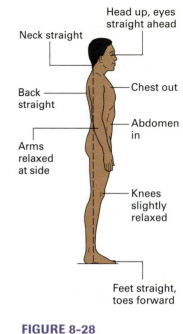

FIGURE 8-28
Body alignment.

Head up, eyes straight ahead
Neck straight
Back straight
Chest out
Abdomen in
Arms relaxed at side
Knees slightly relaxed
Feet straight, toes forward

alignment to put in a straight line

TABLE 8-2:	Positioning Devices			
DEVICE	**PURPOSE**	**USERS**	**PRECAUTIONS**	
Pillows Sandbags	To assist in positioning, provide support and alignment; used to elevate, pad, protect	All residents who require assistance with positioning	Pillows or sandbags should be placed to support joints and to provide comfort. Improper placement can cause redistribution of pressure, discomfort, and pain.	
Trochanter roll (placed next to the greater trochanter—the tip of the thigh bone)	To prevent external rotation of the hip, which results in permanent disability and interferes with ambulation	Residents in the supine position—especially the dependent resident	The rolls should be placed properly to prevent external rotation. They must be removed and the area massaged to avoid prolonged pressure. *Note:* A trochanter roll may be made by rolling up a towel or small blanket and placing it against the hip as shown.	

TABLE 8-2: Positioning Devices (continued)

DEVICE	PURPOSE	USERS	PRECAUTIONS
Abduction splint (device designed to keep the thighs apart)	To keep thighs apart to maintain proper alignment of the hip joints, and to prevent skin-to-skin contact	Residents who have had hip surgery or who have skin breakdown on knees or thighs	It is very important to keep this splint properly placed after hip surgery until healing has occurred. The areas of splint contact must be massaged and observed to reduce chance of skin breakdown.
Palmer splint (device designed to keep the hand in a functional position)	To prevent contractures of the hand, fingers, and wrists	Used for residents with paralysis of the hand or wrist	The splint must be properly applied and checked frequently to avoid pressure from straps or frame of splint. The splint must be removed to allow for exercises, cleansing, and massage each shift.
Hand roll (round device made up of different materials, placed in the palm of the hand)	To prevent contracture and to maintain hands in a functional position; to prevent fingers and nails from pressing into palm of hand, creating pressure and skin breakdown	Residents who have contractures of the hand or may develop contractures	Hand rolls must be removed several times daily and the hand area cleaned. Air circulation in the hand area is reduced and moisture collects, which contributes to bacterial growth and skin breakdown.
Foot board (padded board placed or affixed to the foot of the bed)	To prevent foot drop, a type of contracture of the foot that impairs ambulation	Residents in the supine position who are nonambulatory and who are dependent	The bottom of the foot must be placed securely against the board so that pressure is exerted against the bottom of the foot (similar to the pressure the resident would feel if standing). Make sure that pressure is off the heels, to avoid skin breakdown.

Note: Some textbooks refer to right-side-lying and left-side-lying positions. Research has shown that these direct side-lying positions should be avoided in the elderly or chronically ill because of the increased pressure on the bottom leg and hip. The right and left semisupine and semiprone are used in place of any direct side-lying position.

THE SUPINE (FACE UP) POSITION (FIGURE 8-29)

The placement of the pillow is important. It should come to the tip of the shoulder, not under the shoulders. Too many pillows or pillows placed under the shoulders over a prolonged period causes too much flexion of the neck. This results in contracture of the neck and increased pain.

The arms should be placed at the side of the body allowing enough space for air to circulate around the axilla (armpits). They may be up or down. When arms are placed across the chest or against the body, air circulation is reduced and moisture collects, which contributes to bacterial growth and skin irritation.

Rules for positioning:

1. Straighten rather than flex the joints.
2. Avoid skin-to-skin contact by using pillows and pads as well as by positioning the arms and legs away from the body.
3. Change position frequently by making small adjustments to the arms or legs.
4. Ask the resident whether he or she is comfortable.
5. Keep trying to make the resident comfortable until you succeed.

When a resident is in the supine position, there is a natural tendency for the legs to roll outward (called *external rotation*). If this external rotation is allowed to persist over a prolonged period, the hip joint becomes "fixed" and ambulation is very difficult. A rolled towel or blanket (**trochanter roll**) should be placed at the hip joint to prevent external rotation.

A resident who is unable to move the hands and fingers due to paralysis should have a hand roll placed in his or her hand to prevent contractures.

The feet need to be properly placed against a padded footboard to prevent foot drop, a type of contracture that occurs quickly in residents who do not stand.

In bed, the feet tend to point downward. The weight of the bed coverings contributes to this problem. This can be avoided by the use of a foot cradle.

Just as you move the arms slightly away from the body, you should position the legs so they are slightly apart to reduce irritation in the perineal area.

The heels need to be protected from pressure. A small roll, made with a towel, a piece of foam, or sheepskin, can be used to elevate the heels and keep them from touching the bed.

Caution: Never place a pillow or blankets under the heels. These are too large, causing redistribution of body weight and increased pressure on the sacrum or coccyx area and contributing to skin breakdown there.

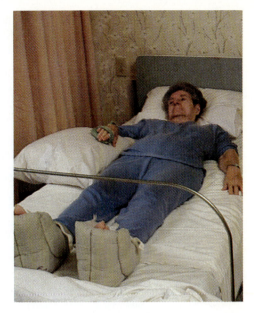

FIGURE 8-29
The supine (face up) position.

trochanter roll   a rolled towel or blanket

FIGURE 8-30
The semisupine (tilt) position.

THE SEMISUPINE (TILT) POSITION (FIGURE 8-30)

In the semisupine or tilt position, the resident is positioned so that body weight is supported by a pillow placed behind the back and another pillow folded in half under the top leg. Both legs are extended (not flexed). The top leg is placed a little behind the bottom leg and supported on the folded pillow so that it is level with the hip joint. Make sure the lower shoulder is brought forward so that pressure is distributed over the back of the shoulder. Place the lower arm away from the body and support the upper arm on a pillow as necessary.

This position replaces the direct side-lying position and can be used on either right or left side. Note how this position prevents pressure on the sacrum and coccyx, yet does not place direct pressure on the hip, where skin breakdown frequently occurs.

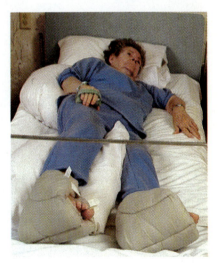

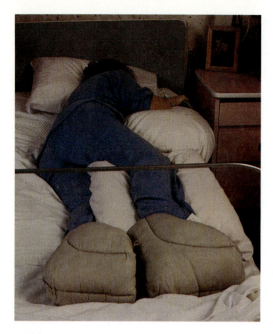

FIGURE 8-31

The semiprone position.

spasticity   tightening of the muscle with short jerking movements

FIGURE 8-32

The prone position.

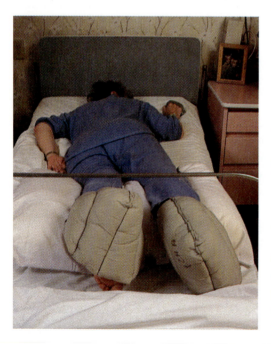

Some residents who have experienced a recent stroke may need to have the paralyzed side flexed due to spasticity. Follow the directions of your physical therapist to determine whether this is necessary.

THE SEMIPRONE POSITION (FIGURE 8-31)

The semiprone position is a reversal of the semisupine. The resident is tilted forward with one pillow supporting the chest and shoulder. Both legs are extended. The lower arm is usually placed behind the resident and the upper arm on a pillow in front of the resident. Semisupine and semiprone are positions that most residents find comfortable. They are excellent positions to reduce pressure and prevent contractures.

THE PRONE POSITION (FIGURE 8-32)

The prone position is an important position that is not used often enough. There are some residents who cannot or will not tolerate this position, so check with your charge nurse if you are unsure.

- The resident's head is turned to one side and placed against the mattress. No pillow is used.
- Position the resident so that the spine is in good alignment.
- Place a small or flat pillow under the lower abdomen to reduce strain on the back. However, some residents are more comfortable without the pillow.
- If the shoulders roll forward, use a small rolled-up towel to support the shoulders.
- The arms may be positioned at the sides with the palms up, or one arm may be flexed and placed next to the head with palm down and the other down at the side with palm up.
Caution: It is generally not advisable to place both arms up next to the head, as this produces strain across the shoulders and causes pain.
- The best way to position the feet is to allow the toes to fall between the end of the mattress and the end of the bed. If this is not possible, place a small rolled-up towel under the ankles to reduce pressure on the toes.

To some residents, the prone position is a little frightening because they feel so dependent. Some even fear suffocation in the face-down position. Explaining the procedure to the resident, having a call light in reach, and leaving the resident in the prone position only for short periods of time at first may make this position more acceptable.

Notice how this position prevents pressure on the major pressure points of the body. For this reason, it is very helpful in reducing pressure on the coccyx, sacrum, heels, hips, and shoulder blades.

Certain residents may require modifications of positioning techniques. These are residents who have **spasticity** (tightening of the muscle with short jerking movements), contractures, or pressure sores. With spasticity, it is more difficult to keep a limb extended, and you will need to reposition more often. With contractures, the joints must always be supported.

When pressure sores exist, care must be taken to avoid pressure on the involved area. This can be done through a technique called **bridging.** Bridging is accomplished by supporting the areas above and below the pressure sore with foam or pillows (Figure 8-33). The involved area is thus free of pressure as it rests between the supports.

Positioning residents properly is a very important nursing responsibility. Good positioning reduces pain and helps to prevent both skin breakdown and joint deformities.

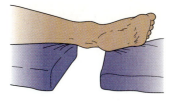

FIGURE 8-33

Bridging.

bridging technique used to support areas above and below a designated area

Summary

SUMMARY People are often residents in nursing homes because they are unable to walk, position themselves, or exercise their joints. In this chapter, you have had an opportunity to understand how the muscular system works as well as what happens when it doesn't.

The consequences of not moving result in further loss of function and in problems including pressure ulcers, pneumonia, infection, contractures, and anky-losed joints. Activities like walking are essential to good health and body functioning. Walking helps the digestive, urinary, muscular, and skeletal systems function better. Bearing weight is essential to reduce osteoporosis and the risk of kidney and bladder stones. Also, the ability to walk is important to feeling independent, which makes residents feel good about themselves. As a result of the aging process, even brief periods of bedrest or inability to walk cause a loss of function that may be impossible to restore. For these reasons, the effort it takes to help residents walk for as long as possible are important to good care of the resident. When assisting the resident to ambulate, safety is the primary concern. Practice both ambulating the resident and the use of the devices you have learned about. Ask your instructor, the physical therapist, or your peers to watch you and give you feedback on easier or safer methods. Be sure to ask for help when the resident is weak or unstable. Report any changes in their abilities to the charge nurse.

Proper positioning of the bedfast resident can do much to promote comfort and minimize the effects of inactivity. Positioning and exercise together can reduce the risk of atrophy, contractures, and pressure ulcers. You need only recall a time when you were on a long trip in a car or plane to remember how uncomfortable you can become if you are unable to stretch, move, and adjust your position. Residents who are confined to a bed or wheelchair rely on you to help them move. Imagine how uncomfortable they must be!

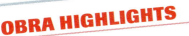

OBRA HIGHLIGHTS

In order for each resident to remain as independent as possible, it is essential that they maintain range of motion. The regulations state: "A resident who enters the facility without a limited range of motion does not experience reduction in range of motion unless the resident's clinical condition demonstrates that a reduction in range of motion is unavoidable; and a resident with a limited range of motion receives appropriate treatment and services to increase range of motion and/or to prevent further decrease in range of motion."

SELF STUDY

Choose the best answer for each question or statement.

1. Which type of muscle tissue makes up the voluntary muscles?
   a. striated muscle tissue
   b. cardiac muscle tissue
   c. smooth muscle tissue
   d. tendon muscle tissue

2. Which type of muscle tissue includes the muscles that push food and water through the gastrointestinal tract?
   a. striated muscle tissue
   b. cardiac muscle tissue
   c. smooth muscle tissue
   d. tendon muscle tissue

3. Paralysis of muscles may be due to injury or illness. The paralyzed muscle does not move because
   a. the transmission of signals from the brain telling the muscles to move no longer occurs
   b. the tissue in the muscle cannot respond to brain messages telling it to move
   c. the brain forgets the muscle is there and does not send messages telling it to move
   d. the muscle does not have enough blood in it to move and produce heat

4. What causes muscles to atrophy, or decrease in size?
   a. lack of exercise   c. limb in a cast
   b. paralysis   d. all of the above

5. When a muscle becomes permanently shortened through lack of use, it is called
   a. an atrophy   c. an ankylosis
   b. a contracture   d. edema

6. You are requested to do passive range-of-motion exercises on Mrs. Green. What will you do?
   a. Instruct Mrs. Green to move each joint through its normal range of activity.
   b. Have Mrs. Green move each of her joints forward and backward three times.
   c. Move each of Mrs. Green's joints through its normal range of activity for her.
   d. Assist Mrs. Green to do stretches and trunk twists.

7. When you flex a joint, you
   a. bend the joint
   b. move it toward the center of the body
   c. move it away from the center of the body
   d. straighten the joint

8. When you adduct a resident's arm you
   a. turn the palm up
   b. turn the palm down
   c. move it toward the center of the body
   d. move it away from the center of the body

9. Which of the following guidelines should you follow when you perform range-of-motion exercises?
   a. Exercise the joints starting at the feet and working toward the head.
   b. Put each joint through each movement six times.
   c. Support the limb at the joint as you exercise it.
   d. All of these guidelines should be followed.

10. Mr. Johnson is able to do his own range-of-motion exercises. What are the nursing assistant's responsibilities?
    a. Verify that Mr. Johnson is doing the exercises.
    b. Compliment Mr. Johnson on his efforts when doing the exercises.
    c. Record that the exercises are being done in Mr. Johnson's chart.
    d. All of these are the nursing assistant's responsibilities.

11. Which of the following is *not* a positive effect of ambulation?
    a. stimulating circulation
    b. strengthening muscles
    c. decreasing function of digestive system
    d. extending and moving joints

12. What should you do if a resident begins to fall while you are assisting with ambulation?
    a. Hold the resident as upright as possible and call for help.
    b. Ease the resident gently to the floor and call for help.
    c. Let the resident fall; you could hurt yourself trying to stop the fall.
    d. Hold the resident by the gait belt and pull him toward a chair.

13. Mr. Melvin is unable to ambulate. He likes to be up in his wheelchair during the day. Which of the following guidelines should you follow for Mr. Melvin?
   a. Assist him to stand hourly, and to bed after three hours to rest.
   b. Allow him to be in the wheelchair for as long as he wishes.
   c. Assist him to elevate his feet to waist level several times a day.
   d. Allow him to be in the wheelchair only for three hours per day.

14. Which of the following is true about placement of pillows for a resident?
   a. Placing several pillows under the head will help keep the neck from becoming fatigued.
   b. Placing the pillow under the head so it comes to the tip of the shoulder prevents excess flexion.
   c. Placing the pillow under the shoulders each evening will help the resident rest better.

d. Placing the pillow under the head so it comes to the tip of the shoulder will cause neck contractures.

15. When you position a resident, you should
   a. flex the joints as much as possible
   b. keep the body in alignment whether it is comfortable or not
   c. avoid skin-to-skin contact by using pillows and pads
   d. place a pillow under the heels to prevent pressure ulcers

16. A resident who is unable to stand should have which of the following equipment?
   a. a trochanter roll
   b. a hand roll
   c. a palmer splint
   d. a padded foot board

Getting CONNECTED
Multimedia Extension Activities

www.prenhall.com/will-black

Use the above address to access the free, interactive Companion Website created for this textbook. Hear the pronunication of the key terms in the chapter. Get instant feedback to a variety of chapter-related questions. Link to other interesting sites.

Video

Watch the video *Body Mechanics* from the Care Provider Skills series.

CASE STUDY

Eleanor Amy is an 83-year-old woman with rheumatoid arthritis and heart disease. Because movement is so painful, she refuses to get out of bed or to participate in physical therapy. She is becoming weaker and weaker due to lack of activity. She believes the cure for weakness is rest in bed. You have heard of her but have never been assigned to her.

1. What actions can be taken by the staff to prevent her from developing contractures?
   a. Insist that she get up in spite of her wishes.
   b. Agree to provide her with range-of-motion exercises while in bed.
   c. Ask the director of nursing to get involved.
   d. Leave her alone—it was her choice to refuse.

2. When you are caring for her, she agrees to get up long enough for you to change the bed. In order to transfer her to a chair, you will need
   a. assistance from another staff member or use of a mechanical lift
   b. help from a therapist
   c. no help since she isn't very heavy
   d. a registered nurse

3. When giving Mrs. Amy range-of-motion exercise, she yells every time you touch her hands or arms. You should
   a. avoid touching her hands or arms
   b. ask the charge nurse to give her pain medication
   c. report to the charge nurse and ask for guidance
   d. tell her "no pain, no gain"

4. Because Mrs. Amy continues to refuse to get out of bed, she is at risk for which of the following complications?
   a. contractures, pressure ulcers, and loss of ability to perform activities of daily living
   b. heart attack
   c. cancer
   d. falls with fractures

Chapter 9

THE DIGESTIVE SYSTEM

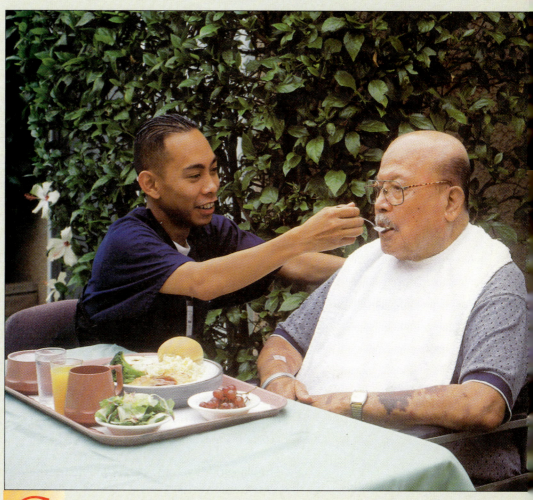

CARING TIP

Mealtime can be the highlight of the day. Savor the opportunity to visit with the resident as you feed them.

Joan M. Scribner, RN, BSN
Affiliate Faculty
Penn Valley Community College
Kansas City, Missouri

OBJECTIVES
What You Will Learn

When you have completed this section, you will be able to:

- List three basic functions of the digestive system
- Label the components of the digestive system
- Match the organs in the digestive system with their functions

KEY TERMS

alimentary tract	dysphagia	liver
appendix	enzymes	peristalsis
aspiration	feces	rectum
bile	gallstones	sigmoid colon
cirrhosis	gastritis	sphincter muscles
duodenum	GERD	ulcer
	hemorrhoids	villi

THE DIGESTIVE SYSTEM

The digestive system (Figure 9-1) is composed of:

- Teeth
- Tongue
- Salivary glands
- Esophagus
- Stomach
- Pancreas
- Appendix
- Liver
- Gallbladder
- Small intestine (including duodenum)
- Large intestine (including colon)
- Anus

Functions of the digestive system are to:

- Ingest food
- Prepare food for use by the body
- Excrete body wastes

alimentary tract route taken by food as it passes from the mouth to the anus

The digestive system is responsible for the process of breaking down food that is eaten and changing it so that it can be used by the cells of the body. This process is both chemical and mechanical. The **alimentary tract** (route taken by food as it passes from the mouth to the anus) is about 30 feet long. Each part of the alimentary tract has special functions.

Digestion begins in the mouth, where food is chewed and mixed with saliva secreted by the salivary glands. When we swallow, moisturized food travels down the esophagus to the stomach. The stomach churns and mixes the food while it is being changed chemically by special digestive secretions **(enzymes).**

enzymes digestive secretions

duodenum first loop of the small intestine and most major area of digestion

Water is essential to the chemical process of changing food into its final form. Most of the digested food particles are absorbed (taken into the bloodstream for use by the body) in the area of the **duodenum,** the first loop of the small intestine and the most important area of digestion. Here partially digested food from the stomach mixes with digestive secretions from the duodenum, the pancreas, and the liver to complete the process of digestion. One of the liver's many functions is to manufacture a substance called **bile,** which

bile substance stored in the gallbladder that aids in the digestion of fats

The digestive system includes the digestive tract and various supportive structures and accessory glands. The tract begins at the oral cavity with the teeth and tongue. The salivary glands release saliva into the mouth to moisten food for swallowing. The tract continues down the throat to the esophagus, through the cardiac sphincter, and into the stomach. Acid and digestive enzymes are added to the food to produce chyme. The chyme passes through the pyloric sphincter to enter the small intestine. Digestive enzymes from the pancreas and bile from the liver are added to the chyme. The process of digestion and absorption are completed in the small intestine. Wastes are carried through the ileocecal valve into the large intestine. The wastes are moved to the rectum, from where they can be expelled through the anus.

Liver, Stomach, and Pancreas

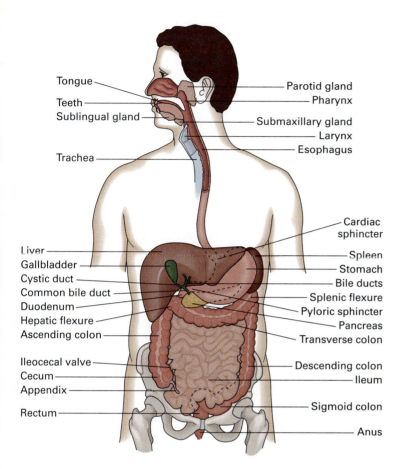

Organs of the Digestive System

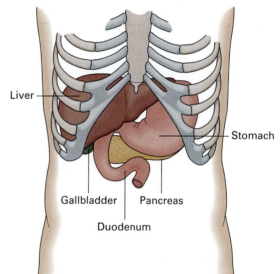

Large Intestine

Small Intestine

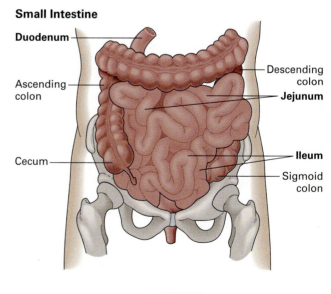

FIGURE 9-1

The digestive system.

is stored in the gallbladder and released into the duodenum to be mixed with other digestive enzymes. Bile is important in breaking down fats eaten so that the digestive enzymes of the pancreas and liver can further complete the digestive process.

THE DIGESTIVE PROCESS

The duodenum is composed of thousands of fingerlike projections called **villi.** Each of these projections (villus) absorbs digested food particles and releases them into the bloodstream. Some digestion continues to occur in other parts of the small intestine.

The remainder of the digested food is moved by rhythmic contractions **(peristalsis)** through the large intestine.

The **appendix** is a small projection of tissue located where the small and large intestine meet. The appendix has no digestive function but frequently becomes infected, causing fever and pain. An appendectomy is the surgical removal of the appendix.

The lower portion of the large intestine curves in an 'S' shape. This area is called the **sigmoid colon.** The sigmoid colon leads directly into the rectum. In the large intestine, water is reabsorbed by the body. Excess water is removed from the remaining digested material. Semisolid waste **(feces)** is created. Feces are excreted from the body through the rectum. The **rectum** is composed of delicate tissues surrounded by **sphincter muscles** (muscles that squeeze down). This allows the contents of the rectum (feces) to remain in the rectum until voluntary elimination (bowel movement) occurs.

Another organ important in the digestive process is the **liver.** The liver is a very complex organ and has many functions. The most important functions of the liver are:

- Storage area for simple sugar (glucose). This form of sugar is stored and released in large amounts when the cells need it.
- Storage of vitamins and proteins essential for proper circulation of the blood.
- Removal of poisons or toxins from the blood through a filtering function.
- Carrying out metabolic functions essential for the blood-clotting process.

ABNORMALITIES OF THE DIGESTIVE SYSTEM

Abnormalities of the digestive system include the following:

- **GERD,** or gastroesophageal reflux disease, is common in adults and the elderly. The symptoms include heartburn, sour-tasting fluid in the throat, and difficulty swallowing. The symptoms are caused by acid that escapes from the stomach through a weakened one-way valve called the lower esophageal sphincter located near the top of the stomach. Smoking, caffeine, and alcohol all increase the level of acid, causing even more heartburn. Residents are instructed to avoid eating carbonated drinks, fried and fatty foods, spicy foods, citrus fruits and tomatoes, onions, peppermint, and chocolate. In addition, it is recommended that the resident eat several small meals each day and sleep with the head of the bed raised. Avoidance of tight-fitting clothing and bending over are also suggested. GERD can progress and lead to inflammation, ulcer, and narrowing of the esophagus.

villi small fingerlike projections of the duodenum that absorb digested food particles and release them into the bloodstream

peristalsis rhythmic contractions that assist in moving food through the intestines

appendix small projection of tissue located where the small and large intestines meet

sigmoid colon lower portion of the large intestine which curves in an 'S' shape

feces solid human waste

rectum lowest section of the large intestine adjacent to the outside of the body

sphincter muscles type of muscle that contracts to close a body opening

liver the largest gland of the body and one of its most complex organs; is part of the digestive system and performs about 500 functions

GERD gastroesophageal reflux disease—a condition with backflow of contents of the stomach into the esophagus, producing burning pain

- **Dysphagia,** or difficulty swallowing, is more common with advancing age. It is particularly common in the elderly nursing home resident. Residents with dementia are at high risk. Any process that affects the swallowing mechanism can cause dysphagia. This may include inflammation, obstruction, neurological disease, and use of certain drugs such as tranquilizers and antidepressants. Dysphagia can result in pneumonia because of food being taken into the lungs, which is called **aspiration.** Dysphagia can also lead to malnutrition, which often leads to poor wound healing, decreased ability to fight infection, and reduced physical functioning. The signs to watch for include choking, coughing, and even vomiting. Harder-to-recognize symptoms include wheezing, drooling, gurgly speech, difficulty chewing, slow eating, and holding food in the mouth. Usually, it is harder to swallow liquids than solids.

- **Ulcer** is a cavity that develops, creating an open wound. There are many factors related to the development of stomach ulcers, but prolonged stress and pain are the most common. Ulcers are very painful and require special medications, special diets, and sometimes surgical removal.

- **Gastritis** is inflammation of the stomach caused by bacteria, viruses, vitamin deficiency, excessive eating, or overindulgence in alcoholic beverages. Gastritis is often associated with nausea and vomiting.

- **Gallstones** are cholesterol crystals that settle out of the bile stored in the gallbladder. Stones form and often block the secretion of bile. This condition causes pain, nausea, and vomiting, especially following meals. Surgical removal of the gallstones or the gallbladder may be necessary.

- **Hemorrhoids** are enlarged blood-filled vessels that surround the area of the rectum. These enlarged blood vessels are painful, especially during a bowel movement. They may bleed, causing the stool to become blood tinged.

- **Cirrhosis** is an inflammation of the tissue of an organ, particularly the liver. The normal liver tissue is replaced by fibrous (tough) tissue, and liver function is decreased or lost. Cirrhosis is commonly associated with excessive drug or alcohol abuse. Poor nutrition over a long period of time also leads to cirrhosis.

dysphagia   difficulty in swallowing

aspiration   inhaling food or fluid into the lungs

ulcer   break in the skin creating an open wound

gastritis   inflammation of the stomach caused by many different factors

gallstones   cholesterol crystals that settle out of the bile stored in the gallbladder

hemorrhoids   enlarged blood-filled vessels that surround the rectal area

cirrhosis   inflammation of a tissue or organ, particularly the liver

SECTION 2   Basic Nutrition

OBJECTIVES
What You Will Learn

When you have completed this section, you will be able to:

- Describe what a well-balanced diet should contain

- Describe the basic bodily functions of:
  - Carbohydrates
  - Proteins
  - Fats
- Explain why water is considered an essential nutrient

- List the six groups of food items described in the Food Pyramid with the number of recommended servings of each per day
- Correctly calculate percentages of food eaten

KEY TERM   nutrition

PRINCIPLES OF NUTRITION

nutrition   science of food
and its actions or relationship to health

Nutrition is the science of foods and their actions or relationship to health.
The body depends on food for:

- Growth and repair of tissue
- Energy
- Maintenance and regulation of body functions

    In this section, you will learn what a well-balanced diet consists of as well
as how different nutrients (substances) are essential to good health.

NUTRIENTS

The following table of nutrients (Table 9–1), their bodily functions, and food
sources should be studied so that you understand what good nutrition means
to you as well as to the LTC resident.
    Calories in a normal diet are provided through eating:

Carbohydrates	58 percent
Proteins	12 percent
Fatty acids	30 percent
Calories	100 percent

TABLE 9-1   A Well-Balanced Diet

- *Sufficient carbohydrates to meet the individual's energy requirements*

Nutrient Class

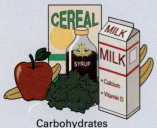

Carbohydrates

Bodily Function

Provides work energy for body activities
and heat energy for maintenance of body
temperature.

There are no essential carbohydrates; however, it is important to have a good balance of
the various carbohydrate sources.

Food Sources

Cereal grains and their products (bread,
breakfast cereals, pasta products),
potatoes, sugar, fruits, milk, vegetables,
nuts.

- *Sufficient protein to supply the body with the nine essential amino acids.* (Amino acids are
the units of structure in proteins.)

Nutrient Class

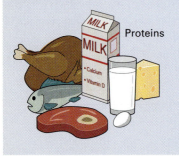

Proteins

Bodily Function

Build and renew body tissues; regulate
body functions and supply energy.
Complete proteins: maintain life and
provide growth. Partially complete
proteins will maintain life, but they lack
sufficient amounts of some amino acids
necessary for growth. Incomplete proteins
are incapable of replacing or building new
tissues and therefore cannot support life.

Food Sources

Complete proteins: derived from animal
foods—meat, milk, eggs, fish, cheese,
poultry. Partially complete proteins: derived
from vegetable foods—soybeans, dry
beans, peas, some nuts, and whole-grain
products. Incomplete proteins: gelatin from
Jello.

TABLE 9-1   A Well-Balanced Diet (continued)

- *Sufficient fatty acids to include the essential fatty acids.*

Nutrient Class

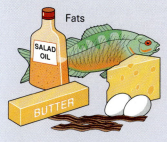

Fats

Bodily Function

Give work energy for body activities and heat energy for maintenance of body temperature. Carriers of vitamins A and D, provide fatty acids necessary for growth and maintenance of body tissues.

Food Sources

Some foods are chiefly fat, such as lard, vegetable fats and oils, and butter. Many other foods contain smaller proportions of fats—nuts, meats, fish, poultry, cream, whole milk.

- *Adequate amounts of vitamins*

Nutrient Class

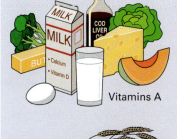

Vitamins A

Bodily Function

Necessary for normal functioning of the eyes, prevents night blindness. Ensures a healthy condition of the skin, hair, and mucous membranes. Maintains a state of resistance to infections of the eyes, mouth, and respiratory tract.

Food Sources

One form of vitamin A is yellow and one form is colorless. Apricots, cantaloupe, milk, cheese, eggs, organ meat (especially liver and kidney), fortified margarine, butter, fish liver oils, dark green and deep yellow vegetables.

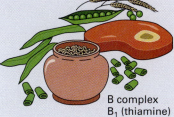

B complex
B₁ (thiamine)

Maintains a healthy condition of the nerves. Fosters a good appetite. Helps the body cells use carbohydrates.

Whole-grain and enriched grain products; meats (especially pork, liver, and kidney), dry beans, and peas.

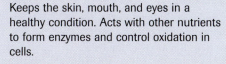

B₂
(riboflavin)

Keeps the skin, mouth, and eyes in a healthy condition. Acts with other nutrients to form enzymes and control oxidation in cells.

Milk, cheese, eggs, meat (especially liver and kidney), whole-grain and enriched grain products, dark green vegetables.

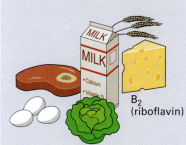

Niacin

Influences the oxidation of carbohydrates and proteins in the body cells.

Liver, meat, fish, poultry, eggs, peanuts, dark green vegetables, whole-grain and enriched cereal products.

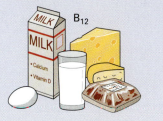

B₁₂

Regulates specific processes in digestion. Helps maintain normal functions of muscles, nerves, heart, blood—general body metabolism.

Liver, other organ meats, cheese, eggs, milk.

TABLE 9-1   **A Well-Balanced Diet (continued)**

Nutrient Class	Bodily Function	Food Sources
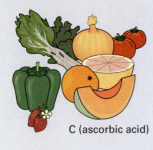 C (ascorbic acid)	Acts as a cement between body cells, and helps them work together to carry out their special functions. Maintains a sound condition of bones, teeth, and gums. Not stored in the body. Protects vitamins A and E. Helps in the absorption of iron.	Fresh, raw citrus fruits and vegetables—oranges, grapefruit, cantaloupe, strawberries, tomatoes, raw onions, cabbage, green and sweet red peppers, dark green vegetables.
D	Enables the growing body to use calcium and phosphorus in a normal way to build teeth and bones.	Provided by vitamin D fortification of certain foods, such as milk and margarine. Also fish-liver oils and eggs. Sunshine allows the body to make its own vitamin D.
K	The vitamin helps the liver produce substances that are essential to blood clotting.	All green leafy vegetables, egg yolk, soy bean oil, liver, alfalfa, lettuce, spinach, cauliflower.

• *Essential elements—minerals.* There are many known essential elements. Some of the most common are shown.

Nutrient Class	Bodily Function	Food Sources
Minerals Iron 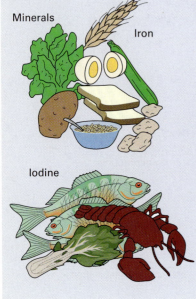	Builds and renews hemoglobin, the red pigment in blood that carries oxygen from the lungs to the cells.	Egg yolks, meat, especially liver and kidney; deep yellow and dark green vegetables; potatoes, dried fruits, whole-grain products; enriched flour, bread, breakfast cereals.
Iodine	Enables the thyroid gland to perform its function of controlling the rate at which foods are oxidized in the cells.	Fish (obtained from the sea), some plant foods grown in soils containing iodine; table salt fortified with iodine (iodized).

TABLE 9-1   A Well-Balanced Diet (continued)

Nutrient Class	Bodily Function	Food Sources

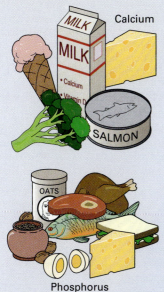

Calcium

Builds and renews bones, teeth, and other tissues; regulates the activity of the muscles, heart, nerves; is important in the clotting of blood.

Milk and milk products, except butter; most dark green vegetables; canned salmon.

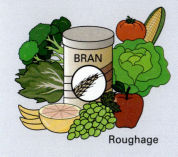

Phosphorus

Associated with calcium in some functions needed to build and renew bones and teeth. Influences the oxidation of foods in the body cells; important in nerve tissue.

Widely distributed in foods, especially cheese, oat cereals, whole-wheat products, dry beans and peas, meat, fish, poultry, nuts, and eggs.

- *Sufficient dietary fiber—roughage or indigestible material.* Only recently has dietary fiber been considered an essential component of a balanced diet.

Nutrient Class

Bodily Function

Associated with prevention of constipation, hemorrhoids, and other digestive diseases, as well as cancer of the colon.

Food Sources

A widely varied diet that contains unprocessed grains, vegetables, nuts, and fruits.

Roughage

- *Sufficient fluid intake.* Although water does not furnish calories or vitamins, it is as essential as any nutrient. Water comprises 70% of an individual's body weight. Six to eight glasses (1 1/2 to 2 quarts) per day are essential to good health.

Nutrient Class

Water

Bodily Function

Regulates body processes. Aids in regulating body temperature. Carries nutrients to body cells and carries waste products away from them. Helps to lubricate joints. Water has no food value, although most water contains mineral elements. More immediately necessary to life than food—second only to oxygen.

Food Sources

Drinking water and other beverages; all foods except those made up of a single nutrient, such as sugar and some fats. Milk, milk drinks, soups, vegetables, fruit juices, ice cream, watermelon, strawberries, lettuce, tomatoes, and cereals.

THE FOOD GUIDE PYRAMID

The Food Guide Pyramid (Figure 9-2) sets the standard for a balanced diet on a daily basis. Foods are placed in categories and arranged in a pyramid. You need to eat more items each day from the bottom of the pyramid than from the top. At the bottom is the bread, cereal, rice, and pasta group. Adults need

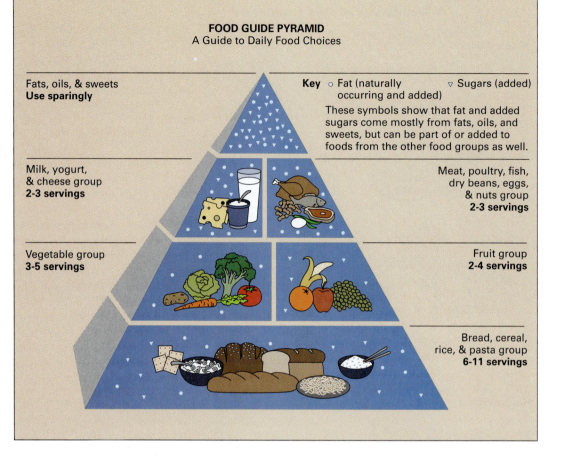

FIGURE 9-2

The Food Guide Pyramid illustrates the fundamentals of healthy nutrition.

Source: U.S. Department of Agriculture/U.S. Department of Health and Human Services.

from 6 to 11 servings from this group each day. An example of one serving from this group would be one slice of bread or one ounce of dry cereal or ½ cup of cooked rice or pasta.

The next food group is the vegetable group. A healthy daily diet would include from three to five servings from this group. Examples of one serving would be 1 cup of raw leafy vegetables or ½ cup of cooked or raw chopped vegetables.

The fruit group requires from two to four servings daily. One serving would be one medium apple, orange, or banana or ¾ cup of fruit juice.

Meat, poultry, fish, dry beans, eggs, and nuts are limited to two to three servings.

One ounce of meat is equal to one serving. (A "quarter-pounder" contains four ounces of meat—more than one day's healthy portion!) In addition, ½ cup of dry beans or peas is equal to one serving from this category.

The milk, yogurt, and cheese group is also limited to two to three servings. One portion would be 1 cup of milk, 2 slices of cheese, or 2 cups of cottage cheese.

At the top of the pyramid is the group including fats, oils, and sweets. You will notice that there are no recommended servings for this group. This is because these foods should be eaten as little as possible. Most are provided in other foods; for example, meats and dairy products often contain fat. In the Food Guide Pyramid, the small circles represent fat, which you will notice is included with all except the fruit group, while the triangles represent sugars that are present in every group except the meat, poultry, fish group.

An easy-to-remember guideline is to eat more from the bottom of the pyramid than from the top.

NUTRITION AND THE ELDERLY

Nutrition for the elderly is not much different from that needed by everyone. However, there are age-related changes that affect their nutritional status:

- The elderly require fewer calories because they are less active.
- Elderly residents require more vitamins and minerals because they have more digestive disturbances, which affect how nutrients are absorbed and utilized.
- Elderly people take more drugs than any other age group in America. Many commonly used drugs affect how nutrients are absorbed and utilized.
- Poor oral hygiene or loose, poorly fitted dentures will contribute to poor nutrition.
- The elderly have a diminished sense of taste, which may make foods less appealing and cause residents to eat less.
- Many elderly suffer from chronic diseases that decrease energy or the ability to eat independently. Studies show that approximately 70 to 80 percent of all residents in skilled nursing facilities require some assistance with eating, and approximately 20 to 30 percent need assistive eating devices.

Some residents are affected by physical conditions that impair the resident's ability to chew and swallow. Others experience states of depression, loneliness, and dependency, which affect appetite. Nutritional deficiencies can lead to changes in behavior such as:

- Anxiety (fear)
- Apathy (lack of interest)
- Fatigue (being overly tired)
- Loss of appetite
- Loss of memory
- Irritability

CULTURAL AWARENESS Food is very important to all of us. We usually get a great deal of pleasure from eating; eating is a social activity for most people. We also associate food with recreational activities, such as hot dogs with ball games and turkey with holidays such as Thanksgiving and Christmas. Food is a source of pride and accomplishment for many—being a good cook and meal planner takes practice and skill. Food has religious importance, and special foods are prepared for certain religious occasions.

Most people follow dietary habits they have established early in life based on their cultural, social, and religious background. Some residents will refuse certain foods that are in conflict with their religious beliefs. These religious preferences should always be honored and a substitution made.

The resident's cultural and religious practice often involve eating or avoiding certain types of food. In many Latin American cultures, for instance, the concept of keeping the body in balance involves the use of foods identified as "hot" foods or "cold" foods. Depending on the illness, which is also considered "hot" or "cold," a resident may prefer to eat a particular food in order to bring the body into balance. An example of a "hot" food among Puerto Ricans might be corn meal or peas, while a "cold" food would be bananas or lima beans. There are also hot and cold medicines and herbs. Similar beliefs are found among Asian cultures who believe in the philosophy of Tao. According to Taoism, harmony is maintained through a balance of yin and yang. Yin represents cold, darkness, and female, while yang represents hot, light, and male. Certain conditions or illnesses are considered either yin or yang and require the opposite types of food or herbs for treatment. A yin food would include mostly fruits and vegetables, while yang foods include meat, chicken, and most but not all kinds of fish.

Some groups avoid certain types of food altogether. A resident may be a strict vegetarian, avoiding not only meat, fish, and poultry, but also all dairy products. Other residents may avoid certain foods on certain religious occasions. Some may fast on religious holidays. Resident's have the right to decide what they will eat and when they eat it. Facilities are expected to make reasonable accommodations in order to satisfy the resident.

When you learn that a resident is avoiding a particular food or wishes to have an alternative, notify the licensed nurse and/or food service supervisor so that special arrangements can be made that respect the choices of the resident.

In order to help the resident adjust to the changes in dietary habits, the staff must be very sensitive to the resident's likes and dislikes. Research has shown that when residents are able to keep their normal food habits, eating behaviors improve, and nutrition is better.

CALCULATING AND RECORDING FOOD INTAKE

It is very important to assist residents in meeting their nutritional needs. You will need to learn how to evaluate the resident's intake accurately and how to report and record intake. Remember that the food percentages you calculate and record must be accurate. Important decisions related to the resident's medical care and treatment may be based on this documentation.

The most accurate way to chart intake is to observe the resident's tray after eating and chart exactly what was eaten. "For the dinner meal, Mr. Jones ate all the roast beef, half the potato, none of the vegetables, all the roll and margarine, dessert, milk, and coffee." However, most facilities require the nursing assistant to chart only the percentage of calories consumed at each meal, utilizing the following guidelines.

If the resident consumes all the food and fluids served, he or she has eaten 100 percent of that meal. If the resident consumes none of the food or fluids served, he or she has eaten 0 percent of that meal.

In order to accurately chart partial percentages of food or fluids eaten, you must use the guides that have been developed by the dietitian for the specific menus used in your facility. The following are samples taken from a typical menu.

At first you may wish to check out your results with your instructor or charge

TABLE 9-2   Percent of Intake

MEAL	PERCENT OF CALORIES	RESIDENT ATE	PERCENTAGE CONSUMED
Roast beef	40	All the roast beef	40
Baked potato	10	Half the potato	5
Mixed vegetables	5	No vegetables	0
Roll/margarine	20	All the roll/margarine	20
Cake with icing	10	All the cake	10
Milk	15	Half the milk	7.5
Coffee	0	All the coffee	0
		Total percent consumed	82.5

Sample Charting Guides

	Food Item	Percent of Calories
Breakfast	Juice	10
	Cereal	20
	Egg	20
	Toast/margarine	30
	Milk	20
		100
Lunch or dinner	Main dish*	40
	Starch	10
	Vegetable	5
	Bread/margarine	20
	Dessert	10
	Milk	15
		100

This breakdown shows the percentage of calories of each food item served in a meal. Simple arithmetic is used to calculate the total percentage of calories the resident consumes each meal. You must observe how much of each food item is consumed and add the percentages together. If the resident eats only half of a food item, add only half of the percentage of that food item.

*Note: When the main dish consists of a casserole or a combination of foods, add the percentages of each item to get the total percentage for the casserole or combination dish. Example: Chicken noodle casserole would be a total of the chicken and sauce (40 percent) and the noodles or starch (10 percent), which equals 50 percent of the calories from the tray. Coffee has no calories and is therefore not counted in the food percentages.

Remember that if the resident ate half of the food on the tray he or she did not necessarily receive half of the calories.

nurse. Be sure to write down the information as soon as possible so that it is not forgotten.

Study Table 9-2 to see how the process works.

Report to the charge nurse any time residents refuse a meal or their eating habits change. You must never ignore poor intake!

SECTION 3 Therapeutic Diets

OBJECTIVES
What You Will Learn

When you have completed this section, you will be able to:

- Define the term *therapeutic diet*
- List two ways the nursing assistant can verify the resident's diet order
- Match the appropriate description of a diet with the correct terminology
- Explain why it is important for each resident to receive the diet ordered by the physician

KEY TERMS

gastrostomy tube

hypertension
nasogastric tube

parenterally
therapeutic

THERAPEUTIC DIETS

Eating properly to provide the body with essential nutrients is always important. When a person has a disease, is weak, or sick, it becomes even more important. Remember, it is through the digestive process that all the cells of the body are nourished!

Many illnesses and diseases interfere with proper nutrition. Because of this, the physician will modify or restrict the resident's diet. The physician determines and orders the kind of diet that will best meet the resident's nutritional needs. These diets are frequently referred to as:

- Special diets
- Modified diets
- Restricted diets
- Therapeutic diets

therapeutic pertaining to or effective in treatment of disease

Therapeutic means pertaining to or effective in the treatment of disease. The purpose of a therapeutic diet is to provide the resident with a diet that will help in the medical treatment of a particular disease or illness.

For example, a resident who has diabetes will generally be on a diet in which the total calories are limited and the amounts of protein, fat, and carbohydrates are specified. You will study more about the diabetic resident in Chapter 14.

hypertension high blood pressure

A resident with heart disease or **hypertension** (high blood pressure) will generally be on a diet that is salt (or sodium) free or salt restricted.

Sodium (abbreviated Na) is contained in salt and is the primary element that is restricted. Therefore, the amount of sodium is specified in the metric system of grams, that is, 1-g Na diet.

The proper diet is a very important part of the resident's treatment plan. You will need to understand the basic difference between the types of diets served so that you can verify that the residents are receiving the diet ordered by their physician.

You can determine what the diet order for each resident is by:

- Checking the diet tray card (Figure 9-3)
- Verifying the diet order on the resident's chart or health care plan

In many facilities, residents who have special diet orders are given different-colored arm bands to remind those providing care of the modified or re-

FIGURE 9-3

A diet tray card.

Resident's name Mary Smith	Rm. No. 210 A
Diet order Regular mechanical soft	
Food allergies Strawberries, green beans	
Breakfast Likes prune juice, scrambled eggs only	
Beverage Coffee	
Lunch Likes soup often and fruit plate	
Beverage Coffee, juice	
Dinner No fish or rice	
Beverage Coffee	
Likes/Dislikes no rice — no fish — no gravy Likes fruit plates, soups	
Special Instructions Needs plate guard each meal	

stricted diet order. Be sure you know what the color-coded arm bands mean in your facility; examples are:

- Red arm band—diabetic diet
- Yellow arm band—low sodium

Type of Diet	Characteristics	How used
Calorie Controlled • Low calorie • High calorie • Diabetic (The American Dietetic Association [ADA], has established specific diets with appropriate balances of carbohydrates, proteins, and fats for diabetic residents)	Specifies the total number of calories allowed and the precise balance between carbohydrates, proteins, and fats.	Frequently ordered for residents who are on a weight reduction program and also for diabetic residents who require restricted calorie intake and balance. In the calculation of the type of calorie-restricted diabetic diet, the intake is balanced with the resident's insulin requirements and exercise. High-calorie diets may be ordered for residents who would benefit from weight gain or residents who are younger or more active and would require additional calories to maintain their weight.
No concentrated sweets and no added sugar	Excludes candies, pastries, and baked goods containing sugar. No sugar is served with meal. Fruit juices and alcoholic beverages are usually avoided.	May be ordered for some residents who do not require a calorie-controlled diet but who, because of adult diabetes, need to control simple carbohydrates. Is easier to follow and closer to a regular or normal diet.
Bland	Nutritionally adequate diet with food mixed in flavor. Does not contain highly seasoned or gas-forming foods (i.e., beans, onions, cabbage). Generally contains foods that are easily digested.	Easily digested foods that avoid irritation of the digestive tract for residents who have ulcers, colitis, or gallbladder disease.
Restricted salt and sodium (*Salt* and *sodium* are sometimes used interchangeably. However, it is the sodium in the salt that is the concern in the salt-restricted diet.)	Limits foods naturally high in salt content (i.e., ham, cheese, canned soups, luncheon meat, etc.). It also limits the amount of foods that contain sodium.	For residents who are hypertensive or have diseases of the circulatory system or kidney disease.
No added salt	Excludes use of salt on tray or table and foods known to be very high in sodium like ham, bacon, and saltine crackers.	Provided for residents who must limit sodium due to hypertension, kidney, or heart disease but who do not need the restriction of a low-sodium diet.
Low fat	Limits foods high in fat (i.e., butter, cream, egg yolks)—such as bacon, pie crust, donuts, fried foods.	Ordered for residents who have difficulty digesting fats (i.e., residents with gallbladder and liver disturbances).
Low cholesterol	Limits foods high in cholesterol: egg yolks, whole milk, animal fats, some meats (i.e., fats found in animal products)	Ordered for residents who have to decrease the level of cholesterol in their blood.
High protein	Provides extra amounts of protein: meat, fish, cheese, eggs, etc.	Ordered for residents who have poor intake or skin breakdown, or for seriously debilitated residents who require additional protein to assist in tissue repair.

Type of Diet	Characteristics	How used
Tube feeding	Liquid form containing all the nutrients required for a well-balanced diet. Can be bought commercially in a canned form or can be made using milk or meat-based formula.	Given through a nasogastric or gastrostomy tube. (Nasogastric tube is a plastic tube put into one nostril and passed through the esophagus into the stomach. Gastrostomy tube is inserted through a surgical opening made in the abdomen directly into the stomach.) Only administered to residents unable to swallow or take adequate oral foods and fluids. Always administered by a licensed nurse so that proper placement of the tube is verified.

ENTERAL FEEDING

Some residents are unable to meet their nutritional needs by eating. They may be depressed or comatose, have a swallowing problem due to stroke, or have other disorders of the digestive system. These residents may receive all or part of their nutrition in a liquid formula given through a tube. The tube may be inserted through the nose and into the stomach (called a **nasogastric tube,** Figure 9-4)

nasogastric tube tube inserted through the nose and into the stomach

FIGURE 9-4

A nasogastric tube is inserted through the nose into the stomach.

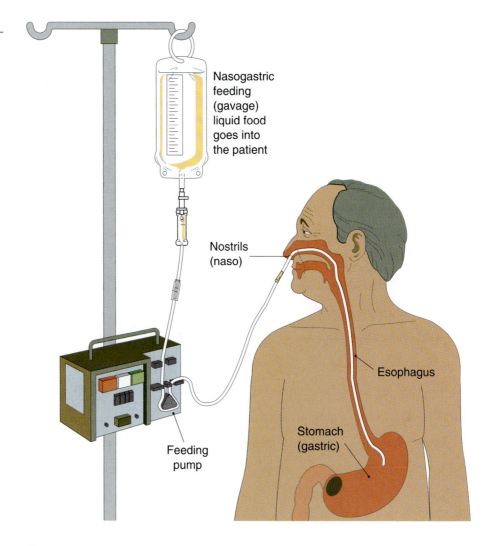

Nasogastric feeding (gavage) liquid food goes into the patient

Nostrils (naso)

Esophagus

Stomach (gastric)

Feeding pump

or directly into the stomach through a small incision or surgical opening (called a **gastrostomy tube,** Figure 9-5).

Residents with problems absorbing sufficient nutrients through the digestive system may receive their nutrition **parenterally** (through a tube inserted into the vein or into the atrium of the heart). This is called *total parenteral nutrition* (TPN). Care of this resident is much like care of the resident with an IV, which is discussed in Chapter 18.

Following a restricted diet is not easy for anyone. Many residents find it very difficult. Some will "cheat" on their diets. Family members may bring in forbidden foods. Be alert and report any failures to follow the prescribed diet to your charge nurse. Sometimes residents and families need help to understand the medical reasons for the special diet.

Some residents may attempt to remove their nasogastric tubes because they are uncomfortable, because they do not wish to be fed, or because they may be confused. The use of mittens to prevent grasping and dislodging the tube may be necessary. Because mittens are a form of restraint, they may never be applied without a physician's order. The mittens must be applied properly so that they are not too tight and the hands are kept in proper alignment. Mittens must be removed to allow for skin care and range-of-motion exercises to the fingers. If possible, these residents should be involved in activities that may distract them from removing the tube. If the resident succeeds in removing the tube, notify the charge nurse immediately.

Residents who have the capacity to make decisions or who have written their decisions in advance may choose to refuse enteral or tube feeding. In most states, tube feeding is considered the same as any other treatment that the resident has the right to refuse. Although a facility may adopt a policy that says that they have moral or religious objections to withholding or withdrawing tube feedings, they have an ethical duty to help the resident to transfer to another facility that does not have such a policy. When a resident and family have made a decision to stop a tube feeding or not to start one, they must receive excellent care even if you disagree with their choice. When a

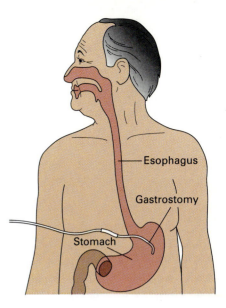

FIGURE 9-5
Gastrostomy tube.

gastrostomy tube a tube inserted directly into the stomach for purposes of providing food, water, and medications for a resident who is unable to swallow

parenterally through a tube inserted into a vein or into the atrium of the heart

PROVIDING CARE TO THE RESIDENT WITH A NASOGASTRIC TUBE

- Keep the head of the bed elevated 45 degrees during and for one hour after each feeding. If the resident is fed using a continuous flow with a pump, they may not have the head of the bed flat at all. This is dangerous to the resident and may cause them to **aspirate** (take into the lungs) the feeding.
- Make sure that there is no tension or pulling on the tube when the resident changes positions.
- Keep the tube clean and free from mucous deposits at the opening of the nostrils.
- Make sure that the tube is securely taped around the entrance to the nostrils to avoid displacement of the tube.

- Check the resident to see that there is no skin irritation around the tube or tape area.
- Fasten the connecting tubing to the resident's clean clothes or gown at the shoulder to prevent strain or tension on the tube.

If the resident has a gastrostomy tube, the principles are the same. Prevent pulling on the tube and provide good skin care to the area around the tube. Report immediately if the tube becomes dislodged. It is not necessary to elevate the head of the bed for a gastrostomy feeding.

Guidelines

resident is not eating or drinking, more frequent oral and skin care and emotional support are needed. It is never appropriate to "abandon" or neglect the resident.

All facilities must provide care and services according to the physician's orders. You may never decide to allow deviations from the physician's diet order. It is as important that each resident receives the right diet as it is that each receives the right medication.

SECTION 4 — Preparing for Mealtime, Serving, and Assisting with Eating

OBJECTIVES
What You Will Learn

When you have completed this section, you will be able to:

• List three ways to prepare the resident's environment for mealtime and to prepare the resident for mealtime

• Explain why it is important for residents to eat in the dining area

• Describe how you can be certain you are serving the right tray to the right resident

• Feed a dependent resident

• List the four precautions to take when feeding a resident with dysphagia.

• Identify the professional consultant who works with residents requiring assistance in performing activities of daily living

PREPARING FOR MEALTIME

As a nursing assistant, you will assist residents in meeting their nutritional needs each day. You will play a major role in creating a pleasant mealtime experience (Figure 9-6).

The following guidelines should be used when preparing the resident for mealtime. Prepare the environment as follows:

• Remove unnecessary supplies or equipment from the resident's room.
• Remove any unsightly or odor-producing articles.
• Clean off the overbed table and straighten the bedside cabinet.
    • Make sure that the dining room tables are clean and that the area is ready for mealtime.
    • Adjust the lighting.
    • Provide privacy for residents who have unpleasant eating habits.

    Prepare the resident:

• Provide residents with the opportunity to use the toilet, bedpan, or urinal prior to mealtime.
• Take care of any personal needs—residents should always be clean and dry before a meal is served. Premoistened towelettes may be used.
• Assist residents in washing hands and face or brushing teeth as necessary.
• Avoid performing major procedures immediately before or after meals. Increased activity just prior to mealtime can interfere with the resident's appetite.
• Observe and report indications that the resident is in pain so that the charge nurse can administer pain-relieving medica-

FIGURE 9-6

A pleasant dining experience.

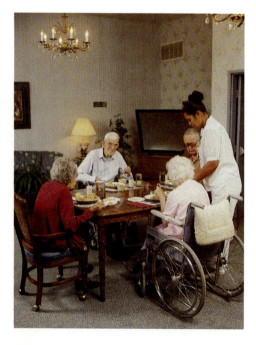

tion prior to mealtime. Residents in pain generally have poor appetites.

- Position the resident in bed in the supine position with the head of the bed elevated as high as is comfortable (Figure 9-7). The upright position is the natural eating position and should be used when possible. The overbed table should be placed at the appropriate height and distance for the resident. Straighten the linens as needed.

- Position the resident in a chair at the bedside. Be sure the resident has shoes or slippers and that the resident's feet are supported by the floor or a stool. The overbed table should be placed at the appropriate height and distance for the resident.

- Position the resident in a wheelchair in the dining room at tables of appropriate wheelchair height (Figure 9-8). Make sure the resident is properly aligned in the wheelchair, with feet supported on foot rests or the floor. If at all possible, walk the resident from the door of the dining room to a chair at the table. This provides good exercise and a more normal eating environment.

- *Note:* Sometimes you will need to use soft protective devices or a pillow to support the resident in order to maintain proper body alignment.

- Provide protection for the resident's clothing when necessary.

- Make sure that any special adaptive eating equipment is available if necessary.

Some residents will need assistance getting to and from the dining room. Encourage residents to eat in the dining areas and help them find compatible social groups. Remember, mealtime should be a pleasant social experience. Some residents develop habits of dining in a particular place and become very upset if their routine is disturbed. When possible, allow the residents to make their own decisions and choices.

SERVING THE RESIDENT

- Wash your hands prior to handling food trays.
- Check the diet card for:
  —Name of the resident
  —The diet order
  —Special instructions
  —Allergies

If you find differences between what the diet card says and what is served, notify the charge nurse at once.

- Remove the tray from the food cart and see that all necessary items are there—silverware, napkins, cups, and so on.

- Take the tray to the resident's room as quickly as possible to ensure that food is served at the appropriate temperatures.

- Before serving the tray, verify the resident's name by checking the arm band against the

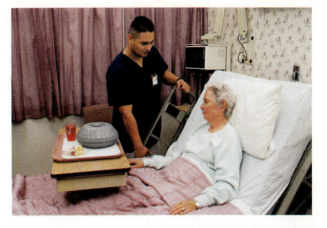

FIGURE 9-7
Positioning for mealtime in bed.

FIGURE 9-8
Positioning for mealtime in a wheelchair.

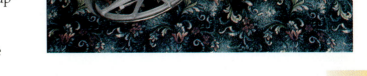

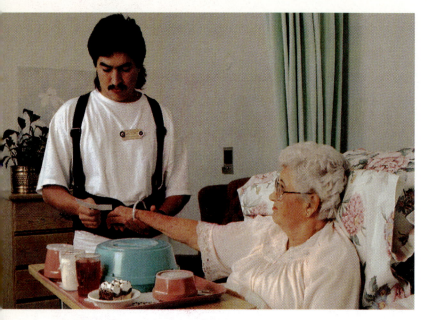

FIGURE 9-9

Checking identification.

name printed on the diet card to ensure that you are serving the right diet to the right resident (Figure 9-9). If the resident is unable to eat at regular mealtime, remove the tray at once and notify the charge nurse so that the tray can be kept hot until the resident is ready.

- If an item on the tray has spilled, return the tray to the dietary department and obtain a replacement. Never serve a meal that looks unappetizing.
- Serve tray and remove plate covers. Arrange dishes and silverware so that they are easy for the resident to use. Arrange the plate so that the main entrée is closest to the resident.
- Observe and provide whatever assistance the resident needs with eating. Cut meat, spread butter, open packets of crackers, pour hot drinks. Make sure that the resident has started eating and does not require more assistance before leaving the room.
- Return to the resident's room periodically during the meal period to check if further assistance is needed. Encourage the resident to eat all of the diet served. Take time to talk with the resident and encourage socialization with other residents. Remember, mealtime is traditionally a social time.
- Make sure that every resident receives a tray each meal. Report any omissions immediately to your charge nurse.
- When you pick up the resident's tray, you must observe and accurately record the amount of food and fluids consumed. Do not trust your memory—write down your observations immediately. Report and record any unusual observations or complaints. For example, when you go in to pick up Mr. Jones's tray, you notice that he has not eaten any fish. He states, "I never eat fish." You will need to report this to the charge nurse so that a substitute can be obtained and the dietitian can be notified of the resident's refusal to eat fish.
- Assist the resident in washing hands and face and remove any food particles from bed linens or clothing.
- Reposition the resident as necessary following mealtime. Residents in bed cannot usually tolerate the upright eating position for long periods and need to be repositioned after every meal.

THE DEPENDENT RESIDENT

Some residents require more than assistance with eating. They may be totally dependent on others to meet their nutritional needs due to disease, illness, or injury. The nursing assistant must be very sensitive to the feelings of the dependent resident. Avoid any word that labels a resident, such as the term *feeder* for a resident who is dependent in eating. A more acceptable phrase would be "the resident who requires assistance with eating." It is not easy for anyone to feel totally dependent on others. It can be very frightening and frustrating. Try to put yourself in the resident's place.

The totally dependent resident is at higher risk for choking than other residents. Many have difficulty chewing and swallowing (dysphagia). Once dys-

ASSISTING THE DEPENDENT RESIDENT IN EATING

When feeding the dependent resident, it is essential to prepare the environment and the resident prior to mealtime as previously described.

- Position the resident in a sitting position either in a chair at the bedside or with the head of the bed elevated.
- When you serve the tray, tell the resident what foods are on the tray.
- Try to seat yourself next to the resident so that you can make eye contact. Talk to the resident and set the mood for a pleasant social experience (Figure 9-10).
- Allow the resident as much independence as possible. Even if the resident requires total assistance with feeding, many can choose how they want their food seasoned or in what order they want to eat their food. Allow them as many choices as possible.
- Use a spoon when feeding. Only fill the spoon half full. Take care to test food temperatures so that residents are not burned by foods that are too hot or startled by foods that are too cold. Do this by feeling the container and testing a small amount of the food against your wrist.
- Feed from the tip of the spoon, using gentle downward pressure in the center of the tongue

(Figure 9-11). If the resident is paralyzed on one side of the body, make sure you place food in the side of the mouth that is not paralyzed so that the resident can chew and swallow more easily.
- If the resident cannot see the tray or is unable to recognize the food items, name each mouthful of food as you offer it.
- Offer foods in logical order, that is, soup or juice before the main course, and alternate between liquid and solid foods throughout the meal.
- Take time—allow the resident time to taste, chew, and swallow. Do not rush the resident. This does not make mealtime a pleasant experience. Given enough time and encouragement, many residents can tolerate regular diets. Too often residents are given mechanically altered diets such as pureed or chopped food, not because they have difficulty swallowing or chewing, but because they are slow. It is never appropriate for the resident's diet to be mechanically altered unless they are physically unable to manage a regular diet
- Accurately document and report food and fluid intake, remove food leftovers, and provide the resident with personal care as necessary. Then reposition the resident as discussed previously.

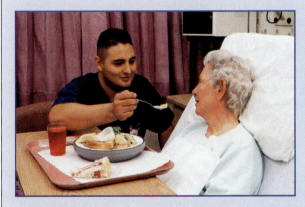

FIGURE 9-10
Seat yourself next to the resident to make eye contact.

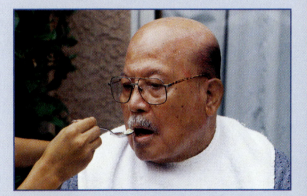

FIGURE 9-11
Feed from the tip of the spoon using gentle downward pressure.

phagia has been identified, the physician, dietitian, speech therapist, and nurse develop a plan. Often, the diet will be changed to include food that requires less effort to swallow. The liquids may be thickened, often to the texture of pudding or mashed potatoes. Solid foods may be softened or even pureed. The feeding technique may be written down and all nursing assistants instructed in how to feed the individual resident. Always follow the plan and feed each resident

Guidelines

as instructed. There are some general guidelines to keep in mind when feeding any dependent resident, including those with dysphagia:

- The resident should be seated upright in a bed or chair.
- The chin is down.
- Feed small amounts.
- Continuously observe the resident to verify that the food is being swallowed.
- If choking and coughing occur, stop. Ask for guidance.
- Feed at a slow pace to allow time for the resident to swallow.

Some residents are positioned at 45 degrees following the meal to prevent aspiration. Never attempt to feed a resident who is unable to chew or swallow. Report to the charge nurse at once. Some facilities use plastic syringes to feed residents who are difficult to feed and slow to eat. This is considered forced feeding and is a dangerous practice because it carries risk of choking and aspiration. The use of a spout cup or spoon to feed the resident who is slow and difficult to feed is more appropriate.

USE OF ASSISTIVE EATING DEVICES

Many assistive devices are available. These are special feeding utensils designed to help residents perform tasks that would otherwise be impossible for them (Figures 9-12 and 9-13). Usually, an assistive eating device is necessary due to lack of mobility or disability due to weakness. Use of any assistive device requires training of the resident and consistent encouragement from the staff. In the beginning, it may take more time for the resident to use an assistive device than it takes for you to perform the task for the resident. Keep in mind the importance of encouraging independence and allow the time necessary for learning.

Most LTC facilities employ an occupational therapy consultant to evaluate and work with residents who require special assistance in performing activities of daily living (Figure 9-14). The occupational therapy consultant will also assist the staff in learning how to help the resident use special assistive devices.

Many residents of LTC facilities require a nutritional supplement. This supplement is frequently necessary for residents to receive adequate nutrition. The most commonly used type of nutritional supplement is a high-protein drink.

FIGURE 9-12

Assistive eating devices.

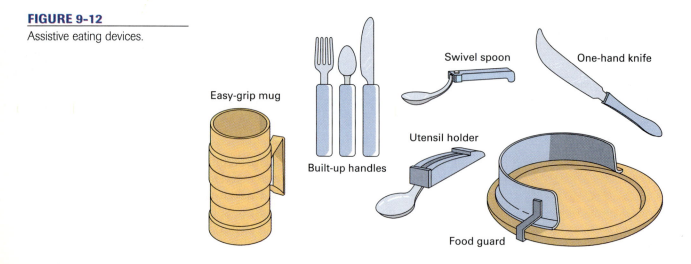

Easy-grip mug

Built-up handles

Swivel spoon

One-hand knife

Utensil holder

Food guard

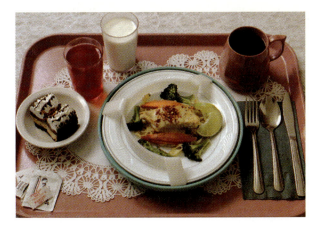

FIGURE 9-13
A plate guard in use.

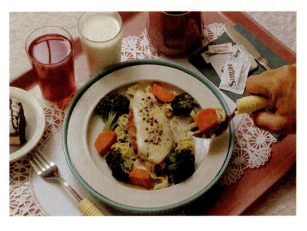

FIGURE 9-14
Resident using assistive devices.

If the resident requires a nutritional supplement, the physician's order will contain:

- The name of the supplement to be given
- The amount to be given
- How often it should be given

Because the nutritional supplement is part of the physician's treatment plan, it is very important to see that the resident not only receives but also eats or drinks the nourishment provided. Residents on restricted diets will also have specific orders for the kinds and amounts of between-meal snacks that they may have.

SECTION 5   Elimination

OBJECTIVES
What You Will Learn

When you have completed this section, you will be able to:

- Define the term **defecation**
- List four important observations related to bowel elimination
- Describe why accurate recording of the resident's bowel function is essential

- List three nursing measures used to decrease constipation in the elderly or chronically ill
- Identify one complication related to constipation that requires the immediate attention of the licensed nurse
- Insert a rectal suppository
- Administer a cleansing enema

- Define the term **colostomy**
- Change the colostomy bag
- Collect a stool specimen
- List four ways the nursing assistant can assist a resident to regain bowel control

KEY TERMS

colostomy
constipation
defecation
diarrhea

enema
enemas until clear
fecal impaction
ileostomy
laxative

suppository
ostomy
stoma
ureterostomy

THE PROCESS OF ELIMINATING WASTES

As you know, the foods you eat contain various nutrients that are absorbed and used by the body. Some elements of food cannot be used and are eliminated as waste material. These various waste products are eliminated through the skin, lungs, kidneys, and the bowel. The bowel is the most important excretor of solid wastes of the body. **Defecation** is the process of eliminating waste material from the bowel. The waste product itself is called feces (stool, BM). Normally, the stool is about three-quarters water by weight and one-quarter solid waste materials. This waste material is about 30 percent dead bacteria and 70 percent undigested roughage from food. The normal color of feces is brown, caused by bile, which is stored and released from the gallbladder. The characteristic odor of the stool is produced by the action of intestinal bacteria on food eaten.

defecation process of eliminating waste material from the bowel

The appearance and composition of feces are important indications of whether or not the digestive system is functioning normally. Changes in bowel habits may also be an indication of illness or disease. If the bowel becomes obstructed or blocked, it is a medical emergency and must be treated immediately.

You should report and chart the following related to bowel elimination:

- Changes in the color of the stool. (*Note:* The color of the feces can change when certain drugs or vitamins are taken. For example, drug preparations containing iron give the stool a black color, and some green vegetables or foods may cause the stool to be green.) You should always report changes in color to the charge nurse.
- Presence of blood. Blood in the stool should always be reported immediately. Save the specimen for observation by the licensed nurse.
- Presence of large amount of undigested foods or mucus.
- Presence of parasites (worms).
- Change in bowel habits.
- Complaints of pain related to bowel movement.
- Constipation or diarrhea.
- Uncharacteristic odors.
- **Diarrhea** is defined as semifluid feces. It may occur as a result of bacterial or viral infections, from eating spoiled and irritating foods, or from emotional upsets. Persistent diarrhea can lead to severe loss of fluids and loss of chemicals necessary for normal body functions. The nursing assistant must report to the charge nurse when any resident has diarrhea.

diarrhea semifluid feces

CONSTIPATION

constipation buildup of fecal material in the large intestine

Constipation is the buildup of fecal material in the large intestine that is not easily passed through the rectum. Constipation occurs as a result of several factors. Nursing measures effective in decreasing the likelihood of constipation include encouraging adequate intake of the right kinds of foods/fluids; encouraging exercise and ambulation, if possible; helping residents protect the need for privacy when toileting; and helping residents to reduce fears of incontinence by responding promptly to their needs.

Constipation is a common problem of the elderly and chronically ill. The nursing assistant must immediately report a lack of bowel movement or complaints of pain or discomfort.

fecal impaction serious and painful condition in which feces remain in the S-shaped area of the colon and rectum, where they may block the intestinal passage

A serious complication related to constipation is the development of a **fecal impaction.** Feces stay in the S-shaped area of the colon and rectum where water is absorbed, causing the feces to become dry and hard. This condition is very serious. It may block the intestinal passages, and it is very painful for the resident. This condition requires the immediate attention of a licensed nurse. Any complaints of pain, absence of bowel movements, or liquid movements should be reported to your charge nurse immediately. Fecal impaction is considered a "sentinel event" in a nursing home, requiring each incident to be investigated to determine how it could have been prevented. It is generally considered an indication of inadequate nursing care of the resident.

Remember, it is the digestive system that prepares food for use by the body. Whenever a disruption in the normal process occurs, it can be very serious. Nausea, which causes a resident to reject food, can be serious and should never be taken lightly by the nursing assistant. Report all complaints of nausea or episodes of vomiting, constipation, or diarrhea to your charge nurse immediately. Episodes of flu, abdominal distress, or diarrhea can be life threatening to a weak or seriously ill resident.

LAXATIVE MEDICATIONS

There are some special medications and treatments ordered by the physician to treat problems related to elimination. The purpose of enemas, laxative medications, and suppositories is to empty the bowel of its contents. A **laxative** is a medication that loosens the bowel contents and encourages evacuation.

laxative medication that loosens the bowel contents and encourages evacuation

Laxative medications and treatments may only be given when the physician orders them, as there are dangers associated with overuse. Frequently, the physician will order laxative medication administered by the licensed nurse. Many times the only way the licensed nurse can determine a resident's need for laxative medication is by the records and reports the nursing assistant makes. For this reason, it is essential to record each bowel movement. You will need to question those residents who have independent bowel function to gather this information.

In some facilities, the licensed nurse will be responsible for insertion of laxative suppositories; in other facilities the nursing assistant is trained to insert them. Make sure you follow your facility's policies and procedures regarding insertion of suppositories.

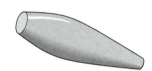

FIGURE 9-15
Rectal suppository.

THE USE OF RECTAL SUPPOSITORIES

A rectal **suppository** is a cone-shaped semisolid medicated substance that frequently contains glycerin (Figure 9-15). It is about 1½ inches long. The rectal suppository works to stimulate the inner surface of the rectal lining, creating an urge to empty the bowel as well as lubricating and coating the stool for easier evacuation.

suppository cone-shaped semisolid medicated substance inserted into the rectum

ENEMAS

An **enema** is the introduction of fluid into the rectum and colon. Enemas are given to stimulate the bowel and cause the contents to be released. The kind of solution and the amount of fluid used for the enema are prescribed by the physician. The most common solutions are:

enema introduction of fluid into the rectum and colon

- Tap water
- Commercially prepared (Fleet, oil retention)
- Saline (salt solution)
- SSE (soap suds enema)

PROCEDURE

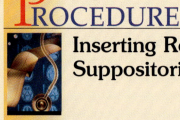

Inserting Rectal Suppositories

Beginning Steps

1. Assemble your equipment:
   - A suppository as ordered
   - Lubricant
   - Bedpan with cover
   - Disposable gloves
   - Toilet tissue

2. Wash your hands.
3. Identify the resident.
4. Provide privacy.
5. Explain to the resident what you are going to do.
6. Raise the bed to a comfortable working position.

Steps

7. Position the resident or ask the resident to turn on one side and raise one knee toward the chest. Assist as necessary.
8. Lift the sheet and expose the buttocks.
9. Put on disposable gloves.
10. Open lubricant and apply to gloved index finger.
11. Apply lubricant around anal area.
12. Holding the suppository between the thumb and index finger, spread the buttocks. Slowly and gently insert the suppository with a rotating motion, as far as your lubricated index finger will reach (2 to 3 inches).
13. It will help the resident relax the anal sphincter if he or she "pants" while you insert the suppository.
14. Withdraw the finger and hold toilet tissue against the anus briefly.

Ending Steps

15. Remove gloves by turning them inside out.
16. Reposition the resident and encourage him or her to retain the suppository as long as possible (15 to 20 minutes).
17. Provide a bedpan for use, if necessary, or assist to the bathroom.
18. Discard disposable gloves, toilet tissue, and suppository wrapper and wash your hands.
19. Monitor the resident every few minutes.
20. Assist the resident to clean up.
21. Reposition and make comfortable, lower the bed, and replace the call signal.
22. Return or discard used equipment appropriately.
23. Wash your hands.
24. Record the time and type of suppository given, as well as the results.
    - Example: 9:15 A.M. Glycerin suppository inserted. S. Smith N/A

       9:45 A.M. Large amounts of soft brown formed stool eliminated, resident stated he feels much better. S. Smith N/A

Commercially prepared enemas are the most common types used in LTC facilities today.

The amount of solution varies between 500 cc (2 cups) to 1,000 cc (4 cups). The solution should be a comfortable temperature (40° to 50°C or 105°F). Always check the temperature against the inside of your wrist. Solutions that are too cold cannot be retained, and solutions that are too hot can cause irritation, pain, and damage to the rectal tissues. The container holding the solution, if not the commercially prepared type, should not be higher than 18 inches above the anus. Any height greater than that creates too much pressure, causes discomfort, and increases the urge to expel the contents immediately.

The resident receiving an enema should be positioned on the side or the back as tolerated. The side-lying position is the most common position. If the resident can be positioned on the left side with the hips slightly elevated, the flow of the solution is better.

Residents should not be given enemas while seated on a toilet or commode, as the sitting position does not allow the solution to flow up into the colon. It merely collects in the rectum, causing dilation and the urge to defecate immediately.

ADMINISTERING THE COMMERCIALLY PREPARED ENEMA

The disposable commercially prepared enema is commonly used. The administration is simple. Whenever you use any disposable product, read the directions printed on the container carefully. You will follow the basic procedure for administering a cleansing enema, with the addition of:

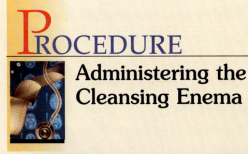

PROCEDURE

Administering the Cleansing Enema

Beginning Steps

1. Assemble your equipment:
   - Disposable enema unit or reusable enema, bucket bag, tubing, clamp
   - Solution ordered by the physician at warm temperature (105°F, 40.5°C)
   - Disposable gloves
   - Toilet tissue
   - Lubricating jelly
   - Bedpan
   - Bed protector

2. Close the clamp on the enema tubing and fill the enema bucket with the specified type and amount of solution.
3. Test the temperature of the solution to ensure that it is neither too hot nor too cold. It should feel warm when run across the inside of your wrist (105°F, 40.5°C).
4. Open the clamp and allow the solution to fill the tubing to remove air. Close the clamp.

5. Wash your hands.
6. Identify the resident.
7. Provide privacy.
8. Explain to the resident what you are going to do.
9. Raise the bed to a comfortable working position.

Steps

10. Position the resident on the left side with the left knee and hip flexed, if possible, or in the supine (back-lying position) with knees flexed, if the side-lying position cannot be used (Figure 9-16A).
11. Protect the bed with disposable pads or linens.
12. Have the bedpan within easy reach.
13. Keep the resident covered, exposing only the buttocks.
14. Put on gloves.
15. Lubricate the tip (2 to 4 inches) of the enema tubing by rotating it in lubricant jelly that has been placed on toilet tissue.
16. Lift the upper buttock to expose the anal area, then gently and slowly insert the tip of the tubing 2 to 4 inches (Figure 9-16B). Never push against resistance. Use a gentle rotating movement. Have the patient "pant" while you insert the enema tubing, as this will help the resident relax.

FIGURE 9-16a

Administering the cleansing enema.

a Assist the resident onto the left side.

PROCEDURE

continued

17. Open the clamp and raise the enema bucket about 12 to 15 inches above the anus and let the solution flow in slowly (Figure 9-16C).

18. If the resident is uncomfortable, you may need to clamp the tubing and wait a minute or so before allowing the flow of solution to continue. Encourage the resident to take all the solution ordered; however, stop if the resident is too uncomfortable.

19. When the solution is almost gone, clamp the tube and slowly withdraw the tubing. Place the tubing into the enema bucket. Avoid bringing the contaminated tip into contact with the bed or floor.

20. Assist the resident onto the bedpan, toilet, or bedside commode. Encourage the resident to retain the solution as long as possible.

21. Monitor the resident every few minutes.

Ending Steps

22. Assist the resident to clean up.

23. Reposition and make the resident comfortable, lower the bed, and replace the call signal.

24. Return or discard equipment appropriately.

25. Wash your hands.

26. Record the time and type of enema given, as well as the results.

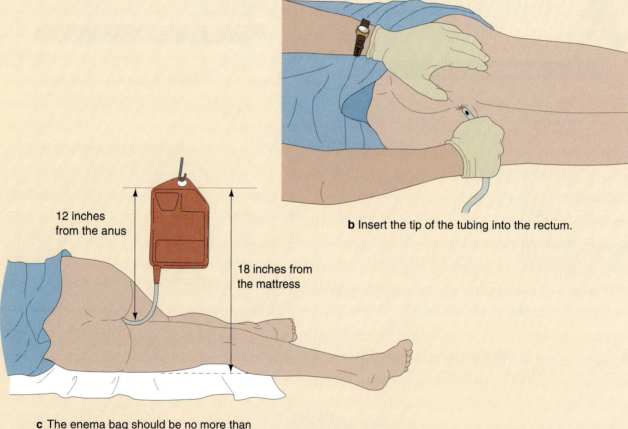

b Insert the tip of the tubing into the rectum.

12 inches from the anus

18 inches from the mattress

c The enema bag should be no more than 18 inches from the bed or 12 inches from the anus.

FIGURE 9-16b & c

Administering the cleansing enema.

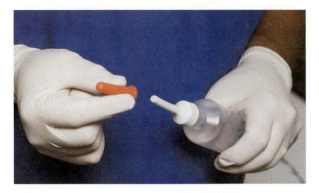

FIGURE 9-17

Remove the cap and expose the tip of the enema container.

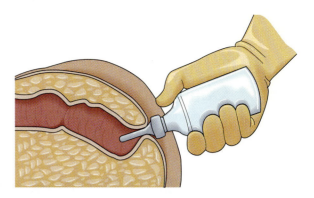

FIGURE 9-18

Insert the lubricated tip of the enema container into the rectum.

- Removing the protective cover (Figure 9-17)
- Inserting the prelubricated tube slowly and gently (Figure 9-18)
- Squeezing the bottle to expel the solution slowly
- Replacing the tube and restoring it in the original container to discard in the appropriate waste container (Figure 9-19)

THE OIL-RETENTION ENEMA

The oil-retention enema is given in the same manner; however, the resident needs to be encouraged to retain the solution for a longer period, 10 to 20 minutes, if possible. Frequently, the physician will order a cleansing enema after an oil-retention enema.

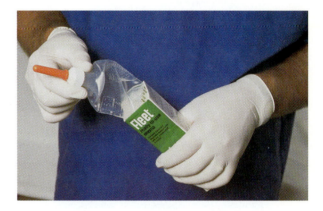

FIGURE 9-19

The tip of the used container is placed into the original container to prevent contamination.

There are occasions when the physician will order laxative medications and "enemas until clear." This is done to cleanse the bowel prior to diagnostic procedures or surgery. You would follow the physician's order for the type of solution and the amount of solution to be used. Clarify any questions regarding this procedure with your charge nurse. **Enemas until clear** means that there is no solid fecal material present when the solution is expelled. The solution, however, will be discolored and particles of feces will be present.

enemas until clear there is no solid fecal material present when the solution is expelled

Elderly or seriously ill residents may become very fatigued after receiving an enema. For this reason, check with the charge nurse before giving more than two enemas, even when the results are not yet clear.

OSTOMIES

An **ostomy** is a surgical opening made on the surface of the abdomen to release waste from the body. The opening is called a **stoma.** An ostomy becomes necessary when the ileum, colon, or urinary tract becomes diseased or injured to the extent that normal passage of waste materials is impossible. The most frequent reason for an ostomy is the removal of tumors or obstructions. Sometimes the surgery is done to permit the colon to heal following an injury. This is referred to as a *temporary ostomy.* Once healing has taken place, surgery is performed to reconstruct the normal passage for the waste materials.

ostomy surgical opening made on the surface of the abdomen to release waste from the body

stoma an opening

PROCEDURE

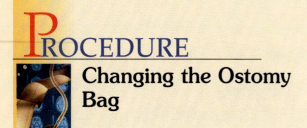

Changing the Ostomy Bag

Beginning Steps

1. Assemble your equipment:
   - Bedpan
   - Clean ostomy appliance, adhesive, and belt (optional)
   - Skin protector or cream as ordered by the physician
   - Bed protector
   - Toilet tissue
   - Basin of water
   - Disposable gloves
   - Washcloth, towel, and soap

2. Wash your hands.
3. Identify the resident.
4. Provide privacy.
5. Explain to the resident what you are going to do.
6. Raise the bed to a comfortable working position.

Steps

7. Position the resident in the supine position with the head elevated, if possible.
8. Protect the bed with a bed protector on the side of the stoma.
9. Place the bedpan within easy reach.
10. Expose the abdomen, taking care to keep the genital area covered.
11. Fill basin with moderately hot water (115°F, 46.1°C), have washcloth and soap nearby. Put on disposable gloves.

12. Carefully open belt and remove the soiled or full ostomy bag, taking care to peel it away from the stoma gently. Use toilet tissue to protect the skin around the stoma from coming into contact with fecal material.
13. Place the soiled ostomy bag in the bedpan. Remove the belt if it is soiled, and cleanse the area around the ostomy stoma with soap and water.
14. Apply lubricant, skin protector, or skin cream, as ordered, around the stoma. Observe for any skin irritation or breakdown.
15. Place a clean belt around resident and place a clean bag over the stoma. Make sure that it is attached securely.

Ending Steps

16. Assist the resident as necessary to clean up.
17. Observe the contents of the ostomy bag for blood, undigested food particles, or for changes in form consistency. Report anything unusual to your charge nurse immediately.
18. Dispose of the full ostomy bag according to your facility's policies. Check to see if stool or feces is considered infectious waste. If fluid blood is present, it is "medical waste" and must be disposed of properly, usually in a special container.
19. Remove your gloves.
20. Return or discard equipment appropriately.
21. Wash your hands.
22. Record changing the bag and any unusual observations.
23. Reposition and make the resident comfortable, lower the bed, and replace the call signal.

---

colostomy opening into the colon

ileostomy opening into the ileum

ureterostomy opening into one of the ureters

Permanent ostomies are performed when reconstruction is impossible due to diseased tissue. The location (site) of the ostomy and stoma depend on where the disorder is located (Figure 9-20):

- **Colostomy**—opening into the colon
- **Ileostomy**—opening into the ileum
- **Ureterostomy**—opening into one of the ureters

There are thousands of people with permanent ostomies who live normal lives. Most residents with ostomies have made their initial adjustment prior to admission to the LTC facility because the surgery and patient teaching is part of most acute hospital programs. For some residents, the adjustment is very difficult. When possible, ostomy residents are encouraged to perform their ostomy care independently.

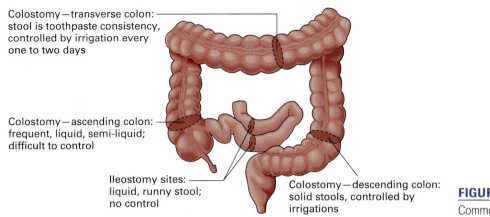

Colostomy—transverse colon: stool is toothpaste consistency, controlled by irrigation every one to two days

Colostomy—ascending colon: frequent, liquid, semi-liquid; difficult to control

Ileostomy sites: liquid, runny stool; no control

Colostomy—descending colon: solid stools, controlled by irrigations

FIGURE 9-20

Common ostomy sites.

Some individuals wear only a small gauze pad over their stoma, but most ostomy residents wear an appliance that covers the stoma and collects waste material released (Figure 9-21). Many different types of appliances are used, depending on the size and location of the stoma as well as the sensitivity of the resident's skin to the various adhesive substances.

Three very important nursing functions are associated with providing care to the resident with an ostomy. They are to:

- Protect the skin around the stoma from breakdown or irritation.
- Assist in reducing odors.
- Observe to ensure that the ostomy is functioning properly.

The ostomy bag may be changed in the bathroom with the resident seated on the toilet. For some residents, this is preferred because the problem of odor is confined to the bathroom and privacy is maintained. The bag itself should not be discarded in the toilet. Follow the basic procedure for changing the bag in bed.

There are occasions when residents may require an ostomy irrigation. This is done to help the resident establish a regular pattern of elimination. Ostomy irrigation is a procedure much like that of giving an enema. Before attempting this procedure, you must find out if nursing assistants in your facility are permitted to perform the irrigation, and you must receive specific instructions and supervision.

FIGURE 9-21

An ostomy device in place over a stoma, and equipment.

COLLECTION OF A STOOL SPECIMEN

There are times when it is necessary to collect specimens for laboratory analysis. You will be instructed by the charge nurse when a stool specimen has been ordered by the physician.

BOWEL INCONTINENCE

When normal nerve pathways that control the release of the contents of the bowel are affected, incontinence may result. This embarrassing condi-

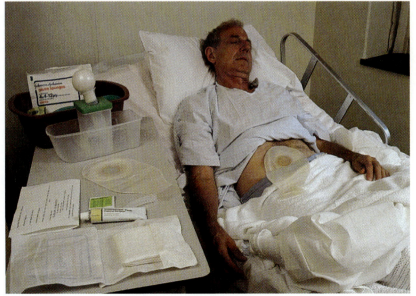

PROCEDURE

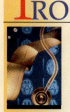

Collecting a Stool Specimen

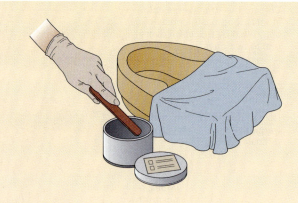

FIGURE 9-22

Place fecal material into the labeled stool specimen container.

Beginning Steps

1. Assemble your equipment:
   - Bedpan and cover
   - Stool specimen container and label
   - Wooden tongue depressor
   - Disposable gloves (optional)

2. Wash your hands.
3. Identify the resident
4. Provide privacy.
5. Explain to the resident that you need to collect a specimen. Ask the resident to call you when he or she feels the need to move the bowels. If the resident is unable to cooperate, check frequently and have equipment ready for collection of the specimen when defecation occurs.

Steps

6. Once the resident has had a bowel movement, take the covered bedpan into the bathroom and use the wooden tongue depressor to remove one to two tablespoons of fecal material from the bedpan. Place this into the labeled stool specimen container (Figure 9-22).

7. Cover the container immediately.
8. Wrap the tongue depressor in a paper towel and discard.
9. Empty the bedpan, clean it, and return it to its proper place.

Ending Steps

10. Wash your hands.
11. Follow the instruction of the charge nurse for storage of a stool specimen prior to collection by the laboratory.
12. Assist the resident as necessary to clean up.
13. Reposition and make the resident comfortable, lower the bed, and attach the call signal.
14. Record and report collection of the stool specimen, along with any unusual observations.

tion may be caused by stroke (CVA), spinal cord, or brain injury, in addition to many other diseases or medications.

Incontinence may occur during an episode of serious illness or hospitalization. Regardless of the cause, it is always important to assist the resident to regain control if possible. Incontinence occurs most often with residents who are not fully aware of their surroundings. However, even residents who are confused or unaware realize when they have soiled themselves. Incontinence promotes feelings of embarrassment and humiliation and loss of self-respect and self-esteem. For these reasons, it is never appropriate to scold or make fun of the incontinent resident. A matter-of-fact attitude is the best way to reduce negative feelings.

The physician and the licensed nurse will evaluate the nature of the resident's bowel incontinence as well as their food and fluid intake pattern and habits of elimination. A plan will then be developed to assist the resident in regaining bowel control. The specific plan for bowel retention should be recorded on the health care plan. Your charge nurse will give you further instructions.

PROVIDING INCONTINENCE CARE

When an incident of bowel incontinence has occurred, it is important to clean the resident as soon as possible. Feces left on the skin becomes dry and hardened and is both damaging to the skin and hard to remove. A resident who remains soiled suffers from a bad odor and loss of dignity. Equipment you will need includes:

- Gloves
- Toilet tissue
- Warm, soapy water or a special solution for incontinence care like Periwash®
- Washcloth
- Towel
- Plastic bag for waste
- Clean clothing and linens as needed

Use the tissue to remove the majority of the fecal material and place in the plastic bag. Then use the washcloth with soapy water or the special spray solution. Always wipe from the top of the buttocks down, making one wiping motion. Never rub up and down or go back and forth because this can cause injury to delicate skin. Wash the skin thoroughly and be sure all the skin is cleaned. Gently pat dry. You may apply lotion. Use only an amount that can be gently rubbed into the skin. If necessary, blot or pat dry. Avoid use of powder because it becomes paste-like when in a moist area, thus increasing the skin irritation. There are also some concerns that the resident and the nursing assistant can inhale particles of the powder.

BOWEL RETRAINING

As a nursing assistant you can play a major role in helping residents regain bowel control by:

- Encouraging the resident to consume adequate amounts of food and fluids. Fluid intake of between 2,000 cc (8 cups) and 3,000 cc (12 cups) daily is needed to provide the average adult with good hydration and to prevent constipation.
- Reporting signs of constipation so that medication can be administered.
- Following carefully and consistently the bowel retraining plan found on the resident's health care plan. *Note:* The bowel retraining plan should be based on the individual resident's problem and his or her bowel habits as well as the resident's ability to communicate and comprehend.
- Answering the call signal promptly as well as checking with residents frequently to assist them to use the bathroom or bedpan. Some residents are considered incontinent because they are unable to get the help they need fast enough!
- Identifying the residents' normal bowel evacuation times and assisting them to use the bathroom or bedpan prior to that time.
- Assisting residents to exercise in and out of bed. Exercise helps maintain muscle tone necessary for good bowel function.
- Helping the resident get adequate rest and sleep is important. Confusion and incontinence result when the resident is overly tired.

- Praising the resident for successful efforts to regain continence and ignoring accidents.
- Providing the resident and family with emotional support and encouragement.

Assisting a resident to regain bowel control is a very important accomplishment. It builds self-esteem and self-confidence.

SUMMARY

The things you have learned about the functioning of the digestive system and about nutrition can contribute to your personal life as well as to your role as a nursing assistant. Healthy living requires good nutrition. Following the Food Guide Pyramid as included in this chapter will help you provide yourself and your family with a healthy lifestyle. You've also learned about the importance of food and eating to the resident's quality of life. Ways that the diet can be used as a treatment for various diseases and conditions were included in the section "Therapeutic Diets." When you serve a therapeutic diet, you are assisting in the treatment of the disease and you are contributing to the resident's comfort and well-being. You'll use the feeding techniques you learned on a daily basis. The most important thing to remember about feeding the resident is to feed slowly and gently. Remember, the way you feed your residents is crucial to their health, safety, and quality of life. This chapter also included bowel elimination and related care and treatment. The key point when providing any treatment related to bowel care procedures is to maintain the privacy and dignity of the resident when performing such intimate and personal care. A professional attitude is a matter-of-fact attitude to make the process as comfortable as possible for the resident.

OBRA HIGHLIGHTS

The regulations address nutrition in several ways. First, residents should not lose their ability to feed themselves, they must maintain adequate nutrition, they must be provided the proper therapeutic diet, and they must not be fed by tubes unless it is unavoidable. Regarding nutrition, the regulation states that a resident "maintain acceptable parameters of nutritional status such as body weight and protein levels, unless the resident's clinical condition demonstrates that this is not possible."

SELF STUDY

Choose the best answer for each question or statement.

1. Which of the following is a function of the digestive system?
   a. It filters toxins out of the blood.
   b. It prepares food for use by the body.
   c. It produces hormones to control functions of glands.
   d. It fights infection that invades the body.

2. Where are most of the digested food particles absorbed into the body?
   a. in the stomach
   b. in the rectum
   c. in the duodenum
   d. in the liver

3. What is the function of bile?
   a. It breaks down fats.
   b. It regulates blood sugar.
   c. It secretes digestive enzymes.
   d. It absorbs digested foods.

4. Which of the following is true of the appendix?
   a. It is located between the duodenum and small intestine and helps digest grains.
   b. It is located near the sigmoid colon and helps digest fats.
   c. It is located between the stomach and small intestine and helps digest meat.
   d. It is located between the large and small intestine and has no digestive function.

5. Which of the following is true of stomach ulcers?
   a. They are very painful.
   b. Residents with stomach ulcers must take special medications.
   c. Residents with stomach ulcers are on special diets.
   d. All of these statements are true.

6. If a resident has liver cirrhosis, his normal liver tissue has been replaced by
   a. fragile tissue that bleeds easily but still functions
   b. tough fibrous tissue that cannot function correctly
   c. tissue blocked by stones that can only partially function
   d. tissue containing enlarged blood-filled pockets that cannot function

7. Which of the following would a resident with gastroesophageal reflux disease (GERD) be allowed to have?
   a. sliced tomatoes
   b. chocolate cake
   c. fried chicken
   d. baked potato

8. You are feeding Mr. Snodgrass. Which of the following would indicate that he has difficulty swallowing?
   a. drooling during the meal
   b. chewing and swallowing food quickly
   c. preference for liquids over solids
   d. all of the above

9. Which of the following are food sources of carbohydrates?
   a. meats, milk, and cheese
   b. vegetable oils, butter, and nuts
   c. cereals, grains, and potatoes
   d. milk, margarine, and egg yolks

10. What amount is considered a serving of vegetables?
    a. one-fourth cup cooked and one-half cup of raw vegetables
    b. one-half cup cooked and one cup of raw vegetables
    c. one-half cup cooked or raw is a serving of vegetables
    d. one cup cooked or raw is a serving of vegetables

11. Mr. Martin will not eat macaroni and cheese. This dish is sometimes on the menu as a meat substitute. What should you do?
    a. Make sure Mr. Martin gets second helpings of other menu items.
    b. Ask Mr. Martin's family to bring him a hamburger when macaroni and cheese is served.
    c. Notify the nurse and food service supervisor so that special arrangements can be made.
    d. Encourage Mr. Martin to eat the macaroni and cheese when it is served in place of meat.

12. What is the most accurate way to chart a resident's intake of food?
    a. Estimate the percent of food left on his plate and chart this amount.
    b. Chart exactly what was eaten during the meal by the resident.
    c. Round the amount eaten to 100 percent unless it is less than 50 percent.
    d. Ask the resident what percentage of the meal he thinks he ate.

13. Ms. McMehan has diabetes. Which of the following diets would be right for her?
    a. low calorie and low fat
    b. no added salt
    c. high protein
    d. no concentrated sweets or added sugar

14. Which of the following items should *not* be served to a resident who is on a no-added-salt diet?
    a. bacon
    b. ice cream
    c. fruit juice
    d. cabbage

15. You have served Ms. McMehan's tray to her. Which of the following should you do before you leave the room?
    a. Tell her when you will back to pick up the tray so she can be finished by then.
    b. Make sure she has started eating and does not require further assistance.
    c. Remove any foods or liquids she does not think she will want.
    d. All of these are appropriate to do for Ms. McMehan.

16. You are feeding Mr. Wong, a resident who has dysphagia. Which of the following actions should you take?
    a. Position him so that his chin is titled upward so he can swallow better.
    b. Place the soft foods and liquids in a plastic syringe and push the food into his mouth.
    c. Check to be sure that he is swallowing each bite of food before giving him another.
    d. If he coughs, give him more fluid to wash down the foods that are difficult to swallow.

Getting C O N N E C T E D
Multimedia Extension Activities

www.prenhall.com/will-black

Use the above address to access the free, interactive Companion Website created for this textbook. Hear the pronunciation of the key terms in the chapter. Get instant feedback to a variety of chapter-related questions. Link to other interesting sites.

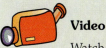

Video

Watch the section on "Handling Infectious Waste" in the video *Infection Control* from the Care Provider Skills series.

CASE STUDY

George Green is 78 years old and has resided in the facility for about 6 months. He has been diagnosed with cirrhosis of the liver due to chronic alcohol abuse. He is on a low-fat diet.

1. Some of the foods that are not permitted on a low-fat diet include
   a. fruits and vegetables
   b. fish and chicken
   c. bacon and eggs
   d. sugar, fruit juice, and cake

2. Mr. Green wants to eat in bed instead of going to the dining room. When serving him, it is important that the nursing assistant
   a. position him in bed sitting at a 90-degree angle
   b. position him lying on his left side
   c. allow his food to cool before serving
   d. insist that he eat in the dining room

3. Mr. Green has a stroke and loses his ability to swallow. He has an advance directive that states that he does not wish to be fed by tube. Your responsibility to Mr. Green is to
   a. tell him he must have a tube or he won't get well
   b. give him excellent care in all ways but honor his wishes
   c. feed him with an oral syringe
   d. avoid contact with him

4. You notice it has been 4 days since Mr. Green had a bowel movement. You report this to the charge nurse. She asks if you believe the resident has a fecal impaction. The signs you would look for include
   a. chills and fever
   b. nausea and abdominal pain
   c. skin rash with itching
   d. burning pain upon urination

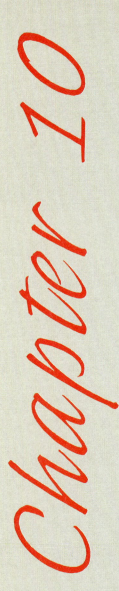

Chapter 10

THE URINARY SYSTEM

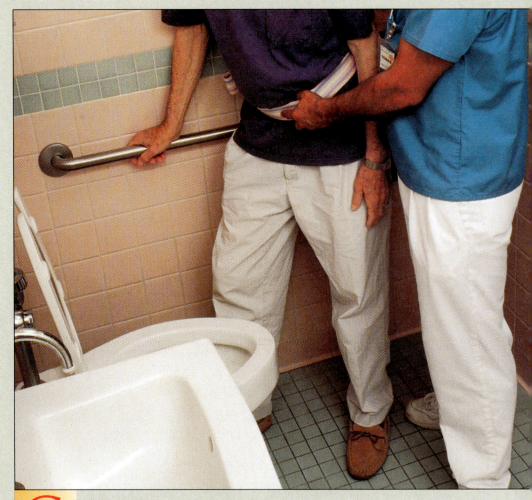

CARING TIP

Respecting the resident's dignity is an essential part of every nursing activity.

Dr. Anne Woodtli
Professor of Nursing
University of Arizona
Tucson, Arizona

SECTION 1 Anatomy and Physiology

THE URINARY SYSTEM

The urinary system (Figure 10-1) is composed of:

- Kidneys
- Bladder
- Ureters
- Urethra

Functions of the urinary system are:

- Remove wastes from the bloodstream
- Produce urine
- Maintain homeostasis

The urinary system removes waste products from the body by producing and eliminating urine. Other organs that assist in the elimination of waste products are the lungs, intestinal tract, and sweat glands.

FIGURE 10-1

The urinary system.

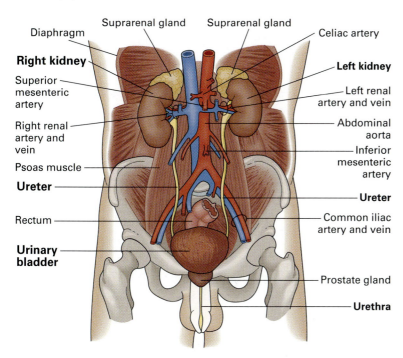

The urinary system is part of the body's excretory structures (urinary system, lungs, sweat glands, and intestine). The kidneys remove the wastes of chemical activities (metabolism) in the body. These wastes are removed from the blood to produce urine. At the same time, the kidneys remove certain excess compounds, regulate the blood pH (acid-base balance), and the concentration of sodium, potassium, chlorine, glucose, and other important chemicals.

THE KIDNEYS

kidneys two bean-shaped organs in the pelvis of the body that act as a filtration system to eliminate waste products

nephrons microscopic filtering units of the kidney

renal artery artery that supplies blood to the kidneys

glomerulus a network of capillaries in the kidney that filters the blood

renal pelvis part of the kidney that serves as a funnel for urine coming from the kidney into the ureter

ureters tubes that extend from the kidneys to the bladder through which urine passes

The **kidneys** are two bean-shaped organs that lie just below the diaphragm and posterior abdominal wall on either side of the lumbar region of the spine (Figure 10-2). In an adult, the kidney is about 4 inches long, 2 inches wide, and 1 inch thick. Each kidney weighs 4 to 6 ounces. In this tiny organ, there are over 1 million microscopic filtering units called **nephrons** (Figure 10-3). One of the amazing examples of the body's reserve is that we can lose large amounts of nephrons to age or disease and still live normally. Many people live with only one kidney.

Blood enters the kidney from the **renal artery,** where it is distributed through arterioles into millions of capillaries that lead to the nephrons. Fluids and other substances pass through the thin capillary walls and are collected in the central part of the nephron, the **glomerulus,** which is found inside Bowman's capsule. This special network of capillaries acts like a filter. Materials not needed by the body are filtered out and carried through a series of tubules. These tubules make up the rest of the nephron. When this filtered material from the blood flows through the tubules, the tiny capillaries surrounding the tubules selectively reabsorb (take back into the blood) substances needed by the body. Other substances not needed, such as drugs, some vitamins, and excessive fluids, are not reabsorbed. Combined with excess water, these substances create the waste product, urine.

Once urine is formed, it moves into a collecting funnel called the **renal pelvis,** where it passes into the right and left ureters attached to the right and left kidneys. The **ureters** are tiny tubes about 10 inches long that start at the renal pelvis and empty into the bladder. Here, special **stretch-receptor** nerve cells in the walls become stimulated when the bladder is full. A message is sent to the brain, which results in **urination** (emptying of the bladder).

The bladder has a tube (the **urethra**) that leads outside the body. It is through the urethra that urine passes from the body. The urethra in the male is about 8 inches long because it runs through the penis. In the female, it is about 1½ inches long. Because this tube opens to the outside, there is always a threat of infection. When infection develops, it travels up into the bladder and sometimes into the kidney itself, causing very serious complications.

FIGURE 10-2

The kidney.

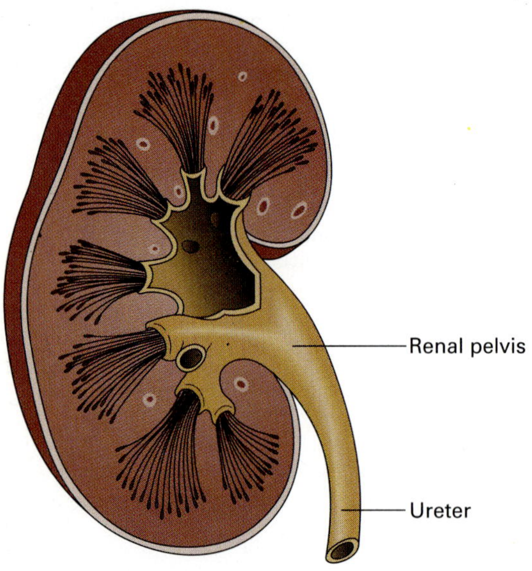

Renal pelvis

Ureter

FIGURE 10-3

The nephron.

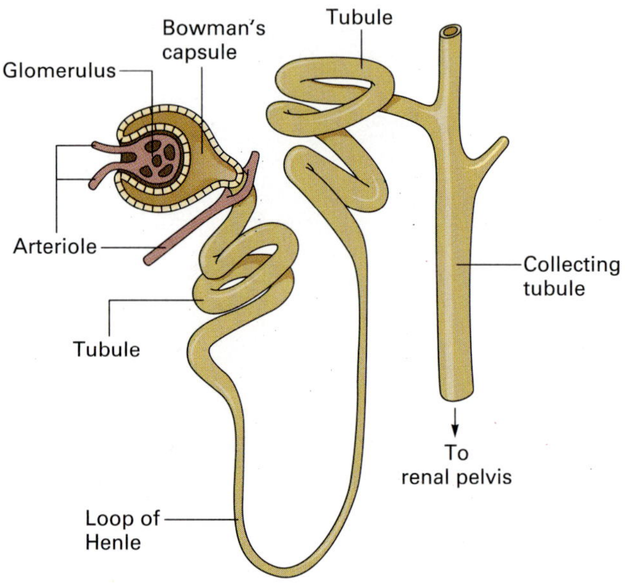

Glomerulus

Bowman's capsule

Tubule

Arteriole

Tubule

Collecting tubule

To renal pelvis

Loop of Henle

In the average adult, about 1½ quarts of urine are produced every 24 hours. The kidney is a very efficient organ when functioning normally. It has the capacity to filter 1 quart of blood per minute or 360 gallons each day. Normal urine is straw-colored and clear. Urine that is dark, bloody, or filled with sediment (flecks or particles) or mucus is not normal and should be reported immediately. Urine has a characteristic odor, but this changes when it is very concentrated or when infection is present. One of the most important factors in maintaining normal kidney function is to ensure that residents have adequate fluid intake. You will study problems related to dehydration and will learn how to measure intake and output later in this chapter.

AGE-RELATED CHANGES

The kidney and its specialized tissues function to maintain homeostasis. The kidney actually determines the water and chemical composition of the blood, which in turn determines the content of the tissue fluid that surrounds the cells.

A number of age-related changes affect the urinary system. As an individual ages, the kidneys function less efficiently. An 80-year-old person will have about half the nephrons of the newborn infant. If only half the nephrons are available, their efficiency will decrease greatly. For this reason, an elderly resident is more likely to have a drug reaction than the middle-aged or young adult. The kidney is less efficient in removing the drug from the bloodstream. Reactions to medications must be observed for and reported to the charge nurse.

Arteriosclerosis can affect the blood vessels that supply the urinary system. When circulation is poor, there is a greater chance of developing infection as well as decreased ability to recover from illness or injury. There are age-related changes that decrease the elasticity of the ureters, bladder, and urethra. The muscle tone decreases, and the amount of urine the bladder can hold is reduced. Sometimes the elderly resident will not be aware of the need to urinate until the bladder is almost full. This leads to:

- **Frequency**—the need to urinate often
- **Urgency**—an immediate need to urinate
- **Nocturia**—waking at night to urinate

These problems, along with chronic illness and some types of medications, may lead to incontinence. **Urinary incontinence** is the inability to control urination. It is a very distressing and embarrassing problem for most residents. Residents with neurological disease or injury frequently have no control of the bladder functions because the brain is unable to receive signals that control urination.

Urinary tract infections are a common problem in all ages. However, the elderly resident who is confined to bed or has an **indwelling catheter** (a tube inserted into the bladder that drains urine into a collection bag) is especially vulnerable. Immobility has serious effects on the urinary system primarily due to the incomplete emptying of urine from the kidneys and bladder. When urine is retained too long, bacteria grow, resulting in infection and development of kidney stones. Stones (called **calculi**) may develop in either the kidneys or the bladder, and they are extremely painful. Incomplete emptying of the bladder may be related to the position of the body when

stretch-receptors nerve cells in the wall of the bladder that send a message to the brain when the bladder is full

urination the process of emptying the bladder of its contents

urethra tube from bladder to the outside of the body

frequency the need to urinate often

urgency an immediate need to urinate

nocturia waking at night to urinate

urinary incontinence inability to control urination

indwelling catheter tube inserted through the urethra into the bladder to drain urine into a collection bag

calculi stones in the kidney or bladder

FIGURE 10-4

Contrast in degree of bladder emptying.

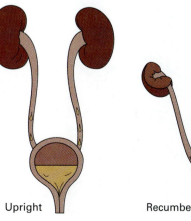

Upright   Recumbent

urinating. When the resident is confined to bed and is in a reclining or semi-reclining position, it is almost impossible to empty the bladder completely (Figure 10-4).

Urinary tract infections will also develop when good hygiene measures are not practiced after urination and defecation. Bacteria normally present in the bowel are very frequently the source of the infection. Poor fluid intake is also a cause of urinary tract infections. Repeated infections damage the kidneys and are a major cause of fever and serious illness in the elderly. Many important nursing measures can help reduce the incidence of infection.

SECTION 2 Fluid Balance—Intake and Output

OBJECTIVES
What You Will Learn

When you have completed this section, you will be able to:

- Describe what is meant by **fluid balance**
- Identify those items that should be calculated as fluid intake
- Compute intake accurately
- Compute output accurately
- List three ways the nursing assistant can help residents meet their fluid needs

KEY TERMS

calibrated
central line
dehydration

dialysis
emesis
fluid balance
fluid intake

fluid output
hemorrhage
imbalance
NPO

FLUID BALANCE

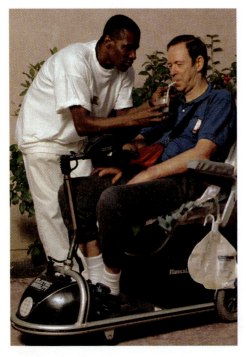

FIGURE 10-5

Fluids are essential to life.

The nursing assistant assists residents in maintaining normal fluid balance. Water is essential to human life. Next to oxygen, water is the most important substance the body takes in (Figure 10-5). A person can lose half of the body protein and almost half of the body weight before death occurs. Yet if an individual loses about one-fifth of the total body fluids, death usually results.

Through eating and drinking, the average healthy adult will consume between 2½ and 3½ quarts in a 24-hour period. **Fluid intake** is the amount of fluid consumed by:

- Mouth
- Special feeding tubes
- The parenteral routes (into a vein and under the skin)

FLUID INTAKE AND FLUID OUTPUT

The same average healthy adult will eliminate between 2 and 3 quarts in a 24-hour period. **Fluid output** is the total amount of fluid eliminated from the body through:

- The kidneys as urination, also referred to as voiding or passing water (approximately 1½ quarts in 24 hours)
- The skin through perspiration and the lungs through respiration (approximately 1 quart in 24 hours)
- The intestinal tract, where fluid is absorbed and discharged as part of the feces or stool (less than 1 cup)

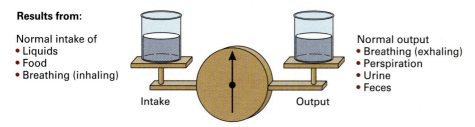

Results from:

Normal intake of
• Liquids
• Food
• Breathing (inhaling)

Intake   Output

Normal output
• Breathing (exhaling)
• Perspiration
• Urine
• Feces

FIGURE 10-6

Fluid balance: intake equals output.

• Other ways, such as **emesis** (vomiting), wound drainage, severe perspiration, severe diarrhea, or **hemorrhage** (bleeding).

Fluid balance means that the person eliminates about the same amount of fluid that is taken in (Figure 10-6).

To determine the minimum amount of fluid a particular resident requires for a day, the following formula has been suggested. The resident's weight in pounds is divided by 2.2 (to convert to kilograms) and then multiplied by 30 (cubic centimeters, cc). The total is the minimum fluid required for that individual for 24 hours. For example:

$$\text{Weight} = \frac{110 \text{ lb}}{2.2} = 50 \text{ kg}$$

$$50 \text{ kg} \times 30 \text{ cc} = 1,500 \text{ cc minimum for 24 hours}$$

If the output is high due to perspiration, wound drainage, or increased urine output, then more fluid would be necessary to replace the lost fluid.

FLUID IMBALANCE

An **imbalance** of body fluids occurs when fluid intake exceeds fluid output (Figure 10-7). Fluid is retained in the body, leading to edema. Symptoms of edema or fluid retention are:

• Swelling of feet, ankles, face, hands, fingers
• Weight gain
• Collection of fluid in abdomen and lungs
• Decreased urine output

Another type of imbalance exists if fluid intake is less than fluid output (Figure 10-8). This results in a condition called **dehydration**. Dehydration is one of the most common medical problems of the long-term care resident. Dehydration is due to consuming insufficient quantities of liquids. Dependent residents may be reluctant or unable to ask for water or may simply forget. Incontinent residents may stop drinking to reduce the chance of having an accident.

fluid intake total amount of fluid taken into the body over a given amount of time

fluid output total amount of fluid eliminated from the body in a given amount of time

emesis vomiting

hemorrhage bleeding

fluid balance the individual takes in and eliminates about the same amount of fluid

imbalance lack of equality

dehydration condition in which fluid output is greater than fluid intake

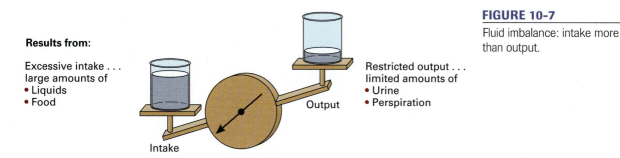

Results from:

Excessive intake . . .
large amounts of
• Liquids
• Food

Intake   Output

Restricted output . . .
limited amounts of
• Urine
• Perspiration

FIGURE 10-7

Fluid imbalance: intake more than output.

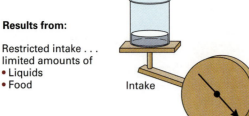

Results from:

Restricted intake . . .
limited amounts of
• Liquids
• Food

Intake

Output

Excessive output . . .
large amounts of
• Urine
• Vomitus
• Blood
• Drainage
• Perspiration

FIGURE 10-8

Fluid imbalance: intake less than output.

Eliminating too much fluid also causes dehydration. Examples are vomiting, bleeding, perspiring profusely, or losing fluid through diarrhea or wound drainage.

The symptoms of dehydration include:

Early	*Late*
• Fatigue	• Thirst
• Weakness	• Decreased urine output
• Lethargy	• Dry skin with reduced elasticity
• Dizziness	• Parched or cracked lips and tongue
• Headache	

Dehydration affects all systems of the body; it is a life-threatening problem. Although the physician will prescribe treatment for the cause of dehydration, you play a vital role in helping residents meet their fluid needs. You do this by:

• Keeping fresh water within the resident's reach at all times.
• Offering fluids and reminding residents to consume fluids. A good habit to follow is to offer residents fluids each time you enter the room unless there is a fluid-restriction order.
• Providing encouragement to the resident so that all fluids served with meals or as between-meal nourishments are consumed. Menus are planned to provide the resident with a substantial portion of their required fluid intake.

Older people generally start with less water than those who are younger, so they are at greater risk for dehydration. Providing adequate fluids benefits the resident by preventing kidney stones and decreasing the risk of urinary tract infection and constipation.

Some dehydration is not treatable. When a resident is dying or when he or she refuses treatment (for the dehydration), he or she may become dehydrated. In this case, your role is to provide oral and skin care that will keep the mouth, lips, and skin from drying out. There are products available that keep the mouth and lips moist for up to 8 hours. The goal is to keep the resident comfortable!

Each facility has established policies and procedures for providing residents with fresh water. This is usually done each shift so that there is a constant supply of fresh drinking water available to residents. In some facilities, each water pitcher is taken to a clean area and filled with ice and fresh water. In other facilities, water pitchers are reprocessed and filled in the dietary department and returned to the resident. You will need to follow the policies and procedures established in your facility.

UNDERSTANDING FLUID INTAKE AND FLUID OUTPUT

To determine the resident's intake, you must measure and record everything a resident consumes by mouth that is a fluid, including water, milk, juice, coffee, tea, soups, and so on. Food items that become liquid at room temperature, such as gelatin and ice cream, must also be included. Although solid foods contain some liquid, most of the fluid intake comes from what a person drinks in the form of actual liquids (Figure 10-9).

Some residents who are unable or unwilling to drink fluids by mouth may receive them parenterally either through a vein (intravenous [IV]) or through a catheter placed into the atrium of the heart (central line). The licensed nurse is responsible for recording fluids administered parenterally.

To determine the resident's fluid output, you must measure and record all urinary output and vomitus and report hemorrhage, excessive wound drainage, or excessive perspiration. You will measure urinary output of the resident with an indwelling catheter by emptying and measuring the contents of the urinary drainage bag. If the resident is incontinent, you will not be able to collect or measure urine output. It is important to record on the intake and output record the number of times the resident is incontinent each shift.

If vomiting, hemorrhage, excessive wound drainage, or excessive perspiration occur, notify your charge nurse at once. The charge nurse will help you estimate the amount of fluid lost and will take other corrective actions. Never discard vomitus or drainage before the charge nurse has a chance to observe it.

Severe diarrhea can result in excessive fluid loss. Any observations or complaints of diarrhea should be reported to the charge nurse at once. When a fluid imbalance is suspected, you may be instructed to measure and record the resident's fluid intake and output. LTC facilities have written policies and procedures on how to measure and record intake and output. Be sure you follow the specific procedures outlined in your facility.

Measuring and recording fluid intake and output is very important! Many times the physician will use the data recorded on the intake and output record to determine which medications or treatments the resident needs.

The time for the nursing assistant to record fluid intake is when the resident consumes it. Fluid output should be recorded when urination or vomiting occurs. Do not try to remember—this is not the time for guesswork. Most facilities total the resident's intake and output at the end of each shift. The 24-hour total is generally calculated and recorded on the night shift.

Another method of finding out if a fluid imbalance exists is by measuring the specific gravity of the urine. This may be done by using a test tape and following the manufacturer's directions or by using a piece of equipment called a hydrometer. The hydrometer includes a glass tube that holds the urine and a measuring device similar to a thermometer that floats in the urine and gives the reading. If your facility uses this equipment, ask for a demonstration and instructions. The specific gravity shows how concentrated or how dilute the urine is. The specific gravity is an indicator of too much or too little fluid in the body.

The most reliable measure of hydration is a blood test that measures the concentration of sodium in the blood. The higher the amount of sodium, the greater the dehydration. The nursing assistant may notice the signs of dehydration early by observing that the urine is dark in color or has a strong odor.

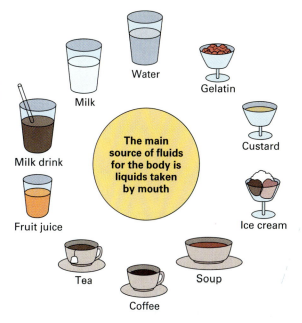

The main source of fluids for the body is liquids taken by mouth

Water
Gelatin
Milk
Custard
Milk drink
Ice cream
Fruit juice
Tea
Soup
Coffee

FIGURE 10-9

Sources of fluid.

central line catheter placed into the atrium of the heart

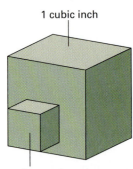

1 cubic inch

1 cubic centimeter

FIGURE 10-10

Size contrast: cubic inch versus cubic centimeter.

calibrated   marked with graduations, as on a thermometer or graduate

dialysis   use of a machine that performs the base functions of the kidney

USING THE METRIC SYSTEM

The most commonly used system of measurement in health care is the metric system. In the past, the facilities in the United States used a system called the U.S. customary system, made up of ounces, pints, and quarts for measuring liquids and inches, feet, yards, and miles for measuring distance. However, there is increasing reason to use the metric system of measurement because scientists, engineers, and health care personnel almost always use this system.

Fluids are measured in cubic centimeters (cc). A cubic centimeter is simply a square block with each edge of the block 1 centimeter long (Figure 10-10). If the block is filled with water, there would be 1 cubic centimeter (1 cc) of water inside the block. The accompanying conversion chart lists the U.S. customary liquid measure with equivalent metric measurements.

Containers, graduates, or measuring cups are used to measure fluid intake and output. Notice that the side of the graduate is **calibrated** (marked) with a row of short lines and numbers. This shows measurement in both cubic centimeters (cc) and ounces (oz).

Some residents are able to assist in keeping track of their fluid intake. Allow the resident to help as much as possible, being sure their accuracy is verified.

ENCOURAGE FLUID INTAKE

When residents need to have their fluid intake increased, the physician or nurse will give instructions to "force fluids." More accurately stated, the term *force fluids* would be "encourage fluids." Sometimes, a resident will need continuous encouragement and persuasion to consume adequate fluids. On some occasions, the physician will even specify the amount of fluids the resident is to receive: "Give 2,000 cc each 24 hours." Ways you can help residents consume more fluids are:

- Follow the plan for carrying out the physician's order. For example: "Give 2,000 cc each 24 hours. Total of 1,300 cc contained on meal trays, encourage to consume all. Give 350 cc additional on 7–3 shift and 350 cc on 3–11 shift."
- Offer liquids each time you enter the room.
- Find out what kind of liquids the resident prefers and notify the charge nurse so that they are available when the diet order permits.
- Have the family assist in encouraging the resident to take more fluids. Suggest that they bring in special fluid treats, as the diet order permits.

RESTRICTING FLUID INTAKE

There are times when it is necessary for the physician to order that fluids be restricted. Residents who have congestive heart failure or kidney disease may need to have their fluid intake limited. Residents on kidney **dialysis** (the use of a machine that performs the basic functions of the kidney) almost always require some type of fluid restriction. The physician's order may read "Give no more than 1,500 cc in 24 hours." It is always important to explain the reasons for fluid restrictions to the resident and family. Follow the instructions of your charge nurse and measure all fluids accurately. If fluid restrictions are not followed, the resident may suffer from fluid overload. Excess fluids may damage the kidneys and the heart by increasing their workload.

MEASURING FLUID INTAKE

- Obtain a list of the most commonly used fluid containers in your facility, along with a listing of how many ounces or cc's each will hold. If this is not available, you will need to measure the amount of liquid each container holds and make a list for yourself.
- Obtain the forms used for recording intake and output in your facility.
- Measure and record all fluids consumed by the resident during your shift of duty. (Calculate the difference between the full amount of the container and the amount left in the container.) Observe and record fluids consumed from the resident's meals, water pitchers, and between-meal snacks.
- Convert (change) amounts such as half a bowl of soup, half a glass of juice, or a quarter cup of coffee into cubic centimeters for recording. For example: Mrs. Jones's water pitcher contained 1 quart (liter), which equals 1,000 cc. At the end of the shift, you would measure what remained (in this case, 250 cc) and subtract the difference: 1,000 cc minus 250 cc equals 750 cc. In addition, Mrs. Jones drank half a glass of juice (4-ounce juice glass equals 120 cc) (120 cc divided by 2 equals 60 cc) and a quarter cup of coffee (8-ounce cup equals 240 cc) (240 cc divided by 4 equals 60 cc).

Water	= 750 cc
Juice	= 60 cc
Coffee	= 60 cc
Total	= 870 cc

- Record intake after each meal before the tray is removed.
- Record other intake as it is consumed.

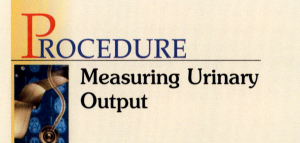

PROCEDURE

Measuring Urinary Output

It is not possible to measure accurately the amount of fluid eliminated through the intestinal tract, the respiratory tract, or the skin. Therefore, the urinary output is the most reliable measurement of fluid output.

Beginning Steps

1. Assemble your equipment in the resident's bathroom:
   - Bedpan, urinal, or special container
   - Disposable gloves
   - Graduate or measuring cup (Figure 10-11)

2. Put on your gloves.

Steps

3. Pour the urine into the measuring graduate.
4. Place the graduate on a flat surface at eye level and read the amount of urine in the graduate.
5. Observe the urine for any abnormalities, such as blood, dark color, large amounts of mucus or sedi-

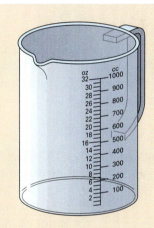

FIGURE 10-11
Calibrated graduate.

ment, or changes in the characteristic odor. Report any abnormalities to your charge nurse immediately before discarding the urine.

6. Discard the normal urine into the toilet or hopper.
7. Rinse the graduate, bedpan, urinal, or special container and return to their proper places.

Ending Steps

8. Remove your gloves.
9. Wash your hands.
10. Record the amount of urine (cc) on the intake and output record. Record the time of each entry.

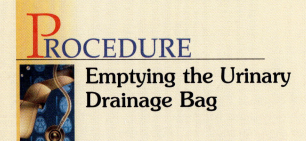

PROCEDURE

Emptying the Urinary Drainage Bag

Beginning Steps

1. Assemble your equipment:
   - Graduate or measuring cup
   - Disposable gloves
   - Bedpan or urinal

2. Put on your gloves.

Steps

3. Carefully open the drain outlet from the urinary drainage bag, making sure the *drain outlet does not touch the container or the floor.* Bacteria can be introduced into the drainage bag, causing infection (Figure 10-12).

4. Allow the bag to drain completely and reattach the drainage outlet securely to the drainage bag.

5. Pour the urine from the bedpan or urinal into the measuring graduate.

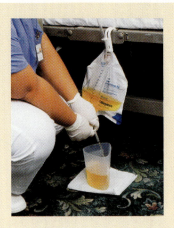

FIGURE 10-12
Emptying the urinary drainage bag.

6. Place the graduate on a flat surface at eye level and determine the amount of urine in the graduate.

7. Discard urine into toilet or hopper.

8. Rinse graduate, bedpan, or urinal and return to their proper places.

Ending Steps

9. Remove your gloves.

10. Wash your hands.

11. Record the amount of urine in cc's and the time collected on the Intake and Output Record.

12. Report any unusual observations, such as blood in the urine, a change in the color, or uncharacteristic odor of the urine, to the charge nurse immediately.

NPO consuming nothing by mouth

There are some occasions when a physician will order a resident to be **NPO** (consume nothing by mouth). NPO is taken from the Latin *nils per os,* which means "nothing by mouth." This is usually ordered prior to surgical or laboratory procedures. The NPO resident may not eat or drink anything at all—not even water! For example, the physician's order might say "NPO until lab work done in A.M." After the lab work has been drawn, normal intake may be resumed. Since residents who are NPO can become irritable, explain why the order is necessary.

SECTION 3 — NURSING MEASURES RELATED TO THE URINARY SYSTEM

OBJECTIVES
What You Will Learn

When you complete this section, you will be able to:

- Place a resident on a bedpan and offer a urinal to a male resident
- Give perineal care to a resident with a catheter

- Identify four places where bacteria can enter the urinary drainage system
- Identify activities necessary for collecting a **clean-catch** urine specimen

KEY TERMS

clean catch   closed urinary drainage system   reflux

PROVIDING PRIVACY

Elimination of waste products is a natural process, and most healthy people have regular elimination habits. When someone becomes ill, these habits are disrupted. Sometimes control is lost. Most people regard elimination as a very personal function, and when it becomes necessary to ask for assistance, they are embarrassed.

Consider the feelings of residents when you are assisting them with their elimination needs. You can help preserve dignity by providing care with an accepting, matter-of-fact attitude. Remember, your body language and facial expressions convey many messages.

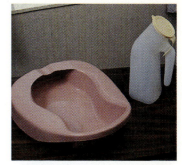

FIGURE 10-13
A bedpan and urinal.

CULTURAL AWARENESS Many cultures have strong views about modesty related to viewing or touching private areas. Some examples are Gypsies and those from Asian countries. In some cases, personal care must be provided by a member of the same sex. In others, no one but the spouse must be allowed to view these areas of the body. In order to properly provide catheter care, assist with toileting and bathing residents, all the staff needs to be aware of the cultural limitations. If necessary, a nursing assistant of the same sex should be assigned. At all times, protect the resident's modesty by uncovering only those areas of the body that are necessary. Carry out the care in a matter-of-fact manner and perform it as quickly as possible.

When you are assisting the resident to use a bedpan, urinal, or bedside commode, provide as much privacy as possible. Put yourself in the resident's place and consider how you would feel.

The female resident will use the bedpan for both urination and bowel elimination, while the male resident will generally use the bedpan for bowel elimination and the urinal for urination. The regular-sized bedpan is most commonly used (Figure 10-13). Some residents who have difficulty moving (especially following hip fracture) will need to use the smaller, flatter "fracture" bedpan.

Assisting the residents to practice good hygiene following urination and defecation is very important in preventing urinary tract infections. The female resident is much more likely to develop infection than the male, due to the shortness of her urethra. It is easier for bacteria to travel up the short urethra into the bladder and kidneys. For residents who provide their own care, help them remember:

- Always wipe from front to back after urination and defecation.
- Wash the perineal area thoroughly with soap and water when bathing.

Some residents have indwelling catheters (Figure 10-14). Catheters may only be inserted on the orders of a physician. An indwelling catheter is a tube inserted through the urethra into the bladder. It is used to drain urine from the bladder. The catheter is connected to the drainage tubing, allowing the urine to flow uninterrupted into the urinary drainage bag or collection unit. This is called a **closed urinary drainage system.**

An indwelling catheter is often necessary for residents with neurological (nerve) injury following a stroke or spinal cord injury. These residents are unable to tell when the bladder is full and have no control of urination. Some incontinent residents may require a catheter to avoid tissue damage or skin breakdown resulting from constant exposure to urine. There is an increased risk of developing infection when a catheter is present, indwelling catheters should only be used when absolutely necessary. First you must understand where bacteria can enter the urinary drainage system. Contamination of any of these areas can lead to urinary tract infection.

closed urinary drainage system method of collecting urine that prevents contamination as it is uninterrupted

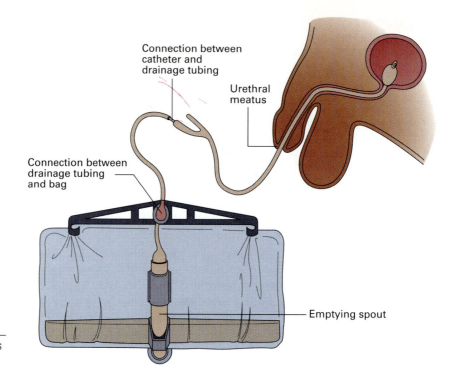

Connection between
catheter and
drainage tubing

Urethral
meatus

Connection between
drainage tubing
and bag

Emptying spout

FIGURE 10-14

An indwelling catheter with sites
where bacteria can enter.

PROCEDURE

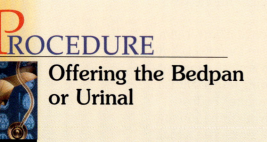

Offering the Bedpan
or Urinal

Beginning Steps

1. Assemble your equipment on the bedside table:
   - Bedpan and cover, or fracture bedpan and cover, urinal
   - Toilet tissue
   - Disposable gloves

2. Wash your hands.
3. Provide privacy.
4. Lower the side rails.

Steps

5. Fold back the top sheets so that they are out of the way.
6. Raise the resident's gown, but keep the lower part of the body covered.
7. Ask the resident to assist by bending the knees and placing the feet flat on the mattress. Then ask the resident to raise the hips. Assist as necessary by slipping your hand under the lower back and lifting slightly. Place the bedpan in position, with the seat evenly under the buttocks (Figure 10-15, left).
8. If the resident is unable to assist, turn the resident to one side and place the bedpan against the buttocks, pushing downward into the mattress as you gently turn the resident back onto the bedpan.
9. Give the urinal to the resident or assist as necessary in placing the urinal between the legs, with the penis inside the opening.
10. Replace the sheets over the resident.
11. Elevate the head of the bed and the knees slightly if allowed, so the resident can assume a sitting position.
12. Put toilet tissue and the call signal within easy reach of the resident (Figure 10-15, right).
13. Ask the resident to signal when finished.
14. Raise the side rails to the up position.
15. Wash your hands and leave the room to provide the resident with privacy.
16. When the resident signals, return to the room. If the resident is unable to signal, *check frequently.* Never leave a resident sitting on a bedpan for a prolonged period or with the urinal where pressure can be created.
17. Put on your gloves.
18. Assist the resident to raise the hips so that you can remove the bedpan.
19. Cover the bedpan or urinal immediately. You can use a disposable pad or a paper towel if no cover is available.

PROCEDURE

continued

20. Assist the resident to clean and wipe as necessary. Make sure the anal area is clean. Turn the resident to the side for easier cleaning.
21. Remove the bedpan or urinal to the bathroom.
22. If a specimen is required, collect it at this time. Measure urine if the resident is on intake and output.
23. Check the feces or urine for abnormal appearance.
24. Empty the bedpan or urinal into the toilet and flush.

25. Follow your facility's procedure for cleaning the bedpan or urinal.

Ending Steps

26. Remove and dispose of your gloves.
27. Wash your hands.
28. Put the clean bedpan or urinal and cover back into the bedside table.
29. Assist the resident with handwashing.
30. Make the resident comfortable. Lower the head of the bed as necessary and replace the call signal.
31. Wash your hands.
32. Report and record when a specimen is collected and any unusual observations.

FIGURE 10-15
Place the bedpan in position; leave the call signal within easy reach.

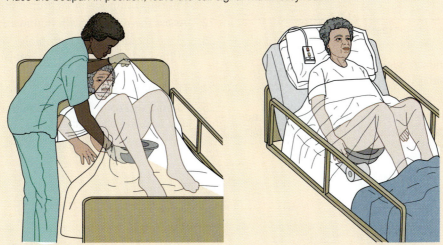

PROCEDURE

Using the Portable Bedside Commode

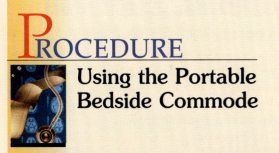

Beginning Steps

1. Assemble your equipment:
   - Portable bedside commode next to the bed
   - Bedpan and cover, or the container used in your facility
   - Toilet tissue
   - Disposable gloves

2. Wash your hands.
3. Provide privacy.
4. Tell the resident you will assist with transferring onto the bedside commode, if necessary.

Steps

5. Place the commode next to the resident's bed. Open the cover and insert the container under the toilet seat (Figure 10-16).
6. Assist the resident to sit on the side of the bed. Put slippers on the resident before transferring onto the bedside commode.
7. Place toilet tissue and the signal cord within the resident's reach.
8. Ask the resident to signal when finished.

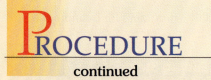

PROCEDURE

continued

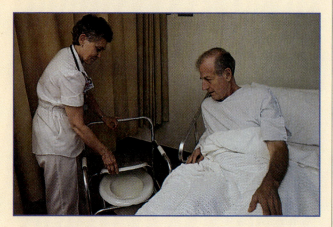

FIGURE 10-16

Place the commode next to the resident's bed.

9. Wash your hands and leave the room to provide the resident with privacy.
10. Put on your gloves.
11. When the resident signals, return to the room and assist the resident as necessary to clean and wipe. Make sure that the anal area is clean.

12. Assist the resident in transferring back to bed.
13. Close the cover on the commode.
14. Remove the container from under the commode. Cover it and take it to the bathroom.
15. Check the feces or urine for abnormal appearance.
16. Measure the output if the resident is on intake and output. If a specimen is required, collect it at this time.
17. Empty the bedpan into the toilet and flush.
18. Follow the procedures for cleaning the bedpan in your facility.

Ending Steps

19. Remove and dispose of your gloves.
20. Wash your hands.
21. Put the clean bedpan back in the bedside table. Put the commode in its proper place.
22. Assist the resident with handwashing.
23. Make the resident comfortable, lower the head of the bed as necessary, and replace the call signal.
24. Wash your hands.
25. Report and record if a specimen was collected and any unusual observations.

PROCEDURE

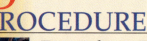

Providing Daily Catheter Care

Beginning Steps

1. Assemble your equipment:
   - Antiseptic solution (packets)
   - Disposable bed protector (optional)
   - Disposable gloves

2. Wash your hands.
3. Identify the resident.
4. Provide privacy.
5. Explain to the resident what you are going to do. *Note:* Make sure that the genital/perineal area is clean. Provide perineal care as necessary prior to providing catheter care. See Chapter 6.

Steps

6. Place disposable bed pad under resident.
7. Observe the area around the catheter for lesions (sores), crusting, leakage, or bleeding. Report any unusual observations to your charge nurse immediately.
8. Open antiseptic solution packet.
9. Put on disposable gloves.
10. Remove the antiseptic applicator from the packet. Apply antiseptic solution around the entire area where the catheter enters the urethra. On female residents, gently separate the labia with your thumb and forefinger and apply the antiseptic solution. On the uncircumcised male resident, retract the foreskin and apply the antiseptic solution to the entire area.
11. Apply antiseptic solution to the 4 inches of catheter tubing nearest the resident (Figure 10-17).

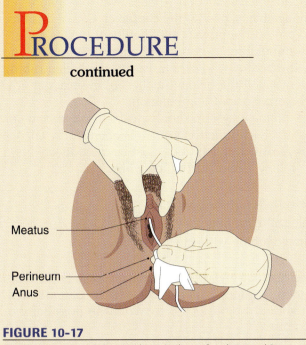

PROCEDURE

continued

Meatus
Perineum
Anus

FIGURE 10-17

Apply antiseptic solution to the 4 inches of catheter tubing nearest the resident.

12. Apply antiseptic ointment (if ordered) around the catheter tube at the urethra according to your facility's policies.
13. Position the resident so that the catheter and tubing are free of kinks or pulling.
14. Remove the disposable bed protector.
15. Cover the resident.

Ending Steps

16. Discard disposable equipment.
17. Remove your gloves.
18. Wash your hands.
19. Reposition and make the resident comfortable and replace the signal cord.
20. Wash your hands.
21. Report and record care given and any unusual observations.

The indwelling catheter (often referred to as a Foley catheter) is designed to be held in position in the bladder by an inflatable balloon located along the tip of the catheter. The catheter is inserted by a licensed nurse using strict aseptic technique, and the balloon is inflated with sterile water so that it will not come out. Once a catheter is inserted, special catheter care must be given daily. There are some very important guidelines that must be understood and followed in order to provide safe care to residents with indwelling catheters.

Make sure that the catheter tubing and drainage tubing are free of kinks or obstruction. Many facilities use a strap that goes around the resident's thigh to secure the catheter and prevent pulling or sliding in and out of the urethra. The strap has a loop or Velcro fastener that attaches to the catheter tubing.

The strap must not be so tight as to injure the skin or interfere with circulation. Always check the strap to be sure that it is not too tight or causing irritation of the skin.

Report to the charge nurse if there is any leaking around the catheter. This is often a sign of infection, bladder spasms, or obstruction. Observe for, report, and document any swelling, discoloration, skin irritation, or complaints of pain in genital or perineal area.

Measure and record urinary output as required as well as the color, odor, and appearance of the urine. As urine collects in the drainage bag and tubing, it begins to break down or decompose. Bacteria multiply very quickly under these conditions. For this reason the collection bag must always be kept below the level of the resident's bladder (Figure 10-18). This prevents urine collected in the bag from running back up the tubing and into the bladder. This is called **reflux.**

When the resident is in a wheelchair, the collection bag should be passed below or under the wheelchair seat and fastened behind the wheelchair at a point below the level of the resident's bladder

reflux return flow of urine back into the bladder from a drainage bag

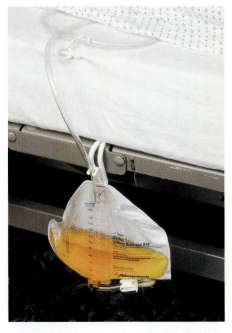

FIGURE 10-18

Positioning of catheter on bed.

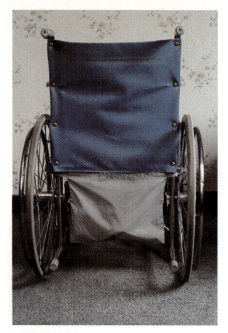

FIGURE 10-19

Positioning of catheter on wheelchair.

(Figure 10-19). There are special decorative bags available that fasten to the chair. The drainage bag slips into the container. Use of this type of container helps to protect the privacy and dignity of the resident.

If the resident is ambulating, carefully disconnect the tubing and collection bag from the bed or wheelchair. Fasten the coiled tubing and bag to the resident's clothing below the level of the bladder. It is important to drain the urine prior to ambulation.

The closed urinary drainage system should not be disconnected unless absolutely necessary. Each time the system is opened, the chance of infection increases greatly. If the system must be disconnected and a catheter plug used, follow aseptic technique while:

- Disconnecting the catheter from the tubing
- Inserting the sterile catheter plug
- Covering the drainage tubing with the sterile cap

The drainage collection bag and drainage tubing should never come in contact with the floor. The floor is always considered contaminated, and this equipment should be protected to avoid the possibility of infection.

Some residents, such as those who have spinal cord injury with neuromuscular loss of bladder control, may prefer to have their catheters attached to a leg drainage bag (Figure 10-20). Notice that the leg drainage bag is positioned so that the inlet of the bag is at the top.

They are applied next to the resident's leg. Be sure that the straps are not applied over the bag preventing it from filling. The straps are always attached to the collection bag prior to applying it to the resident's leg. Review your facility's policy for emptying, cleaning, and storing leg bags if reusable bags are used.

When providing care to residents with indwelling catheters, you must:

- Make sure the system is open (urine is flowing into the collection bag). If the catheter becomes plugged with sediment or mucus, the licensed nurse must be notified immediately.
- Observe for decreased urinary output. This is a serious problem that must be reported to the charge nurse immediately. The normal healthy adult will produce between 1,500 and 2,000 cc in 24 hours (approximately 50 to 80 cc each hour).
- Make sure that the catheter tubing and drainage tubing are free of kinks or obstructions.
- Report to the charge nurse if there is any leaking around the catheter. This is often a sign of infection, bladder spasms, or obstruction.
- Observe for, report, and document any swelling, discoloration, skin irritation, or complaints of pain in genital or perineal areas.
- Measure and record urinary output as required as well as the color, odor, and appearance of the urine.

The entire urinary drainage system (catheter, drainage, tubing, and bag) should be changed together. If the drainage bag is changed by itself, strict aseptic technique must be followed.

The nursing assistant is usually responsible for the collection of urine specimens. It is very important to remember to wash your hands carefully before and after you collect specimens. One of the most frequently ordered

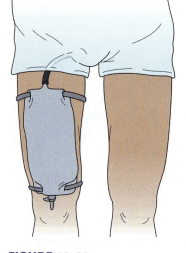

FIGURE 10-20

A leg drainage bag.

USE OF AN EXTERNAL CATHETER

Incontinent male residents may have a physician's order for the application of an external catheter (a condom connected to a tube that drains urine into a collection bag) (Figure 10-21). The collection bag may be a leg bag for ambulatory residents or a urinary drainage bag.

An external catheter must be properly applied to prevent skin breakdown, cutting off circulation, or closing off the urethra, leading to stopping the flow of urine. Use the following guidelines when applying the external catheter:

• Wear gloves.
• Wash and dry the penis.
• Special surgical adhesive may be used.
• Roll the condom over the penis, leaving ½ to 1 inch extending beyond the tip of the penis.
• Apply elastic tape spirally around condom and penis. Never completely encircle the penis, as this could interfere with circulation.
• Apply tape snugly enough to prevent leakage but not tight enough to restrict circulation.

Because the condom is flexible, it tends to twist around itself after application. The nursing assistant

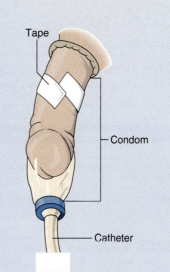

FIGURE 10-21
External catheter.

must check the resident with an external catheter frequently to ensure that the urine flow is not obstructed and there is no injury or cutting off of circulation. Usually, the external catheter is reapplied daily or more frequently if it is necessary.

PROCEDURE

Collecting a Routine Urine Specimen

Beginning Steps

1. Assemble your equipment (Figure 10-22):
   • Resident's bedpan and cover, or urinal
   • Disposable gloves
   • Graduate used for measuring output
   • Urine specimen container and lid
   • Label, if your facility's procedure is not to write on the lid
   • Laboratory request slip, which should be filled out by the charge nurse
   • Paper bag

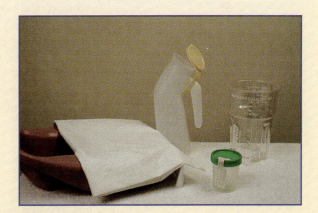

FIGURE 10-22
Urine specimen collection equipment.

2. Wash your hands.
3. Identify the resident by checking the identification bracelet.
4. Provide privacy.

PROCEDURE

continued

5. Tell the resident a urine specimen is needed and explain the procedure. Some residents may be able to collect the specimen themselves.

Steps

6. Have the resident urinate into the clean bedpan or urinal.
7. Ask the resident not to put toilet tissue into the bedpan or urinal and to use the paper bag provided.
8. Prepare the label immediately by copying all necessary information from the resident's identification bracelet. Record the time and date.
9. Put on your gloves.
10. Take the bedpan or urinal to the resident's bathroom and pour the urine into a clean graduated container.

11. Pour urine from the graduate into a specimen container and fill it three-fourths full, if possible.
12. Place the lid on the specimen container. Check to ensure that the correct label is on the container.
13. Pour the leftover urine into the toilet and flush.
14. Clean and rinse the graduate. Put it in its proper place.
15. Clean the bedpan or urinal and put it in its proper place.

Ending Steps

16. Remove and dispose of your gloves.
17. Wash your hands.
18. Make the resident comfortable and replace the signal cord.
19. Assist the resident in handwashing.
20. Take the labeled specimen container to the charge nurse.
21. Wash your hands.
22. Report and record that a specimen was obtained and any unusual observations.

tests is a urinalysis, which requires a routine urine specimen. Use the following procedure when collecting a routine urine specimen.

A special method is used to collect a resident's urine when the specimen must be free from contamination. This kind of specimen is called a midstream clean-catch urine specimen. In most health facilities, a disposable midstream cleaning kit is available.

All the equipment, supplies, and instructions necessary for this type of specimen are found in the kit. Midstream means catching the urine specimen between the time the resident begins to urinate and the time urination stops. **Clean catch** refers to the fact that the urine is not contaminated by anything outside the resident's body. The procedure requires careful washing of the perineal area.

clean catch urine that is not contaminated by anything outside the body

There are a number of ways to recognize abnormal function of the urinary system. You should be familiar with the following in order to report problems promptly:

- Inadequate urinary output—if resident does not void or voids very small amounts frequently, there is a serious problem that requires immediate attention
- Changes in color, consistency, and odor of the urine
- Poor skin turgor—the skin becomes limp or dry and nonelastic
- Fever, complaints of burning, frequency, urgency
- Unusual discharge, swelling, redness at the urethral opening
- Change in excretory habits—a continent resident becomes incontinent

The excretory function is very important. Be sure you observe carefully and report problems promptly!

SECTION 4 CARE OF THE INCONTINENT RESIDENT

OBJECTIVES
What You Will Learn

When you have completed this section, you will be able to:

• Define the term *incontinence*

• List four possible causes of urinary incontinence

• Describe proper use of disposable briefs

• List four nursing measures that can increase a resident's chance of successful bladder retraining

URINARY INCONTINENCE

You will provide care to many residents who are incontinent of urine. Some residents have control of bowel and not bladder function, and others are incontinent only periodically. Urinary incontinence can have many causes:

• Stress, worry
• Anger, frustration
• Anxiety, fear
• Urinary tract infection
• Medications

• Injury to the central nervous system
• Bladder spasms or tumors
• Confusion
• Altered bladder reflexes
• Inadequate fluid intake

Incontinence is not a normal result of the aging process. When recognized and treated early, it can often be treated successfully.

Many residents experience embarrassment, shame, loss of self-esteem, and frustration when they become incontinent. It is important to provide care in a matter-of-fact way to minimize negative feelings. Be sure to:

• Approach the resident in a calm, professional way
• Never tease, scold, or ridicule
• Protect the resident's privacy when you provide care
• Wear gloves when you come in contact with body fluids

Incontinent residents must be checked frequently to ensure they are not left wet or soiled for prolonged periods. Urine or feces are destructive to skin tissue and will cause skin breakdown if not cleaned and removed promptly.

Incontinent residents may use cloth or disposable diapers when retraining is not a possibility. When talking about these "diapers," the terms to use are *briefs, underwear,* or *underpants.* Do not use the term *diaper* because it is disrespectful and takes away the dignity of the resident. When using disposable or cloth briefs, follow these guidelines:

• Use them only for those residents who cannot be toileted or use a bedpan. They may be used temporarily if the resident is going on an outing and is fearful of an accident.
• Select the appropriate size.
• Learn proper method of application for the specific brief used.
• Check the resident often to see if changing is needed. Some briefs include a color change wetness indicator to assist you.
• Always wash the skin with soap and water or Peri-wash® when changing the brief.

- Observe the skin for any signs of irritation and report your observations promptly.
- Dispose of the briefs in the proper container. Do not discard in the trash container in the resident's room or bathroom. Usually, cloth briefs need to be rinsed if they are soiled with feces.

Always be sure that the resident is clean and dry before meals or before taking them to a public area. This helps the resident maintain dignity and self-esteem.

BLADDER RETRAINING

Some residents who are incontinent of urine can be successfully trained to regain bladder control. When successful, regaining continence can be one of the most important elements in helping residents reestablish a positive self-image.

When a resident is placed on a bladder retraining program, all who provide care must follow the established plan consistently! Inconsistency will lead to poor results. The physician and the licensed nurse will evaluate the cause of the resident's incontinence and will develop a plan. The specific approach should be outlined on the resident's health care plan.

The individualized plan will include a schedule for intake that specifies time and quantity of fluids to be consumed and a schedule for elimination that identifies frequency and method. For example: "Offer 100 cc's each hour from 8 A.M. to 8 P.M. Toilet every three hours or when requested. Use a bedpan from 8 P.M. to 8 A.M." Favorite liquids may be included in the plan. Some residents might not be willing to drink water, but they may like coffee, tea, or other drinks.

Success requires commitment and a positive approach. It is a known fact that those people with the greatest potential for influencing another person's behavior are those with whom the person has the most direct and frequent contact. For this reason, the nursing assistant is the most important person in assisting residents in regaining bladder control.

Since people tend to repeat behavior that is rewarded, the nursing assistant should reward any positive steps toward continence made by the resident. Be sure to praise the behavior you want repeated. "Mr. Smith, you are doing so well in asking for and using the urinal. I'm really proud of you." Be sure you reward the resident promptly and consistently.

Other types of rewards in addition to praise include:

- Extra time spent with the resident
- A walk outside
- Special outings

It is easy to give extra attention when good progress is made, but what should you do if the resident is not making progress? The best approach is a matter-of-fact manner. Never scold or reprimand. Certain measures can increase the resident's chance of successful bladder retraining, including:

- Maintaining adequate fluid intake (2,000 cc or more per day).
- Observing and recording times when the resident is incontinent can help establish a schedule for taking the resident to the bathroom or offering the bedpan or urinal.
- Following the established plan carefully and consistently.

- Answering the call light promptly. Some residents cannot wait and become incontinent due to inattention.
- Involving the resident and/or family in the retraining plan so there is a complete support system.
- Documenting and reporting the resident's progress or lack of progress to the plan. If results are poor, the approach may need to be changed.
- Not giving up—it takes time to reestablish continence.

SUMMARY

In this chapter, you have learned about the urinary system, the key to the maintenance of homeostasis and good health. The most important concept to remember is the importance of providing residents with enough water and other fluids to meet their needs and to protect them from the consequences of dehydration. Many elderly are residents in a nursing home because they cannot meet their own basic needs. It is the responsibility of the facility staff, particularly the nursing assistant to offer and encourage adequate fluid intake.

Because the elderly nursing home resident is so vulnerable to infection, the care provided by the nursing assistant must reduce the risk of exposure when handling the catheter or providing incontinence care. This means proper use of gloves and strict use of handwashing.

A common problem related to the urinary system is urinary incontinence. Although statistics vary, there are reports that over 50 percent of nursing home residents are incontinent of urine. This means that much of the care you provide is related to the management and treatment of incontinence. Many residents have a type of incontinence called *functional incontinence* that results from the resident's inability to perform the activities necessary to go to the toilet independently. Sometimes, the rules imposed by the facility to assure safety and prevent falls may actually promote incontinence. The resident may be instructed to call for help before attempting to walk to the bathroom. Because the perception of needing to urinate often may come late, incontinence may result from a slow staff response. It is in these cases that good care based on regular toileting can effectively restore the dignity of the resident.

OBRA HIGHLIGHTS

There are a number of regulations relating to the urinary system. The facility is required to provide care that prevents residents from losing control of their bladder function, avoids use of indwelling catheters unless necessary, and provides each resident with sufficient fluid intake to maintain proper hydration and health.

Choose the best answer for each question or statement.

1. Which of the following is true of the kidneys?
   a. They are cone-shaped.
   b. They lie close to the back below the diaphragm.
   c. They lie close to the back above the diaphragm.
   d. They each contain about a hundred neurons, or filtering units.

2. The two tiny tubes that stretch from the renal pelvis to the bladder are the
   a. ureters
   b. urethras
   c. glomerulus
   d. nephrons

3. What can happen if bacteria enters the urethra?
   a. It can cause incontinence.
   b. It can cause urinary retention.
   c. It can cause a urinary tract infection.
   d. It can cause kidney stones.

4. Which of the following is a description of normal urine?
   a. dark amber with sediment
   b. straw-colored with mucus
   c. straw-colored and clear
   d. dark yellow with blood

5. Which of the following changes occur in the urinary system due to aging?
   a. The ureters, bladder, and urethra become less elastic.
   b. The muscle tone in these structures decreases.
   c. The amount of urine the bladder can hold is reduced.
   d. All of these changes occur with aging.

6. What is the most important action a nursing assistant can take to prevent urinary tract problems in residents?
   a. Ensure that residents have adequate fluid intake.
   b. Turn the resident every 2 hours or more frequently.
   c. Ensure that residents get food and fluids containing vitamin C.
   d. All of these actions are equally important.

7. You notice that Mrs. Joseph's ankles and feet are swollen this morning. She also has a moist-sounding cough and says her pants feel tight. Which of the following problems might Mrs. Joseph be having?
   a. early stages of dehydration
   b. fluid retention (edema)
   c. urinary tract infection
   d. late stages of dehydration

8. If a resident complained of weakness, dizziness, and headache, which of the following problems might be occurring?
   a. early stages of dehydration
   b. fluid retention (edema)
   c. urinary tract infection
   d. late stages of dehydration

9. How will you help residents meet their fluid needs?
   a. Encourage residents to drink fluid only during the morning to prevent incontience at night.
   b. Offer fluids every time you enter a resident's room unless the resident is on a fluid restriction.
   c. Encourage residents to drink fluids between meals only if they did not consume all the fluids served with their meals.
   d. Take residents to the water fountain once every shift.

10. Mr. Taylor is on intake and output. He consumes all of the following during lunch. Which will you record as fluid intake?
    a. soup, tea, gelatin, and ice cream
    b. mashed potatoes, peas, and soup
    c. chocolate cake, chicken breast, and gelatin
    d. soup, chicken breast, and peas

11. Mr. Taylor was incontinent of urine twice during your shift. He also voided 250 mL in the urinal once. What will you write on the output portion of his intake and output sheet?
    a. "Incontinent"
    b. "Unable to measure"
    c. "250 mL urine; incontinent × 2"
    d. "250 mL urine"

12. What is the best way to record intake and output accurately?
    a. Ask the resident how much he had to drink and how many times he urinated since morning.

b. Write the amount of fluid consumed and eliminated as soon as it occurs.

c. Remember the amounts of intake and output for the resident until the end of shift, then record the total amounts.

d. Any of these methods are accurate.

13. Ms. Martinez is on fluid restriction. She can have only 600 cc of fluid on your shift. What could result if she is given more fluids than are allowed?

a. She could develop kidney stones.

b. Her bladder could rupture.

c. Her kidneys and heart could fail to work properly.

d. She could become incontinent of urine.

14. Mr. Melvin is ordered to be NPO until after his fasting blood sugar is drawn. This means that Mr. Melvin

a. cannot eat or drink anything at all.

b. cannot eat or drink anything except water.

c. can eat but not drink anything with sugar in it.

d. can drink water but not eat anything with sugar in it.

15. Which of the following guidelines should you follow to prevent infection in the resident with an indwelling catheter?

a. Observe for and report any leaking around the catheter.

b. Keep the drainage bag above the level of the resident's bladder.

c. Wash the perineal from back to front during bathing and catheter care.

d. When the resident is in a wheelchair, fasten the drainage bag to the arm of the chair.

16. You notice that Mr. Melvin is voiding frequently, but only expels about 60 cc of urine each time. What should you do?

a. Total the amount of urine for your shift; if it is over 250 cc, it is a normal amount of output.

b. Report this to the nurse because it could indicate a urinary tract infection.

c. Encourage Mr. Melvin to drink more fluids so he will have more output when he urinates.

d. Encourage Mr. Melvin not to drink so often, so he won't have to urinate as often.

Getting C ONN ECTED
Multimedia Extension Activities

 www.prenhall.com/will-black

Use the above address to access the free, interactive Companion Website created for this textbook. Hear the pronunciation of the key terms in the chapter. Get instant feedback to a variety of chapter-related questions. Link to other interesting sites.

 Video

Watch the video *Infection Control* from the Care Provider Skills series.

CASE STUDY

Mrs. Myrna Tamayo is an 80-year-old resident who was born and raised in the Philippines. She has a diagnosis of end-stage renal disease. She has an indwelling catheter in place. She leaves the facility for dialysis every Monday, Wednesday, and Friday afternoon.

1. When you are getting her ready for her appointment, she asks you for a soft drink from the machine in the employee lounge. Your response should be
   a. "You can't have soft drinks, you are on a restricted diet."
   b. "Do you have a dollar to pay for it?"
   c. "Let me check with the nurse first to be sure it is okay."
   d. "I'll be right back."
2. You notice that when you give her personal care, she won't look at you or talk to you. This may be because
   a. in her culture, there is a high degree of modesty
   b. she doesn't like you
   c. she is ashamed of her body
   d. she is tired from the dialysis
3. Proper care for Mrs. Tamayo involves
   a. protecting her from development of pressure ulcers
   b. preventing contractures
   c. keeping accurate records of her intake and output
   d. providing a low-calorie diet
4. Providing catheter care for Mrs. Tamayo includes
   a. providing perineal care
   b. positioning the catheter to ensure a free flow of urine
   c. applying antiseptic solution to the 4 inches of catheter nearest the resident
   d. all of the above

Chapter 11

THE NERVOUS SYSTEM

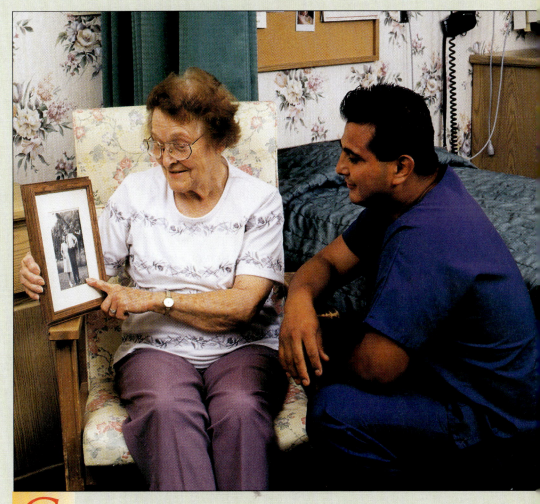

CARING TIP

Sharing the past with the resident brings

happiness to the present.

Nancy Brown, RN, MSN
San Juan Basin Technical School
Durango, Colorado

SECTION 1 Anatomy and Physiology

OBJECTIVES
What You Will Learn

When you have completed this section, you will be able to:

- Describe two functions of the nervous system
- Briefly explain how damage or disease of the nervous system differs from damage and disease of other body systems
- Give the primary function of the four areas of the brain
- Explain the basic function of the spinal cord

KEY TERMS

autonomic nervous system
cerebellum
cerebrum
diencephalon
hemispheres
medulla
midbrain
neurons
parasympathetic nervous system
pons
reflexes
spinal cord
sympathetic nervous system
vertebral column

THE NERVOUS SYSTEM

The nervous system (Figure 11-1) consists of:

- The central nervous system
  —Brain
  —Spinal cord
- The peripheral nervous system
  —31 pairs of spinal nerves
  —12 pairs of cranial nerves

neurons specialized cells of the nervous system

The nervous system controls and organizes all body activities. The nervous system and the endocrine system function together to maintain a balance among the various body activities. The nervous system is composed of billions of specialized cells called **neurons** (Figure 11-2). The neuron is the most complex cell in the body, and it differs from other body cells in a very important way—it does not reproduce. If nerve cells or neurons are destroyed, they are not replaced.

FIGURE 11-1
The nervous system.

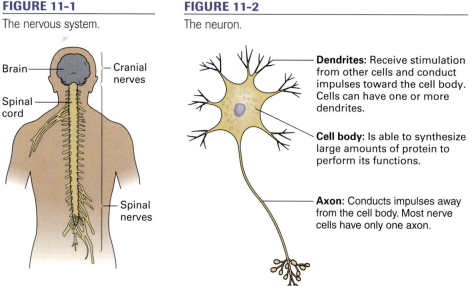

Brain
Cranial nerves
Spinal cord
Spinal nerves

FIGURE 11-2
The neuron.

Dendrites: Receive stimulation from other cells and conduct impulses toward the cell body. Cells can have one or more dendrites.
Cell body: Is able to synthesize large amounts of protein to perform its functions.
Axon: Conducts impulses away from the cell body. Most nerve cells have only one axon.

Neurons and nerve fibers are present all over the body. Special types of neurons work together to carry out their important functions. Remember, it is the nervous system that coordinates and controls all of the body's activity. The nervous system makes it possible for you to speak, hear, taste, smell, see, think, act, learn, and remember.

One of the most important functions of the nervous system is to receive signals from inside or outside the body and send these signals to the brain. The brain interprets these signals and sends a message back to the appropriate body part or system.

THE BRAIN

The brain is a very complex organ that has many functions. It is surrounded by the skull and in an adult weighs about 3 pounds. The brain is divided into specific areas, all of which have specialized functions (Figure 11-3).

The **cerebrum,** in the upper portion of the skull, is divided into **hemispheres** or halves by a deep groove. The right hemisphere controls most of the activity on the left side of the body, and the left hemisphere controls most of the activity on the right side of the body. It is in the cerebrum that all learning, memory, and associations are stored. It is here, too, that decisions are made for voluntary actions. Certain areas of the cerebrum perform special activities.

- Occipital lobe—the place where what you see is interpreted
- Frontal lobe—the primary area of thought, reason, and speech
- Temporal lobe—the auditory (hearing) area

cerebrum part of the brain responsible for thinking, learning, and memory

hemispheres halves

diencephalon area of the brain where control is exercised over body activities, such as regulation of body temperature and the endocrine glands

cerebellum part of the brain that coordinates voluntary movement

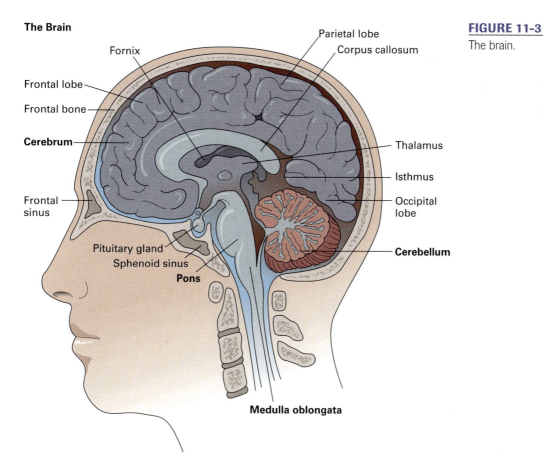

The Brain

- Fornix
- Frontal lobe
- Frontal bone
- **Cerebrum**
- Frontal sinus
- Pituitary gland
- Sphenoid sinus
- **Pons**
- Parietal lobe
- Corpus callosum
- Thalamus
- Isthmus
- Occipital lobe
- **Cerebellum**
- **Medulla oblongata**

FIGURE 11-3
The brain.

midbrain part of the brain through which nerve impulses pass

pons part of the brain through which nerve impulses pass

medulla vital center in the brain that controls breathing, swallowing, sleep, and heartbeat

spinal cord long cable of nerves that extends from below the medulla to the second and third lumbar vertebra

reflexes automatic response to stimulation

FIGURE 11-4

The spinal cord.

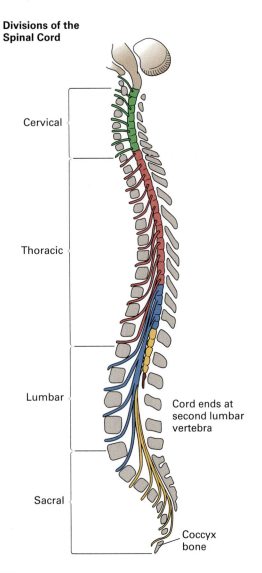

Divisions of the Spinal Cord

Cervical

Thoracic

Lumbar

Cord ends at second lumbar vertebra

Sacral

Coccyx bone

• Parietal lobe—the area for awareness of sensations of heat, cold, touch, pressure, and pain

The **diencephalon** is the area of the brain where a specialized structure (hypothalmus) exercises great control over the body's activities, including regulation of body temperature and the endocrine glands. This area screens all impulses going to the brain, either speeding them up or slowing them down.

The **cerebellum** is the part of the brain that coordinates voluntary movement. It is essential for normal movement and works with parts of the inner ear so that equilibrium (balance) is maintained.

The **midbrain, pons,** and **medulla** are primary pathways through which nervous impulses reach the brain from the spinal cord. The medulla is called the *vital center* because it controls breathing, swallowing, sleep, and the heartbeat.

THE SPINAL CORD AND PERIPHERAL NERVOUS SYSTEM

The **spinal cord** is a long cable of nerves that extends from the area below the medulla to the level of the second or third lumbar vertebra (Figure 11-4). The spinal cord serves to relay messages to and from the brain and is the center for reflex activity. **Reflexes** are automatic responses of the muscles or skin to stimulation. No thought is involved. Most reflexes occur without a message going all the way to the brain. An example would be the knee-jerk reflex. When a doctor taps a particular area of the knee with a rubber hammer, the knee jerks.

The spinal cord is oval in shape and runs through the **vertebral column.** Thirty-one pairs of spinal nerves exit from successive levels of the spinal cord. These nerves have specific functions.

The peripheral nervous system consists of the 31 pairs of spinal nerves and 12 pairs of cranial nerves arising principally from the brain stem. The nerves of the peripheral nervous system have many branches, which extend to all parts of the body.

The peripheral nervous system has a special division called the **autonomic nervous system.** The autonomic division supplies structures and organs of the body not under voluntary control. Some examples of involuntary activities are:

• Digestion
• Heart beating
• Glands secreting

The autonomic nervous system has two divisions, the **sympathetic** and the **parasympathetic.** The neurons that make up the sympathetic division become active during stress, danger, excitement, or illness. These neurons cause the pupils of our eyes to become larger so that we can see more clearly. These neurons also cause the heart to beat more strongly and to send more oxygen to the large muscles of the body in case it is necessary to fight or run. Sometimes when we experience frequent or prolonged stress, the action of the sympathetic system causes changes in the structure or function of some of our vital organs, causing illness.

The neurons that make up the parasympathetic division are in control when we are relaxed or when we are sleeping. They help us conserve energy.

We are fortunate that there is a check and balance system between the two divisions; when one has been active for too long, the other automatically switches on. The autonomic nervous system plays a vital role in maintaining homeostasis.

ABNORMALITIES OF THE NERVOUS SYSTEM

After age 25, there is a gradual and steady loss of neurons. In general, these losses do not cause changes in behavior or performance unless disease, injury, or nutritional deficiencies occur.

Cerebral vascular accident (CVA or stroke), organic brain syndrome, seizure disorders, Parkinson's disease, Alzheimer's disease, and multiple sclerosis are among the more common abnormalities of the nervous system. There are also many long-term care residents who have conditions that they were born with or that resulted from trauma at some other point in their lives. Examples are developmentally disabled residents and residents who have sustained spinal cord or brain injuries. Because the nervous system is so highly specialized, each of these conditions affects people in a unique way. Not only is each condition or disease unique, but each person who has the condition or disease has particular signs and symptoms as well as specialized needs.

vertebral column column of bones of the spine through which the spinal cord passes; spine; backbone

autonomic nervous system part of the nervous system that controls organs not under voluntary control

sympathetic nervous system part of the autonomic nervous system that controls response to stress

parasympathetic nervous system part of the autonomic nervous system that conserves energy

SECTION 2 The Resident with a Nervous System Abnormality

OBJECTIVES
What You Will Learn

When you have completed this section, you will be able to:

- List three common symptoms of Parkinson's disease
- Describe the nursing care of the resident with Parkinson's disease
- Identify the age group most often affected by multiple sclerosis
- Describe why the nature of multiple sclerosis makes adjustment more difficult for the victim
- Define the terms **remission** and **exacerbation** in relationship to multiple sclerosis
- Define the terms **paraplegic** and **quadriplegic**
- Give one example of how spinal cord injury affects each of the body systems
- Describe the measures to be taken when the emergency called autonomic dysreflexia occurs
- Explain the nature of a CVA or stroke
- Select a stroke victim and write a case study
- List four tips for improving communication with the aphasic resident
- List the three goals for care of the resident with impaired consciousness
- Identify five conditions that increase the frequency of seizures
- Identify which statements about epilepsy are true and which are false
- Describe emergency measures to be taken when a resident experiences a seizure

KEY TERMS

absence seizures
aphasia
atonic seizures
autonomic dysreflexia
cerebral vascular accident
coma
complex partial seizures
crede
embolus
emotional lability

encephalitis
epilepsy
euphoric
exacerbation
flaccid
hemiplegia
hyperactive
hypotension
impaired consciousness
level of injury
meningitis

myelin
paraplegic
proprioception
quadriplegic
remission
seizures
spasm
thrombosis
tonic–clonic seizures
tonic seizures

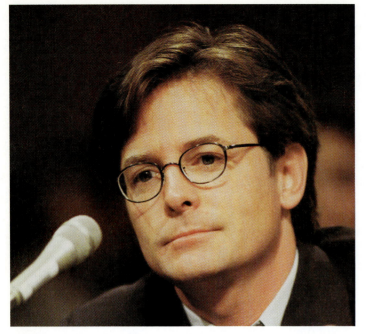

FIGURE 11-5

Parkinson's disease can affect anyone.

PARKINSON'S DISEASE

Parkinson's disease is a degenerative disease of the brain that usually occurs in people in middle to later life. About one million people are affected at this time (Figure 11-5). Parkinson's progresses slowly and does not shorten life. The intelligence is not affected. However, the symptoms may lead to depression. The typical symptoms are:

- Rigid muscles
- Tremor (shaking or trembling)
- Weakness

These symptoms combine to cause the following problems:

- Poor balance, leading to falls
- Slowness of movement
- Poor handwriting
- Problems with speech, swallowing, and eating; may experience drooling and have weight loss
- Lack of facial expression, referred to as a "masklike" face
- Constipation

Although no cure is known, many residents receive medications to reduce or control their symptoms. Nursing care is directed toward preventing complications and managing the disabilities resulting from the condition.

Table 11-1 indicates common problems, goals of care, and nursing measures to be followed with a resident who has Parkinson's disease. This is not a plan of care as you studied earlier because it does not consider each resident's individual problems and needs. In addition, the goals described are nursing goals rather than resident goals.

MULTIPLE SCLEROSIS

myelin insulating material that surrounds the nerve fibers

Multiple sclerosis, or MS as it is often called, is a chronic degenerative disease of the nervous system. The body's immune system attacks and damages the covering surrounding the nerves in the brain and spinal cord. The covering is called **myelin,** which serves as a conductor of nerve signals. Destruction of myelin interferes with normal nerve signals. The particular area in the brain or spinal cord damaged determines the symptoms that result. Although the cause of MS is still unknown, there is a higher incidence in family members. A child or sibling of someone with MS is about 10 times as likely to get MS than someone in the population at large. MS is twice as likely to occur in women than in men. In addition, MS tends to be more common in certain parts of the world where the climate is colder. MS is not contagious and although it may cause severe disability, the disease itself does not shorten life.

MS is called "a disease of young adults" because it usually begins between the ages of 20 and 40. About 250,000 people in the United States have been diagnosed as having MS. The disease is diagnosed by ruling out or eliminating other diseases, studying the history and the symptoms, and using a type of x-ray called magnetic resonance imaging (MRI), which makes it possible to see areas of the brain or spinal cord where the myelin has been destroyed.

TABLE 11-1 Care of Residents with Parkinson's Disease

PROBLEM	GOAL OF CARE	NURSING CARE
Drooling	Protect the skin from breakdown	Keep skin clean; apply protective cream or ointment.
Slowness in eating	To provide adequate nutrition	Keep food from becoming cold by using warming dish. Give time enough to eat. Assist with finishing, if resident becomes too tired.
Difficulty speaking. Speech very slow and without expression	To establish communication	Be patient! Take time to listen. Do not ignore.
High risk for contractures	To prevent contractures	Encourage self-care; give range-of-motion exercises.
Constipation	To eliminate constipation	Encourage to take fluids. Encourage intake of roughage in diet (fruits, vegetables, cereals).
High risk for falls, due to propulsive gait	To prevent falls	If assisting to ambulate, walk in front or have resident push a straight chair. May use pick-up walker. Encourage to stand as straight as possible.
Depression, shown by withdrawal from contact with others	To decrease depression	Promote self-care. Spend time with resident. Encourage to talk about feelings. Listen.

Symptoms include:

- Lack of coordination
- Visual disturbances, such as double vision, blind spots, blurriness, loss of color vision
- Difficulty in speech
- Bowel and bladder disturbances
- Paralysis
- Loss of sexual functioning
- Weakness
- Tremors
- Array of unusual sensations, such as numbness, tingling, burning

Only recently has it been recognized that there are cognitive and emotional problems that occur with MS. They occur because proper thinking and emotional functioning depend on communication between different parts of the brain, which takes place through myelinated nerves vulnerable to attack. Some people with MS experience mood changes, which cause them to be chronically depressed or constantly **euphoric** (experiencing an exaggerated feeling of well-being).

euphoric experiencing an exaggerated feeling of well-being

Generally, there are two types of MS. One type is called chronic–progressive because the person's disability and symptoms become progressively worse. The second type is called relapsing–remitting or exacerbating–remitting. An **exacerbation** is a rapid-onset attack of increasing MS symptoms that is thought to indicate a new attack on myelin. With this type, the symptoms become markedly worse for a period ranging from days to months. This is followed by improvement of function. Recovery may be to previous levels of functioning,

exacerbation return or increase of symptoms

remission   lessening or
disappearance of disease
symptoms

or there may be ongoing impairment. After the exacerbation, there is a period of **remission** lasting weeks, months, or years with minimal symptoms.

There are some things that seem to cause a return of symptoms. They include infections of any kind, especially respiratory (colds, pneumonia) and bladder infections, and very warm weather, fatigue, stress, and anxiety. MS victims are so sensitive to heat that a hot bath may cause return of symptoms, including weakness that prevents them from getting out of the bathtub.

Some special emotional or psychological factors are common with MS. Some of these problems have to do with the difficulty in determining the diagnosis and the lack of predictability about the course of the disease. The MS victim is unable to make plans for the future. He or she may become depressed due to loss of control and the need to be more dependent on others.

Most persons with MS continue to live independently. Usually, those seen in LTC facilities are those whose symptoms have progressed to a point where they require nursing care. They are usually unable to walk and may be wheelchair or bed-bound. Some are blind.

Nursing care of the resident with multiple sclerosis must be individualized due to the great variety of symptoms. The goals include prevention of complications of inactivity (contractures, pressure sores, pneumonia, kidney and bladder infections, and kidney and bladder stones) and helping the person to be as independent as possible for as long as possible.

AMYOTROPHIC LATERAL SCLEROSIS

Amyotrophic lateral sclerosis is referred to as ALS or Lou Gehrig's disease. ALS is a rapidly progressive, fatal neuromuscular disease. It attacks the neurons responsible for transmitting electrical impulses from the brain to the voluntary muscles throughout the body. When these muscles fail to receive messages, they eventually lose strength, atrophy, and die. There is no known treatment. Lou Gehrig, a famous baseball player during the 1930s, became afflicted with ALS at the peak of his career. He had been known for his strength, agility, and excellent health. Gehrig died at the age of 38. Anyone can get ALS. Most people with ALS are between the ages of 50 and 75, although there are cases of teenagers with the disease. The cause, prevention, and cure are unknown. ALS does not affect the mind or the senses of sight, hearing, taste, smell, and touch. Bladder and bowel muscles are generally not affected. ALS seldom causes pain, although some people do have cramps and discomfort from lengthy sitting or lying down. Early symptoms include lack of coordination with frequent falls, loss of use of hands and arms, and difficulty in speaking and swallowing. ALS is a costly disease in its later stages, demanding extensive nursing care. The resident may have a feeding tube due to loss of ability to swallow and a ventilator due to inability to breathe independently. Nursing care is directed toward preventing the harmful effects of immobility and providing the highest quality of life possible. The resident will need end-of-life care, which may include the provision of care from a hospice program.

SPINAL CORD INJURY

Every year more than 10,000 people experience injury to the spinal cord. About 85 percent are men between the ages of 18 and 25. Most spinal cord injuries result from automobile, motorcycle, and sports injuries.

Injury to the spinal cord is one of the most catastrophic events that can affect the human body. Because of the fact that cells within the nervous system do not repair themselves, spinal cord injury is permanent. Scientists are looking for a way to repair injured spinal cord tissue, but they have not been successful so far.

In describing a person with a spinal cord injury, the terms *quadriplegic* and *paraplegic* are used. A **quadriplegic** has paralysis of all four limbs and the trunk of the body (Figure 11-6). A **paraplegic** has paralysis of the lower limbs and lower trunk. The part of the spinal cord that is injured determines the amount of paralysis. The term **level of injury** identifies the location of the injury in relationship to the vertebrae that surround the cord. There are seven cervical, twelve thoracic, five lumbar, five sacral (fused into one sacrum), and five coccygeal vertebrae (fused). The level of injury will be stated in the diagnosis such as "quadriplegia, C5 (cervical 5)" or "paraplegia with injury at the L1 (lumbar 1) level."

Other important terms are *complete* and *incomplete*. These terms describe the degree of damage to the cord itself. If complete, all functions below the level of injury are lost. If incomplete, some functions may be retained.

Because the spinal cord acts as a relay station, sending impulses or messages to and from the brain, injury causes this process to stop. The impulses from the brain to the rest of the body include impulses for fine skillful movement, balance, respiration, and flexor motor activity.

The impulses from the rest of the body to the brain that can be lost include:

- Pain
- Temperature
- Pressure
- Touch
- Vibration
- Knowledge of location of body parts (called **proprioception**)

INITIAL TREATMENT OF SPINAL CORD INJURIES

The first phase of medical treatment of a spinal cord injury is emergency life-saving care. For about the first six weeks after injury, a condition known as spinal shock exists. During this time, all function below the level of injury is lost, including reflex activity. The paralyzed limbs are **flaccid** or limp. The bladder, the bowel, and the sexual organs are also paralyzed and flaccid. All sensation below the injury is also lost. Due to injury to the autonomic nervous system, the blood pressure is low, there is no perspiring below the level of injury, and there is decreased activity in the gastrointestinal tract.

Once spinal shock has subsided, there is a return of reflex activity below the level of injury. This is involuntary movement, which may give the victim false hopes of a return of voluntary activity. Many times the reflexes are overactive or **hyperactive,** which is shown by spasm (sudden uncontrolled jerking movements). These spasms may be so strong that they cause the individual to fall out of a wheelchair or off the toilet. Spasms can be started by touching the bottom of the feet of the paralyzed person such as during dressing or bathing or when placing the feet on the wheelchair pedals.

Individuals who sustain a spinal cord injury have the best chance of recovery when they receive immediate treatment from a physician who is knowledgeable and experienced in treating spinal injuries. There are some medications and treatments that can decrease the damage to the spinal cord if administered promptly.

When a paraplegic or quadriplegic is admitted to an LTC facility, the acute phase of the injury will have passed and some rehabilitation may have begun.

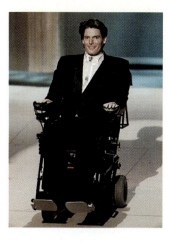

FIGURE 11-6

Christopher Reeve is a quadriplegic.

quadriplegic   person with paralysis of all four extremities

paraplegic   person with paralysis of the lower limbs

level of injury   in spinal cord injury, the location of injury in relationship to the vertebrae that surround the cord

proprioception   knowledge and awareness of the position of one's body parts in space

flaccid   limp

hyperactive   extremely, abnormally active

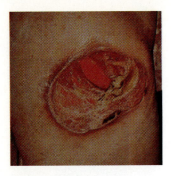

FIGURE 11-7

A pressure ulcer.

Nursing care is difficult and complex, requiring special knowledge and skill. The resident will often know more about the care required than the nursing staff. One important tip is to *listen* to the resident and allow him or her to participate fully in the care.

SPINAL CORD INJURY EFFECTS

Every system of the body is affected when a spinal cord injury occurs. The effects on each system and the required nursing care follow.

INTEGUMENTARY SYSTEM

Due to immobility, the person with a spinal cord injury is at great risk for development of pressure ulcers (Figure 11-7). Lack of sensation prevents awareness that an ulcer is developing, and the message to move or change position because of discomfort does not get through to the brain. Lack of ability to perspire below the level of injury interferes with the maintenance of body temperature. When the temperature outside the body goes up, the temperature inside the body does, too.

Nursing care of the skin not only involves keeping the skin clean, dry, and lubricated, but also includes pressure sore prevention measures. Tub baths are desirable because they improve circulation and reduce spasms. Since sensation may be absent, special care must be taken to avoid burns from hot bath water.

MUSCULAR SYSTEM

Muscles that are not used atrophy (waste away). Below the level of injury, the paralyzed muscles will appear thin and lacking in bulk.

Nursing care related to the muscular system consists of passive range of motion and encouraging maximum independence in activities of daily living. Residents often exercise their unimpaired muscles in order to take over the work done by the paralyzed muscles. A paraplegic often has highly developed arm muscles even though the legs may be atrophied.

SKELETAL SYSTEM

Inability to bear weight on the long bones leads to a loss of calcium. Bones become porous and are weakened. Fractures can occur with only slight trauma. Nursing care related to the skeletal system includes gentle turning and repositioning as well as measures to prevent falls and injuries. Frequently, residents with a spinal cord injury will have a "standing frame" or long leg braces to allow them to bear weight on their legs in order to decrease the loss of calcium from the bones.

DIGESTIVE SYSTEM

The movement in the digestive system is slower and less efficient, leading to constipation. Lack of voluntary control contributes to the problem, making a bowel management program essential.

Residents are urged to eat a high-protein diet with ample bulk. High fluid intake is needed to reduce constipation. In addition, the routine for bowel management may include use of rectal stimulation from a lubricated, gloved finger, a suppository, or occasional enemas. As a rule, frequent enemas tend to stretch the bowel and cause it to lose tone. Due to the chronic nature of the bowel problem, enemas are discouraged.

URINARY SYSTEM

The calcium that leaves the bones is eliminated through the kidneys and bladder. This increases the risk of kidney and bladder stones. The loss of control of urination requires the use of an indwelling catheter, external catheter, intermittent catheterization, or wearing of protective clothing. Some paraplegics empty the bladder by **crede** (pressing on the area of the abdomen over the bladder to push the urine out). Regardless of the method used, the spinal cord injury victim is very likely to retain urine in the bladder and to develop infection. In fact, the most common cause of death of the spinal cord injured is kidney disease.

    Nursing care related to the urinary system begins with encouraging a high intake of fluids. A young, otherwise healthy quadriplegic should consume about 3,000 cc of liquid every 24 hours. This individual may require catheter care to prevent infection if an indwelling catheter is used. Use of external urinary devices or a "Texas catheter" requires thorough care of the skin of the penis as well as frequent observation for impairment of circulation.

crede   pressing on the area of the abdomen over the bladder to push the urine out

NERVOUS SYSTEM

Damage to the nervous system includes paralysis and loss of sensation. In addition to the inability to move independently, the resident is at risk for injury because of lack of ability to recognize pain, temperature, and location of body parts. The person might burn himself with a cigarette or spill a hot liquid and never know it. He may be positioned in a way that restricts the circulation to a part of his body and not notice until damage has been done. Nursing care focuses on protecting the person from harm through careful observation and monitoring.

CARDIOVASCULAR SYSTEM

The blood tends to pool due to the effects of inactivity and gravity. There is a greater risk of blood clot formation, and the person often experiences low blood pressure **(hypotension)**, rapid pulse, and fatigue. Hypotension occurs most often when the person is sitting upright and may even cause loss of consciousness or fainting.

    Nursing care to prevent hypotension includes gradual raising of the head of the bed to increase tolerance, use of antiembolic (TED) stockings or elastic bandage wraps, and, with some individuals, use of a corsetlike abdominal binder. When the resident loses consciousness and is up in the wheelchair, simply pull the chair back against your body, tilting it at an angle. This will raise the blood pressure and return consciousness. If the resident is in bed, lower the head of the bed to raise the blood pressure.

hypotension   low blood pressure

RESPIRATORY SYSTEM

If the level of injury is above the T7 (thoracic 7) area, the respiratory muscles can be involved. Breathing is shallow, and the resident has difficulty coughing. Combined with inactivity, this increases the risk for pneumonia.

    The nursing assistant can help prevent respiratory complications by repositioning the resident and by encouraging deep breathing and coughing. Some quadriplegics are unable to cough or sneeze. There is a technique for assisting these residents to cough by applying manual pressure to the diaphragm. The resident will probably be able to instruct you. This should not be attempted without supervision from a licensed nurse.

REPRODUCTIVE SYSTEM

Men with spinal cord injury are seldom able to father children. Generally speaking, a quadriplegic has erections that are reflex in nature. That is, the penis will become erect when stimulated physically, but not psychologically. There is rarely an ejaculation. Pleasurable sensations are experienced only above and at the level of injury, not below.

Paraplegics, particularly those injured at the lumbar level (L1) or below, often have no erections. Although sexual intercourse may not be possible, they experience the same pleasure of closeness and intimacy as they did before they were injured. There are surgical procedures available called penile implants that either keep the penis permanently erect or have inflatable parts. Although this would permit intercourse, it cannot provide an ejaculation.

Some paraplegics and quadriplegics have injuries that are incomplete; that is, the spinal cord is not completely severed. They may have erections and ejaculations.

Women with spinal cord injury are still able to become pregnant and bear children. They usually do not experience orgasms but, like men, experience other physical and psychological pleasure.

SPINAL CORD EMERGENCY

autonomic dysreflexia in spinal cord–injured victims, a life-threatening condition that is caused by stimuli from the skin, the bowel, and the bladder

The spinal cord–injured victim may experience an emergency condition called **autonomic dysreflexia.** This condition is *life threatening* and results in severe high blood pressure. Causes are stimuli from the skin, the bowel, and the bladder. When the bladder is full, when there is trauma to the skin, or when the bowel is full, the body overreacts, resulting in dysreflexia. The person experiencing dysreflexia develops headache, goose pimples, sweating of the face, and stuffy nose. The blood pressure increases, and the heart rate slows.

This is an emergency and must be acted upon immediately! Treatment includes raising the resident's head (to lower the blood pressure) and finding and removing the cause. Commonly, the catheter is kinked or plugged, an arm or leg is positioned poorly or caught between the bed and side rail, or a fecal impaction exists. Appendicitis, kidney stones, and bowel obstruction can also cause dysreflexia. Report any signs of dysreflexia to the charge nurse immediately. When a resident complains of dysreflexia, believe him!

REHABILITATION OF THE SPINAL CORD–INJURED RESIDENT

Rehabilitation consists of preventing complications and helping the individual to learn to cope with his disability. The resident is taught as much as possible about his or her condition and how best to live with it. The resident who has spent time in a rehabilitation program is usually very well informed. As in all rehabilitation, maximum independence is the goal. The resident should be given as much control as possible over his life. This person may exert his control by directing the nursing assistant in every activity he or she performs. It is best to accept his need for control and do things the resident's way whenever possible.

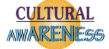

In Hispanic and Asian cultures, independence and self-care may not be highly valued. The older males typically expect to be cared for. They may participate in rehabilitation activities, but when family members come to visit, they expect the family to do things that they can do for themselves. They are not being difficult, lazy, or demanding—they simply have different values and beliefs. Help the family members find ways to care for the resident, focusing on those things the resident cannot do for himself.

CEREBRAL VASCULAR ACCIDENT

The term **cerebral vascular accident** (CVA) means stroke. Stroke is the third leading cause of death in the United States. About 4.5 million persons in the United States are living with disabilities caused by strokes. Each year there are about 500,000 new strokes, while 100,000 are recurrences. The incidence is highest among African Americans. Twenty-eight percent occur in people under age 65.

Stroke is caused by bleeding in the brain or by existence of a blood clot in a blood vessel of the brain (Figure 11-8). This clot may originate in the brain **(thrombosis)** or travel to the brain from elsewhere in the body (called an **embolus**). Usually, the person has high blood pressure and arteriosclerosis, which increase the risk of stroke. Stroke or CVA is actually a disease of the circulatory system but is discussed here because the results of stroke affect the nervous system profoundly.

The type of symptoms and their severity are determined by the location of the problem and the amount of brain tissue destroyed due to lack of oxygen and other necessary nutrients. For our purposes, we will deal with some common results of stroke.

Frequently, the stroke victim is left paralyzed on one side of the body. This is called **hemiplegia.** Depending on whether the person's left or right side is paralyzed, we use the term *left hemiplegia* or *right hemiplegia.* In addition to paralysis, sensation can be lost. This includes loss of ability to feel heat, cold, pressure, and pain in the areas affected. Some individuals seem to forget the paralyzed side and fail to dress, apply makeup, shave, or groom that side.

When the face is involved, there may be drooping of the eyelid or inability to close the eyelid. The eye may become dry and irritated because of decreased or absent tearing. There are often accompanying losses of vision in the affected eye. Drooping of the muscles on one side of the face may cause drooling on that side. There may be problems in chewing and swallowing on the affected side. There is often an inability to feel the food on the paralyzed side, which increases the risk of burns, choking, and accumulating food in the cheek.

cerebral vascular accident stroke

thrombosis a blood clot that originates in the brain

embolus a blood clot that moves within the bloodstream

hemiplegia paralysis of one side of the body

FIGURE 11-8
Causes of stroke.

Thrombosis   Embolism   High blood pressure

Atherosclerosis   Hemorrhage

Spasticity of paralyzed limbs can also occur. **Spasm** is an involuntary contraction of muscles. The stimulation of exercise or bathing and dressing may
cause the muscles to spasm into a position of flexion or extension. Spasms
are increased by nervous tension, cold temperature, and pain. This greatly increases the risk for contractures since the limb remains fixed in one position.

Paralysis of the arm and leg interferes with the ability to perform all activities of daily living, including eating, grooming, dressing, ambulation, and toileting. The inability to move increases the risk of contractures, pressure sores,
pneumonia, urinary stones, and constipation.

Because certain brain functions are located only on one side of the brain,
there are differences between individuals who have right brain injury (left paralysis) and left brain injury (right paralysis). It is important to know these differences so that your care can be most effective.

Right brain injury (left paralysis):

- Partial or complete paralysis of the left face, arm, and leg
- Loss of, or changes in, sensation of pain, touch, and temperature on the
  left side; may not know location of body parts on the left side
- Difficulty in judging size, distance, and rate of movement
- May behave impulsively and unsafely; tends to overestimate abilities

Left brain injury (right paralysis):

- Partial or complete paralysis of the right face, arm, and leg.
- Loss of, or changes in, sensations of pain, touch, and temperature on the
  right side. May not know location of body parts on the right side.
- Loss of language (aphasia) may include speaking, understanding of
  speech, reading, and writing.
  Note: About 50 percent of left-handed people will not have loss of language with left brain injury because their speech area is on the right. That
  group may have loss of language when they have right brain injury.
- Tends to be very cautious and slow. Needs lots of encouragement to keep
  trying.

It has been estimated that out of every 100 people who survive a stroke,
10 will have no impairment, 40 will have mild disability, 40 will be severely disabled, and 10 will need institutional care. Some residents may experience significant recovery with a return of function, while others must learn to adapt
to a permanent disability.

Most gains in a person's ability to function in the first 30 days after a stroke
are due to spontaneous recovery.

NURSING CARE OF THE RESIDENT WITH A CVA

Nursing care of the resident with a cerebral vascular accident is aimed toward
protection from injury, prevention of disability, and achieving the maximum
independence possible for the individual.

Protection from injury involves:

- Eye care—The eye may be taped shut, and a patch may be worn. Physician may prescribe eye drops.
- Supervision of feeding to prevent choking—Place food on unaffected side
  of mouth. Check mouth after meals to be sure food is not stored in the
  paralyzed side.

- Prevention of facial skin breakdown from drooling—Wash and dry gently. Use protective skin creams.
- Supervision of shaving and grooming—Absence of sensation may cause the resident to omit shaving or grooming the paralyzed side or to keep shaving over and over the same place, causing a burn or skin damage.
- Assistance with ambulation to prevent falls—Lack of vision on affected side may cause falls or bumping into objects.
- Supervision of bathing to prevent falls and burns from water that is too hot—The ability to perceive temperature can affect judgment about how hot the shower or bath is.

Prevention of disability involves:

- Positioning in proper alignment using trochanter rolls, hand rolls, foot boards, and foot cradles to prevent contractures—Special positioning splints are often used to prevent contractures of the wrist and fingers.
- Providing good skin care to prevent pressure ulcers—This includes repositioning, keeping skin clean and lubricated, using pressure-reducing devices, and preventing injury.
- Giving passive range-of-motion exercises to strengthen and prevent contractures.
- Providing food and fluids to prevent bowel and bladder complications, such as constipation and dehydration—Food should be adequate in calories to meet needs and should include following the Food Guide Pyramid, with sufficient protein, vitamins, and roughage.
- Preventing withdrawal and loss of hope by treating each individual as a unique, worthwhile person with potential to improve. Louis Pasteur, the famous French scientist of the 1800s, carried on most of his work after suffering a major stroke.

Achievement of maximum independence for the person who has suffered a stroke involves:

- Encouraging involvement in care through decision making and doing as much of the care as possible.
- Teaching self-care techniques such as how to feed, groom, bathe, and dress oneself.
- Obtaining special self-help devices for the stroke resident. These devices allow the resident to be more independent.
- Providing an environment where independence is praised and encouraged.
- Giving the resident time to do things.
- Enhancing ambulation and function through use of braces and splints (Figure 11-9). These devices are used to stabilize the paralyzed limb. They are prescribed and fitted by specialists.

Self-help devices can be a great aid to the stroke victim. Some of these devices can be made by the staff or family, while others may be purchased from medical supply companies. An occupational therapist is an excellent resource for recommending and obtaining self-help devices.

FIGURE 11-9

Positioning a splint.

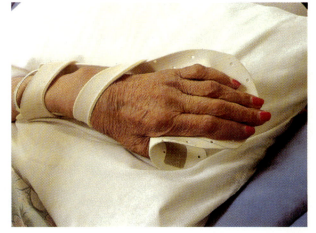

Recovery from a stroke depends on:

- The extent to which the brain is affected
- The survivor's attitude
- The skill of the rehabilitation staff
- The cooperation of family and friends

EMOTIONAL REACTIONS TO STROKE

emotional lability over-reaction of the emotions to a stimulus (e.g., crying or laughing inappropriately)

When individuals experience CVA or stroke, their lives change suddenly and drastically. The person grieves for the lost functions of the paralyzed limbs, loss of ability to communicate, loss of independence, loss of control over his or her life, and lost hopes and dreams for the future.

The denial, anger, depression, and eventual acceptance are often accompanied by emotional lability. **Emotional lability** is the overreaction to a stimulus. The person may burst into tears or laughter for no apparent reason. Crying is more common than laughing. This is both frightening and embarrassing to the person, who may feel that he or she is going crazy. The nursing assistant must accept the behavior in a matter-of-fact way. Usually, it is best to ignore the inappropriate bursts of laughter or tears.

RESIDENTS WITH APHASIA

aphasia loss of language or communication ability

About one-fifth of adult stroke victims experience **aphasia.** The term *aphasia* refers to a loss of language. Aphasia occurs most commonly with the right hemiplegic, as the language area of the brain is on the left in most people. There are many types of aphasia. The resident may have difficulties in understanding what is heard, using numbers, reading, writing, or speaking. Some have difficulty in all these areas. Usually, automatic speech is retained. This means that the resident may swear or sing or use common phrases such as "yes," "no," "thank you," though not always correctly or accurately. These words or phrases just come out automatically.

The ability to communicate is so important to our lives that the loss of this ability has severe effects on the resident. Anger, frustration, depression, and withdrawal are common responses. You must be able to recognize the problem in order to be most helpful. Probably the most important aspect of caring for the aphasic person is patience. Keep trying! Don't avoid the person or attempt to anticipate all his or her needs. Persons with aphasia usually need extra time to understand what is said and often take longer to express themselves. Speech may return completely or partially, but in either case, return takes work. Although a speech therapist may be involved, you, the nursing assistant, deal with the resident for longer periods of time on a continuous basis. You can make the difference!

Techniques for talking with an aphasic resident include:

- Get the attention of the resident before beginning to talk.
- Talk and work slowly.
- Use short sentences. Communicate one idea at a time.
- Repeat or rephrase instructions as often as necessary.
- Describe what you are doing as you perform tasks.
- Use body language (gestures, facial expression, tone of voice) to communicate your message.
- Try writing.

When listening to the resident, remember:

- Encourage writing or using a communication board if the resident is able (Figure 11-10).
- Allow lots of time for a response.
- Avoid scolding the resident for swearing or making mistakes.
- Don't interrupt the resident when he tries to say something.
- Give clues to the words, instead of the words themselves.
- Trigger the word by saying the first sound. For example, "You want cr— in your coffee." If the person can't find the word, tell her.
- Treat the person like an adult.

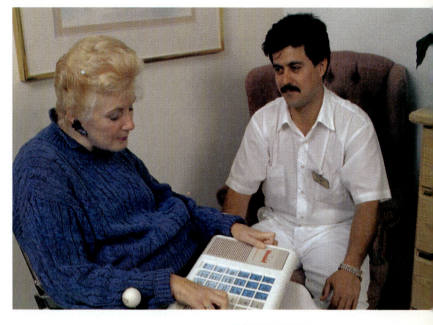

FIGURE 11-10
Using a communication board.

With patience and cooperation, communication may be established. Keys to communication with the aphasic resident should be written on the plan of care so that all staff can benefit from what is known to be effective with the individual resident.

IMPAIRED CONSCIOUSNESS

Some residents may have what is called **impaired consciousness.** This means that they are not awake and alert. They are not aware of their surroundings, nor can they react to their surroundings. Impaired consciousness may be brief or prolonged, mild or severe. In severe impairment, the term **coma** is used. This means that there is an absence of understandable speech, no ability to follow instructions, and no eye opening upon stimulation. The person is not arousable; he or she cannot be "awakened." You may hear the term *semi-comatose* or *lethargic* to refer to less severe forms of impaired consciousness. In defining consciousness, it is important to understand the difference from confusion or dementia. Confusion and dementia have to do with impaired intellectual functioning, not wakefulness and alertness.

Any resident who is unable to respond to his or her surroundings is at risk for developing complications of inactivity. These residents require thorough and complete nursing care to assure their safety, provide stimulation for the senses, and prevent complications.

The priority is to maintain the resident's ability to breathe. This is accomplished through proper positioning and the use of suctioning to remove secretions and may include the use of oxygen. Some residents may require an opening into the trachea called a *tracheotomy.* This opening is maintained by using a tube to keep the breathing passage open. Secretions may be removed by use of a suction tube or catheter. This suctioning is a function of the licensed nurse. However, it is essential that the nursing assistant observe the airway and obtain prompt assistance if it is blocked! Care of the resident with a tracheotomy is described in Chapter 18. Some residents may be positioned on their side to allow secretions to drain from the mouth. Others may have the head of the bed elevated to make breathing easy. Frequent changes of position help prevent pneumonia from occurring from the accumulation of fluids in the lungs.

impaired consciousness the resident is not awake or alert; is unaware of and unable to react to the surroundings

coma severe impairment of consciousness with absence of understandable speech, eye opening, and ability to follow instructions

The resident in a coma is also at risk for the development of skin breakdown and pressure ulcers because of his or her inability to move. Such residents are also incontinent, so the skin may be exposed to urine and feces, contributing to breakdown. Contractures may result from lack of movement, and the risk is increased with brain injury and other types of brain disease that may cause muscle spasm. The physical or occupational therapist may provide splints to the arms or legs to keep contractures from developing. Range of motion must be provided to all extremities.

Because the resident is unable to chew or swallow, he or she will probably be fed through a nasogastric or gastrostomy tube. This places the resident at risk for additional complications described in Chapter 9.

Because of breathing difficulties and the presence of a feeding tube, the resident with impaired consciousness needs frequent and thorough oral care. Keeping the mouth moist will prevent sores from developing in the mouth and will prevent infection. Use of flavored mouthwash or flavored "toothettes" also adds stimulation to the sense of taste.

Although the resident is unable to respond, good nursing care requires treating the person as if he or she could see, hear, and respond to everything going on. It is widely believed that many are still able to hear although they cannot speak or follow commands. Therefore, all staff and visitors should talk to the resident, not about him or her. You should not make remarks or comments that you would not want the resident to hear. It is a good idea to greet the resident upon entering the room, identify yourself, and explain in a step-by-step way everything that you are going to do.

Stimulating the senses of residents with impaired consciousness is part of their care and treatment. Prevention of sensory deprivation is discussed in detail in Chapter 5.

Because the resident is unable to express her or his wants and needs, the nursing assistant along with the licensed nurse must observe the resident often and regularly. Remember that when caring for a resident with impaired consciousness, the health care team has to learn to anticipate the needs of the resident!

SEIZURES

Seizures occur when a group of brain cells overreact, disrupting the normal conduction within the brain. The term *seizure* means "sudden attack." The individual has no control over the seizure, though some have a brief warning before the seizure begins. Seizures occur in all age groups. Sometimes the entire brain is involved; other times only part of the brain is involved.

There are many causes of seizures:

- Injury before, during, or after birth
- Infection—**encephalitis, meningitis** (infection of the brain and surrounding membranes)
- High fever
- Pressure in the brain—from tumor or blood clot or bleeding
- Presence of toxic chemicals in the blood—poisons, drugs
- Lack of necessary substances, such as hormones, calcium, sugar

Everyone is capable of having seizures if their brain cells are irritated enough. There are several types of seizures, partial and generalized. Some individuals experience more than one type.

Generalized, **tonic–clonic seizures** used to be called *grand mal* seizures. The episodes are dramatic. There may be a brief warning, consisting of a feeling in

seizures overreaction of brain cells; a sudden attack

encephalitis inflammation of the brain

meningitis inflammation of membranes surrounding the brain

tonic–clonic seizures Previously called *grand mal.* The limbs first become stiff and rigid and breathing stops. The jaws are clenched and the tongue or lips may be bitten. The tonic phase is followed by the clonic phase in which the body is shaken by violent, rhythmic jerking of the limbs. The person loses consciousness and may be confused and sleepy for an hour or two afterwards

the pit of the stomach or the person may smell a particular smell or hear a particular sound. The arms and legs become stiff and rigid, and breathing stops. The lips may be blue, and there may be a frothy saliva. The eyes roll upward and the jaw is clenched. Sometimes the tongue and lips are bitten. This "tonic phase" is followed within 30 to 60 seconds by the clonic phase, in which the body is shaken by a series of violent, rhythmic jerking of the arms and legs. These usually stop after 2 to 3 minutes. Sometimes, the person loses control of the bowel and/or bladder. The person then recovers consciousness but may be confused for several minutes and may sleep for an hour or two. Headache and muscle soreness are common after the attack. The person does not remember the seizure.

Absence seizures are not dramatic. They often go unnoticed. This form of epilepsy was known as *petit mal* seizures. Absence seizures begin in childhood and may cease at puberty or may continue throughout adult life. Usually, the person stares vacantly for a few seconds, fluttering the eyelids briefly. He appears to be out of contact with his surroundings. The person does not fall and recovers promptly. At times, the person with absence seizures is thought to be "daydreaming."

Other types of generalized seizures are uncommon, but they include myoclonic seizures where there are sudden symmetrical contractions of the arms and legs, which may or may not be followed by loss of consciousness. With **atonic seizures,** there is loss of tone in the muscles, leading to falling to the ground. **Tonic seizures** include stiffening of the body and arching the back. Tonic seizures may be followed by loss of consciousness.

Partial seizures are those in which the activity in one area of the brain does not cause loss of consciousness. They may be simple or complex. Usually, there is a part of the brain that was injured. There may be movement of only that body part controlled by the injured portion of the brain. **Complex partial seizures** may involve alteration of awareness. These attacks may consist of a feeling of intense familiarity with the surroundings but being unable to respond. Automatic chomping movements of the jaw may occur. Each form of partial seizure may lead to a generalized tonic–clonic seizure.

When prone to seizures and no specific cause can be determined, a person is said to have **epilepsy.** Epilepsy can often be controlled by taking certain medications. There are many superstitions about epilepsy and those who have it.

The nursing assistant should know the facts about epilepsy:

- Epilepsy is not disfiguring.
- Epilepsy is not painful.
- Epilepsy does not shorten life.
- Epilepsy does not cause insanity.
- Epilepsy does not cause mental retardation or affect one's intelligence.
- Epilepsy is not contagious.

Many prominent individuals in the arts, science, and politics have had epilepsy. They have lived successful and productive lives.

In addition to taking the prescribed medication, the person with epilepsy can reduce the risk of seizures by avoiding these things:

- Illness of any type
- Lack of physical activity
- Fatigue
- Constipation
- Emotional stress

absence seizures a type of seizure formerly called *petit mal* that involves numerous daily episodes in which the victim may stare vacantly for a few seconds, seeming to be out of contact with surroundings; occurs most often in children

atonic seizures a type of seizure with loss of tone in the muscles, leading to falling to the ground

tonic seizures a type of seizure in which stiffening of the body is the predominant feature; may or may not be followed by loss of consciousness

complex partial seizures a seizure with movement and sensory symptoms and a change in the level of consciousness

epilepsy a disorder in the electrical functioning of the brain, resulting in seizures

In an LTC facility, you will have residents who have epilepsy as well as those who might have a seizure due to tumor, stroke, or high fever. When a seizure occurs, it may frighten all concerned. It is important to rehearse the proper nursing actions.

NURSING CARE DURING A SEIZURE

The major concern is to protect the resident from injury. During a grand mal seizure, the jaw clamps down tightly. Because this results in an occasional biting of the tongue or cheek, "bite sticks" or padded tongue blades were used in the past. It has since been determined that the dangers of using the stick (injury to the teeth, choking, etc.) are greater than any possible benefits.

Do not leave the resident. There is no time. Use the call signal to summon help. Assist the person to lie down to prevent a fall. Move furniture out of the way to prevent injury. Protect the head with a pillow or other soft cushion. Never attempt to restrain the resident from moving. If possible, turn the resident to one side to allow secretions to drain from the mouth and nose.

Observe the seizure so that you can report the length, the presence of any warning, the part of the body where the seizure began, incidence of incontinence, and any injury. When the seizure is over, the resident should rest in bed. Side rails should be up at all times. Sometimes side rails may be wrapped with soft cloth to provide cushioning to prevent injury. Help the resident through the period of amnesia that may follow a seizure. Any seizures must be reported and recorded in the health record.

SEIZURE DOS AND DON'TS FOR GENERALIZED TONIC–CLONIC SEIZURES

What to Do

- Protect from nearby hazards.
- Loosen clothing.
- Protect head from injury.
- Turn on side to keep airway clear.
- Reassure as consciousness returns.
- If there are multiple seizures, or if one seizure lasts longer than 5 minutes, immediate help is needed.

What Not to Do

- Don't put any implements into the mouth.
- Don't try to hold the tongue. It cannot be swallowed.
- Don't attempt to give liquids during or just after a seizure.
- Don't hold the person down or try to restrain movement.

SECTION 3 The Resident with Alzheimer's Disease and Dementias of the Alzheimer's Type

OBJECTIVES
What You Will Learn

When you have completed this section, you will be able to:

- Select the correct definition of Alzheimer's disease
- Identify which statements are true and which are false about Alzheimer's disease
- Categorize symptoms of Alzheimer's disease into appropriate stages of the disease
- Identify the three most important considerations when providing care to a resident with Alzheimer's disease
- List four factors that worsen the behavioral problems in an Alzheimer's disease resident

KEY TERMS

Alzheimer's disease
apathy
catastrophic reaction
dementia
reality orientation
reminiscence
validation

Alzheimer's disease (AD) is an incurable disease affecting the brain. It is the most common cause of progressive *dementia* in older adults. **Dementia** means deprived of reason, mentally deteriorated. Alzheimer's is the fourth leading cause of death in the United States of those over 75, and it affects an estimated 1.5 million Americans. Projections indicate that by the year 2040, one in every three families will be directly touched by this devastating disease. There is no cure and no way to slow the progress of the disease.

Alzheimer's disease incurable disease affecting the brain that occurs predominantly in older adults and affects memory, thinking, and judgment

dementia deprived of reason; mentally deteriorated

Several diseases can cause dementia besides Alzheimer's disease. They include:

- Huntington's disease
- Multi-infarct dementia
- AIDS-related dementia

These diseases of the brain may affect residents in different ways; however, loss of recent (short-term) memory, confusion, and lack of reasoning and poor judgment are the most common indicators (Figure 11-11).

The deterioration of the brain seen in the AD resident is not part of the normal aging process. AD usually begins after age 60; however, it may occur as early as age 40. It is a terminal illness that affects more women than men and is more common in countries where the life expectancy is longer. It was first identified by a German pathologist, Dr. Alois Alzheimer, and bears his name.

FIGURE 11-11
Residents in Alzheimer's unit.

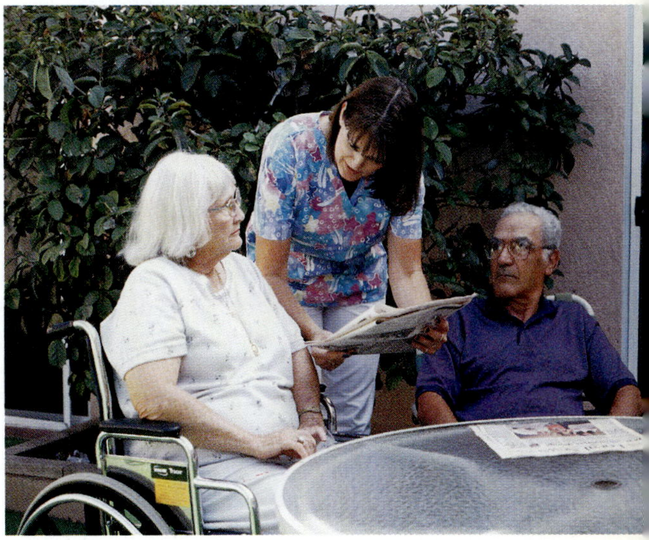

Current research supports the theory that a *genetic* (inherited) mechanism is evident in the development of Alzheimer's disease. There are also, however, many cases of Alzheimer's disease in which there is no previous history of the disease within the family. There is no easy way to diagnose AD except by examining brain tissue after death, so diagnosis is done by excluding all other causes of curable and incurable memory loss.

During the course of the disease, the nerve cells in the brain that control memory, thinking, and judgment are damaged. There is disruption in the ability of nerve cells to transmit messages to one another, and one theory suggests that certain substances (called neurotransmitters) necessary

for this transmission to occur are missing in AD victims. If you think of the brain as the body's master switchboard that processes information, receives calls, and sends calls, you can understand the result if the switchboard were to become defective and inoperable on certain lines; this is what happens to the AD resident.

The early symptoms, which include forgetfulness and loss of concentration, can be easily missed. Memory impairment becomes so severe that the resident is eventually unable to carry on a conversation, follow a line of thought, or even recognize loved ones. Over the course of several years, thinking, personality, and the ability to function are destroyed. This progressively devastating disease is unlike most other terminal illnesses where physical deterioration is the primary concern. The AD victim suffers a kind of psychological death—it is the personality of the AD victim that is lost. Once the AD resident's personality and memory deteriorate, the qualities that make each person a unique individual are gone. The AD resident is unable to provide necessary input, which is essential to sustain any healthy relationship. The "loss of the person" while the body is physically intact is one of the most difficult adjustments for families and loved ones.

The entire health care team should be involved in providing information and support to the family and loved ones. There are community support groups (Alzheimer's Disease and Related Disorders Association, 1-800-621-0379), and many facilities offer special programs for families of the AD victim. The nursing assistant can offer the most important support to families and loved ones by providing the resident with the best possible care. As they have to cope with their loss and grief, there is a lessened burden when they know the resident is receiving professional, compassionate care. It is important to understand that AD affects people in different ways and people react differently and do not progress through the various stages with any kind of uniformity. In some, the deterioration is more rapid than others.

The stages listed next have been adapted (with permission from *Care of Alzheimer's Patients: A Manual for Nursing Home Staff* by American Health Care Association and Alzheimer's Disease and Related Disorder Association). The stages are only a basic road map of the course of the disease, with each person following a slightly different route and time frame.

FIRST STAGE

The first stage lasts from 2 to 4 years. This stage leads up to and includes diagnosis. Symptoms include:

- Recent or short-term memory loss
- Difficulty concentrating
- Inability to remember instructions
- Gets lost and loses things
- Loss of spontaneity or enthusiasm
- Loss of initiative—unable to start things
- Mood and personality changes
- Poor judgment and decision making
- Unable to organize, plan, and follow through
- Difficulty handling money, paying bills
- Thoughts of persecution
- Inappropriate outbursts of anger

SECOND STAGE

The second stage occurs two to ten years after diagnosis. This is the longest stage and will require supervision and assistance. The second stage will include all the symptoms of the first stage plus the following:

- Increasing memory loss and confusion, along with a much shorter attention span
- Loss of some perceptive responses, sight, hearing, and touch
- Makes repetitive statements and/or movements
- Becomes restless, especially in late afternoon and at night
- Experiences occasional muscle twitching or jerking motions, unsteady gait
- Has difficulty with perceptual–motor problems, is unable to get into a chair easily, and may be unable to set the table or use familiar objects correctly
- Has trouble expressing self with the right words and will often make up stories to fill in the blanks
- Finds reading, writing, and working with number combinations very difficult
- May become suspicious, irritable, fidgety, silly, and subject to mood swings, especially tears
- Loses some basic impulse control; may not want to bathe, may undress in public; may forget table manners
- Has weight fluctuation, usually gains and then loses weight; will eat other people's food; will forget when last meal was and gradually loses interest in food
- May see or hear things that are not there and will be convinced they are real
- Often gets fixed ideas about something that is not real or true; repeats things over and over
- Generally requires full-time supervision
- Difficulty speaking, unable to understand and carry on conversation

THIRD OR TERMINAL STAGE

The third stage lasts one to three years and requires constant supervision. The third stage includes all the symptoms of the first and second stages plus the following:

- Cannot recognize family or self in mirror
- Will lose weight even with a balanced diet
- Has very little ability to provide any self-care, such as dressing, eating, and toileting
- Loses the ability to communicate with words; may groan, scream, or make strange sounds
- May revert to behaviors such as putting everything into the mouth or touching everything
- Loses control of bowel and bladder functions
- May experience seizures, difficulty swallowing, skin breakdown, and infection as a generalized debilitation occurs
- Will become totally dependent and will sleep more; gradually, body functions decline until death occurs

CONTROLLING DIFFICULT BEHAVIORS

After reviewing the symptoms of AD, it is understandable that one of the greatest challenges in providing nursing care is to manage difficult and disruptive behavior. It is this behavior that prompts most families to seek placement in a long-term care facility.

It is helpful to remember that the AD resident is not deliberately difficult. The behaviors are a result of the disease, and the resident is often unable to control angry outbursts, irrational, or childish behaviors. Some researchers believe that difficult behavior is related to some type of discomfort and that agitated and combative behavior is always a reaction to a stimulus. Frequently, staff can only guess the event that might have triggered an episode. There is an element of trial and error that allows staff to determine "this works with Mr.—" and "this seems to agitate him more." What is effective in reducing undesirable behavior in one resident may be totally ineffective with another. Remember, it is how the AD resident perceives the event that triggers the behavior. Obtaining a detailed and complete history of the resident can help the staff understand their behavior, their preferences, and those things that add to their quality of life.

Example: You may tell a resident that you are going to take him to the shower, but by the time you get there he has forgotten what you are going to do. Then as you start to undress the resident, he may perceive this as a type of assault and become combative. Remember that combative or resisting behavior may actually be the resident's attempt to protect or defend him from a threat. For example, when taking the resident for a shower, he may have forgotten where he is going, may be afraid of water, or may be afraid of having his body exposed. You may need to provide a bed bath instead or, if you have a hand-held shower hose, the resident can be covered with a sheet and showered underneath.

catastrophic reactions
sudden changes from baseline behavior that are socially unacceptable

The AD resident will often overreact or experience exaggerated responses to many situations. These disruptive reactions are referred to as **catastrophic reactions** (sudden changes from baseline behavior that are socially unacceptable). Four factors seem to worsen behavioral problems with AD residents.

FATIGUE

Residents with dementia tend to get tired easily, and as they fatigue, they are less able to function. The nursing assistant should be alert to signs the resident is getting tired and should plan ways to help conserve energy. Scheduling naps or rest periods and reducing time in activities are just a few of the ways to help the AD resident conserve energy and avoid fatigue.

REALITY ORIENTATION

The person who is disoriented needs an environment that has little change. Room changes should be avoided. If possible, the same staff members should care for the resident all the time. Such items as clocks and calendars should be available and prominently displayed. Sometimes it is helpful to identify the resident's room and bed in a special way. The physical layout of many facilities is confusing even to the staff! In these cases, a picture by the door or a large red bow, for instance, will single out a particular room.

The way you communicate with the resident is extremely important. Despite the resident's unusual or childlike behavior, always show respect. One way we show respect is by avoiding teasing or "playing along" with the disorientation. Residents may have a doll, for instance, that they refer to as their "baby." This baby may have a name and daily routines. Although the resident may never overcome the attachment to the doll, you must never add to the disorientation by saying "How is your baby today?" or "May I hold your baby?"

The concept of **reality orientation** is controversial at the present time. Reality orientation was developed by people working with elderly, mentally ill residents. Some say the results at bringing residents back to reality have been poor. The techniques of reality orientation must be practiced by all staff 24 hours a day. *Repetition is the key.* The disoriented resident usually attends a class daily, during which the day, date, time, weather, place, and person's name are given repeatedly. The information is also written and posted prominently in the facility.

Nursing staff remind residents frequently of who they are, where they are, and the date. Incorrect remarks made by the resident are corrected. For example, "No, Mr. Smith, your wife is not here. She died several years ago." Through consistency and repetition, the resident is supposed to regain orientation. Regardless of whether one believes that the person can regain his or her previous level of orientation, it would certainly never be appropriate to do anything that added to the existing disorientation. The attitude taken should be one of firm kindness. If the resident becomes angry or agitated when attempts are made to correct false statements, it may be best to simply ignore the statements.

reality orientation technique for reducing and eliminating disorientation

VALIDATION

One approach to working with the elderly who exhibit signs of disorientation or malorientation was developed by social worker Naomi Feil. While working with elderly at Montifiore Home for the Aged in Cleveland, Ohio, she recognized the fact that reality orientation not only did not help the resident, but in many cases residents seemed harmed by it, as shown by their withdrawal from others and retreat further into their past. In an effort to give them comfort, she developed validation as an approach. **Validation** is a method of acknowledging the feelings of the resident and accepting those feelings as true. She observed that, when she validated the feelings of the residents, they appeared to be happier. Her basic beliefs include use of empathy to tune into the inner reality of the individual, which builds trust. With trust comes safety, and with safety renewed feelings of worth and the restoration of dignity. Feil believes that the behavior seen in the disoriented resident has meaning and that they are "working through" some of their life issues. Their goal is to die in peace. With this in mind, she developed an approach to helping them by using validation.

validation a method of helping residents with dementia by supporting their feelings rather than reminding them of the day, time, and place

Validation is not an appropriate technique for everyone. Those who do not benefit include those who are oriented (they know the date, time, place, person), those who are mentally ill or who have a history of mental illness, and those who have experienced a physical trauma such as a head injury or a stroke. These people are considered capable of changing their behavior, while those who benefit from validation are unable to change behavior through behavior modification or through insight or confrontation. The decision of the best type of approach to use with a given resident is best made by the resident care planning team with input from those with knowledge of the resident's medical condition and history and those with knowledge of therapeutic techniques.

Ms. Feil describes the validation worker as a nonjudgmental person who accepts and respects the wisdom of old people. They are always honest. The goal is to help the disoriented accomplish their task of dying in peace by

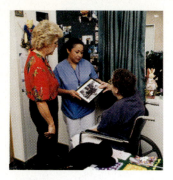

FIGURE 11-12

Reminiscence using family photographs

reminiscence   the act or habit of thinking about or relating to past experiences

listening and respecting their feelings. The effective validation worker does not treat the resident as a child. The worker respects and acknowledges the wisdom of the resident and treats each as a unique individual.

When validation is working, you can expect to see less need for chemical and physical restraints, less aggressive behavior, less crying and pacing and acting out. You will also notice that the resident is more alert (eyes open), sits up straighter, and communicates more.

Current research indicates that there are many benefits to the elderly when reminiscence therapy is used. **Reminiscence** is defined as "the act or habit of thinking about or relating to past experiences." The benefits include reducing loneliness, helping the person feel better about him or herself, and creating a positive attitude toward life. Most elderly residents conduct a type of life review in which they evaluate their past experiences and accomplishments and decide whether or not they reached their life goals. They often take great pleasure in talking about their life experiences. The nursing assistant can assist the resident in reminiscing by showing interest, asking questions, and listening (Figure 11-12).

CHANGE OF ROUTINE OR ENVIRONMENT

The resident with any type of dementia usually finds any kind of change very disruptive. Change requires residents to think about how to do things—the more they have to think about a task, the harder it is for them to accomplish the task. Residents with dementia initially tend to develop specific routines—they do things the same way, at the same time, everyday. This way, function is almost automatic. When routines are changed and disrupted, the resident may experience increased anxiety, leading to behavioral problems. Allowing residents to do things in their own way and minimizing changes in routine and environment are ways the nursing assistant can help the AD resident to avoid behavioral outbursts.

TOO MUCH STIMULATION

As dementia increases, the AD resident has trouble understanding and processing all kinds of external stimuli (sights, sounds). What they see is often misinterpreted, and what they hear is confusing and irritating. Sometimes areas where there is a lot of activity and/or sound will increase the AD residents' anxiety level. Common signs of increased anxiety include fidgeting, picking at clothing, wringing hands, pacing, and wandering.

The nursing assistant can help minimize noise and activity levels when disturbing to the AD resident. Reporting signs of stress and anxiety responses to the charge nurse early may help to avoid episodes of difficult or disruptive behavior. Sometimes medications are ordered to help reduce anxiety.

Family, loved ones, and staff need to understand that it is inappropriate to push the AD resident to perform. AD residents are initially aware of their loss of function or ability. When others challenge them to try harder, they are less able to perform. Pressures and demands that force the resident to think or concentrate on a function almost always result in failure. The more a resident with dementia concentrates or thinks about a task, the more impossible it becomes.

Asking a resident with AD to "try harder" is like asking an amputee to walk without a prosthetic device or assistance. The family and facility staff must become the assistance device and the memory prosthesis for the AD resident.

PHYSICAL PAIN, DISCOMFORT, AND REACTIONS TO MEDICATION

Whenever behavior becomes different or disruptive, the charge nurse should be notified so that a determination can be made whether or not physical problems such as constipation, a full bladder, arthritic pain, upper respiratory, or urinary tract infection exists. Even mild discomfort can cause increased anxiety in the AD resident. Because some medications cause behavioral changes, the licensed nurse should be made aware of any changes in order to assess the resident's response to prescribed medications.

The following principles are generally helpful in dealing with a resident with difficult or disruptive behaviors:

- Remain calm, get the resident's attention, try to establish direct eye contact.
- Touch the resident gently, take his or her hand, speak slowly using as few words as possible.
- Keep communication clear and simple, speak slowly.
- Patting, rocking, and holding hands may help to calm the resident.
- If a resident shrinks away from touch, refrain from touching.
- Assure the resident that he or she is safe.
- Try to redirect or distract his or her attention to a different, less upsetting focus: "Come outside for a walk"; "Sit down and talk with me."
- When possible, remove the resident from the immediate surroundings and take to a quiet, less stimulating environment; because short-term memory is impaired, just the change may cause the resident to forget the reason for the outburst.
- Use a calm unhurried approach; do not make unnecessary demands on the resident.
- Use reflective terms like "you seem upset"—allow the resident to express angry or hostile feelings as long as talking about them decreases the behavior; if this intensifies the behavior, try to distract the resident using familiar words or objects: "It is lunch time, let's go to the table"; "The picture has beautiful flowers"; "What is your favorite song?"
- Avoid approaching the resident from the side or behind; intrusions into what they think of as personal space are viewed as loss of control of their environment and may lead to aggressive behavior.
- Reassure the resident when behavior is related to feelings of persecution: "You are safe, no one can hurt you"; "We would never keep you from visiting with your wife"; "Your dog is safe, he is with your daughter."
- Help out when you observe frustration building such as difficulty buttoning a shirt or dress: "May I help you with that?"
- Avoid verbal battles—never argue or scold residents, for even though they may be confused, they are able to experience feelings of shame and embarrassment; it is not helpful and will not change the undesirable behavior. For example, when a resident takes things from another resident's room:
  Do not say: "You know this is not your room, you should never go into someone else's room!"
  Do say: "Take my hand, I will take you to your room."
- Observe and identify *patterns* of behavior with your charge nurse; look for events or circumstances that might lead to undesirable behavior; when this is possible, removing or eliminating these events can markedly decrease difficult behavior.

apathy lack of feeling or interest in things

Other common behaviors seen in many Alzheimer's residents are depression and **apathy** (a lack of feeling or interest in things). This is particularly true of residents in the earlier stage of the disease as they recognize that something is not right. Alzheimer's residents suffering from depression function below their real abilities and there is a constant feeling of withdrawal and sadness.

The following strategies may be helpful in caring for depressed or withdrawn behaviors:

- Report observations of depressed behavior to the charge nurse so that an assessment can be made to determine if medications might be helpful.
- Identify events that might cause feelings of worthlessness, sadness, or apathy.
- Encourage residents to talk with staff and others. Find opportunities to assist residents in developing social relationships.
- Listen—help residents feel comfortable in your presence. Show them that you are interested in them by listening. Very often they will share their feelings with you.
- Do not deny their feelings. Don't try to "cheer them up." Respect the residents right to feel sad and offer your support and concern.
- Encourage the resident to become involved in activity programs and to do physical exercise as possible.

Recent years have shown a definite trend toward development of special treatment units designed specifically to meet the unique needs of AD residents. Many people believe that AD residents function better longer when they are in a separate environment where special programs are used to maximize their functional abilities. Research on the best care for persons with dementia tells us that the most important element is having staff that is committed to working with demented residents. That staff must also have knowledge about dementia and management of its symptoms. The residents need privacy, adequate stimulation, and maximum decision making.

Because Alzheimer's is an incurable, terminal disease, goals for care of the AD resident must be directed toward improving the quality of life. We can:

- Develop programs to maximize resident's functional abilities—keep them as independent and as much in control of their lives as possible for as long as possible
- Design environments that promote mobility and independence while safeguarding the welfare and safety of the residents
- Reduce the complexity of both the daily routines and environment so that residents can be as effective (successful) as possible each day
- Recognize the uniqueness of each resident and ensure that all residents are treated with respect and dignity
- Provide families with accurate information regarding the resident, the disease process, the plan of care, and the facility routines
- Recognize the family's need for emotional support and understanding as they watch the deterioration and loss of their loved one each day

Three of the most important considerations in providing care to the AD resident will be referred to as the three C's:

Caution: protect from physical harm.
Communication: provide a clear understanding by using simple terms.
Comfort: physical, emotional, and environmental.

PROBLEM	GOAL OF CARE	ACTIONS/APPROACHES
High risk for falls due to unsteadiness	Decreased incidence of falls, no injuries by _____ (date).	Properly fitted nonskid shoes. Remind to use hand rail. Close supervision.
Wanders and rummages through drawers, unable to find room.	Decreased intrusions into other residents room by _____. Will rummage in specially prepared drawer by _____.	Identify room with colored ribbon—tie same color to wrist band. Provide a rummaging drawer. Distract with other activities.
Weight loss due to inability/refusal to feed self and swallowing difficulties.	No decrease in weight by _____.	Report intake less than 80% to charge nurse. Offer substitutes. Offer finger foods. Change consistency of foods to resident's tolerance.
Inappropriate behavior and catastrophic reaction to various daily routines.	Decrease number of catastrophic reactions by _____.	Reduce noise. Reduce contact with crowds. Break down tasks into simple steps. Plan rest periods. Report symptoms of pain or discomfort.
Family distress at resident's inappropriate behavior.	Family verbalizes understanding of disease process and its effect on resident's behavior by _____.	Listen, allow family to express feelings. Refer problems or questions to charge nurse. Invite to family night.

Caring for AD residents and providing the necessary support to the families is one of the most challenging responsibilities of the nursing assistant! The following plan of care was developed by the interdiscipling team for a specific resident with a diagnosis of dementia of the Alzheimer's type.

SUMMARY

Diseases and injuries of the nervous system are among the most serious and debilitating that a person can experience. Most of the diseases studied in this chapter are chronic, with a slow decline in residents' ability to care for themselves. The resident must learn to cope with a series of losses and a constant reminder of the effects of the diseases. Many experience grief over their lost abilities so that depression is common. As a nursing assistant, you can contribute much to the resident's ability to cope by the attitude you display to the resident. It is of great importance that you adjust your care to changes in the resident's abilities. Your attitude needs to be "matter-of-fact" in that you neither ignore nor accentuate the losses of ability. In a gentle, thoughtful way, say things like "May I help you with that?" or "Let me help you."

Because memory loss, impaired judgment, and difficulty communicating also accompany many of the diseases, the nursing assistant must be an excellent observer and protector. Safety of the resident becomes the primary goal. This means that you must supervise the resident, involve them in meaningful activities, and learn approaches to difficult behaviors.

SELF STUDY

Choose the best answer for each question or statement.

1. Which of the following are parts of the central nervous system?
   a. brain and spinal cord
   b. spinal nerves and cranial nerves
   c. peripheral nerves and dendrites
   d. all of the above

2. What does the right hemisphere of the cerebrum control?
   a. most of the activity on the right side of the body
   b. most of the activity on the left side of the body
   c. most of the activity of the upper half of the body
   d. most of the activity of the lower half of the body

3. Which of the following is true of reflexes?
   a. No thought is involved when a reflex occurs.
   b. They are automatic responses of the muscles or skin to stimulation.
   c. They occur without the message going all the way to the brain.
   d. All of these are true of reflexes.

4. Mr. Goldman is a resident in the long-term care facility. His muscles are rigid, he never smiles, and his hands shake and tremble a great deal. He is unable to walk because his legs are so weak. Which of the following disorders of the nervous system might he have?
   a. multiple sclerosis
   b. Parkinson's disease
   c. cerebrovascular accident (stroke)
   d. seizures

5. Which of the following is true of multiple sclerosis (MS)?
   a. It affects the person's memory and understanding.
   b. It causes tremors and a masklike expression.
   c. It usually affects young adults between the ages of 20 and 40.
   d. It occurs because of an injury to the spinal cord.

6. Ms. Kravitz is a resident who is quadriplegic. This means that she is paralyazed
   a. on one side of her body
   b. from the waist down
   c. in both arms
   d. in all four limbs

7. Ms. Kravitz will benefit from a tub bath because it will
   a. help her sit up for awhile
   b. improve circulation and reduce muscle spasms
   c. increase nerve function in her limbs
   d. prevent muscle atrophy in her limbs

8. Which of the following urinary problems result from spinal cord injuries?
   a. kidney and bladder stones
   b. urinary retention
   c. kidney disease
   d. all of the above

9. Ms. Kravitz must be watched closely for autonomic dysreflexia. This condition is life threatening because it causes
   a. aspiration and pneumonia
   b. prolonged seizures
   c. severe high blood pressure
   d. chest pain and heart failure

10. Ms. Kravitz complains of a headache and stuffy nose. You notice goosebumps on her arms and sweat on her face. What should you do?
    a. Report these symptoms to your charge nurse immediately.
    b. Cover her with a blanket and take her temperature.
    c. Ask the nurse if she can have an allergy pill.
    d. Lower the room temperature and elevate her head.

11. Which of the following is *not* a cause of CVA (stroke)?
    a. blood clot originating in the brain
    b. blood clot traveling to the brain from another part of the body
    c. hemorrhage
    d. severe emotional shock

12. Mr. Washington has had a CVA. He has left hemiplegia. This means that
   a. his left side is paralyzed
   b. he may have no sensation in his left side
   c. he may forget his left side when he shaves
   d. all of the above

13. Mr. Washington often begins to cry when you are assisting him with his care. Your best response to him is to
   a. tell him that everything will be all right and not to be sad
   b. ask him what is making him feel so sad
   c. ignore his tears and treat him in a matter-of-fact way
   d. tell him you understand how depressed he must be

14. Ms. Mattingly was in a car accident and is now in a coma. This means that she is
   a. unconscious and cannot be aroused
   b. confused and does not know who she is
   c. disoriented and does not know where she is
   d. very sleepy but can wake up with difficulty

15. The resident you are with has a seizure in the dining room. What should you do?
   a. Go to the nurse's station and use the intercom to get help.
   b. Move furniture out of the way to prevent injury.
   c. Hold the resident tightly to keep him from moving.
   d. Find something to put in his mouth to keep him from biting his tongue.

16. Mrs. Baker has Alzheimer's disease and is confused. Her husband died several years ago and she gets very upset when his death is mentioned. She asks if her husband is coming to visit today. What should you do?
   a. Tell her that he can't come today but probably will come tomorrow.
   b. Tell her that he died several years ago and won't be coming to visit.
   c. Tell her that she will get to visit him again in heaven, but not today.
   d. Tell her you know that she must miss him and ask what they liked to do together.

Getting C O N N E C T E D
Multimedia Extension Activities

www.prenhall.com/will-black

Use the above address to access the free, interactive Companion Website created for this textbook. Hear the pronunciation of the key terms in the chapter. Get instant feedback to a variety of chapter-related questions. Link to other interesting sites.

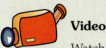

Video

Watch the video *Dealing with Dementia* from the Care Provider Skills series. Also watch the section on "Dealing with Anger" from the video *Focus on Professionalism.*

CASE STUDY

George Gonzales is a 70-year-old man who had a stroke about 6 months ago. He has been in the facility for 3 months and is no longer receiving therapy. He has frequent visitors, including his four sons. He is unable to communicate in English or Spanish due to the effects of his stroke. He is right handed.

1. Because he is aphasic, his paralysis is probably on the
   a. right side
   b. left side
   c. both sides
   d. lower extremities
2. He is participating in the self-feeding program. You observe his wife feeding him his lunch. You should
   a. report it to the charge nurse immediately since she is not supporting his rehabilitation
   b. accept it as part of his culture and notify the therapist so she can be instructed in safe feeding techniques
   c. inform her that she should not feed him
   d. none of the above
3. You notice that Mr. Gonzales is slow and very cautious when walking with his cane. This is probably due to
   a. the part of his brain affected by the stroke
   b. his stubborn personality
   c. his impulsive and unsafe behavior
   d. his cultural beliefs
4. Because of the effects of his stroke, your care needs to include
   a. safety precautions
   b. prevention of pressure ulcers
   c. lots of encouragement to keep trying
   d. nothing in particular—all residents with strokes are the same

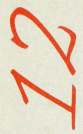

Chapter 12

THE RESPIRATORY SYSTEM

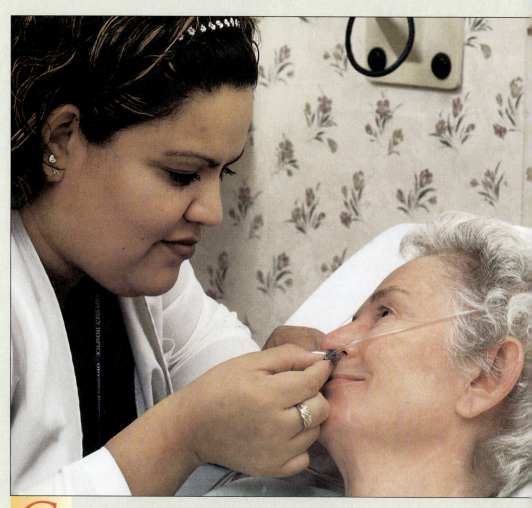

CARING TIP

The caring nursing assistant understands the connection between the mind, body, and spirit, and helps the resident to draw from his or her internal resources to bring about relaxation, acceptance, and slower, easier breathing.

Neva Babcock, BSN, RNC, CDONA, CIC
Performance Improvement/Infection Control Director
St. Thomas More Nursing and Rehab Center
Hyattsville, Maryland

KEY TERMS

alveoli	diaphragm	metabolism
aspiration	epiglottis	respiration
bronchi	larynx	trachea

RESPIRATORY SYSTEM

The respiratory system (Figure 12-1) is composed of:

- Nasal cavity
- Oral cavity
- Pharynx
- Larynx
- Trachea
- Bronchi—right and left
- Bronchioles
- Alveoli
- Lungs—right and left
- Diaphragm

Functions of the respiratory system are to:

- Provide oxygen to the cells of the body
- Remove waste products in the form of carbon dioxide

The respiratory system provides a route or pathway for oxygen to get from the air into the lungs. In the lungs it is picked up by the blood and carried to the cells. The word **respiration** means an exchange of gases between an organism and the environment in which it lives.

The most vital work of the respiratory system is done at the cellular level, where the exchange of oxygen and carbon dioxide occurs. The respiratory system is mainly responsible for getting oxygen into the blood where it is carried to the cells of the body.

Breathing is regulated by a center in the medulla of the brain. If there is an injury or disease to this area, the respiratory function is affected.

The process of respiration consists of one inhalation (breathing in) and one exhalation (breathing out) (Figure 12-2). Oxygen (O_2) is essential to life. When you inhale you take in air containing oxygen through the air passages into the lungs. Oxygen enters the blood through the millions of tiny air sacs called **alveoli** in the lungs.

The body uses this oxygen as well as food ingested as the fuel to supply energy for the activities of living. Carbon dioxide (CO_2) is formed as the waste product of the **metabolism** (breakdown) of food and oxygen at the cellular level.

The respiratory system is structured to help us keep the respiratory passages open at all times. The **trachea** and **bronchi** are kept open by incomplete cartilage rings that give structure to those important air passages.

respiration process of inhaling and exhaling

alveoli tiny air sacs in the lungs where oxygen enters the blood

metabolism complex processes of the living cells in which oxygen is used and carbon dioxide is given off (called the work of the cell)

trachea windpipe; the passage that conveys air from the larynx to the bronchi

bronchi two main branches of the windpipe

The airway consists of structures involved with the conduction and exchange of air. Conduction is the movement of air to and from the exchange levels of the lungs. Air enters through the nose (primary) and mouth (secondary) and travels down the pharynx to enter the larynx. After passing through the larynx, air enters the trachea. At its distal end, the trachea branches into the right and left primary bronchi. These bronchi branch into secondary bronchi, which then branch into the bronchioles. Some of the bronchioles end as closed tubes. Air movement in them helps the lungs expand. The rest of the bronchioles carry the air to the exchange levels of the lungs.

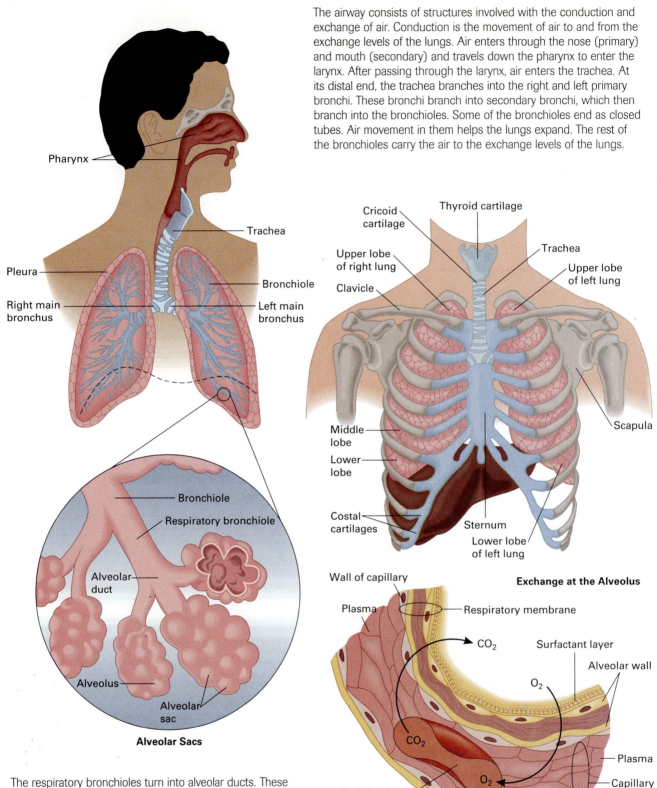

Alveolar Sacs

The respiratory bronchioles turn into alveolar ducts. These form alveolar sacs that are made up of the alveoli. Gas exchange takes place between the alveoli and the capillaries in the lungs.

Exchange at the Alveolus

FIGURE 12-1

The respiratory system.

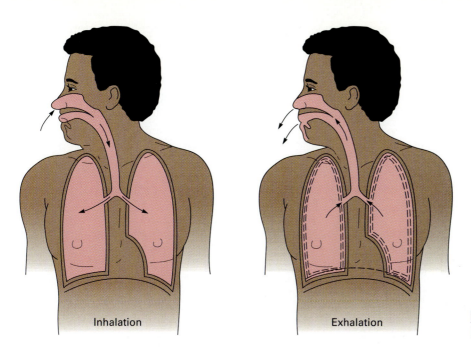

Inhalation   Exhalation

FIGURE 12-2

Inhaling and exhaling.

The **larynx** or voice box contains the vocal cords that make speech possible. There is an important piece of cartilage that covers the opening to the trachea, called the **epiglottis.** It covers the trachea when foods or fluids are swallowed. This prevents substances from entering the trachea and causing choking, obstruction, or aspiration into the air passages. **Aspiration** occurs when small pieces of food or fluid, mucus, or vomitus are taken into the air passages.

The lungs almost stand on the **diaphragm.** The diaphragm is a muscular organ that separates the thoracic (chest) and abdominal cavities. The diaphragm flattens during inhalation, which increases the size of the chest cavity and allows the lungs to expand. The diaphragm expands or pushes up into the chest cavity on exhalation, reducing the size of the chest cavity.

larynx   voice box

epiglottis   cartilage that covers the opening of the trachea when foods and fluids are swallowed

aspiration   inhaling food or fluid into the lungs

diaphragm   muscular organ that separates the chest and abdominal cavities

AGE-RELATED CHANGES

Respiratory problems are among the more common and life-threatening problems facing our elderly population. Pneumonia and various types of influenza are the fourth leading cause of death in those 65 and older. Other diseases of the respiratory system, emphysema, bronchitis, and asthma, rank eighth. Respiratory disease can be very debilitating, preventing people from leading full and active lives. A number of age-related changes affect the respiratory system:

- Respiratory muscles weaken.
- Lung tissue becomes less elastic.
- The rib cage becomes more rigid and the cartilage between the ribs becomes calcified (hardened). This limits full expansion of the chest during inspiration.
- The muscles of the abdomen become weaker, affecting the movement of the diaphragm.
- Generalized weakness may result in inability to cough and clear the upper airway of secretions.
- Postural changes may occur that produce a stooped effect, thereby limiting the expansion of the chest.

All these changes can lead to decreased exchange of oxygen and carbon dioxide, the major function of the lung. Elderly residents without respiratory disease are usually able to meet the ordinary respiratory demands despite these changes. However, once a respiratory problem develops, they are less able to adapt and slower to recover and they require aggressive treatment. It is very important to recognize and treat respiratory conditions early!

SECTION 2   The Resident with Respiratory Disease

OBJECTIVES
What You Will Learn

When you have completed this section, you will be able to:

- Identify the single most important factor contributing to respiratory disease

- Explain why residents confined to bed are at risk for pneumonia
- Describe two nursing measures to prevent pneumonia
- Identify correctly statements related to providing oxygen therapy

- List four ways the nursing assistant can help reduce the resident's fatigue

KEY TERMS

asthma
chronic obstructive pulmonary
   disease (COPD)

cilia
emphysema
humidifier
influenza

pneumonia
postural drainage
purulent material
sputum

DISEASES OF THE RESPIRATORY SYSTEM

Smoking is the most important factor contributing to respiratory disease in all ages (Figure 12-3). Many older adults started smoking in the years before the health hazards associated with smoking were recognized. Smoking is the major cause of chronic bronchitis and the most common cause of emphysema. Smokers are twice as likely to develop lung cancer as nonsmokers. Research statistics show a direct parallel between the increase in cigarette smoking and an increase in lung cancer rates.

FIGURE 12-3

Some of the destructive results of smoking.

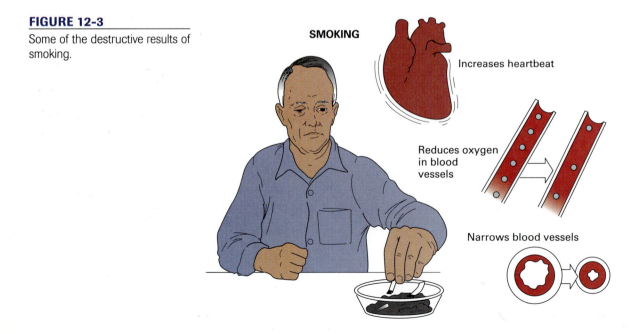

SMOKING

Increases heartbeat

Reduces oxygen in blood vessels

Narrows blood vessels

Stopping smoking leads to a rapid decline in the incidence of lung cancer, reaching the level of a nonsmoker within 13 years. For this reason, it is important that the elderly population be made aware of the dangers of cigarette smoking and the benefits of quitting at any age.

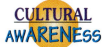 In some parts of the United States and in some cultures such as Asian cultures, smoking is still prevalent. Those who believe that disease is caused by an upset in body balance, for example, will not believe that smoking can harm them. They may see smoking as a sign of sophistication or as something they are entitled to based on their position in society. It would not be effective to attempt to convince them to stop for health reasons.

Smoking habits are not easy to change. Many local health departments, the American Heart Association, the Lung Association, and the Respiratory Diseases Association will provide specific information on various antismoking programs. As a nursing assistant, you can help residents become aware of these programs.

Common respiratory diseases of the elderly are:

- Pneumonia
- Emphysema
- Influenza
- Asthma
- Tuberculosis

INFLUENZA

Influenza ("flu") is a contagious disease caused by a virus. Although the virus may affect many parts of the body, it is considered a respiratory disease. Influenza may be spread through an affected person who coughs, sneezes, or even talks.

influenza a contagious respiratory disease caused by a virus

The person with influenza usually becomes very ill with fever, chills, and weakness, loss of appetite and aching of the head, back, arms, and legs. The person may also have a sore throat and cough, nausea, and burning eyes.

For your residents, influenza can be very severe and even fatal. Although anyone can get influenza, certain people are at high risk and should be immunized.

Those at risk include those who:

- Have chronic respiratory disease such as asthma, emphysema, tuberculosis, or chronic bronchitis
- Have heart disease
- Have chronic kidney disease
- Have diabetes
- Have diseases that depress the immune system
- Live in a nursing home or other type of health care institution
- Are over 50 years old
- Provide care for high-risk persons

Influenza can be prevented by receiving the current influenza vaccine (flu shot). The vaccine is made each year so that it can contain viruses that are expected to cause illness that year. The viruses used are inactivated so that the vaccine cannot cause the flu. It causes the person's body to develop antibodies against the disease.

The vaccine works best if received between October 15 and November 15 each year. The vaccine has been found to be about 74 percent effective in preventing influenza. It may also reduce the severity of influenza in those cases in which it doesn't actually prevent it.

As a nursing assistant, it is important to protect your residents and yourself by obtaining a flu shot each year. Some facilities provide it for their staff and residents. You may be asked to sign a consent form that points out some of the possible side effects. If you have many allergies or are allergic to eggs, you should contact your doctor first. Most facilities have found that absenteeism during flu season decreases when the staff is vaccinated. Although most people have no noticeable reaction to the shot, some have a swollen, red area where the vaccine was given. Others may have a slight fever, chills, or headache. Usually, the reaction lasts less than a few days.

For those who develop influenza, the treatment is mainly directed at controlling the symptoms and providing rest. Antiviral drugs may be part of the treatment along with drugs for reducing fever and aching.

PNEUMONIA

pneumonia acute infection of the lung

Pneumonia is an acute inflammation or infection of the lung. Until the discovery of antibiotics, most elderly people who developed pneumonia died. Pneumonia can be caused by either bacteria, viruses, aspiration, or immobility. The microorganisms that commonly cause pneumonia are always present in the upper respiratory tract and are not disease producing unless resistance is severely lowered. Age and immobility are contributory factors. When a resident is in a reclining position, the chest does not expand completely and fluids and mucus pool in the lungs, causing congestion (Figure 12-4). Many bedridden residents are too weak to cough up these pooled secretions, which provide a good medium for bacterial growth, resulting in infection.

Signs and symptoms associated with pneumonia include:

emphysema disease in which tiny bronchioles become plugged with mucus, making breathing difficult, especially during exhalation

- Cough
- Congestion
- Fever
- Rapid, labored, or shallow respirations
- Noisy respiration such as wheezing, gurgling, and rattling
- Confusion, which can occur as a result of decreased oxygen
- Restlessness, which can occur as a result of decreased oxygen
- Complaints of pain in the chest

FIGURE 12-4

When a person is in a reclining position, fluids pool in the lungs.

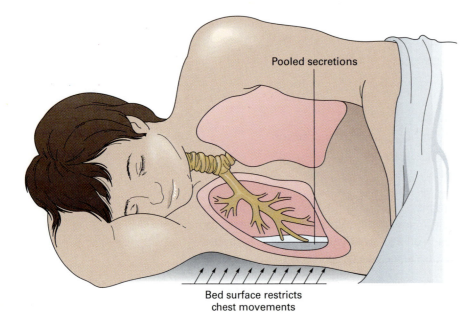

Pooled secretions

Bed surface restricts chest movements

EMPHYSEMA

Emphysema is a disease that begins with the destruction of the air sacs (alveoli) in the lungs where oxygen from the air is exchanged for carbon dioxide. The walls of the alveoli are thin and fragile. Damage is irreversible and results in permanent holes in the tissues of the lungs. As the alveoli are destroyed, the lungs are able to transfer less and less oxygen to the bloodstream, causing shortness of breath. The lungs also lose their elasticity. The resident has greatest difficulty with exhaling. Chronic emphysema takes the lives of over 10,000 Americans each year, and the death rate is increasing sharply. Currently, there are about 2.0 million Americans who have emphysema. Emphysema ranks 15th among chronic conditions that limit daily activities. Many of the people with emphysema are older men, but the condition is increasing among women. Many times, emphysema results after prolonged respiratory problems such as bronchitis, asthma, tuberculosis, or prolonged irritation from pollutants. Individuals who smoke are at high risk for development of emphysema. The disease can be extremely debilitating. Some residents require continuous oxygen and must severely limit their activity. Others are able to pace their activities according to their tolerance.

Emphysema is a diagnosis established by the physician based on pulmonary (lung) function tests and x-ray. Residents with emphysema generally exhibit the following signs and symptoms:

- Persistent cough (moist coughing and wheezing)
- Fatigue
- Loss of appetite
- Weight loss
- Anxiety (due to difficulty breathing)
- Coughing up thick secretions, especially in the morning
- Resident sits leaning forward with shoulders hunched to facilitate breathing
- Breathing with "pursed lips"

ASTHMA

Asthma is another common respiratory disease that affects the elderly. Some elderly have been affected with asthma all their lives; others develop asthma during their later years. Asthma is a disease of the bronchi, characterized by difficulty breathing, wheezing, and a sense of tightness or constriction in the chest due to spasm of the muscles (Figure 12-5). This causes narrowing of the air passages.

Asthma is often the result of an allergic reaction. The person has developed a sensitivity to a particular substance and, when exposed, the body reacts, sometimes in a life-threatening manner. More than half the cases of asthma are related to allergies. For this reason, it is essential that residents are protected from being exposed to substances to which they are allergic.

The resident's medical record will contain a notation related to allergies. The diet card will identify any foods to which the resident is allergic. Some residents are allergic to certain kinds of tape, soap, medications, animals, fabrics, and pillow fillings. You must be aware of residents' allergies.

Some types of asthma are related to the resident's emotional state. Nervous tension, stress, and emotional upsets all can bring on an asthma attack or make an attack worse. You can help protect the resident from sources of emotional excitement and provide a quiet, relaxed atmosphere.

There are specific drugs and special medicated inhalers used to treat the resident with asthma. Observing for the symptoms of an asthma attack and reporting these observations promptly to the charge nurse are very important.

asthma a disease of the bronchi characterized by difficulty breathing, wheezing, and a sense of tightness or constriction in the chest due to spasm of the muscles

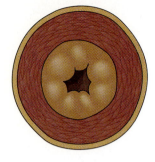

Spasm of muscles

Cross-section of small air tube

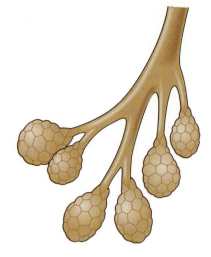

FIGURE 12-5

Bronchial asthma.

Symptoms of an asthma attack are:

- Difficulty breathing (dyspnea)
- Shortness of breath
- Wheezing
- Coughing
- Blue/grey skin color (cyanosis)
- Rapid pulse
- Increased perspiration

Frequently, if medication is administered in the initial phase of the attack, the severity of the reaction is reduced.

Emphysema, asthma, and chronic bronchitis are often referred to as **chronic obstructive pulmonary disease (COPD).** You may see this term used on a health care plan identifying problems related to these diseases.

NURSING CARE OF THE RESIDENT WITH RESPIRATORY DISEASE

All nursing care should be focused on improving the exchange of oxygen and carbon dioxide to prevent respiratory insufficiency leading to respiratory failure. Most residents with respiratory disease require respiratory therapy and oxygen therapy.

RESPIRATORY THERAPY

The respiratory therapist is a health care professional with special expertise in the treatment of respiratory disease. The therapist will assess the resident with respiratory problems and make recommendations to attending physicians for special respiratory treatments and medications. Some treatments may be performed several times a day until the resident's condition improves. Special equipment may be used (see Chapter 18).

The nursing assistant is never responsible for administering respiratory therapy but may have specific assignments related to appropriate handling or cleaning of the equipment. Always follow your facility's policies and procedures.

OXYGEN THERAPY

Every cell requires oxygen to live, and death will occur within 4 minutes if a person stops breathing. There is a delicate balance between the supply and the body's demand. If the demand is greater than the body's ability to supply it, additional oxygen may be administered.

Oxygen is a tasteless, odorless, and colorless gas that may be administered by several different methods. The physician will specify the method, rate, and length of time for oxygen therapy to continue. Some residents with respiratory disease can be harmed by too much oxygen. Therefore, the nursing assistant should not adjust the oxygen flow rate; this is the responsibility of the licensed nurse.

One-way oxygen is administered through a nasal cannula or tubes (Figure 12-6). The cannulas are inserted into the resident's nostrils. The cannula, which is made of soft plastic, is a half-circle of tubing with two openings in the center. It fits about ½ inch into the resident's nostrils. Nasal cannulas are held in place by an elastic headband secured around the back of the resident's head and connected to the source of oxygen by a length of plastic tubing. The nursing assistant should be sure that the cannulas are in place and that the tubing does not create pressure over the ears.

Another method of administering oxygen is through a plastic face mask. The mask is used when cannulas do not stay in place and/or the resident breathes through the mouth. The mask delivers a higher concentration of oxygen (Figure 12-7). The mask is placed over the mouth and nose and is fitted to the nose with a metal nose piece. The mask is held in place by an elastic headband secured around the resident's head and connected to the source of oxygen by a length of plastic tubing. Residents generally prefer the nasal cannulas as they feel less confined.

Oxygen can be supplied through a portable oxygen cylinder or tank (Figure 12-8), through a wall outlet at the bedside delivered from a central oxygen source, or through a portable machine referred to as an oxygen concentrator. Oxygen flowing from the cylinder passes through water, producing bubbles, to reduce its drying effect and then flows into the cannula or mask. The water container is called a **humidifier.** If it appears to be running dry or no bubbles are present, notify the licensed nurse immediately.

Oxygen is essential to life; however, it must always be considered a potential hazard when stored because it supports combustion. Review Chapter 2 dealing with oxygen safety. Remember, a NO SMOKING sign must be posted at the resident's door. Make sure that visitors understand the safety requirements when oxygen is in use.

POSTURAL DRAINAGE

The resident with respiratory disease may require special positioning to assist in draining of collected secretions from the respiratory passages. **Postural drainage** is a form of physical therapy that is often carried out by nursing personnel. The resident is always placed in a position in which the upper trunk is lower than the rest of the body (Figure 12-9). The force of gravity, along with the small hairlike projections of the respiratory passages **(cilia),** moves secretions from the lungs and the bronchial tree into the trachea to be coughed up. The position for the postural drainage depends on the individual resident's tolerance as well as the portion of the lung affected.

Postural drainage is ordered by the physician or planned by the licensed nurse when a resident has excessive secretions. You will need to consult with the licensed nurse before you start position drainage procedures.

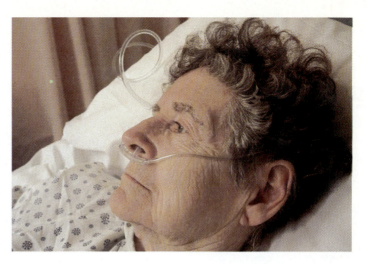

FIGURE 12-6

Oxygen administered through a nasal cannula.

humidifier water container through which oxygen is passed to reduce its drying effect

postural drainage physical therapy in which the resident is positioned so that the upper trunk is lower than the rest of the body, forcing secretions from respiratory passages to be coughed up

cilia small hairlike projections of the respiratory passages

FIGURE 12-7

Oxygen administered by a face mask.

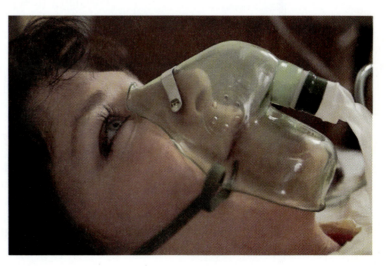

PROVIDING CARE TO THE RESIDENT RECEIVING OXYGEN

- Make sure that the elastic band does not create pressure on the ears or head.
- Adjust the face mask so that it fits snugly to help the resident receive the amount of oxygen ordered.
- Check the nasal prongs to ensure that they are clean and not irritating to the nostrils.
- Wipe collected moisture out of the face mask each shift.
- Give oral hygiene frequently because oxygen dries the mucous membranes of the mouth and nose, resulting in cracking of the lips and mouth.
- Keep the oxygen tubing free of kinks so that the flow is not obstructed.
- Observe the flow rate and the oxygen humidifier to ensure that it is operating properly.
- Report any problems to the charge nurse immediately.
- Always make sure that rules for oxygen safety are followed by residents, visitors, and facility employees.

sputum mucus from the lungs, usually mixed with saliva

purulent material liquid inflammation product containing cells and other fluid

Some residents cannot tolerate some of the positions and may even find the procedure frightening. You will be instructed how to position each resident who requires postural drainage. Postural drainage is generally performed two to three times each day when the stomach is empty so that vomiting, gagging, and discomfort are less likely. The treatment lasts approximately 20 to 30 minutes, or less if the resident is unable to tolerate it. The older resident will need to change positions slowly and rest between position changes.

You should encourage the resident to assist in bringing up the secretions by coughing. Make sure you provide the resident with good mouth care following this procedure. Take care to dispose of sputum and tissues properly. **Sputum** is the substance collected from the resident's lungs that contains mucus, saliva, and sometimes blood or purulent material. **Purulent material** is a liquid inflammation product containing cells and other fluid. Be sure to follow your facility's infection control procedures for handling body secretions.

You will need to chart the result of the procedure: the color, amount, and consistency of the sputum and how the resident tolerated the procedure.

Some residents with chronic respiratory disease need assistance with breathing exercises. We generally take breathing and coughing for granted, but this simple process becomes difficult and ineffective for some residents. Most residents with respiratory disease tend to breathe in rapid shallow breaths that do not allow full expansion of the lungs. The respiratory therapist or physician will order the use of an Incentive Spirometer. This hand-held piece of equipment looks like a child's plastic toy with a mouthpiece connected to plastic tubing attached to a cylinder with a ball in it. The resident is instructed to inhale and hold the inspiration as long as possible; as the sustained inspiration increases the ball moves up the scale on the cylinder. This maneuver helps to open closed alveoli and therefore increase oxygen exchange.

FIGURE 12-8

An oxygen cylinder or tank.

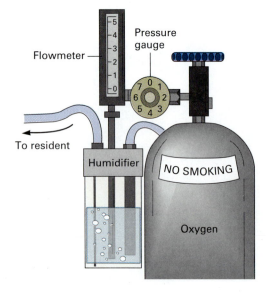

SPUTUM SPECIMENS

At times the physician will order that a sputum specimen be collected for laboratory analysis. Sputum specimens are most easily obtained in the early morning when secretions have collected throughout the night. If you are instructed to collect a sputum specimen, follow the directions on the container package or your facility's procedure. The nursing assistant should have the licensed nurse observe any sputum that appears abnormal; report any sputum tinged with blood, having a dark or colored appearance, or that produces a foul odor.

If certain medications are given early, before respiratory symptoms worsen, serious respiratory emergencies may be prevented. The nursing assistant must be attentive to changes in the resident's respiratory function in order to report these observations to the licensed nurse promptly.

FATIGUE AND WEAKNESS

Almost all residents with respiratory disease complain of weakness and fatigue. There is no drug that restores strength. Sometimes, mild exercise can help, especially if fatigue is due to lack of activity.

When fatigue is caused by lack of oxygen due to respiratory disease, residents may benefit from learning energy conservation methods and by accepting help from others. Occupational therapists are expert at helping residents learn to save their energy by pacing themselves, learning breathing techniques, and learning ways to perform their activities of daily living (ADLs) more efficiently.

The nursing assistant plays a crucial role in helping residents save their energy for those things only they can do. By helping with bathing, grooming, dressing, and all personal care, the resident may have energy to spend time with family and friends and doing things they enjoy. In a rehabilitation setting, the nursing assistant would be encouraging the resident to do as much as possible for him- or herself. With a resident who has fatigue, that may not be important. The charge nurse will give you instructions on how much activity is appropriate for your resident. Other things the nursing assistant can do for residents to preserve their energy include:

- Scheduling care with rest periods
- Avoiding excessively tiring activities (e.g., a bed bath may be a better choice than a shower)
- Paying attention and responding appropriately when signs of fatigue are present (knowing when to allow time for rest)
- Helping the family and other visitors become aware of the resident's need for rest

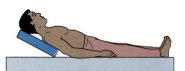
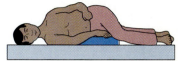
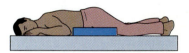
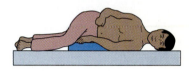

FIGURE 12-9
Postural drainage.

LOSS OF ABILITY TO PERFORM ACTIVITIES OF DAILY LIVING

You have learned that the activities of daily living (ADLs) include eating, bathing, dressing, toileting, and ambulating. Some or all of these abilities may be lost when one is experiencing fatigue. The nursing assistant plays the key role in stepping in to perform many or all of these tasks when a resident loses the ability to be independent.

It is important to provide care in a matter of fact way that doesn't blame or criticize residents for their lack of ability to care for themselves. As you provide care and assistance in ADLs, give the resident as much control as possible. For example, ask the resident what she wants to wear versus choosing the clothing for her. Think of as many ways as you can to give choice about each activity you are performing. Sometimes the only choice may be "yes" or "no" or "now" or "later," but that is still a choice. Be aware that inability to perform ADLs represents a significant loss to the resident and often to his or her family.

ANXIETY

Most residents with respiratory disease have serious anxiety. Difficulty breathing is one of the most distressing symptoms they can experience. Their entire focus is on taking each breath. Usually, residents have certain ways they want things done. They may seem to be very "picky" or critical. It is important not to take their remarks personally but to recognize the behavior as related to their respiratory difficulties. Often, residents become very attached or even cling to a certain caregiver. It is not unusual for residents to beg you not to leave them, particularly when their breathing is most difficult. While medications sometimes are helpful, there are many things the nursing assistant can do to help increase the comfort of the resident and reduce the anxiety:

- *Positioning*—The head of the bed should be elevated. Some residents like to sit on the side of the bed and lean over the overbed table. The overbed table should have as many pillows on it as needed to allow the resident to place their arms on top of the pillows. This allows for the chest to expand and makes breathing easier.
- *Temperature*—The resident may be more comfortable if the room is cool.
- *Use of a fan*—Even with air conditioning, a fan may help improve the air circulation.
- *Reassurance and support.*
- *Convenient environment*—Place needed objects within reach to reduce the amount of energy needed.
- *A calm atmosphere*—Go about your care in a calm, slow way.

SUMMARY

A healthy respiratory system is essential to good health. The energy needed to care for oneself in the most basic ways requires that the cells of the body have enough oxygen. Although with advancing age the body slows its pace, most of the respiratory problems are due to disease rather than aging alone. One of the key factors you have learned about is the impact that smoking has on the function of the respiratory system. Although in many cases, the damage has been done, stopping smoking can improve the health of your residents.

Because of the fatigue and weakness and inability to perform ADLs, residents depend on the knowledge and skills of the nursing assistant even more than with most illnesses. Residents with respiratory disease pose a real challenge to most nurses and nursing assistants due to the high level of anxiety. All the caregiving must slow down to a pace that is comfortable for the energy of the resident. Care must be provided according to their desires to decrease their anxiety and inspire their confidence. On those occasions when you become annoyed and frustrated, you may need to briefly leave the room, talk to a co-worker or supervisor, and "count to 10" before returning. Extreme patience is a must!

OBRA HIGHLIGHTS

One of the rights that all residents are entitled to is that of the right to make choices about their care and daily activities. Just because residents need to live in a long-term care facility, they don't need to give up the choices that we are all able to make in our daily lives. It is the nursing assistant more than any other staff member who is in the position to honor or violate this particular right. The choices involve simple things like what to wear, what to eat, when to get out of bed, and what activities to attend. When a resident says "No, I don't want a shower now," you must honor his or her wishes. If you are unsure about what to do, ask your charge nurse immediately. You can make a great contribution by remembering to offer a choice every time you can. Place the residents' personal items where they want them. Ask how they want things done and do them that way. This is not the time to insist that things are done your way. This right is particularly important when a resident is suffering from a respiratory disease and has to cope with the anxiety that comes with it. Giving choice and control reduces anxiety. The nursing assistant will benefit by having a more positive interaction with the resident.

SELF STUDY

Choose the best answer for each question or statement.

1. What is the main function of the respiratory system?
   a. delivering oxygen into the blood so it is carried to the body cells
   b. expanding the lungs to their full capacity
   c. removing excess water from the body through exhaled vapor
   d. removing part of the carbon dioxide from the body as waste

2. What is the function of the epiglottis?
   a. make speech possible
   b. provide exchange of oxygen and carbon dioxide
   c. cover the trachea during swallowing
   d. divide the chest and abdominal cavities

3. Which of the following explains the effects of smoking on the heart and blood vessels?
   a. Smoking increases the heart rate.
   b. Smoking decreases the oxygen level in the blood.
   c. Smoking causes blood vessels to narrow.
   d. All of these are true of smoking.

4. When a resident's resistance to illness is severely lowered, the microorganisms normally found in the respiratory tract cause which respiratory disease?
   a. influenza
   b. pneumonia
   c. asthma
   d. emphysema

5. What is influenza?
   a. a contagious respiratory disease caused by a virus
   b. an acute infection of the lungs caused by bacteria
   c. a contagious illness that causes nausea and vomiting
   d. an infection in the lungs caused by inhaling food or fluid

6. What can you do to help protect your residents and yourself from influenza?
   a. Obtain a pneumonia vaccination each year.
   b. Obtain a flu shot each year.
   c. Take preventative antibiotics during the winter months.
   d. Get plenty of rest and exercise, and eat balanced meals.

7. Which of the following is true of emphysema?
   a. It is caused by normal microorganisms in the respiratory tract.
   b. It causes pus to build up in the lungs, requiring surgery to remove.
   c. It destroys the walls of the air sacs, making permanent holes in the lung tissue.
   d. It causes the person to have great difficulty inhaling air.

8. Asthma is frequently caused by
   a. emphysema
   b. allergic reactions
   c. heart failure
   d. pneumonia

9. Mrs. Johnson is a resident where you work. After her shower, she complains of difficulty breathing. You can hear wheezing when she breathes, and she is coughing frequently. What will you do?
   a. Notify your charge nurse immediately since she might be having an asthma attack.
   b. Assist her back to bed so she can rest, and check on her in about an hour.
   c. Encourage her to cough up mucus and spit it in a cup; then show the cup to the nurse.
   d. Encourage her to participate in a purposeful activity to get her mind off of her breathing.

10. Which of the following is the responsibility of the nursing assistant?
    a. administering respiratory therapy treatments
    b. increasing the flow rate of oxygen if the resident is short of breath
    c. ensuring that the oxygen cannula is in place in the resident's nose
    d. filling the oxygen humidifier bottle if it runs dry or gets low

11. What should you do after a resident coughs up sputum after receiving postural drainage?
    a. Give good mouth care.
    b. Dispose of sputum and tissues properly.

c. Document the color, amount, and consistency of the sputum.

d. All of these actions should be taken.

12. Which of the following actions can you take to help a resident with respiratory disease conserve her energy?

a. Notice when the resident becomes tired and allow her to rest.

b. Schedule all care at one time so the resident can rest the remainder of the day.

c. Encourage the resident to do just a little bit more when she complains of fatigue.

d. Encourage family members to visit for long periods to prevent loneliness.

13. Mr. Marconi is short of breath and has become increasingly anxious. He begs you not to leave him. Which of the following actions can you take to help reduce his anxiety?

a. Encourage him to think about something else besides his shortness of breath.

b. Position him so his head and shoulders are elevated.

c. Cover him with blankets and keep the room warm.

d. Tell him you have other residents to care for and will let him rest for awhile.

14. Why does a resident who is bedridden have a greater risk for pneumonia?

a. The chest expands more fully while the resident is in bed.

b. Fluids and mucus pool in the lungs while the resident lies in bed.

c. The bedridden resident can cough up secretions as effectively as others.

d. All of these cause the resident to have a greater pneumonia risk.

15. Which of the following respiratory diseases are considered to be a chronic obstructive pulmonary disease?

a. emphysema

b. asthma

c. chronic bronchitis

d. all of the above

16. What effect does stress have on asthma?

a. Stress can bring on an asthma attack or make it worse.

b. Stress has little effect on the frequency of asthma attacks.

c. Stress can cause side effects to asthma medications.

d. Stress is not connected with asthma; it is caused by allergic reactions.

Chapter Review

Getting C O N N E C T E D
Multimedia **Extension** Activities

 www.prenhall.com/will-black

Use the above address to access the free, interactive Companion Website created for this textbook. Hear the pronunciation of the key terms in the chapter. Get instant feedback to a variety of chapter-related questions. Link to other interesting sites.

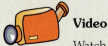 **Video**

Watch the section "Measuring Respirations" in the *Vital Signs* video from the Care Provider Skills.

CASE STUDY

Mildred Jones is an 85-year-old resident who has been in the facility for several years. Every month when you weigh her, you notice she has lost 2 or 3 pounds. She has a cough and has stopped attending activities due to fatigue and weakness. She seems to breathe best when sitting on the side of the bed leaning forward.

1. Her symptoms describe
   a. emphysema
   b. influenza
   c. pneumonia
   d. asthma

2. In order to help her cope with her fatigue and weakness, the nursing assistant should
   a. insist that she continue to perform all ADLs
   b. help with those activities that are the most tiring for her
   c. urge her to stay in bed at all times
   d. tell her that she will get better and then will be able to care for herself

3. Mrs. Jones uses her call signal frequently. She seems to make up reasons to call you into her room. She grabs your hand when you try to leave. She is showing signs of
   a. being spoiled
   b. not trusting you
   c. anxiety because of her difficulty breathing
   d. competing with her roommate for attention

4. Your best course of action is to
   a. tell her you like her better than the roommate
   b. provide a calm and reassuring atmosphere
   c. ask for a change of assignment
   d. try to find a way to make her like you

Chapter 13

THE CARDIOVASCULAR SYSTEM

CARING TIP

While taking a resident's pulse, the nurse assistant should be observant to know how fast the pulse is and whether it is skipping any beats. Be sure to report anything unusual to the nurse.

Sue Archer, RNC
Health Occupations Instructor
Puxico, Missouri

OBJECTIVES
What You Will Learn

When you have completed this section, you will be able to:

- Describe the two basic functions of the cardiovascular system

- Identify the most important function of the red blood cells and white blood cells

- Match types of blood vessels with their descriptions

- Describe why elderly people tire more easily and have less reserve energy

- Match the correct term with the symptoms described

KEY TERMS

aorta	cardiac pacemaker	pulmonic valve
arteries	electrocardiogram (EKG)	septum
arterioles	heart	tricuspid valve
atrium	hypertension	veins
blood pressure	lymph vessels	ventricle
capillaries	plasma	venules
	platelets	

CARDIOVASCULAR SYSTEM

The cardiovascular system (Figure 13-1) is composed of:

- Blood
- Blood vessels
- Lymph vessels
- Heart

Functions of the cardiovascular system are to:

- Carry nutrients and oxygen to body cells by way of the blood vessels
- Remove waste products from the cells

THE BLOOD

Blood is considered a specialized type of connective tissue. The average adult has about 5 quarts of blood in circulation. The fluid portion of the blood is called **plasma.** When separated, it is clear and straw-colored. It composes one-half the total blood volume. Plasma contains proteins, sugars, and chemical substances.

plasma fluid portion of the blood

The formed elements of the blood are:

- Red blood cells
- White blood cells
- Platelets

The most important function of the red blood cells is to carry oxygen from the lungs to the cells. There are 5,000 red blood cells for every 8 white blood cells.

The most important function of the white blood cells is to fight infection. These cells work to block bacteria, viruses, and other foreign agents from causing disease and infection in the body.

Blood **platelets** come from bone marrow cells and are essential to the clotting of the blood. When bleeding occurs, platelets change their shape, cling together, and release substances essential to stop bleeding.

Some important functions of the blood are:

- *Nutrition*—Nutrients from the digestive system are absorbed in the bloodstream and distributed to cells of the body.
- *Respiration*—Blood collects oxygen as it passes through the lungs and gives off carbon dioxide. Oxygen is delivered to body cells, and carbon dioxide is removed by exhalation.
- *Excretion*—The waste products of cellular metabolism are carried by the blood to the kidneys, lungs, and sweat glands for removal.
- *Protection*—The blood contains certain types of cells and chemicals that work to protect the body.
- *Temperature regulation*—The blood plays a major role in temperature through dilation and contraction of blood vessels.
- *Distribution of endocrine secretions*—The endocrine glands secrete hormones directly into the blood, which carries them to various cells of the body.
- *Fluid balance*—Fluids move in and out of the blood to help maintain a normal *viscosity* (the blood is not too thick or too thin).

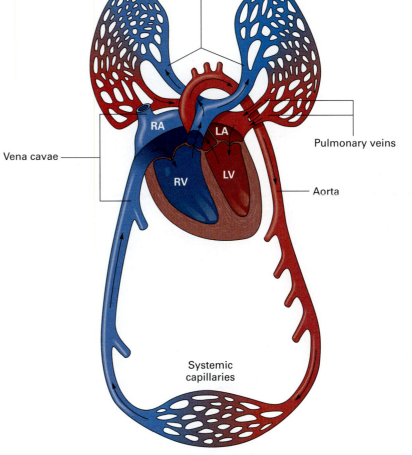

FIGURE 13-1
The cardiovascular system.

BLOOD VESSELS

Blood is distributed through the body by means of blood vessels (Figure 13-2). Blood vessels are cylindrical tubes carrying blood. The types of vessels are:

- **Arteries** are the blood vessels that always carry oxygen-rich blood away from the heart (with the exception of the pulmonary artery). Arteries have the ability to constrict or relax due to their elastic nature.
- **Arterioles** are the very tiny arteries of the body that do not have an elastic nature. They carry blood from the large arteries to the capillaries.
- **Capillaries** are the smallest blood vessels in the circulatory system. They have very thin walls, which are one cell thick. They allow exchange of oxygen, carbon dioxide, and other substances through their thin walls. Capillaries nourish all body cells.
- **Veins** are the blood vessels that always carry oxygen-poor blood back to the heart, lungs, and kidneys (with the exception of the pulmonary vein).

platelets   cells in the blood that are essential for clotting

arteries   blood vessels that carry blood away from the heart

arterioles   tiny arteries that carry blood from the large arteries to the capillaries

capillaries   smallest blood vessels in the circulatory system; they nourish all body cells

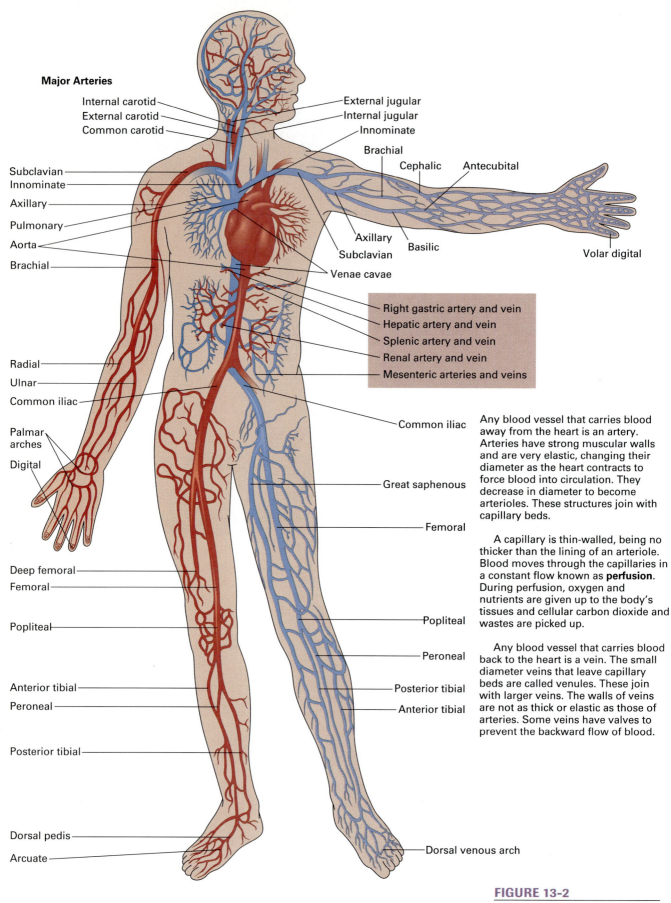

Major Arteries

Internal carotid
External carotid
Common carotid

External jugular
Internal jugular
Innominate

Brachial

Cephalic   Antecubital

Subclavian
Innominate
Axillary
Pulmonary
Aorta
Brachial

Axillary
Subclavian

Basilic

Volar digital

Venae cavae

Right gastric artery and vein
Hepatic artery and vein
Splenic artery and vein
Renal artery and vein
Mesenteric arteries and veins

Radial
Ulnar
Common iliac

Palmar arches
Digital

Common iliac

Any blood vessel that carries blood away from the heart is an artery. Arteries have strong muscular walls and are very elastic, changing their diameter as the heart contracts to force blood into circulation. They decrease in diameter to become arterioles. These structures join with capillary beds.

Great saphenous

Femoral

A capillary is thin-walled, being no thicker than the lining of an arteriole. Blood moves through the capillaries in a constant flow known as **perfusion**. During perfusion, oxygen and nutrients are given up to the body's tissues and cellular carbon dioxide and wastes are picked up.

Deep femoral
Femoral

Popliteal

Popliteal

Peroneal

Anterior tibial
Peroneal

Posterior tibial
Anterior tibial

Any blood vessel that carries blood back to the heart is a vein. The small diameter veins that leave capillary beds are called venules. These join with larger veins. The walls of veins are not as thick or elastic as those of arteries. Some veins have valves to prevent the backward flow of blood.

Posterior tibial

Dorsal pedis
Arcuate

Dorsal venous arch

FIGURE 13-2
Blood vessels.

- **Venules** are the tiny veins of the body. They carry blood from the capillaries to the large veins of the body.
- **Lymph vessels** are tiny capillarylike structures that collect lymph (tissue fluids) from the tissue spaces (areas between the cells). The lymph vessels follow the veins of the body and eventually empty into the large veins. Lymph is a colorless fluid with a salty taste circulating through the system. It is 95 percent water. Lymph is called tissue fluid when it is surrounding the cells. It is called lymph when it is drained from the tissues and collected by the lymph vessels. Along the course of the lymph vessels are lymph nodes. The main lymph nodes are in the neck, under the arms, and in the groin. These nodes often become enlarged when infection or disease occurs.

THE HEART

The heart receives blood through the veins and pumps it out through the arteries to all cells of the body. As blood circulates through the blood vessels, a force called **blood pressure** is created. Blood pressure is the measurable force of the blood against the walls of a blood vessel.

The **heart** is a cone-shaped muscle about the size of a fist. It is located a little to the left of the midline of the chest (Figure 13-3). This efficient pump beats 100,000 times a day to circulate the blood through approximately 100,000 miles of blood vessels. The heart is divided into right and left halves by a tissue called the **septum.** Each half consists of two chambers—a right **atrium** and right **ventricle** and a left atrium and left ventricle. The heart is composed of cardiac muscle, and the ventricles have thick muscular walls.

The heart has a specialized "conduction system" that is responsible for the initiation of the heartbeat. The cardiac muscle is capable of continuous rhythmic contraction. There is a place in the right atrium called the **cardiac pacemaker** that transmits an electrical impulse through the atrium to another specialized area, which sends impulses into the ventricles. This causes them to contract. An **electrocardiogram** (EKG) records the heart's electrical conduction system on a graph for analysis by the physician. Through the EKG, disturbances in the normal conduction system can be identified.

BLOOD FLOW THROUGH THE HEART

Blood flows through the heart in one direction because of four heart valves that prevent backflow. Knowing how the blood flows through the heart and lungs will help you understand some of the changes that occur when heart disease is present (Figure 13-4). The right atrium (2) receives unoxygenated (oxygen-poor) blood through the largest veins in the body, the superior and inferior venae cavae (1)(3). Blood passes from the right atrium (2) through a valve **(tricuspid)** (4) into the right ventricle (5). The right ventricle (5) contracts (squeezes) and pumps blood up through another valve **(pulmonic)** (6) into the pulmonary artery (7). The blood passes through the pulmonary artery (right and left) (7) to the lungs, where waste products in the blood and carbon dioxide are disposed of and oxygen is taken into the blood.

This oxygenated (oxygen-rich) blood returns to the left of the heart through the pulmonary veins (8) into the left atrium (9). The blood drains from the left atrium (9) through a valve (mitral) or bicuspid (10) into the left ventricle (11). The left ventricle (11) contracts and pumps the blood up through

veins blood vessels that carry blood back to the heart

venules very tiny veins that carry blood back to the heart

lymph vessels tiny capillarylike structures that collect lymph

blood pressure measurable force of the blood against the walls of a blood vessel

heart muscle that pumps blood through the vessels

septum tissue that divides the heart into right and left chambers

atrium one of the two upper chambers of the heart

ventricle thick muscular walls of the heart

cardiac pacemaker part of the conduction system of the heart that creates the stimulus for the heart to beat

electrocardiogram (EKG) tracing of the heart's electrical conduction system

tricuspid valve valve between the right atrium and right ventricle of the heart

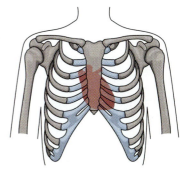

FIGURE 13-3

The position of the heart in the chest cavity.

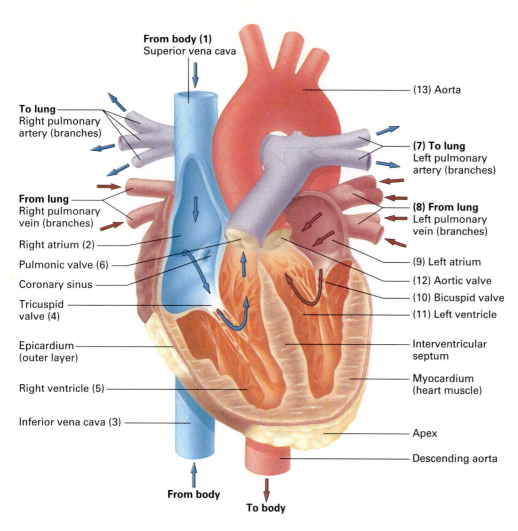

From body (1)
Superior vena cava

To lung
Right pulmonary
artery (branches)

From lung
Right pulmonary
vein (branches)

Right atrium (2)

Pulmonic valve (6)

Coronary sinus

Tricuspid
valve (4)

Epicardium
(outer layer)

Right ventricle (5)

Inferior vena cava (3)

From body

To body

(13) Aorta

(7) To lung
Left pulmonary
artery (branches)

(8) From lung
Left pulmonary
vein (branches)

(9) Left atrium

(12) Aortic valve

(10) Bicuspid valve

(11) Left ventricle

Interventricular
septum

Myocardium
(heart muscle)

Apex

Descending aorta

The heart is a hollow, muscular organ that pumps 450 million pints of blood in the average lifetime. Its superior chambers, the atria, receive blood. Both atria fill and then contract at the same time. The inferior chambers are the ventricles. They pump blood out of the heart. Both ventricles fill and then contract at the same time. When the atria are relaxing, the ventricles are contracting.

The right side of the heart receives blood from the body and sends it to the lungs (pulmonic circulation). The heart's left side receives oxygenated blood from the lungs and sends it out to the body (systemic circulation).

The heartbeat originates at the sinoatrial node (pacemaker) and spreads across the atria to stimulate contraction. After a slight delay, the impulse is sent from the atrioventricular node, down the bundles of His, and out across the ventricles. This stimulates the ventricles to contract while the atria are relaxing.

The heart muscle (myocardium) receives its blood supply by the way of the right and left coronary arteries. These vessels are the first branches of the aorta.

FIGURE 13-4

Blood flow through the heart.

pulmonic valve a valve in the heart between the right ventricle and the pulmonary artery

aorta largest artery in the body

hypertension low blood pressure

another valve (aortic) (12) into the **aorta** (13), the largest artery in the body. The aorta branches into smaller arteries leading to all areas of the body, which in turn branch into arterioles (Figure 13-5).

The arterioles deliver blood to the tiniest blood vessels of the body, including capillaries. The capillaries surround all the cells in the body. They deliver nutrients and oxygen to the cells and remove waste products. They in turn pass the blood into the large veins so that the waste products can be disposed of through the lungs, the kidneys, and the sweat glands. The heart itself receives its oxygenated blood from the coronary arteries, the first branches from the aorta.

AGE-RELATED CHANGES

There are numerous age-related changes to the cardiovascular system. Some are not serious, while others can lead to acute illness. The heart muscle may become enlarged in the older adult with **hypertension** (high blood pressure). When hypertension is present, the heart muscle has to work harder to circulate the blood through vessels that are more rigid and less elastic. When you increase the work of a muscle, it becomes larger. When you decrease the work of a muscle, it becomes smaller. In some older adults, when physical activity has been drastically reduced, the heart muscle can decrease in size.

The heart rate in the older adult is decreased, and the amount of blood pumped out into the circulatory system with each heart contraction is generally lessened (called cardiac output). It is estimated that cardiac output decreases as much as 40 percent between the ages of 25 and 65. This explains why older people tire more easily and have less reserve energy. With advancing age, a number of factors may cause the heart muscle to decrease its ability to pump adequately to maintain normal circulation. Hypertension and myocardial infarction are the most common causes; when these occur, fluids back up in the lungs, producing congestion in the tissues, evidenced by swelling (edema), difficult breathing, and extreme fatigue. This condition is known as congestive heart failure. Other age-related changes occur in the blood vessels themselves; they become thickened and less elastic. Some of the changes may cause blockage or rupture of a vessel, resulting in a cerebral vascular accident (stroke), as described in Chapter 11.

In Chapter 18 you will learn the basics of cardiopulmonary resuscitation; however, it is always recommended that you complete a certified course available through your local Red Cross or American Heart Association where you will have the opportunity to actually practice these life-saving techniques.

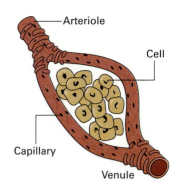

FIGURE 13-5
An arteriole.

SECTION 2 The Resident with Heart Disease

**OBJECTIVES
What You Will Learn**

When you have completed this section, you will be able to:

- Identify three types of heart disease and signs and symptoms associated with each

- Apply antiembolism stockings
- Identify three important measures associated with providing care to the resident with an amputation

- List three guidelines for providing care to the resident with heart disease

KEY TERMS

amputation
angina pectoris
arteriosclerosis
atherosclerosis
cardiac angioplasty
cardiac bypass surgery
cardiac pacemaker

cardiovascular insufficiency
congestive heart failure
demand pacemaker
embolus
fixed rate pacemaker
gangrene
infarct
myocardial infarction

nitroglycerine
peripheral vascular disease
plaque
sodium chloride
stasis ulcers
thrombus
triggered pacemaker
varicose veins

TYPES OF HEART DISEASE

Heart disease is the number one cause of death in the United States. Although heart disease is associated with all ages, as age increases so does the incidence of heart disease. Approximately 18 percent of those over 65 years of age must limit their daily activities due to various heart conditions.

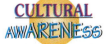

Risk factors for heart disease include increasing age, male gender, smoking, high blood pressure, and high blood cholesterol. Other factors that significantly increase the risk of heart disease are excessive alcohol consumption, individual response to stress, physical

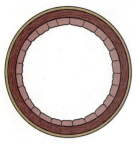

Plaque

Normal blood
vessel

Partially
closed

Closed

FIGURE 13-6

Arteriosclerosis.

**cardiovascular insuffi-
ciency**   type of heart disease in which there is
decreased blood supply to
the major organs of the
body

arteriosclerosis   thickening and loss of elasticity in
the arteries

atherosclerosis   clogging
of the arteries with plaque
and deposits of calcium or
fat

plaque   substance that
clogs arteries producing
atherosclerosis

FIGURE 13-7

The coronary arteries.

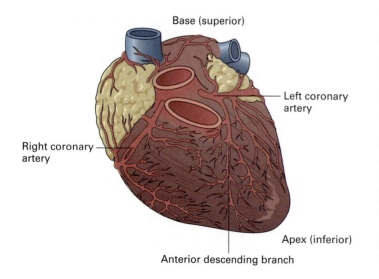

Base (superior)

Left coronary
artery

Right coronary
artery

Apex (inferior)

Anterior descending branch

inactivity, obesity, and diabetes mellitus. Some ethnic and racial groups have a higher risk of heart disease. These include African Americans, Mexican Americans, American Indians, Native Hawaiians, and some Asian Americans. This higher incidence is considered due to higher rates of obesity and diabetes.

There is a great deal of interest and public education concerning ways to prevent heart disease. Being a nonsmoker, maintaining a proper diet, getting regular exercise, keeping weight within normal limits for height and build, along with regular physical examinations are the more important preventative measures that people can take to guard against heart disease.

New techniques for the treatment of various types of heart disease along with a health-conscious society are major factors in the reduction of deaths due to heart disease in recent years. It is helpful to understand what heart diseases are most common and how you can assist residents with heart disease to lead healthy, productive lives.

Cardiovascular insufficiency is a form of heart disease in which there is decreased blood supply to the major organs of the body. The most important cause of cardiovascular insufficiency is associated with arteriosclerosis or atherosclerosis.

Arteriosclerosis is a thickening and loss of elasticity in the arteries of the body (often referred to as a *hardening of the arteries*). **Atherosclerosis** is a form of arteriosclerosis in which the arteries become clogged or blocked with various substances, such as **plaque** and deposits of calcium and/or fat (Figure 13-6).

Arteriosclerosis is the major cause of heart disease and cerebral vascular accident (CVA or stroke). It is estimated that 1 million deaths occur in the United States each year that are directly related to arteriosclerosis or atherosclerosis. Both conditions result in an inadequate blood supply to the heart muscle and other vital organs, such as the brain, kidneys, lungs, stomach, and intestine. The heart muscle receives its blood supply from the coronary arteries, which branch off the aorta (Figure 13-7).

Deaths from heart disease are decreasing due to earlier diagnosis and effective surgical and nonsurgical techniques designed to improve blood flow throughout the heart muscle by restoring circulation through the coronary arteries. **Cardiac bypass surgery** is becoming more and more common. The surgeon removes a blood vessel from the patient's leg and replaces a portion of the coronary blood vessel that is clogged or blocked, thereby restoring cardiac circulation. The patient is placed on special equipment to maintain circulation while surgery is performed on the heart itself. This type of surgery has proved to be very successful.

The procedure is named according to the number of arteries replaced. For example, a double bypass is one in which two arteries were blocked. A quadruple bypass means four arteries were replaced.

Another procedure called **cardiac angioplasty** is being used to open clogged coronary arteries. A special pressurized balloon is threaded through the clogged portion of the artery and pressure is used to open the artery.

When the heart muscle does not receive an adequate blood supply, parts of the heart muscle die **(infarct).** This is called a **myocardial infarction,** often referred to as an MI, or a heart attack. Heart attack can also occur when the conduction system of the heart fails.

PACEMAKERS

A **cardiac pacemaker** (Figure 13-8) is an electronic device that delivers direct stimulation to the heart. The purpose of the pacemaker is to initiate and maintain the heart rate when the special node in the heart that normally does so fails. When this node does not function properly, the heart rate may become very slow or irregular.

In emergency situations, pacemaker wires are inserted through a catheter into the heart and an external pulse generator is worn until a permanent pacemaker can be implanted. Many people have permanently implanted pacemakers.

There are different types of pacemakers:

- **Fixed rate:** Consistently delivers a pacing stimulus at a preset rate, usually between 60 and 70 beats per minute.
- **Demand:** This pacemaker has the ability to sense when the heart rate falls below a preset rate limit and "kicks in" only when needed.
- **Triggered:** This pacemaker has the ability to sense several kinds of cardiac events and will deliver its pacing stimulus based on what is needed.

Due to the many advances and sophistication of today's pacemakers, there is an international five-letter code to describe their function. The physician and licensed nurse will have this important information. There are new methods of testing pacemaker function through telephone telemetry; a call is made to a determined source and the pacemaker can be checked on a regular basis. The licensed nurse is responsible for checking the pacemaker at the frequency ordered by the physician.

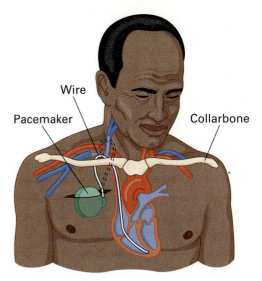

Wire

Pacemaker

Collarbone

FIGURE 13-8

The pacemaker.

cardiac bypass surgery procedure in which a blood vessel is removed from the leg to replace a portion of a coronary blood vessel that is clogged or blocked

cardiac angioplasty procedure used to open clogged coronary arteries

infarct death of part of the heart muscle

myocardial infarction heart attack in which part of the heart muscle dies

CARE OF THE RESIDENT WITH A PACEMAKER

- Review the resident's plan of care to determine what special care is required.
- Report irregular pulse or a rate below the preset rate of the pacemaker.
- Report any complaints of dizziness, shortness of breath, or heart palpitations.
- Report any episodes of hiccups as this could indicate that the pacemaker is not in its proper place.

- Report any expressed concerns about pacemaker function to the licensed nurse.
- Report immediately any signs of swelling, redness, or pain at the site of the insertion to the licensed nurse.

Guidelines

cardiac pacemaker part of the conduction system of the heart that creates the stimulus for the heart to beat

fixed rate pacemaker emits a stimulus to contract the heart muscle at a set rate

demand pacemaker a device used to stimulate the heart. It senses the interval between the heart's natural beats and fires at a programmed interval.

triggered pacemaker senses cardiac events and delivers its pacing stimulus based on what is needed

angina pectoris acute chest pain caused by decreased blood supply to the heart

nitroglycerin medication that, when placed under the tongue to dissolve, will act rapidly to increase blood flow to the heart

SIGNS AND SYMPTOMS OF HEART ATTACK OR MYOCARDIAL INFARCTION

A myocardial infarction (MI) is caused when there is a lack of blood supply to the heart muscle (myocardium). *Infarction* is the term used to describe tissue death. Other terms commonly used are *coronary occlusion* and *coronary thrombosis.* When the blood flow is interrupted, tissue death occurs; the damaged area of the heart muscle may be large or small. An MI is a cardiac emergency and requires immediate medical intervention. The nursing assistant must be alert and quickly identify the following signs and symptoms of heart attack or MI:

- Chest pain, described as a heavy, squeezing, or crushing sensation in the chest, sometimes confused with indigestion
- Pain may radiate through left of chest, left arm, neck, and jaw
- Irregular, weak, thready pulse
- Light-headedness, feeling faint or dizzy, nausea
- Difficulty breathing, shortness of breath
- Shocklike symptoms; pale, cool, clammy skin; decreased blood pressure
- Intense perspiration
- Apprehension, fear, feelings of doom

Not all the symptoms described will be present in most cases, but in varying combinations. The nursing assistant should notify the licensed nurse immediately so that further assessment can be made.

ANGINA PECTORIS

Some residents experience frequent chest pain; **angina pectoris** is the medical term used to describe acute chest pain caused by a decreased blood supply to the heart. Physical exertion, emotional stress, or excitement will increase the heart's need for oxygen and may cause angina.

Residents who have been diagnosed with angina frequently have a medication prescribed by the physician called **nitroglycerin.** Some residents may receive their medication through the skin by wearing a nitro patch or pad. This patch is usually applied to the chest (Figure 13-9). Notify the licensed nurse immediately if the resident removes the patch or if it falls off while you are giving a bath or dressing the resident. This medication is one of a very few that residents may keep at their bedside. The nitroglycerin tablet is taken when chest pain occurs; it is placed under the tongue to dissolve quickly because it causes an increase in blood flow to the heart. Review the resident's plan of care to identify those residents who keep nitroglycerin at the bedside. Assist the resident as instructed and notify the licensed nurse immediately when you observe a resident taking this medication. Angina will usually be relieved by rest and nitroglycerin within 3 to 15 minutes. The licensed nurse will need to take vital signs and observe the resident closely to be sure that the problem is angina and not an MI, because the symptoms are similar. Residents who require nitroglycerin should keep the tablets with them at all times, during therapy sessions, in the dining room, or on trips outside the facility.

FIGURE 13-9

A nitroglycerin patch. Notify nurse if the patch falls off.

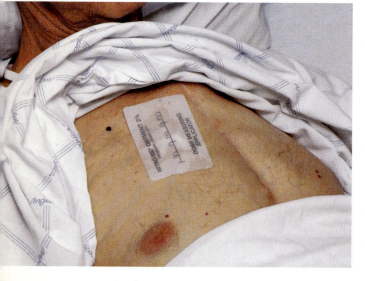

HYPERTENSION

Hypertension is a condition in which the blood pressure is too high. Hypertension is a natural partner of arteriosclerosis; when the blood vessels become rigid, less elastic, or partially blocked, the heart has to work harder to propel the blood through the vessels. The increased resistance of the vessels increases the blood pressure. Other disorders can also contribute to high blood pressure, such as head injuries, kidney disease, tumors of the adrenal gland, and some complications of pregnancy.

Hypertension often leads to heart failure, stroke, kidney failure, and blindness, regardless of its primary cause. A person is considered to be hypertensive if the systolic pressure is consistently above 160 mm and diastolic pressure is over 90 mm. Hypertension is very common in the older adult, and medications will be ordered to lower the blood pressure. The resident will be advised to quit smoking, exercise regularly, balance activity and rest, and reduce salt intake. Signs and symptoms of hypertension are:

- Feeling faint or dizzy
- Headache
- Difficulty with vision or speech
- Nosebleed
- Flushed red face
- Sudden changes in behavior, orientation

SIGNS AND SYMPTOMS OF CONGESTIVE HEART FAILURE

Congestive heart failure is an abnormal condition characterized by circulatory congestion caused by cardiac disorders. Signs and symptoms of congestive heart failure are:

congestive heart failure inability of the heart to pump out all the blood returned to it from the veins

- Congestion in the lungs
- Difficulty breathing
- Restlessness, anxiety
- Edema of legs, feet, hands, face
- Weight gain
- Weakness, fatigue
- Dizziness, confusion
- Chest pain

Congestive heart failure is treated by prescribed medications, treatments, and skilled nursing care. Commonly used medications are digitalis preparations and diuretics. Digitalis preparations slow the heart rate and increase the force of the contraction. Diuretics decrease the workload of the heart by ridding the body of excess fluids. Because these fluids are eliminated through the urinary system, a resident receiving diuretics will urinate frequently. With less fluid to move through the blood vessels and a slower, stronger heartbeat, the heart works more effectively. The licensed nurse administers these drugs. However, you should know if the resident is being given these medications in order to observe and report special problems. Other treatments for congestive heart failure include periods of rest and oxygen therapy.

SIGNS AND SYMPTOMS OF PERIPHERAL VASCULAR DISEASE

peripheral vascular disease poor circulation in the extremities

Residents with heart disease very often experience poor circulation, called **peripheral vascular disease,** especially of the lower extremities (legs and feet). Due to changes in the blood vessels resulting from arteriosclerosis, blood supply to the area decreases, causing tissue death. Signs and symptoms of peripheral vascular disease are:

- Edema or swelling of extremities—hands, fingers, legs, feet, toes
- Changes in skin temperature—infection produces red, warm skin and poor circulation produces cold, pale, or bluish skin
- Shiny, dry, flaky skin
- Pain
- Absence of pulse in legs and feet

stasis ulcers open wounds or sores on the legs caused by stoppage of blood flow

When peripheral circulation is impaired, the development of open wounds or sores on the legs is referred to as **stasis ulcers.** *Stasis* means a stoppage of flow. Stasis ulcers are caused by a stoppage of blood flow. Residents with heart disease and diabetes are particularly likely to develop stasis ulcers. These ulcers heal very slowly if at all. The wounds require special treatment and dressings. The affected area needs to be protected from further injury by bumping or hitting. The resident will be instructed by the licensed nurse to keep the feet and legs elevated to improve the circulation to the wound. Be sure to report to the nurse if there is a new wound, drainage from the wound, or a bad odor to the drainage.

varicose veins swollen (distended) veins especially prominent in the leg caused by lack of exercise, prolonged standing, and loss of elasticity associated with aging

Varicose veins are another type of vascular disease (Figure 13-10). These swollen (distended) veins are especially prominent in the legs. Varicose veins can be caused by lack of exercise and prolonged standing as well as loss of elasticity associated with aging. The resident will experience dull pain and cramp-

FIGURE 13-10

Varicose veins.

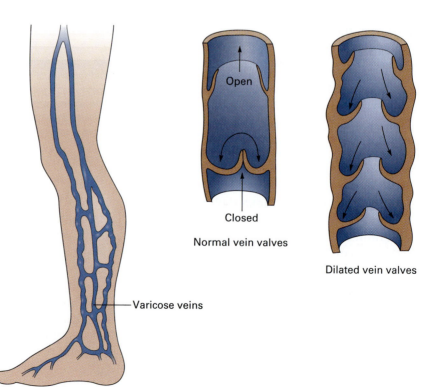

Open

Closed

Normal vein valves

Dilated vein valves

Varicose veins

ing of the legs. Pain is relieved by elevation of the limb and rest. Elastic stockings are used to reduce the pooling of blood in these distended veins and to reduce the possibility of a blood clot formation. A blood clot (called a **thrombus**) is more likely to form in the veins than in arteries because the blood flow is slower. If a blood clot breaks loose from the wall of a vessel and moves within the bloodstream, it is called an **embolus.** If an embolus enters a major organ such as brain, heart, kidney, or lungs, death is likely. Elastic stockings (Ace wraps, "TED" stockings, or antiembolism stockings) may be applied to compress and smooth out the distended walls of the veins. The blood moves through them without pooling. These stockings also help blood return to the heart more efficiently, reducing the workload of the heart. On some occasions, they may be used to provide support and comfort in the event of a sprain or strain at a joint.

thrombus   blood clot

embolus   a blood clot that moves within the bloodstream

APPLYING ANTIEMBOLISM STOCKINGS AND ELASTIC BANDAGES

Antiembolism stockings can be knee length or full length (Figure 13-11). You should always apply antiembolism stockings with the resident in bed. The legs should be elevated briefly prior to application. This helps drain the limb of blood, increasing the efficiency of the stocking when applied. Gather the stocking up and slip over the toe and heel, taking care to smooth out wrinkles. Gently stretch the stocking over the ankle and leg. The stocking should fit snugly. A stocking that is loose is ineffective. One so tight as to impair circulation is dangerous. Elastic stockings must be removed and reapplied at least once every day or more frequently if the physician orders it. Some physicians will order "out of bed only with antiembolism stockings."

Elastic bandages (often referred as Ace wraps) are long strips of elasticized cotton. They are wound into rolls and secured with a metal clip or a strip of Velcro. They are used for the same purpose as antiembolism stockings or to provide support or to hold a dressing in place. The antiembolism stocking is much more effective because it is not apt to slip and wrinkle and cannot be wrapped in such a way as to impair circulation. If you are instructed to apply elastic bandages, several precautions must be kept in mind:

- Never wrap a limb so tightly that you impair circulation. You must check toes or fingers to ensure adequate circulation.

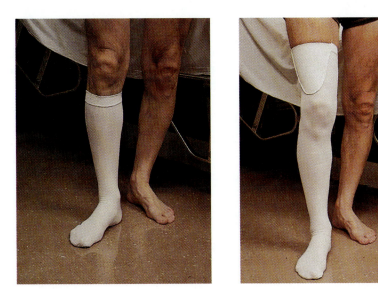

FIGURE 13-11
Antiembolism stockings.

- Never wrap in a way that pinches or applies undue pressure as this can cause tissue injury or skin breakdown.
- Check the resident often since elastic bandages slide as the resident moves and can become dislodged or bunch up, causing pressure and discomfort.
- Never tie an elastic bandage. The wrap should be smooth and even. Ask your charge nurse for assistance when you are unsure on how to wrap an elastic bandage.

gangrene a disease where tissue dies and amputation is often necessary

Probably the most important nursing function related to peripheral vascular disease is observation for changes. If circulation is severely impaired, skin breakdown will occur, and **gangrene,** a disease causing tissue death, develops. Gangrenous extremities almost always require amputation. Gangrene is very painful to the resident. The extremity needs to be handled gently and protected from injury or from bumping. A foot cradle may be used to keep the bed covers off the feet. If the resident is able to endure a surgical procedure and if he or she consents, an amputation may be needed to treat the gangrene.

CARING FOR THE RESIDENT WITH AN AMPUTATION

amputation cutting off a body part, usually an arm or leg

Amputation (cutting off) of any body part is traumatic, both physically and psychologically. Traumatic amputations occur from accidents. Surgical amputations occur because of severe circulatory impairment, infection, or bone tumors. The change in body image requires a great adjustment. Each person has an image or a mental picture of how his or her body looks. We think of ourselves as fat or thin, tall or short, young or old, attractive or unattractive. We visualize ourselves with all of our body parts present and working properly. When there is an image change, such as an amputation, it can take a long time to adjust and form a new body image. When a body part is removed, most individuals also experience feelings of increased dependence and decreased value. The person loses both the part and the function performed by that part, resulting in a need to be more dependent on others.

Emotional or psychological support includes:

- Listening to the resident
- Giving the resident opportunities to make decisions about his care
- Encouraging maximum independence
- Having a matter-of-fact attitude about the amputation

Usually, by the time the new amputee has arrived in an LTC facility, the surgical wound is almost healed. There may still be some sutures in place covered with a dressing. Nursing measures should include:

- Promoting healing of the wound
- Preventing infection
- Preventing contractures
- Decreasing swelling in the "stump" (remaining part of the amputated limb)
- Protecting the stump from injury

The nursing assistant should report any sores, bleeding, or drainage from the wound. The resident should be positioned to prevent contractures. If the amputation is below the knee (BK), the knee joint should be kept in extension (straight out) as much as possible. If the amputation is above the knee (AK), the hip should be regularly extended by positioning the resident onto his abdomen (proning) every day, as tolerated. Swelling is usually controlled by wrapping the stump with an elastic wrap or by using a "stump sock," a cone-shaped elastic stocking that fits snugly over a stump.

The stump must be conditioned prior to the use of a prosthesis; this involves shrinking and shaping the stump into a cone shape. Physical therapy may perform certain exercises to strengthen the stump and other limbs. Occupational therapy may be ordered if the resident has to relearn to perform any activities of daily living.

It is not uncommon for the elderly, debilitated resident to reject the use of a prosthesis. Residents who are very confused will rarely understand and accept the use of a prosthesis. Since crutches are difficult to use, requiring considerable strength and coordination, the elderly debilitated amputee is usually confined to a wheelchair.

Some amputees experience pain in the amputated limb. These pains are called *phantom limb pains.* Although the limb is gone, the resident actually feels pain in the absent part. The pain is not only real but can be quite severe. Report any complaints of pain to the charge nurse immediately. The nursing care you give and the emotional or psychological support you provide can greatly affect the adjustment of the resident who has had an amputation.

NURSING CARE OF THE RESIDENT WITH HEART DISEASE

The nursing care of residents with any kind of heart disease or circulatory impairment is primarily devoted to decreasing the amount of work the heart has to do and to observing and reporting changes in condition. The following guidelines should be followed when providing care to residents with heart disease.

Plan and organize care to assist the resident in balancing activity with rest (Figure 13-12).

The activity of the resident with heart disease must be limited to what he or she is able to tolerate. If the resident's activity causes chest pain or difficulty breathing, the pace must be slowed. Rest periods should be planned throughout the day, and activities should be scheduled around the rest periods. Too often, the needs of residents for adequate rest are placed in a secondary

FIGURE 13-12

Activity and rest should be kept in balance.

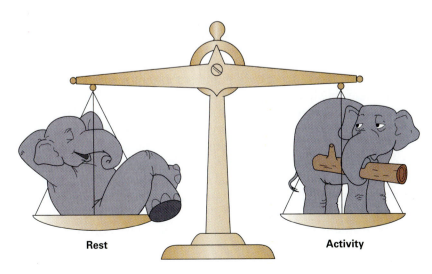

Rest   Activity

position to facility routines and schedules. The nursing assistant must plan rest periods for all residents and especially those with heart disease.

When a resident is acutely ill, even a bed bath can be exhausting. Be observant; listen to the resident. Remember, rest needs to be both physical and emotional. The resident with heart disease and hypertension needs an environment that is non–anxiety producing. Anger, frustration, and emotional upsets all increase the work of the heart and raise blood pressure.

You can help promote rest and reduce anxiety by assisting residents as needed. Many residents with heart disease have difficulty breathing and require special positioning to help them breathe easier. Some will need to sleep in a semisitting position supported with pillows.

Take time to evaluate how the resident rests best. This is particularly important to the totally dependent resident who is unable to communicate his or her needs. Residents with edema also require special positioning. Edema interferes with circulation, which leads to skin breakdown. When the resident has edema of the feet and legs, you should keep the limbs elevated as much as possible to reduce the edema. Elevating a limb improves the flow of blood back to the heart.

In order to decrease the workload of the heart, the resident needs to be at a weight that is appropriate for his or her body height and build. Many times the physician will order a calorie-restricted diet. The resident may need a good deal of support, encouragement, and teaching in order to follow the diet.

Assist the resident to follow the diet ordered by the physician.

sodium chloride table salt

Most residents with heart disease have a problem with fluid retention. Fluid retention causes the heart to work harder and produces edema. An important factor related to fluid retention is sodium intake. Sodium is contained in **sodium chloride** (table salt). Sodium causes tissues to hold onto water. If the average adult did not add salt to food, they would lose approximately 10 pounds of fluid in a year. There are many foods that are naturally high in sodium, such as baking soda (and items made with baking soda—bread, cake, etc.). Milk, cheese, ham, bacon, cold cuts, and soft drinks are all foods high in sodium content. The physician will order a sodium-restricted diet for many residents with heart disease. Salt restriction is not easy to live with. Residents complain the food is bland and tasteless. When the physician's orders permit, a salt substitute can be used, but the taste is still poorly accepted by most residents. You will need to watch the food intake closely and report any departure from the physician's order to your charge nurse. Helping the resident and family understand the reasons for dietary restrictions or modifications helps them to follow the physician's orders.

Be alert for signs and symptoms of heart disease or changes in the resident's condition.

When you recognize the signs and symptoms of various forms of heart disease, you are able to notice subtle changes and report them immediately. Medications and treatments can then be started before an emergency arises. Develop good observational skills and be accurate! Take vital signs carefully. Pay attention to the rate, rhythm, and strength of the pulse. Observe and report sudden changes in behavior, orientation, sleeping and eating patterns. Pay particular attention to circulatory changes such as the presence of edema.

Never assume that the symptoms are due to "old age" or that the resident is just a "complainer." All symptoms of chest pain, difficulty breathing, or even the resident's report that he or she feels "different" or "strange" must be taken seriously and acted upon.

SUMMARY

In this chapter, you have learned about the heart and its functions. You've also learned about the causes and symptoms of the number one cause of death in the United States. The information can help you to live a healthier life and prevent heart disease in yourself. Some of the important principles of caring for a resident with heart disease are the balancing of rest with activity, observing and reporting symptoms, and helping the resident adjust to the lifestyle changes required. This includes not only rest but following the prescribed diet and reducing stress and anxiety. You can learn more about heart disease by asking the licensed nurse or your instructor to help you listen with a stethoscope to the heart of a resident with heart disease. Find out which of your residents have pacemakers, and read the medical record to learn what type of pacemaker they have.

OBRA HIGHLIGHTS

Some residents may refuse a recommended amputation. It is important to remember that every individual capable of decision making may refuse any unwanted medical treatment. Some residents may refuse hospitalization, cardiopulmonary resuscitation, surgery, medications, or artificial nutrition or hydration. When treatment is refused, residents receive all the other good care needed. They are simply exercising their rights. The nursing assistant may disagree with their choices, but their right to make decisions must be respected. It is never appropriate to avoid or neglect residents because they have decided to refuse certain treatments.

SELF STUDY

Choose the best answer for each question or statement.

1. What is the function of white blood cells?
   a. to carry oxygen from the lungs to the cells
   b. to fight infection
   c. to help stop bleeding
   d. to regulate temperature

2. Which blood component is able to change shape, cling together, and cause the blood to clot?
   a. red blood cells
   b. white blood cells
   c. platelets
   d. plasma

3. Which blood vessels always carry blood away from the heart?
   a. arteries
   b. veins
   c. capillaries
   d. lymph vessels

4. Which blood vessels have walls that are one cell thick and allow oxygen and carbon dioxide exchange to occur?
   a. arteries
   b. veins
   c. capillaries
   d. lymph vessels

5. What does blood pressure measure?
   a. the rate at which the heart beats
   b. the force of the blood against the walls of a blood vessel
   c. the difference between the apical and radial pulse
   d. the force of the blood against the walls of the heart

6. What causes lymph nodes to become enlarged?
   a. low levels of oxygen in the blood
   b. a blood clot
   c. too much lymph fluid
   d. infection or disease

7. Where does the blood flow after it leaves the right ventricle?
   a. to the lungs
   b. to the left atrium
   c. to the body
   d. to the inferior vena cava

8. Which valve is found between the left atrium and the left ventricle?
   a. tricuspid
   b. mitral
   c. pulmonic
   d. aortic

9. Which of the following is the number one cause of death in the United States?
   a. asthma
   b. emphysema
   c. heart disease
   d. cancer

10. When arteries become clogged or blocked with plaque and calcium deposits, the condition is called
    a. atherosclerosis
    b. arteriosclerosis
    c. multiple sclerosis
    d. dermal sclerosis

11. Mrs. Melvin has had a myocardial infarction, or heart attack. This means that
    a. part of her heart muscle has died due to lack of blood supply
    b. part of her brain has died due to lack of blood supply
    c. her heart has stopped beating and must be restarted with cardiopulmonary resuscitation (CPR)
    d. her heart is no longer able to pump blood effectively through her body

12. When a resident has chest pain caused by a decrease in oxygenated blood to the heart, the condition is called
    a. cerebrovascular accident (CVA)
    b. congestive heart failure (CHF)
    c. angina pectoris
    d. hypertension

13. Mr. Jefferson has an artificial pacemaker. Which of the following actions should you take when caring for Mr. Jefferson?
    a. Report a pulse lower than the preset pacemaker rate.
    b. Report any episodes of hiccups.
    c. Report complaints of dizziness or heart palpitations.
    d. All of these actions are appropriate to take.

14. Mrs. Melvin complains of chest pain after lunch and takes a nitroglycerin tablet from the bottle at her bedside. What should you do?
    a. Check on Mrs. Melvin again in about 15 minutes to see if the pain is gone.
    b. Notify the licensed nurse immediately that Mrs. Melvin has taken a nitro tablet.
    c. Take a set of vital signs and record them and the chest pain in her chart.
    d. Remove the nitroglycerin patch from her chest since she has taken a nitro tablet.

15. Which of the following blood pressure readings, if found consistently, would indicate hypertension?

    a. 128/88
    b. 146/74
    c. 118/90
    d. 166/92

16. Mr. Morgan's feet and legs are swollen. The skin on them is shiny, dry, and flaky. His feet are both cold and appear bluish. These are all signs and symptoms of
    a. peripheral vascular disease
    b. congestive heart failure
    c. stasis ulcers
    d. gangrene

Getting C O N N E C T E D
Multimedia **Extension** Activities

www.prenhall.com/will-black

Use the above address to access the free, interactive Companion Website created for this textbook. Hear the pronunciation of the key terms in the chapter. Get instant feedback to a variety of chapter-related questions. Link to other interesting sites.

Video

Watch the *Vital Signs* video from the Care Provider Skills series.

CASE STUDY

Roger Jackson is 86 years old. He has had two heart attacks, with each one leaving him weaker and with increased shortness of breath upon activity.

1. In caring for Mr. Jackson, your primary concern is to
   a. ensure vigorous daily exercise
   b. help him to balance rest and activity
   c. keep him confined to bed
   d. none of the above

2. Diet is important to the resident with heart disease. Which kinds of foods should Mr. Jackson avoid?
   a. foods containing lots of salt, such as potato chips, bacon, ham, canned soups
   b. fruits and vegetables
   c. meat, fish, and poultry
   d. dairy products

3. Which of the following complaints may be signs that Mr. Jackson is having another heart attack?
   a. anxiety and fear
   b. pain in the left arm, neck, and jaw
   c. pale, cool, clammy skin
   d. all of the above

4. Because of swelling in his legs and feet, the doctor has ordered elastic stockings. Because they must be ordered, you were told to apply elastic bandages today. Which of the following precautions apply?
   a. Never wrap a limb so tightly that the circulation is impaired.
   b. Wrap the entire leg, including the feet and toes, for even pressure.
   c. When finished, tie the end to the upper portion of the leg.
   d. If the resident complains of discomfort, it must be tight enough.

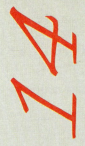
THE ENDOCRINE SYSTEM

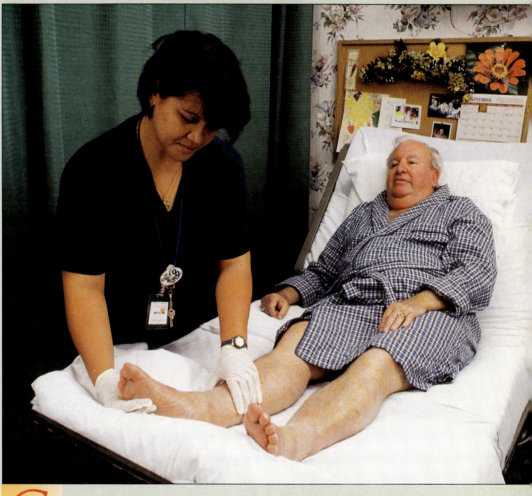

CARING TIP

Observing and reporting foot conditions is very important when caring for a diabetic resident.

Barbara Magrel, RN, MS
Horizon Career Center
Munster, Indiana

OBJECTIVES
What You Will Learn

When you have completed this section, you will be able to:

- Identify the endocrine glands
- Match the functions of the glands with their names

- Identify and describe the most common endocrine disease

KEY TERMS

adrenal glands
bulbo-urethral glands
exocrine
hormones
mammary glands

ovaries
ovulation
pancreas
parathyroid glands
pituitary gland

salivary glands
sweat glands
testes
thymus gland
thyroid gland

The endocrine system (Figure 14-1) is composed of:

- Endocrine glands
  —Pituitary   —Adrenal
  —Thyroid   —Pancreas
  —Parathyroid   —Ovaries
  —Thymus   —Testes

FIGURE 14-1

The endocrine system.

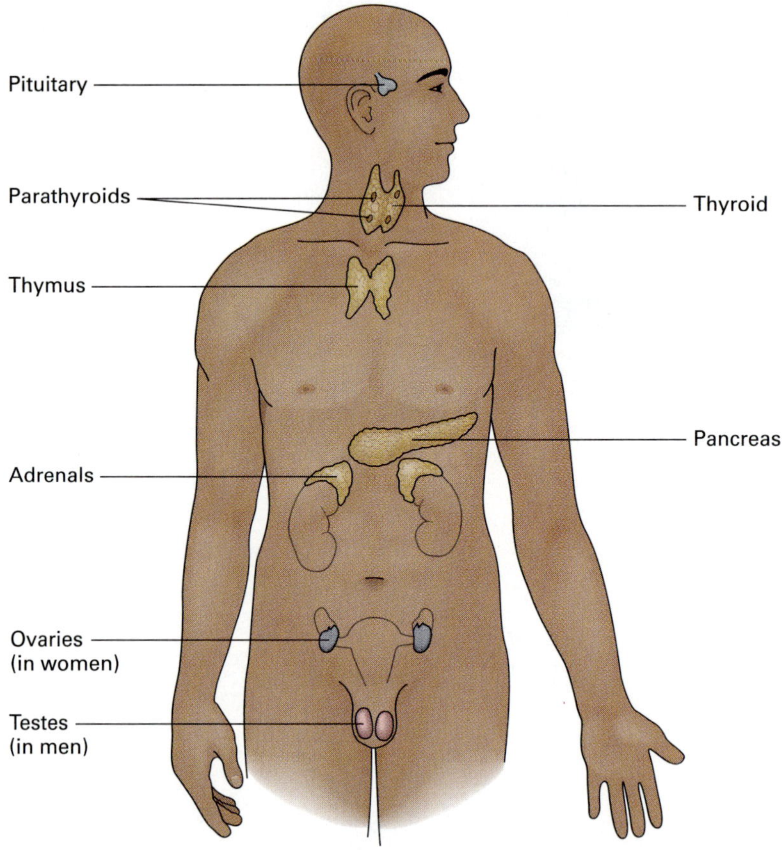

Pituitary

Parathyroids

Thymus

Adrenals

Ovaries
(in women)

Testes
(in men)

Thyroid

Pancreas

- Exocrine glands
    —Sweat glands of the skin
    —Salivary glands of the mouth
    —Other glands that secrete digestive juices

    The functions of the endocrine system are to:

- Secrete hormones to regulate body functions related to growth and development
- Regulate body functions of metabolism and reproduction

    The endocrine glands of the body secrete fluids called **hormones** (hormone is a Latin term meaning to arouse or set in motion).

- The **pituitary gland** is considered the master gland of the body. The hormones secreted regulate metabolism (the work of the cell). The hormones secreted by the pituitary gland affect other endocrine glands, stimulating them to secrete their hormones.

- The **thyroid gland** is the largest of the endocrine glands. It produces hormones that regulate growth and the metabolic rate. Hormones secreted by the thyroid are mainly responsible for the individual's energy level. They influence skeletal growth and sexual development, as well as skin texture and hair luster.

- The **parathyroid glands** are two pairs of small glands located within a capsule of the thyroid gland (one on each side of the thyroid gland). They produce a hormone that together with the thyroid regulates the level of calcium and phosphorus in the body.

- The **thymus gland** is a two-lobed ductless gland, larger in childhood than in adulthood. It has the structure of a lymph node. The exact function is not understood, but it is believed to play a role in the immune system of the body.

- The **pancreas** is the large gland located below and behind the liver and stomach. It is both an endocrine and exocrine gland. The endocrine portion secretes two very important hormones, insulin and glucagon. Insulin decreases the level of sugar in the blood. Disturbances of the insulin-producing gland lead to the disease known as *diabetes mellitus*. Glucagon increases the level of sugar in the blood.

- The **adrenal glands** are two small glands located on the top of each kidney. They are important in the metabolism of proteins, fat, and carbohydrates. They influence the levels of sodium and potassium in body fluids and are important in fluid and electrolyte balance. They produce hormones that help the body react and adapt to stress.

- The **ovaries** are the primary female reproductive organs and have two basic functions (see Chapter 15):
    —**Ovulation,** the process by which an ovum (egg) is discharged from an ovary at regular intervals.
    —Production of the hormones estrogen and progesterone. These two hormones are essential in the reproductive processes and also influence a woman's feminine physical characteristics.

- The **testes** are the primary male reproductive organs and have two basic functions:
    —Production of sperm, which are ejaculated during sexual intercourse.

hormones fluid secreted by an endocrine gland

pituitary gland master gland of the body, which regulates metabolism

thyroid gland largest of the endocrine glands; regulates growth and metabolic rate

parathyroid glands two pairs of glands located within the thyroid that produce a hormone to help regulate the level of calcium and phosphorus in the body

thymus gland two-lobe ductless gland believed to play a role in the immune system of the body

pancreas large gland located in the abdomen; secretes insulin and glucagon

adrenal glands two small glands located on top of each kidney; produce hormones that help the body react and adapt to stress

ovaries primary female reproductive organs

ovulation process in which an ovum is discharged from an ovary at regular intervals

testes primary male reproductive organs that produce sperm

—Production of the hormone testosterone, which is responsible for the masculine physical characteristics and which stimulates the production of sperm.

The hormones secreted by the endocrine system interact with the nervous system to organize and control many activities of the body. These glands are ductless, which means they empty hormones directly into the bloodstream. This makes secretions immediately available to cells in all parts of the body.

The hormones secreted by the exocrine glands are secreted through ducts into a body cavity or to the surface of the body. **Exocrine** means secreting externally. These glands do not secrete directly into the bloodstream.

Functions of the exocrine glands are varied.

exocrine secreting externally

sweat glands glands that produce moisture to cool the body and excrete waste products

salivary glands glands that produce saliva to moisten the mouth and begin the digestion of food

mammary glands glandular tissue of the breast

bulbo-urethral glands exocrine glands located near the prostate in males

- The **sweat glands** are located over the surface of the skin, with approximately 2 million in the body. The largest sweat glands are in the axilla (underarms) and groin. Sweating produces an evaporative cooling of the body. Some waste products are excreted as sweat.
- The **salivary glands** secrete saliva from various areas of the mouth. Saliva is necessary to moisten the mouth and to lubricate the food, making it easier to chew and swallow. Saliva contains enzymes essential to begin the process of food breakdown. The salivary glands produce approximately 3 pints of saliva each day.
- Other exocrine glands are the **mammary glands,** located in the breast in females, the **bulbo-urethral glands,** located near the prostate in males, and various intestinal glands associated with the digestive processes.

A number of diseases are associated with malfunctions of the endocrine system. Such diseases are usually a result of overproduction or underproduction of a hormone. Not many disorders of aging are related directly to malfunctions of the endocrine glands. An older person can develop malfunctioning glandular problems just as a young person can. Some age-related changes do occur naturally—a gradual decrease in thyroid, parathyroid, and adrenal hormone secretions are examples of this.

The most common endocrine disease is diabetes mellitus. Diabetes is not just a disease of the elderly; it affects people of all ages. According to the National Center for Health Statistics, diabetes is the seventh leading cause of death listed on death certificates in 1996. Diabetes is believed to be underreported on death certificates both as a condition and as a cause of death.

There are four groups of people who are most susceptible:

- Those who are obese or who have a history of obesity
- Those over age 45
- Women
- Those who have a history of diabetes in their family

In people over age 65, diabetes is the seventh leading cause of death. There are over 6 million people over 65 in the United States with diabetes. In those age 20 or over, 15.6 million have diabetes. Another way to say it is that of all people over 65, 18.4 percent of them have diabetes. Understanding the nature of diabetes and how to provide nursing care to the resident with diabetes is important to the nursing assistant.

SECTION 2 Care of the Resident with Diabetes Mellitus

OBJECTIVES
What You Will Learn

When you have completed this section, you will be able to:

- Describe diabetes mellitus

- List the two most common types of diabetes
- Define four terms related to diabetes mellitus
- List four common complications associated with diabetes mellitus

- Describe nursing actions that prevent complications of diabetes
- Explain why you should report what is **not** eaten by the resident who takes insulin

---

KEY TERMS

acetone
acidosis
aneurysm
diabetes mellitus

diabetic coma
diabetic shock
glucose
glycosuria
hyperglycemia

hypoglycemia
insulin
insulin shock
ketonuria
lancet

Diabetes mellitus is a disorder of carbohydrate metabolism in which the ability to break down and use carbohydrates is lost due to disturbances in insulin production. Diabetes affects almost all the body systems and is a complex disease process. If insulin protection is too low or absent, the carbohydrates eaten cannot be utilized to nourish the cells of the body. Cells must be nourished in order to live!

diabetes mellitus disease in which the pancreas secretes insufficient amounts of insulin

NORMAL CARBOHYDRATE METABOLISM (FIGURE 14-2)

- Carbohydrate types of food are eaten.
- The food is digested in the stomach.
- The food is converted to a simple sugar (glucose), which is an essential nutrient of the cell.
- The glucose enters the bloodstream for distribution to the millions of cells in the body.
- **Insulin** is secreted into the bloodstream. It is the "key" that opens the door to allow the right amount of glucose to leave the bloodstream.
- Glucose leaves the bloodstream and provides nourishment to the cells.
- Cells metabolize glucose and give off waste products, which are excreted through the kidneys, lungs, and skin.

insulin hormone secreted by the pancreas

Remember, if nutrients (glucose) cannot get to the cells, they are undernourished and may deteriorate or die no matter how much a person consumes.

DIABETIC CARBOHYDRATE METABOLISM (FIGURE 14-3)

- Carbohydrate types of foods are eaten.
- The food is digested in the stomach.
- The food is converted to a simple sugar **(glucose),** which is an essential nutrient of the cell during digestion.
- The glucose enters the bloodstream for distribution to the millions of cells in the body.
- There is no insulin or too little insulin, so there is no "key." The door

glucose simple sugar to which food is converted

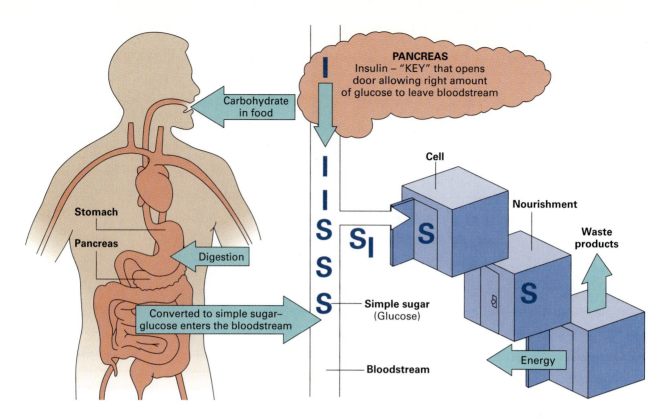

FIGURE 14–2

Normal carbohydrate metabolism.

FIGURE 14–3

Diabetic carbohydrate metabolism.

remains locked, and glucose accumulates in the bloodstream (called **hyperglycemia**).

- The kidneys spill some of this excess glucose into the urine (called **glycosuria**).
- The cells are starving. They have no nourishment, so the body begins to use fats for nourishment. When fats are metabolized abnormally, there is

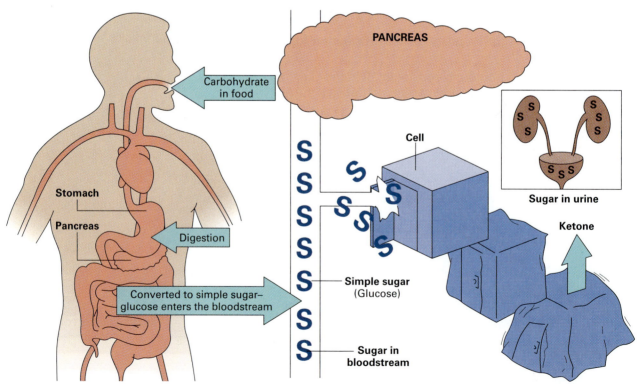

a by-product created called **acetone.** Acetone is a type of ketone. Some ketones may be excreted in the urine (called **ketonuria**). When the acetone ketone buildup is excessive, the body is unable to excrete these toxic substances safely, and they can reach dangerous levels. The condition is called **acidosis.** Severe acidosis leads to coma and death.

Markedly elevated blood sugar and acidosis are the basis of the diagnosis of **diabetic coma.** Diabetic coma is a life-threatening problem that requires immediate diagnosis and treatment. For these reasons you will need to be familiar with signs and symptoms of diabetic coma. They are:

- Gradual onset
- Fruity odor to breath
- Skin hot and dry, face may be flushed
- Deep, labored breathing
- Loss of consciousness
- Nausea
- Glycosuria (sugar in urine)
- Hyperglycemia (high blood sugar)
- Drowsiness and lethargy

There are two primary types of diabetes: Type 1, or insulin-dependent diabetes mellitus, and Type 2, or non–insulin-dependent diabetes mellitus. In addition, gestational diabetes mellitus occurs in pregnancy.

The treatment for diabetes depends on the type of diabetes diagnosed. Type 2 diabetes rarely requires insulin treatment. Risk factors for Type 2 include obesity, physical and emotional stress, certain medications, age over 40, and family history. Treatment includes diet and exercise. Often, an oral medication is taken once or twice a day. These medications work by preventing the body from sending glucose into the bloodstream when insulin is not working properly, releasing more insulin into the bloodstream, and helping the body's own insulin move glucose from the bloodstream into the cells. Some residents may need insulin in addition to oral medications. Some residents may no longer need medication if they lose weight. Regular exercise is important. It helps control the amount of sugar in the blood and helps burn excess calories to achieve optimal weight.

Residents with Type 1 diabetes will require insulin to control their disease. Insulin is a hormone given by injection. It is not available by mouth. Some residents may have an implanted pump that delivers the insulin on a regular basis. However, most require injections. The type and amount of insulin to be given depends on the amount of glucose present in the resident's blood. The nurses and physician monitor this amount by testing a drop of blood one to four times a day if the resident's blood sugar is unstable. Although the nursing assistant is not responsible for the injections or for testing the blood, your observations are essential to good care of the diabetic resident. You will learn the symptoms of too much insulin and the symptoms of not enough insulin. The presence of these symptoms must be reported immediately to the charge nurse. Because the intake of food is balanced with the insulin, any changes in the resident's eating patterns must also be reported. For example, if a resident with Type 1 diabetes refuses to eat breakfast or eats very little, it must be reported immediately.

One of the most common and serious complications associated with diabetes is **diabetic shock** or **insulin shock.** When insulin shock occurs:

1. Insulin is administered. Different types of insulin have their peak effect at different times—some are relatively fast acting; others are slow.

hyperglycemia high blood sugar

glycosuria sugar in the urine

acetone by-product of the metabolism of fat; a type of ketone

ketonuria presence of ketones in the urine

acidosis a dangerous condition related to diabetes when toxic substances build up in the body

diabetic coma high blood sugar with presence of ketones in the urine

diabetic shock very low blood sugar with symptoms of shock

insulin shock low blood sugar, usually from too much insulin or not enough food intake

2. Carbohydrate types of foods are eaten.
3. The food is digested in the stomach.
4. The food is converted to simple sugar (glucose), which is an essential nutrient of the cell during digestion.
5. The glucose enters the bloodstream for distribution to all the cells of the body.
6. If the resident has *received too much insulin or failed to eat enough food,* too much glucose leaves the blood. The central nervous system must have a certain blood sugar level to function normally. Too low a blood sugar is called **hypoglycemia.**
7. Severe hypoglycemia leads to coma and death.

hypoglycemia low blood sugar

Signs and symptoms of insulin shock or diabetic shock:

- Sudden onset
- Perspiration; pale, cold, and clammy skin
- Shallow breathing
- Hunger
- Mental confusion, strange behavior
- Nervousness
- Double vision
- Loss of consciousness
- Low blood sugar (hypoglycemia)

It is often difficult even for the experienced licensed nurse to differentiate between diabetic coma and insulin or diabetic shock. Therefore, it is very important to recognize the little changes and report them before loss of consciousness occurs. If severe, *both diabetic coma and insulin shock can result in irreversible brain damage.*

Hypoglycemia (too *little* sugar) and hyperglycemia (too *much* sugar) are serious emergency conditions related to diabetes. However, there are many long-term complications that must be recognized in residents with diabetes.

Complications related to diabetes include:

- Frequent, chronic infections
- Sores (usually in the feet and legs) that heal poorly
- Impaired vision or blindness (diabetic retinopathy)
- Poor circulation
- Pain in the feet (diabetic neuropathy)
- Arteriosclerosis
- Heart disease
- Stroke

Residents with diabetes are at high risk to develop arteriosclerosis, heart disease, and stroke due to poor fat metabolism. Peripheral vascular disease is very common, resulting in poor circulation to the legs and feet. The poor circulation and elevated blood sugar make the diabetic very susceptible to infection. Once infection or injury occurs, the diabetic has decreased ability to heal or recover. For this reason, many amputations of the lower extremities become necessary due to ulceration and gangrene associated with the resident's diabetic condition.

Impaired vision and blindness are common complications of diabetes. The capillaries that supply blood to the retina of the eye develop weakened areas **(aneurysms)** and rupture, leading to detachment of the retina and blindness.

aneurysm bulging out of the wall of an artery, creating a weakened area subject to rupture

In most cases diabetes can be controlled, although there is no known cure at the present time. The treatment and control of diabetes is a team effort that involves the physician, the licensed nurse, the nursing assistant, and the resident (Figure 14-4).

The physician will order a calorie-restricted diet designed to limit the amount of carbohydrates consumed. The resident, the licensed nurse, and the nursing assistant must monitor the resident's intake carefully to ensure that the amount of carbohydrates consumed does not exceed that ordered by the physician.

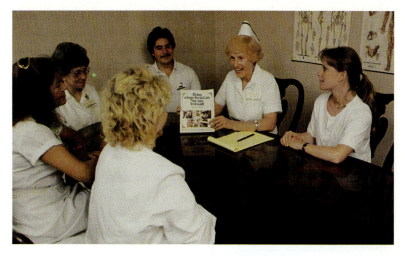

FIGURE 14-4

Understanding diabetes.

CULTURAL AWARENESS When managing a diabetic resident's diet, you must consider his or her cultural beliefs. An individualized plan is required because the standard diet may not fit with the resident's beliefs. It could be that some foods that are served are considered either hot or cold (see Chapter 9) and may upset the balance of the body. Other foods are simply preferred because the resident is accustomed to them. It is important to ask the resident what foods he likes and to observe those things that he avoids. This information should be given to the dietitian so she can adjust the diabetic diet accordingly.

Remember, insulin shock can occur when either *too much insulin is given or too little food is consumed.* If the resident refuses a meal and has taken insulin, there is a danger of insulin shock.

- Physical activity of the resident must be coordinated with the carbohydrates consumed and the insulin given. The licensed nurse and nursing assistant must observe and report changes in physical activity to the physician so that dosages of insulin can be adjusted accordingly. Generally, whenever exercise or heavy activity is planned, the diabetic must either increase carbohydrates or cut down on the insulin.
- Complications such as injury or infection must be prevented. Special skin care is essential. Any break in the skin can lead to severe infection. A small cut or laceration of the legs or feet can, and often does, lead to amputation of the limb. Diabetic residents require special foot care.
- Never attempt to trim the toenails of the diabetic resident. This is done by the podiatrist or licensed nurse only.
- Never cut corns or callouses.
- Note and report any signs of irritation.
- Make sure that the resident's feet are protected with well-fitting shoes and stockings.
- Make sure that there is never any restriction of circulation from elastic hose, garters, or bed covers.
- Protect the resident from overexposure to heat or cold.
- Report any complaints of pain, redness, discoloration, or changes in skin temperature to your charge nurse immediately!

To monitor the resident with diabetes, it is necessary to measure the amount of glucose in the blood (Figure 14-5).

Most facilities check the blood in place of checking the urine of diabetic residents. Many different types of kits are available. This procedure is performed

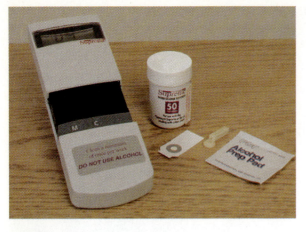

FIGURE 14-5

Checking the residents' blood glucose level.

lancet sharp object used to prick the skin of a fingertip or earlobe to obtain a small sample of blood

by the licensed nurse since it involves pricking the skin of the resident to obtain the blood sample. The kits contain a sharp object, called a **lancet,** that is used to pierce the skin of a fingertip or earlobe to obtain a drop of blood. This drop of blood is then placed on a treated strip, which is then inserted into the reading device. This device reads the glucose content of the blood and displays the results.

Remember that proper care of the resident with diabetes requires team effort. Your continuing observations and proper nursing care contribute significantly to the team. The resident is the most important member of that team. Many residents have managed their diabetes for decades and are expert in knowing about their disease and its management. They can often tell by the way they feel if their blood glucose is high or low. Be sure to listen to them and to involve them in their care.

SUMMARY

In this chapter, you have had an opportunity to learn about a disease that affects millions of people in the United States. You learned that some of the complications of diabetes can be reduced or even prevented by good care and treatment. This good care includes following a prescribed diet, exercising as much as possible, measuring the blood sugar, and taking medications as ordered. Those who follow the plan of care may live a long and healthy life. As a nursing assistant, your observations, your care, and your reporting make a significant difference in the life of the diabetic resident. You must not only monitor and record the resident's eating but be aware of changes in behavior and any signs of infection or injury. Residents with diabetes require protection from injury, especially to the feet and legs, and protection from infection. Those with impaired vision will also require extra care to make up for the loss of vision. You, the nursing assistant, are critical to providing proper care to the diabetic resident.

OBRA HIGHLIGHTS

One of the rights assured by the OBRA regulations is: "The resident has the right to be fully informed in language that he or she can understand of his or her total health status, including but not limited to, his or her medical condition." In the case of the resident with diabetes, this means that the resident is informed of his or her blood sugar measurements on a regular basis. The resident must be taught a great deal about his or her diabetes in order to make good decisions. Many residents come to a long-term care facility after many years of living with diabetes. They are accustomed to managing their disease and have the knowledge and right to continue to do so. That means that the facility staff provides them with all of the information needed to make good choices. Remember, whether or not you agree with their choices, they have the right to determine their own care without fear of retaliation.

SELF STUDY

Choose the best answer for each question or statement.

1. Which of the following is considered the "master gland" of the body?
   a. pituitary
   b. parathyroid
   c. pancreas
   d. thyroid

2. The thyroid gland produces hormones that
   a. regulate the level of calcium and phosphorus in the body
   b. regulate the level of sugar in the blood
   c. regulate growth, metabolic rate, and energy level
   d. play a role in the immune function of the body

3. The gland that secretes insulin and glucagon is the
   a. pituitary
   b. parathyroid
   c. adrenal
   d. pancreas

4. Which of the following is the most common endocrine disease?
   a. hyperthyroidism
   b. diabetes mellitus
   c. hypothyroidism
   d. adrenal insufficiency

5. What causes hyperglycemia?
   a. little or no insulin to allow glucose to get into the body cells
   b. too much insulin, which causes high sugar in the blood
   c. too much thyroid hormone in the blood, which causes a strain on the heart
   d. little or no thyroid hormone in the blood, so sugar stays in the blood instead of the cells

6. When sugar does not enter body cells, they have no nourishment. When the body begins to use fat for nourishment instead, it causes a condition called
   a. psychosis
   b. shock
   c. acidosis
   d. hypoglycemia

7. You are caring for Mrs. Pearson, a resident who has diabetes. She has not felt well for several days. When you check on her, you find her face flushed, her skin hot and dry, and her respirations deep and labored. She does not respond when you try to arouse her, and you notice a fruity smell on her breath. What will you do?
   a. Report this to your charge nurse immediately because she may be in a diabetic coma.
   b. Report this to your charge nurse immediately because she may be in insulin shock.
   c. Give her good mouth care and allow her to rest because she has not been feeling well.
   d. Check her temperature, give good mouth care, and report this at the end of the shift.

8. Mr. Bernstein is a resident with diabetes. He is given insulin injections twice each day. He only ate 25 percent of his lunch today. What should you do?
   a. Encourage him to eat more at dinner so he will get enough food for the day.
   b. Give him a snack of ice cream and fruit at 2 P.M.
   c. Report his lack of intake immediately so he won't go into insulin shock.
   d. Do not be concerned about him—he ate a good breakfast this morning.

9. Why should the nursing assistant never trim the toenails of a diabetic resident?
   a. because diabetics' feet are very sensitive to pain
   b. because diabetics can bleed to death from a small cut
   c. because any small cut in the foot can lead to amputation of the leg
   d. because there are no pulses in the feet of diabetic residents

10. Mr. Bernstein is a fairly new resident to the long-term care facility. He tells you that he must eat his breakfast within 30 minutes of his insulin injection or he becomes ill. Breakfast is not usually served at this time. What should you do?
   a. Report this to the charge nurse, since he knows about his diabetes and its management.
   b. Explain the breakfast schedule to him and let him know you will bring his meal as soon as it is time.

c. Tell him he can eat breakfast when everyone else does and that he will not become ill.

d. Explain that although he is used to the routine he had at home, he can adapt to the routine here.

11. Mrs. Green is a resident with diabetes. When you answer her call light, you find her pale and sweaty. Her skin is cold and clammy. Although she is normally oriented, she is saying things that do not make sense to you. What will you do?

a. Report the situation to the charge nurse because she might be having a stroke.

b. Report the situation to the charge nurse because she may be in insulin shock.

c. Give her a good bed bath and reorient her to the date, time, and location.

d. Talk with her for a while and ask questions to determine what she is talking about.

12. Which of the following groups of people are most at risk for developing diabetes?

a. those who are obese

b. those over age 40

c. females

d. all of the above

13. Mrs. Green, who is diabetic, has a reddened area on her left little toe. You notice a small blister in the middle of the red area. What should you do?

a. Wash the toe well, then cover it with a bandage.

b. Wash and dry the foot well, then apply a clear adhesive dressing to the toe.

c. Notify the charge nurse about the toe, since it could become infected.

d. Place a cotton ball between the little toe and the next toe, then put slippers on her.

14. Which of the following is true of endocrine glands?

a. They secrete hormones directly into the bloodstream.

b. They secrete hormones through ducts into a body cavity or to the body surface.

c. They secrete saliva from different areas in the mouth.

d. All of these are functions of the endocrine glands.

15. Carbohydrate types of foods are

a. converted into protein

b. converted to glucose

c. converted into insulin

d. broken down by bile

16. Which of the following is a treatment for diabetes?

a. carbohydrate- and calorie-restricted diet

b. oral drugs that stimulate the pancreas to secrete more insulin

c. insulin injections given to replace insulin no longer produced by the pancreas

d. all of the above

Getting C O N N E C T E D
Multimedia Extension Activities

 www.prenhall.com/will-black

Use the above address to access the free, interactive Companion Website created for this textbook. Hear the pronunciation of the key terms in the chapter. Get instant feedback to a variety of chapter-related questions. Link to other interesting sites.

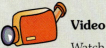 **Video**

Watch the section related to foot care in the video *Personal Care* from the Care Provider Skills series.

CASE STUDY

Sally Richards is a 68-year-old woman with Type 1 diabetes. She has had both legs amputated below the knee. She is overweight and loves to eat candy. She gets her insulin injection at 6:30 every morning. You pick up her breakfast tray and notice she ate very little.

1. You need to report her lack of eating to the charge nurse immediately because
   a. she may become hypoglycemic
   b. she may become hyperglycemic
   c. she may become anemic
   d. none of the above
2. She asks you to bring her a candy bar from the vending machine in the employee lunch room. You tell her
   a. "I'd be happy to. What kind would you like?"
   b. "I need to check with the charge nurse. I am not sure if it is allowed on your diet."
   c. "Are you kidding? You can't have candy!"
   d. "Sure, as long as we keep it our little secret."
3. Because of her diabetes, Mrs. Richards is at risk for all of the following complications *except*
   a. chronic infections
   b. tuberculosis
   c. blindness
   d. stroke
4. You notice when bathing her that Mrs. Richards has a small open sore on the end of her stump. Your responsibility is to
   a. ask the charge nurse for a bandage
   b. wash the area gently and leave it open to the air
   c. notify the nurse immediately
   d. tell Mrs. Richards to be more careful

Chapter 15

THE REPRODUCTIVE SYSTEM AND HUMAN SEXUALITY

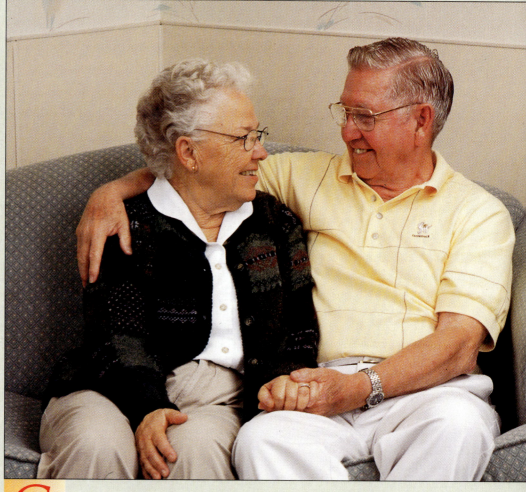

CARING TIP

Providing privacy during a visit with a spouse or significant other is very important to the self-esteem and overall well-being of the resident.

Sue Archer, RNC
Health Occupations Instructor
Puxico, Missouri

SECTION 1 Anatomy and Physiology

KEY TERMS

benign prostatic hypertrophy	nocturia	sperm
clitoris	ova	testes
estrogen	ovaries	testosterone
fertile	ovulation	transurethral surgery
hysterectomy	penis	uterus
impotence	prolapse	urethra
menstruation	prostate gland	vaginitis
menopause	scrotum	vaginal irrigation or douche
	semen	vulvitis

THE MALE REPRODUCTIVE SYSTEM

The reproductive system in the male (Figure 15-1) is composed of:

• Testes
• Scrotum
• Penis
• Seminal vesicle
• Prostate gland

Functions of the male reproductive system are to:

• Reproduce an organism like itself
• Achieve sexual pleasure and release

In the male, the primary reproductive organs are the **testes.** The testes produce **sperm** (reproductive cells released upon ejaculation). The two testicles lie in a sac called the **scrotum** (outside the body and posterior to the penis). The **penis** is the primary male sex organ. The penis is capable of enlargement and erection upon stimulation. It is an important organ for sexual arousal in the male. The hormone **testosterone** influences both sexual activity and reproduction.

During intercourse, sperm travel up the vas deferens to enter the urethra. The sperm mix with secretions from other glands in the male reproductive system, seminal vesicles, prostate gland, and Cowper's gland. These glands contribute water, nutrients, and vitamins that, when added to sperm, make up **semen.** This is the fluid that is *ejaculated* (expelled) at the time the male experiences orgasm.

The **urethra** is the only duct in the penis. It expels urine and ejaculates semen. During the process of intercourse, the internal sphincter of the male's urinary bladder closes tightly so that urine is not mixed with semen.

testes primary male reproductive organs that produce sperm

sperm male reproductive cells released upon ejaculation

scrotum sac outside the male containing the testes

penis primary male sex organ

testosterone male hormone related to sexual activity and reproduction

semen fluid expelled through the penis during ejaculation: contains sperm, water, and nutrients

urethra tube from the bladder to the outside of the body

The reproductive system consists of the organs, glands, and supportive structures that are involved with human sexuality and procreation. In the male, spermatozoa and the hormone testosterone are produced in the testes. The female produces ova (eggs) and the hormones estrogen and progesterone in her ovaries. The union of ovum and sperm produce a single cell called a zygote. Through growth, cell division, and cellular differentiation (the formation of specialized cells), the new individual develops and matures.

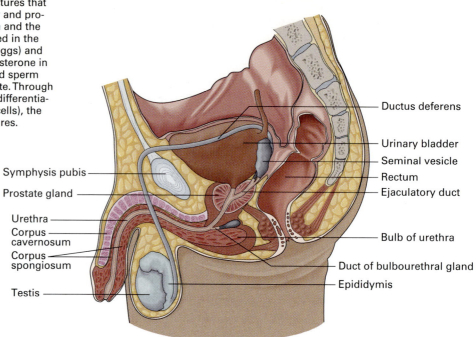

Symphysis pubis

Prostate gland

Urethra

Corpus cavernosum

Corpus spongiosum

Testis

Ductus deferens

Urinary bladder

Seminal vesicle

Rectum

Ejaculatory duct

Bulb of urethra

Duct of bulbourethral gland

Epididymis

FIGURE 15-1

The male reproductive system.

benign prostatic hypertrophy   noncancerous enlargement of the prostate gland

prostate gland   a firm muscular gland that encircles the male's urethra like a donut

nocturia   waking at night to urinate

transurethral surgery   a procedure that removes some of the prostate tissue

impotence   inability to engage in sexual intercourse

AGE-RELATED CHANGES IN MEN

Probably the most significant age-related change that affects the male reproductive system is enlargement of the prostate. A majority of all elderly men develop some degree of **benign prostatic hypertrophy** (noncancerous enlargement of the prostate gland). The **prostate gland** encircles the urethra like a donut and is a firm, muscular gland. When it becomes enlarged, it squeezes against the urethra, causing painful urination, hesitancy, decreased force of the urinary stream, and frequency of urination, which usually results in **nocturia** (the need to get up at night to urinate).

If the condition persists and goes untreated, dribbling, poor urinary control, bleeding, obstruction, and kidney damage may occur. Some men are embarrassed and do not seek medical attention until the condition is advanced. A number of treatments can help resolve the problem. One of the most common is **transurethral surgery.** This type of surgery involves removing some of the prostate tissue. It is compared to "coring an apple" because the part of the prostate surrounding the urethra is removed. This surgery does not cause **impotence** (loss of sexual function).

Tumors of the penis, testes, and scrotum also occur but not more often than in younger males. Any lesion, growth, or lump should be reported at once so that the proper medical examination can be scheduled.

Older men, in general, do experience a slowing down process of sexual desire and function that results in needing more time to achieve an erection. Usually, the erection is not as firm as it was in younger years, but the erection lasts longer.

THE FEMALE REPRODUCTIVE SYSTEM

The reproductive system of the female (Figure 15-2) is composed of:

- Ovaries
- Uterus
- Clitoris
- Vagina
- Fallopian tubes

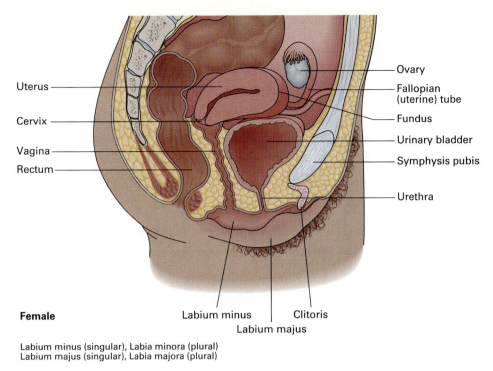

Uterus

Cervix

Vagina

Rectum

Ovary

Fallopian
(uterine) tube

Fundus

Urinary bladder

Symphysis pubis

Urethra

Female

Labium minus

Labium majus

Clitoris

Labium minus (singular), Labia minora (plural)
Labium majus (singular), Labia majora (plural)

FIGURE 15-2

The female reproductive system.

Functions of the female reproductive system are to:

- Reproduce an organism like itself
- Achieve sexual pleasure and release

In the female, the primary reproductive organs are the two **ovaries.** The main function of the ovary is to produce **ova** (eggs). These specialized cells are able to unite with the sperm cell released from the male during intercourse. This fertilized ovum grows for a period of 40 weeks into a human being.

The primary sex hormone in the female is **estrogen,** which enters the bloodstream during ovulation. **Ovulation** is a cyclical process that occurs monthly. An ovum is released from one ovary into the fallopian tube, where it may or may not be fertilized before it moves to the **uterus** (womb). This occurs once each month, usually 14 days prior to the first day of the next menstrual period. It is during this time that a woman is **fertile** (able to become pregnant). The estrogen released during ovulation causes a buildup in the lining of the uterus, preparing it for pregnancy. If pregnancy does not occur, menstruation starts. The hormones from the pituitary gland are involved in the development of the ovum and in maintaining pregnancy.

Menstruation is simply the monthly release of blood and the lining of the uterus. This bloody discharge flows out of the vagina generally for between four and seven days.

The human female has three openings in the perineal area: the urethra, the vagina, and the anus (Figure 15-3). The **clitoris** is the primary female sex organ. It is capable of enlargement and erection upon stimulation. It is an important organ related to sexual satisfaction in the female.

AGE-RELATED CHANGES IN WOMEN

A number of age-related changes affect the female reproductive system. Many of these problems could be managed more easily if regular physical examinations were done.

ovaries   primary female reproductive organs

ova   eggs

estrogen   primary female sex hormone

ovulation   process in which an ovum is discharged from an ovary at regular intervals

uterus   womb

fertile   able to become pregnant

menstruation   monthly shedding of the lining of the uterus

clitoris   primary female sex organ

menopause   the period of time when menstruation stops, ending reproductive ability and resulting in decreased hormone production

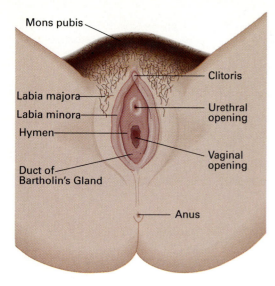

FIGURE 15-3

External female genitalia.

Mons pubis

Clitoris

Labia majora

Urethral opening

Labia minora

Hymen

Vaginal opening

Duct of Bartholin's Gland

Anus

One of the most significant age-related changes in the female is the ending of menstruation, or **menopause.** The menopause, which usually occurs from age 42 to 50, ends the reproductive ability and results in decreased hormone production. This decrease in estrogen is thought to contribute to the other changes described here.

The vulva of the elderly female loses hair, and the labia (fatty tissue) have a flat and folded appearance. These changes cause the vulva to be more sensitive and susceptible to infection called **vulvitis.** For this reason, great care must be taken to ensure that the perineal area is kept clean and free from irritation. When irritation occurs, the resident can scratch and cause more irritation and inflammation. Good personal hygiene, adequate hydration, and good nutrition will help eliminate this problem.

Vaginitis is an inflammation of the tissue of the vagina, which is a common problem due to loss of elasticity of the vaginal tissue and decreased secretions. These changes make the elderly female resident particularly susceptible to irritation and infection. Because of the decrease in secretions, some women experience painful intercourse. This can be remedied by use of water-soluble lubricants. Sometimes the physician will order special vaginal creams or suppositories, and sometimes a vaginal douche or vaginal irrigation is ordered.

PROCEDURE

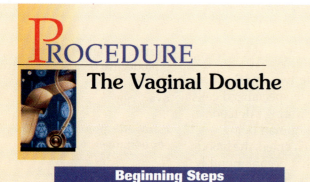

The Vaginal Douche

Beginning Steps

1. Assemble your equipment:
   - Disposable douche kit—irrigating container, tubing clamp, douche nozzle
   - Solution
   - Bedpan and cover
   - Disposable bed protector
   - Disposable gloves

2. Wash your hands.
3. Identify the resident.
4. Provide privacy.
5. Explain the procedure to the resident.
6. Put on gloves.

Steps

7. Offer the bedpan—explain the results of the douche will be better if the bladder is empty.

8. Remove bedpan and measure urinary output if the resident is on intake and output.
9. Empty and rinse the bedpan and change gloves.
10. Place a disposable bed protector under the resident's buttocks.
11. Raise the bed to its highest horizontal position.
12. Open the douche kit, clamp the tubing, and pour the solution into the irrigating douche container.
13. Pour the cleansing solution over the cotton balls.
14. Place the bedpan under the resident's buttocks.
15. Cleanse the vulva using the saturated cotton balls. Separate the folds of the labia (lips) and wipe with cotton ball from front to back on one side. Discard cotton ball in bedpan. Wipe the other side with a cotton ball, again from front to back, and discard the cotton ball into the bedpan. Wipe down the middle from front to back with a cotton ball and discard.
16. Open the clamp to expel air. Allow the solution to flow over the vulva—do not touch the nozzle to the vulva.
17. With solution flowing, insert the douche nozzle tip into the vagina 2 to 3 inches with a gentle upward, then downward, and backward movement.
18. Allow the solution to flow, holding the douche container no more than 12 inches above the vulva or 18 inches above the mattress.
19. Rotate the nozzle until all the solution has been given.

PROCEDURE
continued

20. Clamp the tubing and remove the nozzle gently. Wrap in tissue to prevent contamination and place the tubing inside the douche container for disposal.

21. Assist the resident in sitting upright on the bedpan. This will help drain the solution from the vagina.

22. Assist the resident to dry the perineal area as necessary with tissue and discard into the bedpan.

23. Remove the bedpan—place on chair.
24. Remove the bed protector.
25. Lower the bed.
26. Empty the bedpan, clean, rinse, and return to bedside cabinet.
27. Discard used equipment appropriately.
28. Remove gloves.
29. Make the resident comfortable.
30. Wash your hands.
31. Assist the resident to wash her hands.
32. Wash your hands.
33. Report and record any unusual observations.

The introduction of a solution into the vaginal canal with an immediate return of the solution by gravity is called a **vaginal irrigation** or **douche.** This irrigation is generally ordered to clean the vaginal canal or to relieve inflammation. If this procedure is overused, it will wash away the natural protective secretions, leaving the area more susceptible to irritation and infection. In an LTC facility, a vaginal douche would be administered only when ordered by the physician. In some facilities, the licensed nurse may administer the douche.

The uterus, fallopian tubes, and ovaries are connected to each other by ligaments that normally hold each in their proper place. Sometimes these ligaments are stretched during childbirth and cause the uterus to **prolapse** (fall down into the vagina). This can cause problems in urination and also makes good hygiene more difficult. Sometimes surgery is done to repair the ligaments, or in other cases the uterus is surgically removed (called **hysterectomy**). A hysterectomy is usually necessary when tumors are present or when persistent bleeding occurs.

CULTURAL AWARENESS In many cultures, talking about sexuality or about one's reproductive organs is not done. It may be particularly inappropriate for an older person to speak about it with a younger person or to speak about sexuality with a member of the opposite sex. Because this is such a sensitive topic with many people, simple problems may develop into more serious ones. Observe carefully for abnormalities, symptoms, or complaints and report them promptly.

vulvitis inflammation of the vulva

vaginitis inflammation of the tissue of the vagina

vaginal irrigation or **douche** introduction of a cleansing solution into the vaginal canal with immediate return by gravity

prolapse protruding of the uterus into the vagina

hysterectomy surgical removal of the uterus

SECTION 2 Human Sexuality

OBJECTIVES
What You Will Learn

When you have completed this section, you will be able to:

- Define the term **sexuality**
- List two common myths associated with sex and the elderly
- Describe three ways you can acknowledge the resident's sexuality as you provide care

KEY TERMS

masturbation   sexuality

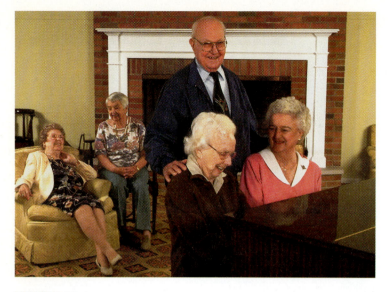

FIGURE 15-4

Needs for meaningful relationships continue throughout life.

In addition to physical problems, there are age-related sexual concerns that require a sensitive, informed approach by the health care team. Residents of LTC facilities have sexual feelings and needs that are frequently ignored due to reluctance to deal with this very natural and normal aspect of life.

In years past, health care professionals have often overlooked the sexual rights and needs of residents. Discussion and education regarding sex have been avoided and discouraged. The reluctance to deal openly and intelligently with our own as well as our resident's sexuality has led to ignorance, prejudice, and misinformation.

Sexuality is defined as the quality of being male or female. Sexuality includes the warm, loving, caring feelings shared between people. Sexuality is not age limited. We are sexual beings during our entire lifespan. Individuals who have over their lifetime established patterns of sexual behavior will generally continue these patterns into old age.

When the topic of sex and the elderly is presented, many social prejudices appear. For example, when a 70-year-old man shows a healthy interest in sex, he may be regarded as a "dirty old man," while the 35-year-old man is considered a "swinger" or "playboy." It is acceptable for young women to be concerned with fashion, sexy lingerie, and makeup, but eyebrows are raised if a grandmother shows interest! The aging process does not take away one's sexuality or one's need for meaningful relationships (Figure 15-4).

sexuality quality of being male or female

masturbation sexual self-stimulation apart from intercourse

SEX AND THE ELDERLY

Common myths associated with sex and the elderly are:

- Older women have lost all interest in sex.
- Older men are not capable of sexual intercourse.
- Older people don't need sexual satisfaction or pleasure.
- Older people don't care how they look and are not concerned about being attractive to the opposite sex.

FIGURE 15-5

Help the resident prepare for special occasions.

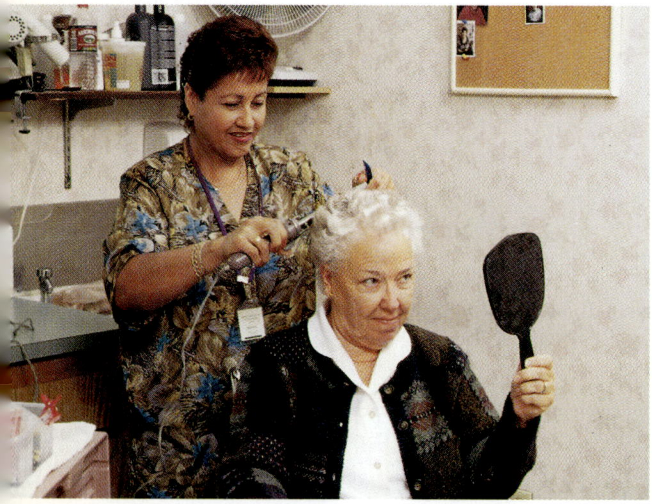

These misconceptions are often imposed on the elderly to the point that they either give up warm, meaningful sexual experiences or they harbor feelings of guilt and shame about having them. They are often deprived of the joy and comfort of feeling important and wanted by someone else.

One of the common reasons residents may not experience sexual fulfillment is the lack of an appropriate partner. They may have lost a spouse through death or divorce and feel that sex without marriage is immoral. For this reason, some may meet their needs for release of tension and sexual satisfaction through **masturbation.** Masturbation is sexual self-stimulation. Contrary to myths surrounding it, masturbation is a normal means of sexual satisfaction that does not harm the individual. You may observe one of your residents in the act of masturbation. If so, provide privacy by drawing the curtain or closing the door. It is never appropriate to ridicule or embarrass the resident. Some disoriented residents or those with dementia may masturbate without seeming to know what they are doing. In that case, be sure to take them to a private place and emphasize that what they are doing is not appropriate in public. Emphasize the inappropriateness of the place, not the activity itself.

Some residents may express their sexual frustration by reaching out to you. They may pat you or grab you where you don't wish to be touched. Handle the situation calmly and without anger. Simply state, "I don't like it when you do that," or "I don't like it when you touch me there." Show the resident af-

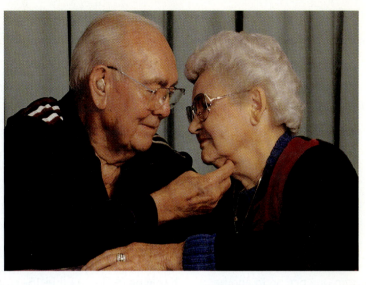

FIGURE 15-6

Show acceptance when the residents show affection for one another.

fection in ways that you feel are appropriate. If your efforts to stop the inappropriate touching are not successful, ask the charge nurse if you can have a conference on how to handle the behavior. You may also obtain the help of the social worker or other members of the health care team.

There are a number of ways that members of the health care team can acknowledge the sexuality of each individual. Helping residents understand the effects of aging on sexual function is a beginning. A willingness on the part of the nurse to discuss sex openly demonstrates concern, acceptance, and respect for the resident's sexuality. Be observant and report special concerns to the charge nurse so that positive steps can be taken to deal with the resident's sexual needs.

You can recognize and accept the resident's sexuality as you provide care by following these guidelines:

- Assist as necessary with personal hygiene and grooming.
- Allow the residents to choose attractive clothing, cosmetics, and hairstyles. Help them to prepare for special occasions or outings (Figure 15-5).
- Assist them to maintain their sexual identity by dressing them in appropriate masculine or feminine attire.
- Always consider the resident's feelings and need for privacy. Take care not to expose residents unnecessarily. Close privacy curtains and doors.
- Help them establish a positive self-image. Never discuss their incontinence or episodes of confusion in the presence of others. Treat them as valued members of society.
- Show understanding and acceptance when they show interest and affection for each other (Figure 15-6).
- Residents should never be made to feel foolish or guilty for their expressions of love or sexuality.
- Consider the individual's right to privacy by allowing residents time alone, knocking before entering, and—when requested—assisting residents to find areas where privacy can be assured (Figure 15-7).

The nursing assistant has an important role in helping the residents realize the full potential of sexuality in their later years.

FIGURE 15-7

Consider the residents' right to privacy.

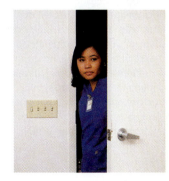

SECTION 3 Sexually Transmitted Diseases

OBJECTIVES
What You Will Learn

When you have completed this section, you will be able to:

- List the diseases described as sexually transmitted diseases
- Describe three measures that will help protect you from sexually transmitted diseases
- Match characteristics of four common diseases with the name of the disease

KEY TERM

Sexually transmitted diseases

---

sexually transmitted diseases a disease passed on from one person to another through vaginal, rectal, or oral sex

Diseases that are passed through sexual activity, including vaginal intercourse, anal intercourse, and oral intercourse, are referred to as **sexually transmitted diseases** (STDs) (Table 15-1). The causes of the diseases vary and include bacteria, viruses, parasites, and fungi. It is believed that over 10 million people in the United States are afflicted with one of the 20 or more sexually transmitted diseases! Although symptoms may be mild at first, the consequences of unrecognized and untreated disease are severe. Not only is the patient at risk, so also are their sexual partners and, for women, their unborn children.

You can reduce your risk of acquiring these diseases by:

- Knowing the signs and symptoms of STDs
- Avoiding sexual contact with persons who have these signs and symptoms

TABLE 15-1 Sexually Transmitted Diseases

DISEASE	SYMPTOMS	TREATMENT
TRICHOMONAS VAGINITIS	For males—none. For females—white, foul-smelling vaginal discharge.	Drug treatment for both sexual partners
HERPES GENITALIS, caused by herpes simplex virus type 2. When victim is stressed, has inadequate diet, or when the immune system is overworked, the virus reactivates. Especially dangerous to the pregnant woman—can infect the baby during birth. Also high risk for cervical cancer.	Vesicles on genitalia that rupture to form painful ulcers. Lesions resolve without scarring. Tends to clear up, then recur. Is not transmissible all of the time. Because it is incurable, there are psychosocial issues about disclosing to a sexual partner that they are at risk.	*There is no known cure.* Antiviral drugs may be given to reduce symptoms and to control the disease.
CHLAMYDIA, the most common STD among heterosexual white Americans. It is estimated that over 3 million Americans have chlamydia, including over 10 percent of all college students. If untreated, males can suffer damage to the prostate, blood vessels, and heart. They may develop arthritislike symptoms. Females may develop pelvic inflammatory disease, sterility, and painful recurring infections. If a female becomes pregnant, her risk for stillbirth and spontaneous abortion is high.	For males—painful urination, urinary frequency, and urethral discharge. For females—a yellowish vaginal discharge, spotting between periods, may have spotting with intercourse. Some females have no symptoms!	If detected early, 2 to 3 weeks of antibiotic medications.

TABLE 15-1 **Sexually Transmitted Diseases (continued)**

DISEASE	SYMPTOMS	TREATMENT
GONORRHEA, one of the most prevalent STDs in the United States. Called "clap" or "drip" by some. If a woman is untreated and gives birth, the disease may cause conjunctivitis in the infant. Newborn infants are routinely treated with eye drops to prevent this.	For males—milky white discharge from the penis, painful urination. For females—many have no symptoms. A few may have a discharge or painful urination. If untreated, may cause sterility in both males and females.	Antibiotic medications
SYPHILIS, a well-known STD. Caused by delicate bacterium that dies upon exposure to air, cold, or dryness. Occurs in four stages if untreated. Often undetected in females. Can be transmitted to a fetus, leading to congenital blindness, deafness, or other birth defects, including death.	For males—often develop a sore called a chancre at site of infections, which is painless, oozing, dime-sized. Occurs 3 to 4 weeks after contact. Secondary symptoms: rash on skin or membranes of mouth or throat, may lose hair, may have fever. Latent (2 to 4 years), not transmitted to others. May affect any organs, especially the nervous system, causing blindness, paralysis, deafness, etc.	Antibiotics, usually penicillin

- Avoiding multiple sexual partners and other persons with multiple sexual partners
- Using condoms with a spermicide
- Following STANDARD PRECAUTIONS

SUMMARY

This chapter has focused on the resident as a human being with the wants, needs, and desires shared by all humans. Living in a long-term care facility makes it more difficult for the resident to satisfy these needs and desires. As a nursing assistant, it is important for you to accept the resident's feelings as normal and provide privacy and respect. It is never appropriate to ridicule a resident for acting on their sexual desires. Because of your opportunity to provide intimate, personal care to your residents as you bathe, dress, and groom them, they may choose to discuss their feelings with you. They may also act out sexually toward you, so it is important to decide what you will do and what you will say before the need arises. Be matter-of-fact and nonjudgmental. Do not personalize the behavior. If you are uncomfortable and unsure about how to handle a situation, ask for help.

SELF STUDY

Choose the best answer for each question or statement.

1. Which of the following are produced by the testes?
   a. sperm
   b. ova
   c. semen
   d. urine

2. Semen leaves the penis during ejaculation through the
   a. ureter
   b. urethra
   c. prostate
   d. seminal vesicle

3. When a male resident has an enlarged prostate, it causes
   a. painful urination
   b. nocturia
   c. frequency of urination
   d. all of the above

4. Which of the following are produced by the ovaries?
   a. sperm
   b. ova
   c. urine
   d. uterus

5. Which of the following is true of ovulation?
   a. It is the time that a women is least likely to become pregnant.
   b. It occurs on the 28th day of each month.
   c. It is when an ovum is released from the ovary into the fallopian tube.
   d. all of the above

6. Which of the following openings are found in the human female's perineal area?
   a. anus and urethra
   b. anus and clitoris
   c. anus, urethra, and vagina
   d. vagina and anus

7. Which of the following can be done by the nursing assistant to prevent vulvitis in female residents?
   a. Give good perineal care, given adequate fluids and nutrition.
   b. Bathe the perineal area three times per day and apply lotion.

   c. Soak the perineum in a tub each day and do not dress the resident in underwear.
   d. all of the above

8. Which of the following is true about the sexual needs of the elderly?
   a. The need for meaningful relationships and sex decreases after age 65.
   b. Residents older than 65 who are interested in sex have a problem accepting aging.
   c. The aging process does not erase the need for meaningful relationships and sex.
   d. The elderly no longer are interested in sexual satisfaction or pleasure.

9. You walk into a resident's room and observe him during masturbation. What should you do?
   a. Tell the resident quietly and firmly that such behavior is unacceptable.
   b. Provide privacy by drawing the curtain or closing the door.
   c. Ask him what he is doing and insist that he stop it immediately.
   d. Inform the charge nurse of this behavior immediately.

10. Mr. Melvin often tries to touch you inappropriately. Several of the staff call him "a dirty old man." How should you handle the situation?
    a. Tell Mr. Melvin that he needs to think about other things and act his age.
    b. Refuse to care for Mr. Melvin because he makes you uncomfortable.
    c. Tell Mr. Melvin's family what he is doing and ask them to make him stop.
    d. Tell Mr. Melvin that you do not like for him to do that and to please stop.

11. Two residents in your facility are attracted to one another and are spending more and more time together. Neither of the residents have spouses. Which of the following guidelines should you follow when dealing with this situation?
    a. Try to keep the two residents apart as much as possible so you do not encourage the relationship.
    b. Allow the residents to have privacy and do not make judgments about the relationship.
    c. Discuss the situation with other staff members and decide how it should be handled.
    d. Ask the families of the two residents for permission to allow them to spend time together.

12. Which of the following is true about a vaginal douche?

   a. It is ordered to clean the vagina or to reduce inflammation.

   b. It can be done anytime a female resident complains of vaginal itching.

   c. It is used only if vaginal creams and suppositories do not reduce inflammation.

   d. An enema kit is used to perform a vaginal douche.

13. When you give perineal care to Mrs. Chester, you notice that her uterus has fallen down into her vagina. This is

   a. a medical emergency and must be treated immediately

   b. vaginal prolapse and is caused by stretched out ligaments

   c. an indication that she has internal bleeding and pressure

   d. common after menopause and requires no treatment

14. Transurethral surgery is used to correct which of the following reproductive conditions?

   a. vaginal prolapse

   b. impotence

   c. testical tumors

   d. enlarged prostate

15. Surgery to remove the uterus is called

   a. hysterectomy

   b. uterusectomy

   c. ureterectomy

   d. vaginectomy

16. Which of the following is true about menopause?

   a. It usually occurs from ages 42 to 50.

   b. It ends the female's reproductive ability.

   c. It results in decreased hormone production.

   d. All of these are true about menopause.

Getting C O N N E C T E D
Multimedia Extension Activities

 www.prenhall.com/will-black

Use the above address to access the free, interactive Companion Website created for this textbook. Hear the pronunciation of the key terms in the chapter. Get instant feedback to a variety of chapter-related questions. Link to other interesting sites.

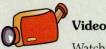 **Video**

Watch the video *Age-Specific Competencies* and the section on perineal care in the *Bed Bath* video from the Care Provider Skills series.

CASE STUDY

Mr. Leo Schwartz has been a resident in your facility for 6 months. Mrs. Hilda Schwartz experienced a stroke and has just been admitted. You find Leo sitting by Hilda's bed at 11 P.M. just as you are going off duty.

1. What do you do?
   a. Wave and tell him you'll see him tomorrow.
   b. Insist that he return to his own room.
   c. Offer to take him to his room, reminding him that he needs his rest.
   d. Report to the charge nurse.
2. Leo asks you why he can't share a room with Hilda, his wife of 55 years. You answer
   a. "That may be possible if the doctor thinks it is okay."
   b. "We don't have any empty beds."
   c. "We keep men on one wing and women on another wing."
   d. "I don't think it is a good idea."
3. You find Mr. Schwartz in bed with Mrs. Schwartz. Your response is:
   a. close the door as you leave the room
   b. tell the other CNAs to come see how cute the Schwartzes are
   c. Say, "Mr. Schwartz, you should be ashamed of yourself."
   d. report it to the charge nurse immediately
4. Today is the Schwartzes 56th wedding anniversary. It would be appropriate for you to
   a. plan a party
   b. be sure both of them look their best by taking extra time with grooming and dressing
   c. ignore the event
   d. call the family and suggest that they plan a party

Chapter 16

DEVELOPMENTAL DISABILITIES

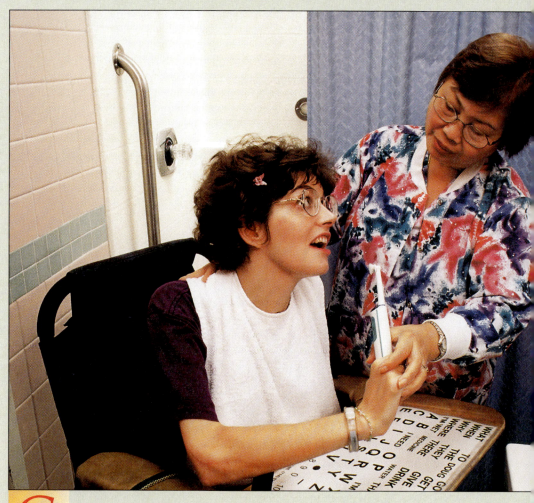

CARING TIP

Enhance communication by using gestures as well as words.

Gail Diffley
RN Inservice Educator
Wesley Health Care Center
Saratoga Springs, New York

SECTION 1 Introduction to Developmental Disabilities

OBJECTIVES
What You Will Learn

When you have completed this section, you will be able to:

- Define the term **developmental disability**

- List three causes of developmental disability
- Define the term **mental retardation**
- Describe what is meant by the concept of normalization, giving examples of a normalized environment

- Define the terms *age appropriate,* **developmental model, least restrictive alternative,** and **active treatment**

KEY TERMS

active treatment

autism

cerebral palsy

developmental disability

developmental model

epilepsy

fine motor skills

functional life skills

gross motor activities

IPPs

least restrictive alternative

mental retardation

normalization

perinatal

postnatal

prenatal

QMRP

sensory-motor activities

Certain long-term care facilities are established for the care of the developmentally disabled. Nursing assistants play a vital role in these facilities. The nursing assistant functions as both a teacher and a caregiver. You may be called a trainer, a developmental aide, or a direct care staff member. Special knowledge and skills are required. In addition to the many nursing skills you have learned, you will need behavior management, teaching, and data collection skills.

The term **developmental disability** (DD) is a legal definition mandated by Congress in 1970 and revised in 1978. *Developmental disability* means a severe, chronic disability of a person that:

developmental disability
a chronic condition related to or needing treatment similar to mental retardation

1. Is attributable to a mental or physical impairment or combination of mental and physical impairments
2. Is manifested (shown) before the person attains age 22
3. Is likely to continue indefinitely (chronic)
4. Results in substantial functional limitation in three or more of the following areas of major life activity:
   —Self-care (activities of daily living)
   —Receptive and expressive language (understanding others and making self understood)
   —Learning (ability to acquire new skills and new knowledge)
   —Mobility (ability to move from place to place without assistance)
   —Self-direction (ability to make decisions about one's own life)
   —Capacity for independent living
   —Economic self-sufficiency (ability to support oneself)
5. Reflects the person's need for a combination and sequence of special, interdisciplinary, or generic care, treatment, or other services that are of lifelong or extended duration and are individually planned and coordinated

Four categories or diagnoses account for the majority of the individuals who are developmentally disabled. They are mental retardation, cerebral palsy, epilepsy, and autism. The new definition does, however, include accident victims and those who sustained brain damage due to illness.

MENTAL RETARDATION

More than 6 million people are believed to be mentally retarded. More than 100,000 babies born each year are likely to join this number. One out of every ten Americans has a mentally retarded person in the family.

mental retardation a significantly subaverage general intellectual functioning existing with deficits in adaptive behavior

Mental retardation is defined as "significantly subaverage general intellectual functioning existing along with deficits in adaptive behavior and manifested during the developmental period."* Although this definition sounds complex, it becomes clear when broken into parts. *General intellectual functioning* refers to the IQ (intelligence quotient) or score obtained on a standard test. The average IQ is 100. Significantly below average is considered to be an IQ of 70 or below. About 3 percent of the population would be classified as mentally retarded based on IQ alone.

Deficits in adaptive behavior are limitations in the person's ability to learn, to be independent, and to be socially responsible (Figure 16-1). The person is evaluated based on what is considered normal or average for his or her age and cultural group. The *developmental period* is the period of time between conception and the eighteenth birthday.

prenatal during pregnancy

Causes of mental retardation are usually divided into three categories: prenatal, perinatal, and postnatal. **Prenatal** causes are those that are hereditary or occur during the pregnancy of the mother. Examples of hereditary causes include Down's syndrome and Tay–Sachs disease. An example of retardation caused by an event during pregnancy would be an instance when the mother abuses drugs or alcohol during the pregnancy, and the baby is born mentally retarded. **Perinatal** causes are those that occur during the birth process. There may be a problem that cuts off the supply of oxygen to the baby, such as an umbilical cord around the neck or physical injury to the brain from difficulty going through the birth canal. **Postnatal** causes include any event that occurs after the birth, including illness, accidents, or physical abuse.

perinatal during the birth process

postnatal after birth

Mental retardation is divided into levels based on IQ scores:

Level	IQ Range
Mild mental retardation	50–55 to approximately 70
Moderate mental retardation	35–40 to 50–55
Severe mental retardation	20–25 to 35–40
Profound mental retardation	Below 20 or 25

FIGURE 16-1

Communication may be difficult.

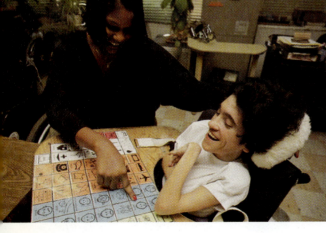

Most of the mentally retarded persons you will care for in a facility for the developmentally disabled will be either severely or profoundly retarded. The *profoundly retarded* person rarely is able to speak. Often this person will have sensory, skeletal, and other physical abnormalities. Most are either bedfast or chairfast. Fifty percent live in institutions. Research shows that they are placed in institutions earlier, are least often visited by family and friends, and die at the youngest age. One study showed that the average age of death of the profoundly retarded is 38. The major cause of death is pneumonia.

* From H. Grossman, ed., *Manual of Terminology and Classification in Mental Retardation.* Washington, DC: American Association on Mental Deficiency, 1973.

The *severely retarded* person will generally have some useful speech by adolescence. The severely retarded have fewer multiple physical handicaps, and their life span is longer than the profoundly retarded.

CEREBRAL PALSY

Cerebral palsy is a developmental disability caused by damage to the brain that results in the person having difficulty controlling the muscles of the body. Because the muscles often include those used in speech, a capable individual can be hidden within a body that cannot be controlled or understood. About 750,000 people in the United States have cerebral palsy. The causes of cerebral palsy are similar to the causes of mental retardation. They occur during pregnancy or birth and may be due to prematurity, lack of oxygen, or injury to the head. Many persons with cerebral palsy live active, successful lives in the community. Examples include a successful rock singer and a well-known comedienne. The person with cerebral palsy who is living in a facility for the developmentally disabled will probably have severe or multiple handicaps and may also be mentally retarded. Never assume, however, that someone with cerebral palsy is mentally retarded. Cerebral palsied persons are unique individuals who should not be labeled, categorized, or treated as part of a group.

cerebral palsy a developmental disability caused by damage to the brain

AUTISM

Autism is a condition occurring in young children before the age of 3 years, characterized by unresponsiveness to human contact, deficits in language development, and bizarre responses to environmental stimuli.

autism a disability related to lack of organization in the functioning of the brain

Autism affects about 60,000 children under 18 years of age in the United States. Boys are affected three to four times as often as girls. Although very little is known about the cause of autism, it is thought to be a disability that results from a lack of organization in the functioning of the brain. Autistic children appear to be aloof and withdrawn from contact with others. They seem to live in their own world. The name *autism* comes from a Greek word *autos,* meaning self. The autistic person seems to respond in unpredictable ways to things he sees and hears. Some never develop speech. Some seem unaware of pain. Although some may become friendly and cheerful, many have severe behavior problems that include violence toward themselves, others, or their immediate environment.

Some of the signs of autism include:

- Rigid or flaccid muscle tone while being held
- Little or no interest in human contact
- Lack of attachment to parents or caretakers
- Language impairment
- Bizarre or repetitive behavior patterns such as head banging, screaming, arm flapping
- Self-destructive behavior
- Overreaction or underreaction to sensory stimulus
- Delayed mental and social skills

Autism may be diagnosed by the behavior and a test showing delayed development, especially of language and social skills.

EPILEPSY

Epilepsy is a condition or disorder in the electrical functioning of the brain that results in various kinds of seizures. Epilepsy does not cause mental retardation

epilepsy a disorder in the electrical functioning of the brain, resulting in seizures

nor is everyone with epilepsy mentally retarded. In fact, the vast majority of those with epilepsy are *not* retarded. (Chapter 11, "The Nervous System," includes information on seizures and epilepsy; review that information now.) Epilepsy is, however, often present along with mental retardation and cerebral palsy because it may be caused by the same event that caused the other conditions.

NORMALIZATION

normalization creating an atmosphere that is as close to normal as possible

A facility providing care to the developmentally disabled adopts guiding principles or a philosophy of care that establishes not only how care will be given, but also the kind of environment in which it will be given. The most basic concept is called normalization. **Normalization** means creating an atmosphere that is as close as possible to the atmosphere provided those citizens who are not mentally retarded (Figure 16-2). It means offering the same opportunities and kind of treatment. Principles of normalization require that positive attributes or qualities of the individual be emphasized while negative qualities are eliminated. For example, if a developmentally disabled resident or client has a physical abnormality such as crossed eyes that would make the client appear unusual or abnormal, the crossed eyes should be corrected with surgery or special glasses. Great care should be taken in the grooming and dressing of your clients so that any negative physical traits are either disguised or offset by attractive, age-appropriate clothing and good grooming (based on chronological age, not mental or developmental age). With older clients, make special effort to select an appropriate hairstyle as well as clothing. For example, an older woman might look absurd in a ponytail with childlike bows or barrettes. There are, however, ways to pull the hair back that are more adult. A child's ponytail is placed high on the back of the head while an adult's is secured lower, at the back of the neck.

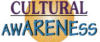

One aspect of normalization is to recognize and to acknowledge the culture of the client. Each client brings an ethnic, racial, or cultural history. Even though the client cannot express his or her culture, the staff must keep it in mind. For example, if the family is Hispanic, it would be important to offer some Hispanic foods. If the family holds certain religious practices, the family may want the client to observe them too. Ask other staff and the family members what their practices and beliefs are so that you can help the client to follow them.

In order to create a normalized environment, it is essential that every staff member hold a particular belief: that all human beings are worthy of being treated with dignity and respect. If you believe that you are somehow "better" than those you serve, you will have difficulty treating your clients or residents as they deserve to be cared for.

Some of the ways you will know normalization when you see it are:

FIGURE 16-2

Example of normalization.

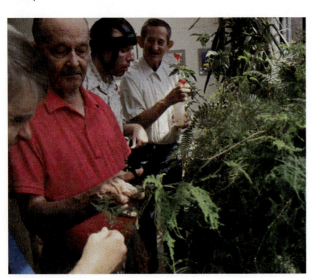

- Staff members treat people under their supervision with dignity and respect.
- Staff members do not exert undue power over the resident.
- Staff play the role of an associate or assistant, not a parent.
- Residents are encouraged to do all they can for themselves.
- Residents' rooms contain many personal items.

- Residents are encouraged to have personal belongings that are age appropriate.
- Residents' clothing is individualized and age appropriate (not "uniform").
- Privacy is available for all residents. This means both visual privacy and privacy of information about the resident.
- Residents are encouraged to make choices about their lives (when to get up, when to go to bed, how to spend leisure time, what to wear, etc.).
- Residents are encouraged to become involved in the community. They are taught skills that will allow them to function successfully away from the facility. For example, if possible they should learn to use the telephone, take a bus, manage money, shop, and so on.

If you are now working in a facility for the developmentally disabled, use the list to see how your facility measures up when it comes to the principle of normalization. If you are seeking employment in this rewarding field, ask questions and observe for these concepts in action.

THE DEVELOPMENTAL MODEL

Another important factor for those working in this setting is a belief in the developmental model. The **developmental model** is based on the philosophy that all human beings have potential. Human beings thrive only to the extent that they are allowed and encouraged to change and to develop. The change and growth you see can seem very small, but to the resident it may be enormous. Your role will be to help each resident achieve as much growth as possible for that person.

developmental model a model of care that is based on the belief that human beings thrive only to the extent that they are allowed to develop.

LEAST RESTRICTIVE ALTERNATIVE

Another guiding principle is that of choosing the **least restrictive alternative.** Whenever there is a choice to be made in method of treatment or selection of activities or living arrangements, the goal is to choose the option that least limits the freedom and independence of the individual resident. In terms of medical care, this means that the physician orders the lowest dosage of a drug that will effectively manage the problem, or it means that, instead of using a medication for a behavior problem, behavior management is attempted first. The least restrictive alternative principle is also shown when residents are taught skills that allow greater independence and the ability to live in an environment where they can experience greater freedom and a more "normal" living situation.

least restrictive alternative a choice of treatment, activities, or living arrangement that least limits the freedom and independence of the individual

PROGRAMMING

Each facility for the developmentally disabled has a program or program plan that describes in writing how the principles of normalization, least restrictive alternative, and the developmental model will be made a reality. You might think of the program as parallel to a curriculum in a school. In fact, that's a good way to think of a DD facility. It is like a boarding school in that it serves as both home and school. The main purpose of the school is to teach skills that maximize or accentuate the positive aspects of each individual client and eliminate the negative aspects. The curriculum is designed to provide individual educational plans, which are called **IPPs** or individual program plans. A team of skilled professionals develop the individualized plan based on assessment of each client's abilities. The team includes the client, the parents of

IPPs the individual program plans used with developmentally disabled clients

the client (if appropriate and possible), any agency that monitors the client's care, professionals including a registered nurse, physical therapist, speech therapist, psychologist, social worker, occupational therapist, special education teacher, and the program director of the facility. This team is referred to as the ID team or interdisciplinary team. The team is headed by a person called the **QMRP** or qualified mental retardation professional. The QMRP may have education and training in any of the professional disciplines mentioned previously. For example, the QMRP might be a psychologist, physical therapist, nurse, and so on. This person must have knowledge and experience beyond the basic training in their particular field or discipline. Most often they must be approved by a state agency to serve as the QMRP.

QMRP   the qualified mental retardation professional who heads the interdisciplinary team for developmentally disabled clients

Your role is to assist in carrying out the IPP as you work with the client individually and in small groups (Figure 16-3). Clients are usually grouped according to ability, common interests, and common learning activities. In order to carry out the IPP, it is essential that you know what the objectives or goals and activities are for each client in your assigned group. At first, you may have to memorize the goals and plans. Normally, these written plans are readily available to you in the classroom where you carry out your activities.

The program plan includes descriptions of all the activities involved in assisting each client to reach her or his individual goals. Activities may be grouped under categories such as functional life skills, fine motor skills, gross motor skills, and sensory-motor skills.

functional life skills
skills necessary to allow an individual to function as independently as possible

fine motor skills   skills that require use of fine muscles such as those of the hands for writing, buttoning, and eating

gross motor activities
involves use of the large muscles such as those used in walking, dancing, and swimming

sensory-motor activities
activities designed to improve the thinking of the client

- **Functional life skills** are the skills necessary to allow the person to function as independently as possible. These may be ADL skills for some or activities such as making change or using the telephone.
- **Fine motor skills** require use of the fine muscles such as those of the hands. Fine motor skills would include such tasks as buttoning, writing, and feeding oneself.
- **Gross motor activities** involve the use of the larger muscles of the body. For example, physical fitness exercises or activities such as walking, swimming, or dancing are gross motor activities.
- **Sensory-motor activities** are designed to improve the thinking of the client by improving the information coming into the brain through all the senses, including sight, sound, smell, and touch. For example, in order to develop understanding of what "round" means, the resident might feel a ball, watch it roll and bounce, and even listen to a sound it makes. The concept of round would be important to learning about money (coins are round) or to learning certain types of jobs.

FIGURE 16-3
(a) Learning to weigh himself;
(b) learning to give insulin.

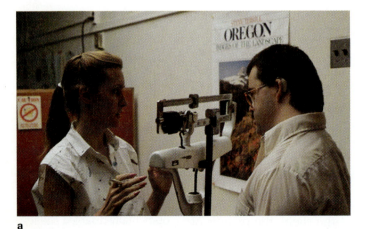

a

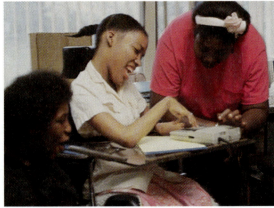

b

LEAST RESTRICTIVE ENVIRONMENT

Whatever the category of skills in the program, the goal is to provide skills that will allow the client or resident to live in the *least restrictive environment* possible. This means that of all the choices available for the living arrangements, the one chosen is as close as possible to "normal." This means that the client is in an environment that allows maximum use of his or her living skills and the most personal freedom (Figure 16-4). To better understand the term *least restrictive environment*, imagine that all the possible places that the client could live were ranked and listed in order of those that allowed for the most independence down to those that allowed the least independence. The list might look something like this:

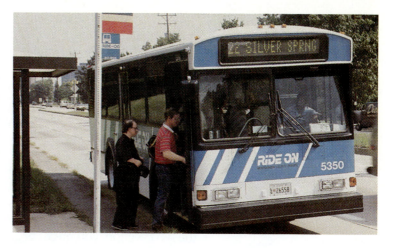

FIGURE 16-4
Least restrictive environment.

1. Living alone in a home or apartment, doing one's shopping, having a job, planning own leisure, and so forth.
2. Living with others in a home or apartment; shopping and household duties are shared by the group. May leave and go to work or school.
3. Living in a small home with others and a caregiver. The caregiver may do some of the household tasks, such as shopping and money management.
4. Living in a small institution with a 24-hour staff. Meals, housekeeping, and laundry are done for the residents by the staff.
5. Living in a larger institution with a 24-hour staff, programs, scheduled activities, and so on. May leave for outings or work.
6. Living in a state hospital where permission has to be given to leave the grounds and where virtually all activities take place on the hospital property.

The type of living that would meet the least restrictive environment test would be different for each client. The goal of programming is to provide training in those skills that would allow the client to live in the least restrictive environment possible for that client. Ideally, all skills should be building the independence of the individual. There are still some settings where individuals are doing things such as sorting shapes of blocks rather than more functional or useful skills such as returning silverware to the right drawer. Both are sorting activities. Sorting silverware is a functional skill; sorting blocks is not.

ACTIVE TREATMENT

The program plan must provide active treatment for each client. **Active treatment** means that each client:

- Has an interdisciplinary professional evaluation
- Has an individual written plan of care that includes measurable goals and an integrated program of activities, experiences, or therapies necessary for the client to reach those goals

active treatment program plan including interdisciplinary evaluation and an individual plan of care with measurable goals and an integrated program of activities

- Participates in the implementation of the plan of care in professionally supervised activities
- Is reevaluated medically, socially, and psychologically at least annually

Facilities for the developmentally disabled are surveyed and evaluated yearly by the government to assure that clients are indeed receiving active treatment as described above. Each part of the process is essential, but emphasis is on whether the program is being carried out and whether clients are reaching the goals set forth.

One goal on a client's IPP might be: "John will be able to put on his pants independently on four out of five days." Your role in training this resident can be broken down into specific steps that include all the activities involved in putting on a pair of pants. Through concepts of behavior shaping described in the next section, you might begin by simply getting John to put his feet through the pant leg and praising him for that step. The plan will be written by an expert in the process of behavior shaping, but your role is to follow the plan. It may be tempting in this case to "help" John by putting his pants on for him. This will only keep him from being as independent as he can be and, in the long run, will harm rather than help him.

SECTION 2 Behavior Management Principles and Techniques

OBJECTIVES
What You Will Learn

When you have completed this section, you will be able to:

- Describe the ABCs of behavior modification

- Match the definitions to the terms **shaping, prompting,** and **fading**
- List the three components of graduated guidance
- Give examples of verbal, gestural, and physical prompts

- Identify types of reinforcers that are appropriate for the nursing assistant to use

KEY TERMS

advocates
aversive
backward chaining
behavior

behavior modification
behavior shaping
fading
forward chaining
graduated guidance

modeling
prompting
reinforcer
shadowing

behavior   action that can be observed and measured

Before you learn about behavior management, the concept of behavior has to be defined and separated from attitudes, feelings, and thoughts. **Behavior** is action. Behavior can be observed and measured. For example, you can measure the *frequency* of a behavior (how often the behavior takes place), the *duration* of the behavior (how long it occurs), or the *intensity* of the behavior (how strong it is). There are both desirable and undesirable behaviors. Generally, we want to increase the frequency of desirable behaviors and decrease the frequency of undesirable behaviors. In a facility for the developmentally disabled, the determination of what is desirable and what is undesirable is important. The key is always in the best interest of the client. Behaviors are desirable if they promote independence, normalization, and the concept of least restricted environment. In other words, behaviors such as self-care activities and courtesy to others would be desirable. Tantrums, violence against self or others, and habits such as spitting or making babbling noises would be undesirable behaviors.

Scientists have learned that behavior that is rewarded will be repeated. They have also noted that the closer in time the reward is to the behavior, the more power it has to cause the behavior to be repeated. A third important principle is that behavior that is punished or ignored decreases or disappears. Using these basic principles, an entire science called behavior management has been developed. Usually, there is a person on the staff at a DD facility who is an expert in the field of behavior management. This is often the psychologist, but may be another consultant or employee. This knowledgeable person will develop the specific management program for the staff to follow. Your help will be essential in measuring the behavior, identifying the best reward, giving or withholding the reward at the right time, and recording the results.

Behavior modification is the process of changing behavior patterns or habits by eliminating ineffective (useless) behaviors and teaching effective (useful) behaviors. Once a specific behavior has been chosen (targeted) to be increased, careful observation is needed to construct a plan. This client must be watched in order to determine what events occur before the behavior and what things occur afterward. These are called the ABCs of behavior modification. The A stands for the event occurring before the target behavior. The A is called the *antecedent to the behavior*. The B represents the *behavior,* and the C stands for the *consequence* or result of the behavior.

behavior modification a process of changing behavior patterns by eliminating useless behaviors and teaching or reinforcing useful ones

INCREASING BEHAVIORS

Increasing behavior is accomplished by following the behavior with a reward or **reinforcer.** There are three types of reinforcers: primary, social, and physical (Figure 16-5). *Primary reinforcers* are food such as raisins, candy, soft drinks, fruit, and so on. *Social reinforcers* are praise, smiles, and so forth. *Physical reinforcers* include touch, such as hugs and pats on the shoulder or arm. When primary reinforcers are used, they are usually given along with social and physical rewards. Primary reinforcers are not always available or effective, so an effort is made to use more social and physical reinforcers. In a normal setting, people are not given food for good performance; they are given praise, smiles, and "thank you's." If our philosophy is that of normalization, we should—whenever possible—choose reinforcers that will occur normally in the environment. In addition, some practical limitations exist using primary reinforcers. For example, food would not be a successful reinforcer if the person just ate

reinforcer   a reward

FIGURE 16-5

Types of reinforcers.

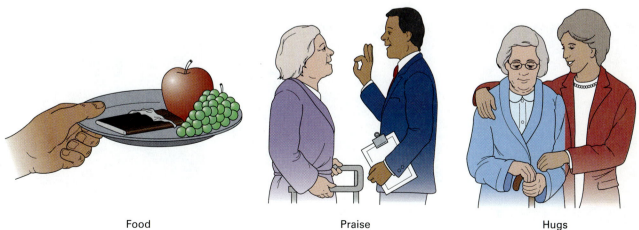

Food   Praise   Hugs

or if the person did not like a particular food. Praise, on the other hand, is always available, and we never lose our appetite for it.

A simple example would be if the resident made his bed. The staff member would reinforce the behavior by saying, "George, you made your bed. Good work!" The praise or positive reinforcer has to be given in a sincere way that fits the person. Use language and gestures that are suited to preferences of the person being rewarded. There should not be too much or too little reinforcement given. Praising desirable behavior as it occurs is less difficult than trying to create a new behavior so that you can reinforce it.

BEHAVIOR SHAPING

The process of creating a new set of behaviors is called **behavior shaping.** This technique is commonly used when teaching clients self-help skills or activities of daily living (ADLs). When teaching new skills or shaping behavior, instead of reinforcing only the final desired skill or behavior, we reinforce or reward steps toward the final behavior. The task is broken down into stages or steps, and the completion of each is rewarded. The process always starts at or below the level where the client is currently performing the skill. In order to cause the behavior to occur, you can use several techniques. These techniques include modeling and graduated guidance. **Modeling** is a powerful technique that is simply showing the person how to perform the task; in other words, the skill is demonstrated for the client. **Graduated guidance** refers to the amount of assistance or prompting necessary (Figure 16-6). During *full graduated guidance,* the staff member maintains thumb and forefinger contact with the client's hands. During another technique, **shadowing,** the hands are kept within one inch of the client's hands while he or she is performing the entire task.

The process of gradually decreasing the amount of guidance is called **fading.** Throughout the training, **prompting** may be gestural, physical, or verbal. You might think of the prompts as techniques a coach uses to get his team to perform. The coach stands at the sidelines and makes gestures (uses signals) to give a player a little push in the direction of the field (physical contact). Once the behavior has been established, the cues are no longer needed, so the cues or prompts are gradually withdrawn. To achieve faster results, it is important for all staff to use the same prompts or cues for the same client. For example, a common prompt is "hands down." Clients will learn the meaning of the phrases and respond more promptly and consistently if each staff member uses the same words for the same prompt.

behavior shaping process of creating a new set of behaviors

modeling a technique of behavior management in which the client is shown how to perform a task

graduated guidance a technique of behavior management in which the amount of assistance or prompting that is necessary is gradually decreased

shadowing a technique of behavior management in which the staff member's hands are kept within one inch of the client's hands while he or she performs a task

fading a technique in behavior management in which the amount of guidance is decreased

prompting a technique used in rehabilitation programs in which the staff verbally reminds the resident what to do next

FIGURE 16-6

Degrees of guidance:
(a) full guidance,
(b) partial guidance,
(c) verbal prompting.

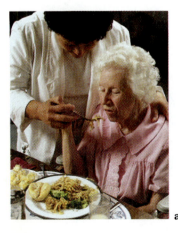
a

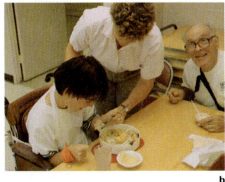
b

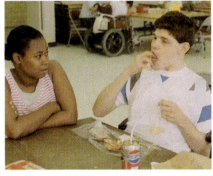
c

Complex skills that are broken down into specific steps can be taught in the order in which they would normally be completed, like links in a chain. This is called **forward chaining.** The same task can also be taught backward. This is called **backward chaining.** Backward chaining is teaching the last step in a skill first, then the next to the last, and so on. The most common example of backward chaining is when teaching a resident to put on his pants. The staff member may do everything except pulling the pants up from the thighs to the waist. The client then completes the task by pulling the pants the rest of the way up. This provides the client with a successful experience and an idea of what the final result or goal is like. The training then proceeds to the skills earlier in the normal sequence. Breaking any task down into the steps required for completion is not simple. It requires time, knowledge, and skill. Usually, the interdisciplinary team will establish the goal and select the task; the QMRP, with help as needed from the occupational therapist or physical therapist, will break the task down and plan the training sequence. The role of the direct care staff is to carry out the plan consistently and accurately.

ELIMINATING UNDESIRABLE BEHAVIORS

Eliminating undesirable behaviors can be accomplished in many ways, some more appropriate than others. The methods can be ranked in order of least restrictive to the most **aversive** (unpleasant or painful). In keeping with the least restrictive alternative principle, the behavior therapist would begin with the least restrictive and progress only if successful. Any plan to modify undesirable behavior must be discussed and approved by a committee in the facility called the Human Rights Committee. This group includes residents, family members, staff members, and client **advocates** (persons who represent residents and act to protect their interests). It is important that the rights of the individual client not be violated. The least restrictive method of modifying an undesirable behavior is to reinforce other behaviors. Another technique considered more restrictive is called *extinction.* When reinforcers are withdrawn and a behavior is ignored, it is eliminated or extinguished. It is important to note here that when a reinforcer is withdrawn and a behavior is ignored the behavior tends to get worse before it gets better. If you are trying to teach your child to sleep through the night, for example, and decide to ignore crying that occurs at four every morning, you'll notice that the first night or two the crying gets worse. If you give in and pick the child up after 45 minutes, you teach the child that if *he or she persists,* you'll eventually give in. If *you* persist instead, the child will begin sleeping through the night. This example assumes of course that there is nothing wrong with the child except a habit of waking up at four in the morning.

In some cases, it is impossible to control the reinforcer since other residents or clients may inadvertently be reinforcing the undesirable behavior. For example, if the client screams, it is natural for others to respond by jumping or turning toward the sound. Some behaviors that are harmful to the client or welfare and safety of others cannot be ignored. In this case, and when all other approaches fail, physical restraint may be necessary. Physical restraint is only used when there is no other alternative. You will receive very strict, specific guidance from your supervisors when there is a need for physical restraint.

Punishment is also rarely used and only under very special, approved circumstances. When aggressive behavior occurs, a procedure called "time-out" may be used. Time-out is not isolation or seclusion. Seclusion (placing a person in a locked room) is not allowed in facilities for the developmentally disabled. Time-out is removing the resident from a reinforcing situation for a brief

(2 to 5 minutes) period of time when the person is engaging in a specific undesirable behavior. As with all behavior-modification techniques, a specific behavior must be identified and a plan written to manage the behavior.

DATA COLLECTION

In addition to providing input into the behaviors in need of change and suggesting reinforcers and carrying out the plan, you will serve a vital role in data collection. The only way a plan is known to be successful is to measure the results. To do this, behaviors are actually counted and recorded in the client's record. Since you are the one with the client most of the time, counting and recording may be your responsibility. Depending on the behavior and the frequency with which it occurs, you may use a tally sheet or a special form for recording.

Remember, the purpose of modifying a client's behavior is to enhance her or his ability to function in a normal environment. Specific behaviors are targeted, observed, and measured. Then a plan is developed, carried out, and evaluated.

SUMMARY This chapter has included many new skills that can be useful in any health care setting. You may never actually work in a home or facility for the developmentally disabled, but the skills of behavior management and reinforcement apply to other situations even as you raise your own children. Should you choose the option of working with the developmentally disabled, you have had the opportunity to learn the basics. You will be provided with more in-depth training once employed by such a facility. Some of the most important concepts you have learned include:

- Protection of the rights of the individual.
- Providing the least restrictive environment possible.
- Promoting normalization.

The Developmental Disabilities Assistance and Bill of Rights Act identified the following core principles in care for the developmentally disabled.

1. *Independence*—Individuals with developmental disabilities and their families are the primary decision makers regarding their lives.
2. *Productivity*—Individuals with developmental disabilities enjoy the opportunity to work, to contribute to society, and to pursue meaningful and productive lives.
3. *Integration and inclusion*—Individuals with developmental disabilities have access to opportunities and the necessary support to be included in community life, have interdependent relationships, live in homes and communities, and make contributions to their families, communities, state, and nation.

OBRA HIGHLIGHTS

Although the OBRA regulations do not pertain to intermediate care facilities for the mentally retarded (ICFMR facilities), some older mentally retarded individuals may live in a skilled nursing facility. According to OBRA, "the facility must promote care for residents in a manner and in an environment that maintains or enhances each resident's dignity and respect in full recognition of his or her individuality." This includes dressing and grooming the resident in an age-appropriate manner. Even though the resident may have a mental age of four and a chronological age of 65, she must be dressed and provided a hairstyle appropriate for a 65-year-old.

SELF STUDY

Choose the best answer for each question or statement.

1. The major causes of developmental disabilities are caused by mental retardation, autism, epilepsy, and
   a. cerebal palsy
   b. car accidents
   c. prenatal events
   d. respiratory illnesses

2. Which of the following is true of a person with mental retardation?
   a. The person's IQ is between 70 and 100.
   b. The person affected is older than 18.
   c. The person has a limited ability to learn.
   d. The person can never be independent.

3. The causes of mental retardation occur during
   a. the prenatal period
   b. the perinatal period
   c. the postnatal period
   d. all of these periods

4. If a person is profoundly retarded, he will
   a. have an IQ of 50 to 70
   b. probably be unable to speak
   c. probably live to be 60 years old
   d. have no physical handicaps

5. Jimmy K. is a resident with cerebral palsy. This means that he
   a. has difficulty controlling his muscles
   b. is severely mentally retarded
   c. will respond in unpredictable ways
   d. will never develop the ability to speak

6. Epilepsy is often present in those with mental retardation or cerebral palsy because
   a. these illnesses cause epilepsy
   b. epilepsy may be caused by the same event that caused these illnesses
   c. people with epilepsy are always mentally retarded
   d. the same part of the brain is affected by all of these illnesses

7. Which of the following would occur in an atmosphere of normalization for developmentally disabled residents?
   a. Staff members assume the roles of parents to the residents.
   b. Residents are dressed in uniforms so they can be easily identified.
   c. Residents are kept separate from the rest of the community.
   d. Residents have personal belongings and items in their rooms that are age appropriate.

8. What is meant by the term *least restrictive environment* when discussing the developmentally disabled person?
   a. The person is in a living environment that allows him to function with the most independence.
   b. Restraints and chemical restraints are prohibited in the living environment of the person.
   c. The person is living with others in a group home or apartment and functioning independently.
   d. The person is living at home with his family or extended family.

9. Which of the following is a behavior?
   a. thinking about a problem
   b. feeling sad about a story
   c. putting on your clothes
   d. desiring to work for money

10. In the ABCs of behavior modification, what does the C stand for?
    a. controlling the behavior
    b. consequences or results of the behavior
    c. the concept of behavior
    d. the client performing the behavior

11. What is the purpose of behavior modification?
    a. Change behavior patterns to eliminate ineffective and teach effective actions.
    b. Punish the resident for performing ineffective behaviors.
    c. Give rewards for performing good behaviors.
    d. Teach a resident how to perform a task such as weighing herself.

12. Which of the following is an example of a social reinforcer used to increase behaviors?
    a. soft drink
    b. pat on the arm
    c. praise
    d. giving a hug

13. When you model how to perform a task, you may use shadowing. This means that you would keep your hands
   a. in contact with the client's hands during the task
   b. on the client's shoulders during the task
   c. away from the client completely during the task
   d. within one inch of the client's hands during the task

14. How is time-out used to decrease aggressive behavior?
   a. The person is placed in a locked room for a specified period of time.
   b. The person is removed from the situation for 2 to 5 minutes.
   c. The person goes to specific place of punishment for a 5-minute stay.
   d. An unpleasant stimulus is given to the person for 2 to 5 minutes.

15. You have been asked to count and record the frequency of a yelling behavior in a resident. You are doing this so that eventually the resident will be able to
   a. function in a normal environment
   b. realize how many times he yells each day
   c. be punished for yelling more than a few times in a day
   d. teach himself not to yell

16. Which of the following is an example of a gross motor activity?
   a. threading a needle
   b. using the telephone
   c. using all the senses
   d. swimming

Getting C O N N E C T E D
Multimedia **Extension** Activities

 www.prenhall.com/will-black

Use the above address to access the free, interactive Companion Website created for this textbook. Hear the pronunciation of the key terms in the chapter. Get instant feedback to a variety of chapter-related questions. Link to other interesting sites.

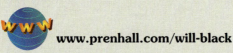 **Video**

Watch the video *Patient Rights* from the Care Provider Skills series.

CASE STUDY

Charlie Sims is a 9-year-old boy who was born with Down's syndrome and multiple physical anomalies including heart, liver, and kidney problems. His parents brought him to the facility when he was 5. They have three other children, all of whom are normal and healthy.

1. Which of the following would be age appropriate to decorate Charlie's room?
   a. pictures of the latest hot musical group
   b. picture of Barbara Streisand
   c. pictures of cars, trucks, and airplanes
   d. pictures of bunnies, chicks, and kittens
2. Charlie is participating in a program to teach functional life skills. This means he will be learning
   a. to dress himself
   b. to work in a sheltered workshop
   c. to speak Spanish
   d. to do math calculations
3. You are told that Charlie needs to develop his gross motor skills. The IPP instructs you to be sure that each day, Charlie
   a. handles money and makes change
   b. goes for a walk
   c. feeds himself
   d. buttons his shirt
4. You are assigned to help at mealtime with clients who need partial guidance. This means that
   a. you must feed the client
   b. you must supervise the clients as they feed themselves
   c. you place your hand on their hand as they bring the spoon to their mouth
   d. you gently touch their hand intermittently to prompt them to bring the spoon to their mouth

Chapter 17

THE RESTORATIVE NURSING ASSISTANT

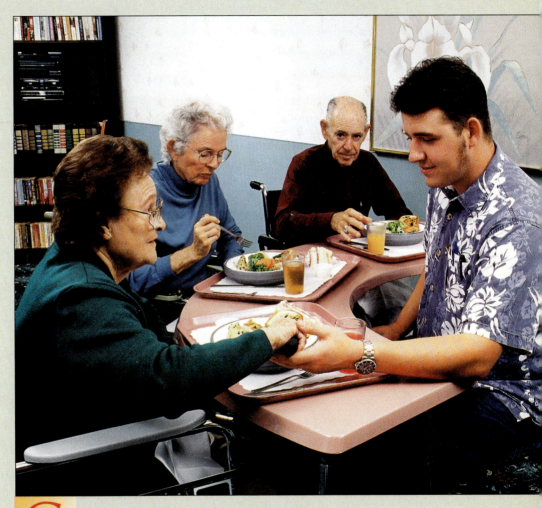

CARING TIP

Regaining lost skills adds to a resident's feelings of self-worth.

Gail Diffley
RN Inservice Educator
Wesley Health Care Center
Saratoga Springs, New York

HEALTH PROMOTION

There is a great need for LTC facilities to focus their efforts toward health promotion and prevention of disease and disability in addition to the treatment of existing and chronic illnesses. Health-promotion activities are programs designed to encourage good health practices. Components might include:

• Exercise
• Good nutrition
• Antismoking
• Discouraging substance abuse

• Health screening
• Immunization
• Socialization

Many of these programs can be offered in the LTC facility through in-house activity, social service, and nursing staff participation as well as through community agencies. When providing care and services to the elderly, prevention of disease and disability must be one of the primary goals!

RESTORATIVE NURSING PROGRAM

In most LTC facilities, there are one or more nursing assistants assigned as restorative nursing assistants (RNAs). These nursing assistants are usually certified nursing assistants who have received additional training in rehabilitation and restorative programs. This training is most often provided by licensed nurses, physical therapists, occupational therapists, and speech therapists.

In other LTC facilities, each nursing assistant will perform specific restorative services as part of her or his daily routine of providing care. Even when the restorative nursing program is delegated to RNAs, the rehabilitative care cannot be isolated and designated as the responsibility of a few. It is the responsibility of the *entire* health care team to continue to focus and direct their care toward maximum rehabilitation of the resident (Figure 17-1). The National Council on Rehabilitation defines **rehabilitation** as follows: "Rehabilitation means the restoration of the individual to the fullest physical, mental, social, vocational, and economic capacity of which he is capable."

rehabilitation the restoration of the individual to the fullest physical, mental, social, vocational, and economic capacity of which he or she is capable

Throughout the book, the importance of preventing disease and deformity as well as maintaining abilities and restoring lost functions has been stressed. It is important to remember that rehabilitation programs should never be limited to physical disabilities or conditions alone. The resident's psychological and social needs must also be included for any program to be successful. These concepts combined are the essential elements of any rehabilitation program.

Nursing assistants selected to work in the restorative nursing program must have a positive attitude about the potential for restoring and retraining residents in basic activities of daily living. This positive attitude should be based on knowledge as well as specialized skills.

The RNA will use all of the restorative skills expected of any nursing assistant, but will also learn additional techniques related to activities of daily living in order to teach and motivate residents to do as much as they are physically capable of doing by themselves.

The physician, licensed nurses, and various therapists will assess the resident's special needs and develop a plan of care that should be followed in order to prevent further disease or deformity. The specific restorative care to be provided is communicated to the resident's physician and a physician's order is given. When you understand that providing restorative care according to the physician's orders is as important as giving the resident the right medication and diet, you will begin to see what an important responsibility the RNA assumes.

The restorative nursing plan will be found on the resident's care plan along with all the other care that is to be provided for the resident. It is helpful for the nursing assistant to understand specifically the goals established for the resident so that all care provided is goal directed. Take time to review the goals and approaches for the resident for whom you will provide restorative nursing care.

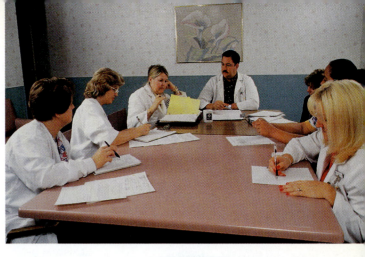

FIGURE 17-1
The rehabilitation team.

DOCUMENTATION BY THE RNA

All the principles of observation and charting previously studied are applicable to the RNA. Accurate documentation is very important due to the fact that the RNA is the only nonprofessional staff member who documents progress or lack of progress to established resident goals in the resident's health record. The RNA will chart care given or attendance at special retraining programs each day by initialing in the appropriate place. Daily programs may require specific narrative charting describing what was done for the resident and the resident's response to the care provided. Notes that would be useful in writing the weekly summary should be kept daily. At a minimum, the resident's progress or lack of progress toward specific goals should be summarized weekly. This weekly summary should be specific, clearly reflecting resident's progress toward goals in behavioral and measurable terms:

Correct: Resident able to stand at bedside with assistance of one for 3 minutes. Balance and strength improving as minimum steadying support is now necessary.

Incorrect: Resident is doing better.

Correct: Resident feeding self using spoon 50 percent of the time versus only 25 percent of the time last week. Requires fewer reminders to use spoon than last week.

Incorrect: Resident using her spoon more, is doing better.

There may be times when residents fail to cooperate with the RNA by refusing to participate in a program or any specific care ordered. When this occurs, it is essential that you:

- Notify the charge nurse of the resident's refusal.
- Chart the resident's refusal as well as the stated reason for refusal: "I'm too tired to walk today"; "My son is coming today, I want to get ready for him early."

SECTION 2 Restorative Nursing Procedures

OBJECTIVES
What You Will Learn

When you have completed this section, you will be able to:

- Demonstrate teaching a resident to perform range-of-motion exercises independently
- Demonstrate teaching a resident to transfer independently
- Select from a given list those statements that are true regarding achieving balance and increasing strength for ambulation
- Demonstrate special positioning techniques to prevent pressure, contractures, and foot drop
- Demonstrate the correct procedure for giving a whirlpool bath
- Describe why performing activities of daily living (ADLs) independently is an important goal for most residents whose functional abilities have been lost or are impaired
- Describe the proper positioning for feeding a resident with dysphagia

KEY TERMS

aspiration   dysphagia

RESTORATIVE NURSING PROCEDURES/GOALS

RANGE-OF-MOTION (ROM) EXERCISES

FIGURE 17-2

Steady the patient by holding the belt at the patient's back.

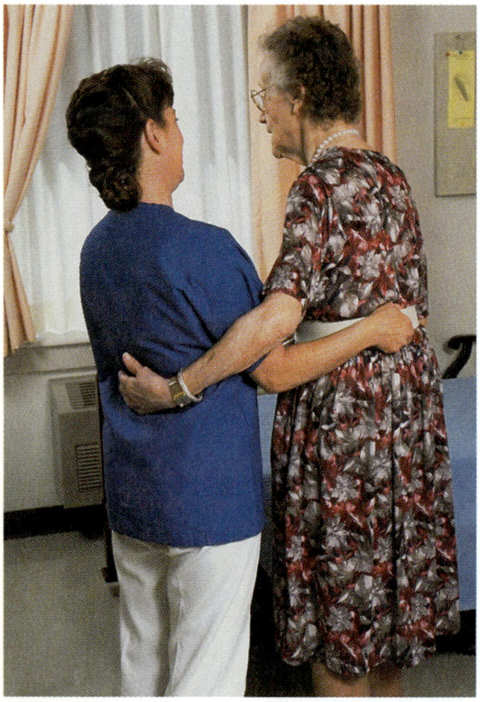

The restorative goal is to preserve the resident's present range, thereby preventing further deterioration, and when possible teach the resident to assist and eventually do ROM exercises independently. The resident may require both active and passive ROM exercises with varying degrees of assistance from the RNA. The physical therapist will provide the RNA with specific instructions if resistive types of exercises are to be used with residents.

TRANSFER TRAINING

The restorative goal could be to achieve independence in transferring from wheelchair to various objects or to transfer with minimal assistance.

ACHIEVING BALANCE IN STANDING, SITTING, OR WALKING

The restorative goals could be to achieve balance in standing, sitting, and walking through increasing strength and practice with the RNA (Figure 17-2).

AMBULATION DEVELOPMENT

The restorative goals could be achieving independence in ambulation, independent ambulation with the use of assistive devices, or increasing ambulation strength and endurance through practice with RNA. Remember to use the safety belt while assisting residents to ambulate (Figure 17-3).

USE OF SPECIAL ASSISTIVE DEVICES

The RNA should be very familiar with how assistive devices can increase independence for residents. The occupational or physical therapist will provide the RNA with additional training in the use of assistive devices. The RNA should observe and monitor the use of these devices with all residents as well as make recommendations to the charge nurse whenever a resident seems to need additional assistive equipment. It is very important that these assistive devices are properly measured and fitted for the resident. The occupational or physical therapist will make necessary recommendations regarding specific equipment. The restorative goals would almost always relate to the resident being able to function independently or with less assistance.

The following are basic guidelines for measuring, fitting, and adjusting assistive devices used in ambulation:

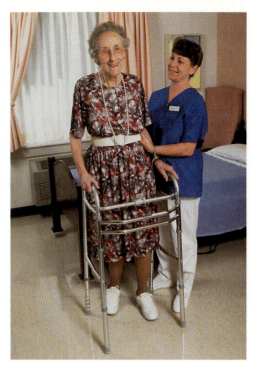

FIGURE 17-3
Ambulating the resident.

- *Walkers*—When the resident is standing erect with hands resting on the hand grips (Figure 17-4), the walker should be at the height of the greater trochanter (straight across from the pubic bone; review the location on the skeletal diagram). There should be approximately 20 degrees flexion at the elbows when the walker is moved forward. The resident should be able to stand erect when moving the walker forward.
- *Crutches*—should be measured from the axilla (arm pit) to the floor and then add 2 to 4 inches. You should be able to insert two to three fingers between the axillary pad on the crutch and the axilla when the crutches are forward 4 and 6 inches out to the side. The hand-grip level should be adjusted to allow 20- to 30-degree flexion of the elbow when moving forward.
- *Canes*—The highest part of the cane should be at the height of the greater trochanter when the cane is at the side. The shoulders should not be elevated or depressed when walking with the cane; they should be level. There should be 20- to 30-degree flexion of the elbow upon movement forward.

The following guidelines should be followed when assisting a resident to relearn how to walk using a walker:

FIGURE 17-4
The walker should be at the proper height.

- *Pick-up walker* (Figure 17-5)—used in non-weight-bearing with progression to full-weight-bearing gait. It is better than crutches for most elderly residents as they feel more secure, and the walker requires less strength and coordination than crutches.
- *Four-wheeled walker*—used to take pressure off the lower back when only moderate or minimal balance impairment exists. It may be used when the resident's upper body strength is poor and she or he is unable to physically pick up and move a walker. It is frequently used when the resident is very close to full weight bearing.
- *Semiwheel walker* (Figure 17-6)—This is the same as a pick-up walker but used when the resident lacks enough strength or endurance.

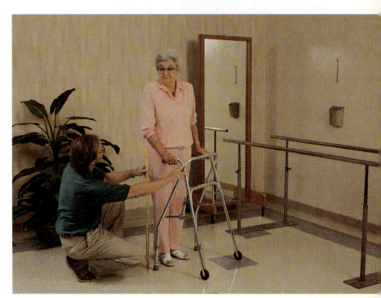

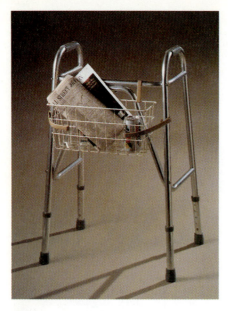

FIGURE 17-5
The pick-up walker.

FIGURE 17-6
The semiwheel walker.

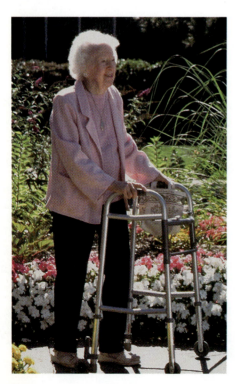

Essential steps to follow when walking a resident with a walker:

- Verify the physician's or physical therapist's order.
- Instruct/inform the resident about the procedure.
- Check joint range of motion and muscle strength.
- Check standing balance.
- Measure and adjust height of walker properly.
- Instruct resident regarding standing and balancing before taking any steps.
- While assisting ambulation with a walker, stand behind the resident and slightly to one side with one hand grasping the safety belt and the other hand ready to grasp the resident's shoulder.

  Note: The gait to be taught will be determined by the physical therapist, based on the disability and its severity. The physical therapist should instruct and initially observe as you assist residents with gait retraining to ensure that proper technique is used. Be sure to follow the therapist's directions.

- *For non-weight-bearing gait:* Stand with weight on uninvolved extremity assisted by walker and use of both upper extremities. Move walker forward and shift weight to upper extremities. Have resident hop forward with uninvolved extremity. Many elderly residents are unable to hop and will use a forward shuffling motion. This is acceptable as long as there is no weight placed on the involved extremity.

- *For partial-weight-bearing gait:* Stand with weight on the uninvolved lower extremity, resting involved extremity on the floor but applying no pressure by supporting the body with the upper extremities on the walker. Move the walker forward, keeping the weight on the upper extremities. Step forward with involved lower extremity, allowing partial weight bearing as ordered by the physician or therapist. Then bring uninvolved lower extremity forward. Repeat.

  - *For full-weight-bearing gait:* Stand with weight evenly distributed or balanced on both extremities, resting hands on walker. Move walker forward, and shift weight to upper extremities. Step forward with involved extremity, and then bring uninvolved extremity forward.

SPECIAL POSITIONING/PREVENTATIVE TECHNIQUES

The restorative goals could be to prevent development of pressure areas or contractures, to use protective devices to position residents so range of motion is not impaired, to prevent foot drop, and to position residents to promote comfort and reduce pain.

WEIGHING, MEASURING, AND REPORTING CHANGES

The RNA is commonly assigned to weigh and measure height of residents on admission as well as on a monthly basis. Because monitoring the resident's weight is an important nursing responsibility, it is often assigned to one person who has demonstrated competence in weighing and measuring residents and who is familiar with balancing the scales when necessary.

The RNA should understand the importance of weighing residents under the same conditions and at approximately the same time of day. Most facilities have the RNA report the monthly weights to the charge nurse for evaluation and recording in the resident's health record. The licensed nurse is responsible for notifying the physician, dietitian, or family of significant fluctuations in the resident's weight.

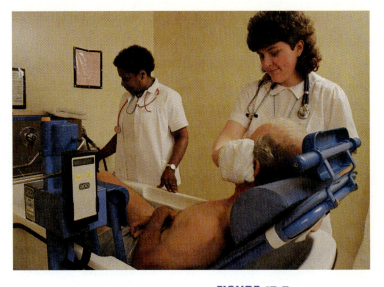

FIGURE 17-7

Giving a whirlpool bath.

GIVING WHIRLPOOL OR MEDICINAL BATHS

The RNA works closely with licensed nursing personnel and the physical therapist when the physician orders whirlpool baths. Specific types of whirlpool therapy may be ordered to achieve a desired effect. Restorative goals could be:

- To stimulate circulation to a particular limb or area
- To cleanse a wound through circulation of water and antiseptic additives ordered by the physician
- To loosen and remove dead, necrotic tissue through the agitation of water against the area
- To relieve tension and discomfort as a relaxation technique
- To apply soothing medications

In some facilities, a mechanical lift will be used to place the resident in the whirlpool tub (Figure 17-7). Water temperature should be the same for a regular bath, 105°F. The physician may order a specific type of antiseptic solution to be added to the bath. The RNA should follow the directions of the licensed nurse or the physical therapist when adding solutions or medications to the whirlpool.

Review the procedures for giving baths in Chapter 6 and make sure to take all safety precautions. The whirlpool bath differs in that the water is agitated through a mechanical device. As with any equipment, it is essential that you understand the exact procedure to be followed for the equipment you are using. Follow manufacture's guidelines and clarify any questions or concerns. Special infection control procedures must be followed to properly clean and sanitize the whirlpool between baths. Due to the fact that open wounds are treated with whirlpool therapy and there is a potential for cross-infection, the policies for cleaning and disinfection of the whirlpool must be followed strictly.

BEHAVIOR MANAGEMENT

The restorative goals of any behavior management program are directed toward changing behavior and replacing undesirable behavior with desirable or more acceptable behavior. The multidisciplinary health care team will develop a plan of care designed to change or modify behavior. It may be the responsibility of the RNA to monitor the implementation of the plan along with the licensed nurse. Sometimes, it takes several kinds of approaches to the problem before behavior changes.

The following is an example of what a behavior management care plan might include:

Problem: Resident yells "help me" continuously.

Approach: Identify times when yelling behavior is increased or decreased. Identify any possible "triggering" factors that initiate the yelling behavior. Identify any factors that decrease yelling behavior. Have staff spend time with resident when he or she is not yelling. Implement factors identified that decrease yelling behavior. When resident is yelling, decrease communication to essential needs only.

Goal: Yelling behavior will decrease from continuous yelling to extend to periods of 30 minutes without yelling by date _____.

Throughout the book are many references to appropriate ways to deal with residents who have behavior problems. Be sure you review and understand the basic principles outlined. See the behavior management section in Chapter 16.

COMMUNICATION DEVELOPMENT

Assisting residents who have difficulty speaking, expressing themselves, and making their needs known is one of the most challenging tasks of any nursing assistant. Probably the most important nursing skill that can be developed is *patience!* There is nothing more frustrating to residents or staff than the inability to communicate; taking time to listen as well as making every attempt to understand that meaning is essential to the emotional well-being of the resident (Figure 17-8).

The speech therapist will generally work with residents who have speech problems and will make specific recommendations to the staff regarding appropriate ways to communicate with the resident. Understanding the different types of speech problems outlined in Chapter 11 will assist you in working more effectively with these residents.

Frequently, the RNA will take the restorative program over from the speech therapist at the appropriate time. The speech therapist will instruct the RNA in exactly how to practice various speech patterns with the resident and how best to communicate with the resident. The communication development program will be outlined in the resident's plan of care so that all who provide care can consistently use the same approach with the resident. When communication can be reestablished for a resident, you will find this event one of the most rewarding experiences in providing nursing care.

FIGURE 17-8

Assisting a resident to communicate requires patience.

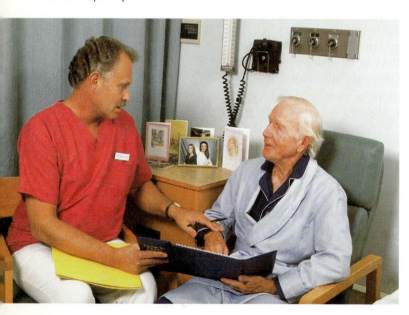

ACTIVITIES OF DAILY LIVING

For those who are well and have no functional impairments, performing activities of daily living is almost automatic. However, when these basic functions are lost, it is frustrating and devastating to residents (Figure 17-9). The loss of control and then dependence on others is both frightening and humiliating. Because ADLs are so basic to our independent lifestyle, these are often the first problems to be addressed in therapy with the impaired resident.

Each resident should be evaluated to determine if he or she could benefit from the ADL program. The evaluation may be done with the physical and/or occupational therapists. Often, a form is completed and placed in the resident's chart. The evaluation includes how much assistance is needed to perform each of the ADL skills.

Commonly used terms are *supervision, standby assistance,* and *minimal, moderate,* and *maximum assistance.* Supervision refers to the need to have a staff member present to provide encouragement and verbal guidance. Standby assist means that a staff member is present to observe and be readily available if help is needed. Minimum assistance usually means that the resident performs about 75 percent of the task and the nursing assistant performs the remaining 25 percent. Moderate assist means that the resident performs about half or 50 percent and the nursing assistant performs the other 50 percent. Maximum assist usually refers to the resident performing 25 percent and the nursing assistant performing 75 percent of the task.

Figure 17-10 is an example of an evaluation that might be used to select candidates for an ADL program and to help set individual goals and approaches.

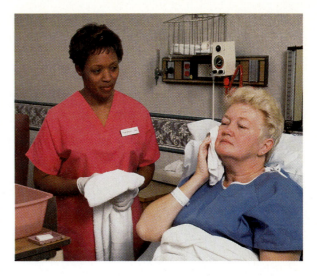

FIGURE 17-9

Encourage indepedence in all ADLs.

RESTORATIVE DINING OR SELF-FEEDING PROGRAMS

The restorative dining program is one of the most important aspects of the restorative nursing program. The major purpose of the program is to assist residents to attain their highest level of independence in eating (Figure 17-11). Each resident should be evaluated by the occupational therapist prior to entry into the program. The resident must have some restorative potential for retraining. The resident who requires feeding and has little restorative potential should be identified and grouped with other residents with similar needs. You need to think of "feeding" and "restorative eating" differently.

CULTURAL AWARENESS You may notice that some residents are less able to feed themselves when family members are visiting or some family members seem to interfere with your program by feeding the resident when they visit. It is important for you to understand that in some cultures, the family is expected to provide care for their elderly family members. In those same cultures, independence may not be highly valued or considered important. Knowing this will help you to set realistic goals and to avoid becoming frustrated or annoyed by the actions of the family.

Residents who are assigned to this program should be those who *do not* have swallowing difficulties but who have difficulty in eating independently. Residents with swallowing problems or other eating difficulties are at high risk for aspiration, and they require special therapeutic assessment as well as a specific plan of care that should be developed by the licensed nurse or occupational therapist. Special feeding techniques to be used for residents with swallowing difficulties should be reviewed and practiced under the direction of the occupational or speech therapist.

Candidates for the program include those who have recently lost some of their self-feeding skills, who have physical disabilities that would benefit from learning to use adaptive equipment, or who have recently completed an

ADL EVALUATION

Name _____ Date of Birth _____
Date of Admission _____ Physician _____
Diagnosis _____
_____

MENTAL STATUS	yes	no
Able to make needs known		
Able to follow one- and two-step commands		
Can attend for at least 5 to 10 minutes		

HEARING
Normal _____
Wears prosthesis _____
Hard of hearing _____
Able to hear best in   Right _____ Left _____ ear.

VISION
Normal _____
Wears glasses _____
Blind _____

RANGE OF MOTION	Able R L	Partially Able R L	Unable R L
Reach hands above head			
Cross arm across chest			
Reach down toward floor			
Bend knees			
Straighten legs			
Move leg away from the body			
Right-handed _____ Left-handed _____ Able to use nondominant hand			
Tremor	mild	moderate	severe
Contractures	mild	moderate	severe
Specify joints involved _____			

Pinch	good	fair	poor
Grasp	good	fair	poor

BALANCE/MOBILITY			
Sitting	good	fair	poor
Standing balance	good	fair	poor
Transfers	light	moderate	severe
Mobility	fully ambulatory	amb. with equip.	nonambulatory
Sitting tolerance _____			minutes.

DRESSING	SUPERVISE	STANDBY	MIN.	MOD.	MAX.	UNABLE
Put on shirt						
Line up buttons						
Button/fasten						
Unbutton/remove						
Get undergarments						
Pull pants over feet						
Stand to pull up						
Put on socks/shoes						
Tie/fasten shoes						
BATHING						
Wash face						
Wash upper body						
Wash perineal area						
Wash legs/feet						
GROOMING						
Brush teeth/dentures						
Brush/comb hair						
Shave						
Apply deodorant						
Apply makeup						

FIGURE 17-10

Sample evaluation form to select candidates for an ADL program.

occupational therapy program and need more practice. Some programs also include residents who take a long time to eat (more than 45 minutes) or who have been refusing to eat.

Residents participating in the restorative eating program may be able to feed themselves but have other eating behaviors that are not socially acceptable such as food stealing, throwing food, making noises, or using hands to eat inappropriately. The format/structure of a dining program should include the following:

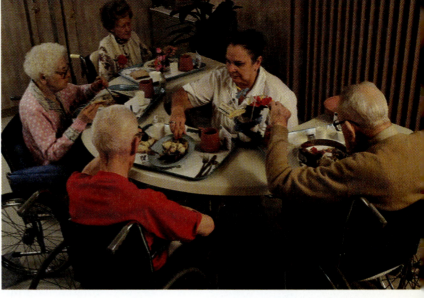

FIGURE 17-11

Assisting residents to attain their highest level of independence in eating.

- Class size should be small with no more than four to six residents assigned for each RNA. (Class size should take into consideration the amount of assistance each participating resident needs.)
- The room for the program should be attractive, well-ventilated, with good lighting, and free from distractions. Making the environment as inviting as possible with tablecloths, flowers, and the like, sets the stage for a positive dining experience.
- Residents participating in the dining program should be grouped together according to their functional abilities. When high-level functioning residents are placed with low-level functioning residents, they regress. If more than one seating is not possible, segregate seating by placing the groups at different tables.
- Each resident who participates in the program should have program goals as well as the appropriate actions and approaches identified on the care plan. This is usually coordinated by the occupational therapist and the licensed nurse. The RNA should follow the plan and report changes in condition or progress to the charge nurse immediately.
- Make sure that any necessary adaptive equipment that has been recommended for the resident is available at each meal. (The occupational therapist is generally responsible for recommending the type of adaptive equipment most appropriate for the resident.)
- Residents must be clean, dry, and properly positioned for mealtime.

RESTORATIVE DINING CARE PLAN ENTRIES

The interdisciplinary team will assess the resident and develop specific care plan goals based on each resident's identified needs. Sample care plan entries are shown below.

Problem: J. Jones uses her fingers for all foods and does not use appropriate utensils.

Approach: Hand spoon to Mrs. Jones when she is given her food. If she begins to use fingers, place your hand across the hand gently and say, "No Mrs. Jones, use your spoon," and hand her the spoon again. Repeat this process as often as necessary during a meal period. Praise when using spoon.

Goal: Mrs. Jones will use a spoon rather than fingers to eat by date _____.

Problem:	Mr. Smith gets up and leaves table many times during meal period.
Approach:	Sit Mr. Smith at table when tray is ready to be served. Set up tray for meal and get him started. When he starts to get up, place hand on shoulder and encourage him to finish minimum of 50 percent before getting up. After getting up, return him to table and repeat until 100 percent has been consumed. Praise for staying seated.
Goal:	Mr. Smith will consume 100 percent of food getting up only one time by date _____.
Problem:	Mr. Hall has left-sided paresis and is unable to use left hand to stabilize dish while eating.
Approach:	Use adaptive dish with suction cup to stabilize on table. Use plate with an inner lip to make scooping food onto spoon or fork easier. Praise successful attempts.
Goal:	D. Hall will feed self 50 percent of meal using suction dish with inner lip by date _____.

Residents who fail to make progress toward established goals need to be reevaluated by either the licensed nurse or occupational therapist. Report lack of progress immediately.

FEEDING A RESIDENT WITH DYSPHAGIA

dysphagia difficulty in swallowing

aspiration inhaling food or fluid into the lungs

Dysphagia means difficulty in swallowing. Residents participating in a restorative nursing program may be experiencing dysphagia due to a recent stroke. Many recover their ability to swallow while others must adapt their way of eating and the kinds of foods they eat for the remainder of their lives. Other factors that may increase the risk for dysphagia include Parkinson's disease, Alzheimer's disease and other forms of dementia, and use of certain kinds of medications. Special feeding techniques are required to prevent the resident from choking and from aspirating food. **Aspiration** means to take material such as food or liquids into the lungs. This is a serious complication that may lead to pneumonia and result in the death of the resident. Residents with dysphagia are also at risk for malnutrition, poor wound healing, and reduced ability to fight infection.

Signs of dysphagia include choking, coughing, and vomiting. Some have difficulty chewing, eat slowly, and hold food in their mouth. Their swallowing may be difficult or slow. Usually, it is easier to swallow solid food than liquids. If you notice any resident with these signs, report to the charge nurse immediately.

Often, a speech therapist or occupational therapist will perform an evaluation to determine the safest way to feed the resident with dysphagia. He or she may use the information provided from a video fluoroscopy—a procedure showing the entire swallowing process. This is done in a hospital setting.

Some possible treatments include use of a feeding tube, either permanently or temporarily, and modification of the diet and eating techniques. You may notice that there is a sign over the bed or a note in the resident's care plan that says "thickened liquids only." There are substances available to be added to liquids that thicken them and make them easier to swallow. Be sure you are aware of which of the residents require their liquids to be thickened or those who have no liquids. In addition to specific instructions for each individual resident, follow the guidelines listed below when feeding a resident with dysphagia (Figure 17-12).

GUIDELINES

- Review the instructions/plan of care.
- Provide a pleasant environment.
- Sit down.
- Position the resident sitting up with the hips at a 90-degree angle.
- The neck should be flexed at about 45 degrees.
- Encourage the resident to keep her head down, swallow, then rest.
- Use a spoon to place about ½ teaspoon of food on the tongue.
- Avoid offering dry foods.
- Be patient!
- Offer encouraging comments.
- Observe the swallowing process.
- Check for food left in the mouth.
- Record the amount eaten as well as observations about the process.

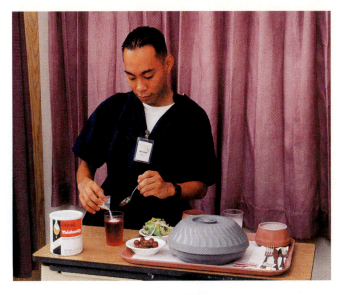

FIGURE 17-12

Feeding a resident with dysphagia; CNA adding a thickening agent to liquids.

BOWEL/BLADDER RETRAINING PROGRAMS

Bowel and bladder retraining programs cannot be delegated to the RNA alone because a successful program must involve all those who provide care to the resident. However, once a plan has been developed, the RNA may be assigned to assume responsibility for:

- Monitoring its implementation
- Teaching other nursing assistants basic elements of the program
- Monitoring daily documentation of nursing assistants
- Monitoring completion of accurate intake/output records

The key to a successful retraining program is consistency. The staff must follow the plan developed and chart the resident's progress or lack of progress each day. If a plan is not working, report this information to the licensed nurse, who can reassess and change the plan if necessary.

SELF-GROOMING PROGRAMS

The development of a self-grooming program can be fun, and residents generally respond positively to programs designed to improve their appearance. Sometimes, it is easier to motivate them toward improved self-grooming than toward improved personal hygiene, which always needs to be included with any self-grooming program. Because self-grooming tasks are usually performed along with the A.M. care or the bath/shower, group classes are not as appropriate as an individualized approach.

The RNA along with the licensed nurse and the occupational therapist can develop a plan for self-grooming after assessment of the resident's functional abilities. The RNA as well as the assigned nursing assistants will be responsible for the implementation of the plan. Documenting the resident's progress or lack of progress each week in the weekly summary is essential. The RNA frequently becomes the "coordinator" of the self-grooming program, working with the assigned nursing assistants to see that the plan is implemented consistently. Remember, the primary purpose of the program is to teach the resident to perform self-grooming and personal hygiene tasks as independently as possible.

Appearance is generally important to all of us; however, if residents do not have access to mirrors, they may not be as motivated to improve their appearance. Having hand mirrors and wall mirrors in residents' rooms has a positive impact on their willingness to work at improving their appearance.

Teaching residents to brush their teeth again, to shave, and to comb their hair is not difficult if you are able to carry out these basic procedures competently for a dependent resident. Review these procedures and make the necessary adaptations to allow the resident to perform independently if possible or with minimal assistance. Remember, regaining skills takes time and patience in addition to accepting the reality that the end result may not be as good as if the task were performed by someone else. Some residents particularly enjoy having makeup applied for them or having someone give them a manicure. Reward residents who are working toward self-grooming goals with these "extras" when possible.

SELF-DRESSING PROGRAMS

Again the RNA along with the licensed nurse and the occupational therapist will need to assess the resident's special needs in order to set up a plan of care. The plan must be very specific because the assigned nursing assistant will most often be responsible for implementing the plan. The RNA can review the plan as well as special dressing techniques with the nursing assistant and monitor the resident's progress several times a week in order to document in the weekly summary specifically what progress has been made.

Relearning to dress oneself takes time! At first, it may take a resident up to 1 hour to complete the task. Later, after much practice, dressing may be completed in 15 minutes. Your patience in allowing as much time as needed makes the difference between a resident who is frustrated by what he can't do and the resident who is proud of what he can do!

Remember the goal is to teach the resident to dress independently if possible. If the resident needs to use assistive devices to reach the goal, be sure that they are available consistently. If you have any questions regarding the need for or use of special assistive devices, talk with the occupational therapist.

EXERCISE PROGRAMS

Physical fitness and group exercise programs are among the most well-received restorative nursing programs offered. Groups of residents with similar abilities can be brought together to perform exercises. In a group they encourage one another and work harder to keep up with the group. Music is used to create an atmosphere of fun and energy. The program usually includes active range of motion beginning with the head and working down to range each of the joints about three times. Sometimes the exercise is provided by kicking and tossing a beach ball or by using a parachute to wave up and down. There are also simple dance records such as "the Hokey Pokey" that provide fun and exercise. The exercise program is an opportunity for almost every resident to participate regardless of mental status, ability to communicate, or ability to perform ADL skills. Residents feel good about themselves when they participate in an exercise program.

The restorative nursing program must be a total program that involves all who provide care. When a program can be developed that directly involves each nursing assistant providing the above-mentioned kinds of care every day, the facility can be proud of its commitment to restorative and rehabilitative philosophies.

SUMMARY

Helping to restore the resident to a previous level of functioning contributes to the quality of life and the morale of the resident. Doing things for himself and not needing to depend on others makes the resident feel better. It also gives more control over daily living. The resident who can feed himself can eat in the order he wants, in the time he wants, and the amount he wants to eat. This feeling of being in control is one that many residents value greatly, particularly if they have been in control all of their lives. Many people feel less worthy when they must depend on others to help them meet their daily needs. Whether you are in the role of being a restorative nursing assistant or not, it is important to use the skills and techniques learned in this chapter to provide each of your residents with the best care possible. Using a positive approach, encourage the resident to do as much as possible for himself. Be aware of the limitations and don't demand that the resident go beyond what is safe or possible to do. Remember to praise all successes with words like "Good job," or "You did that very well," or "You are doing better every day." The praise must, of course, be honest and sincere. Helping restore the resident to a prior level of functioning requires you to:

- Work as a member of a team.
- Be consistent.
- Follow the plan of care.
- Be patient!

Restoring function takes time. It does not happen overnight. Learn to notice and praise even the smallest progress. If there is no progress, praise the effort. If the resident refuses to try, drop the subject and bring it up later.

By using these approaches to the care of residents, you will be able to make a positive difference in their lives.

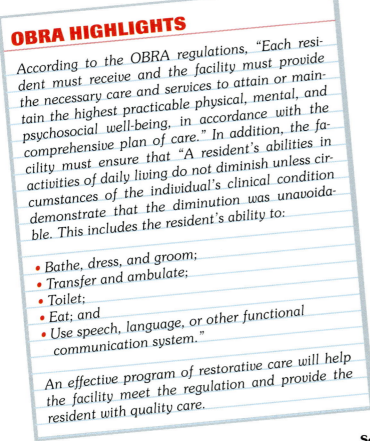

OBRA HIGHLIGHTS

According to the OBRA regulations, "Each resident must receive and the facility must provide the necessary care and services to attain or maintain the highest practicable physical, mental, and psychosocial well-being, in accordance with the comprehensive plan of care." In addition, the facility must ensure that "A resident's abilities in activities of daily living do not diminish unless circumstances of the individual's clinical condition demonstrate that the diminution was unavoidable. This includes the resident's ability to:

- Bathe, dress, and groom;
- Transfer and ambulate;
- Toilet;
- Eat; and
- Use speech, language, or other functional communication system."

An effective program of restorative care will help the facility meet the regulation and provide the resident with quality care.

SELF STUDY

Choose the best answer for each question or statement.

1. Who is responsible for focusing and directing care toward maximum rehabilitation of the resident?
   a. the admitting nurse
   b. the restorative nursing assistant (RNA)
   c. the physical therapy department
   d. the entire health care team

2. Which of the following is the responsibility of an RNA?
   a. assisting the resident with ADLs
   b. teaching residents to be as independent as possible
   c. motivating residents to do all they are capable of doing
   d. all of the above

3. Which of the following is the correct method for documenting a resident's progress toward rehabilitation goals?
   a. Resident is standing better, but still needs help to transfer.
   b. Resident stands alone for short periods, but can fall if left alone.
   c. Resident is able to stand at bedside with minimal assistance for 2 minutes.
   d. Resident shows improvement in standing and is trying hard to transfer without help.

4. You are assisting Mr. Melvin with his walker. How can you tell if the walker is the correct height for him?
   a. The hand grips should be at the height of his greater trochanter when he is standing.
   b. The hand grips should be even with his waist when he is standing.
   c. The hand grips should be at the height of his greater trochanter when he is sitting.
   d. The hand grips should be even with his waist when he is sitting.

5. Mr. Melvin has a partially paralyzed left arm. Which assistive device would be the best choice for him?
   a. a pick-up walker
   b. a semiwheel walker
   c. crutches
   d. a four-wheeled walker

6. You are an RNA assigned to weigh each resident monthly. Which of the following principles should you follow when you weigh the residents?
   a. Weigh only the residents who are able to stand.
   b. Weigh the residents at approximately the same time of day each month.
   c. Report only weight changes of 5 pounds or more to the charge nurse.
   d. Weigh residents immediately after a meal.

7. Which of the following is *not* a reason for whirlpool therapy?
   a. to stimulate circulation to an area
   b. to loosen and remove necrotic tissue
   c. to decrease the frequency of giving baths
   d. to relieve tension and discomfort

8. The ADL evaluation form shows that Mrs. Adams needs moderate assistance with bathing. This means that Mrs. Adams can
   a. complete about 25 percent of her bath alone
   b. complete about 50 percent of her bath alone
   c. complete about 75 percent of her bath alone
   d. bathe herself complete with a staff member providing verbal guidance

9. The nursing facility where you work is establishing a restorative eating program. Which of the following residents would *not* be an appropriate candidate for the program?
   a. Mrs. Gray, who used to feed herself, but has recently lost the use of her left arm
   b. Mr. Brown, who has just completed occupational therapy, but needs practice feeding himself
   c. Mrs. White, who can feed herself, but likes to take food from the trays of other residents
   d. Mr. Green, who chokes very easily and cannot feed himself

10. Mr. Borders is on a bowel and bladder retraining program. Who is responsible for documenting his progress or lack of process each day?
    a. the RNA
    b. the charge nurse
    c. the physical therapist
    d. the nursing staff

11. Which of the following could improve self-grooming of residents?
    a. establishing self-grooming group classes
    b. color-coordinating each resident's clothing
    c. hanging wall mirrors in each resident's room
    d. establishing a wall chart with stars for excellent grooming

12. Mr. Borders is relearning to dress himself after a stroke. Which of the following is appropriate restorative care for him?
    a. Allow him 1 hour to dress himself; after that, finish anything he has not accomplished.
    b. Allow him one-half hour to dress himself, and after that finish for him.
    c. Allow him to take as much time as he needs to dress himself and praise his efforts.
    d. Allow him to try a new dressing task each day until he can dress himself completely.

13. Which of the following would be included in a group exercise program?
    a. music for an atmosphere of fun and energy
    b. active ROM exercises
    c. opportunity for almost every resident to participate
    d. all of the above

14. What happens when high-level functioning residents are grouped with low-level functioning residents in a dining program?

    a. They help teach lower-functioning residents to feed themselves.
    b. They regress to lower-functioning behavior.
    c. They eat less because of the atmosphere.
    d. All of the above will happen.

15. After completing a whirlpool bath for a resident, what should the RNA do next?
    a. Follow special infection control procedures to sanitize the tub before bathing the next resident.
    b. Bathe remaining residents, then sanitize the whirlpool at the end of the shift.
    c. Rinse the tub well with 120° water, then bathe the next resident.
    d. Squirt a disinfectant into the bath water for the next resident to prevent cross-infection.

16. Mr. Goldfarb is beginning to use a walker. He is able to bear weight fully on both legs, but his left leg is weak. When you work with him using the walker, you will remind him to move the walker forward, then
    a. move his right foot forward, followed by his left foot
    b. move his left foot forward, followed by his right foot
    c. move both feet forward at once, supporting his weight on the walker
    d. move his left foot forward but do not touch it to the ground, then move his right foot forward

Getting CONNECTED
Multimedia **Extension** Activities

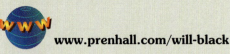 **www.prenhall.com/will-black**

Use the above address to access the free, interactive Companion Website created for this textbook. Hear the pronunciation of the key terms in the chapter. Get instant feedback to a variety of chapter-related questions. Link to other interesting sites.

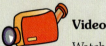 **Video**

Watch the section on assisting with dressing in the *Personal Care* video from the Care Provider Skills series.

CASE STUDY

You are assigned to fill in for the RNA while she takes 2 days off.

1. You are told that Mrs. Anderson has dysphagia and needs to be fed. You immediately begin to plan what you will need to do. You remember that
   a. you will be feeding her liquids only
   b. you must feed her slowly
   c. you will take her to the dining room to have a private dinner with her husband
   d. you will be feeding her with a syringe

2. The most serious potential complication from dysphagia is
   a. pressure ulcer
   b. contracture
   c. aspiration
   d. elopement

3. You remember from your training that the positioning of Mrs. Anderson is important. You will position her
   a. on her left side
   b. with her neck flexed at 45 degrees
   c. next to her husband
   d. sitting at a 60-degree angle

4. You also remember that you must
   a. offer encouraging comments
   b. check for food left in her mouth
   c. be patient
   d. all of the above

Chapter 18

SUBACUTE AND EMERGENCY CARE

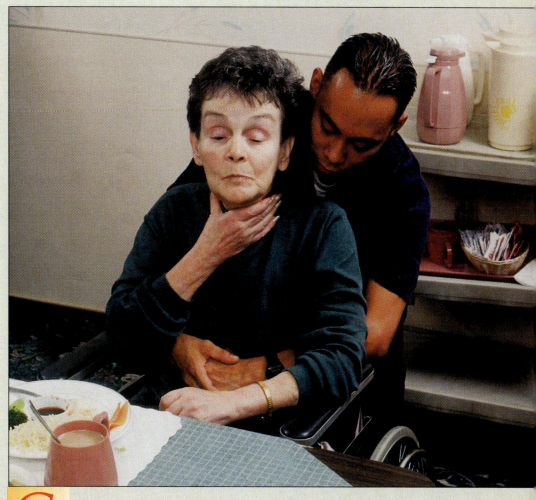

CARING TIP

A person never knows when this skill may be needed but when it is, it leaves a good feeling to know that you performed it correctly and saved someone's life.

Sue Archer, RNC
Health Occupations Instructor
Puxico, Missouri

SECTION 1   The Subacute Unit

OBJECTIVES
What You Will Learn

When you have completed this section, you will be able to:

- Identify the types of services provided in a subacute unit
- Describe in your own words why the nursing assistant working in a subacute unit must be very well trained

KEY TERMS

intensive rehabilitation programs   medical subacute

medical subacute care for medically complex patients requiring specialized services

intensive rehabilitation programs services provided at a fast pace often involving several kinds of therapy requiring 2 to 3 hours per day

FIGURE 18-1

Intensive rehabilitation.

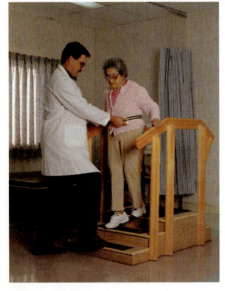

Many long-term care facilities offer subacute care. The care is often provided in a special part of the facility that has been designed or remodeled to allow for more advanced nursing, rehabilitation, and medical services. The unit allows patients to leave the acute hospital sooner and prepares them to be sent home or to a lesser level of care. Usually, the person is referred to as a patient because his or her length of stay is about 30 days and the care is "hospital-like."

Included in subacute care are the following types of services:

- **Medical subacute**—for medically complex patients requiring specialized treatment or services such as:
  —Intravenous therapy
  —Postoperative/postsurgical care
  —Complex wound care
  —Tracheostomy care
  —Head/brain injury care
  —Respiratory care
  —Ventilator care
  —Specialized cancer care
- **Intensive rehabilitation programs**—physical, occupational, and speech therapies are offered. Because the patients may be younger and in better physical health, the rehabilitation may be more intense in duration and frequency than in the elderly rehabilitation patient.

When patients no longer require the services of an acute hospital, but the care is too complex to be provided in most long-term care facilities, the subacute unit may be utilized. Some facilities offer specialized subacute services for those with severe brain injuries and for those in a vegetative state in which the care is complex. These patients may have extended lengths of stay and may be younger than the traditional long-term care resident. Also, patients who require intensive rehabilitation following traumatic injuries are frequently admitted to subacute units for short-term stays prior to going home. The subacute unit provides the long-term care facility with the ability to provide expanded services to its long-term residents when the need arises. The hospital stay can be shortened by sending the resident from the acute hospital to the subacute unit. Following completion of their intensive rehabilitation or improvement in their medical or surgical condition, they may then return to their "home" in the long-term section.

The nursing assistant working in a subacute unit must be very well trained and have developed advanced skills in order to provide quality care to the patients (Figure 18-1).

OBJECTIVES
What You Will Learn

When you have completed this section, you will be able to:

- Select from a given list those statements which are true related to infusion therapy
- List four important observations that should be reported to the charge nurse immediately when providing care to a patient with an intravenous line
- Describe the primary role of the nursing assistant in providing care to a patient with an intravenous line or a Port-a-cath
- State in your own words why the nursing assistant must report any changes of condition to the charge nurse immediately when caring for a resident with head and brain injuries
- Identify specific nursing actions which will promote wound healing
- List the signs of respiratory distress which should be reported immediately to the licensed nurse when caring for a patient with a tracheostomy

KEY TERMS

first intention healing
increased intracranial pressure
patient-controlled analgesic
  (PCA) pump
peripherally inserted central
  catheter (PICC line) and
  Port-a-cath
second intention healing
wound

INTRAVENOUS INFUSION THERAPY

The responsibility of the nursing assistant in providing care to a patient receiving intravenous therapy is to give safe care. To do this, you need to have a basic understanding of the goals of infusion therapy and your role and responsibilities in providing care.

The goal of infusion therapy is to maintain or replace the water electrolytes, vitamins, proteins, fats, and calories needed by the body when a patient is unable to maintain adequate intake by mouth. Intravenous (IV) therapy includes any medication or fluid that is prescribed by a physician to be given directly into a person's bloodstream. Intravenous infusion is also used to deliver certain kinds of medications.

The fluid to be given is contained in a plastic bag that hangs on a pole above the patient's bed or is suspended on a pole next to the bed. Usually, infusions are delivered through a pump or rate-control device to ensure that the rate of infusion is accurate as ordered by the physician (Figure 18-2).

The substance ordered by the physician is infused through either a plastic needle, plastic tube, or surgically implanted catheter that allows repeated use of a site without having to insert a new catheter. These catheters are usually implanted in the upper chest area and may be referred to as a **peripherally inserted central catheter (PICC line)** or a **Port-a-cath** (Figure 18-3). Another advantage of this type of line is that the patient is not always hooked up to an infusion bag, pump, and pole, which limits mobility. Some medications can actually be given directly into the Port-a-cath by the registered nurse.

peripherally inserted central catheter (PICC line) and **Port-a-cath** devices implanted under the skin to give easy access to the veins for medication administration

FIGURE 18-2
Intravenous infusion therapy.

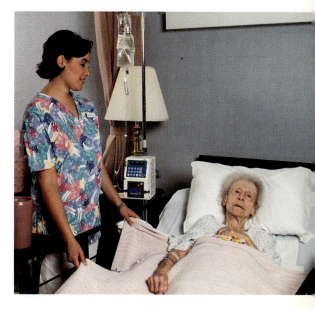

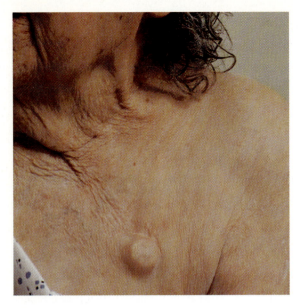

FIGURE 18-3

A Port-a-cath implanted under the skin.

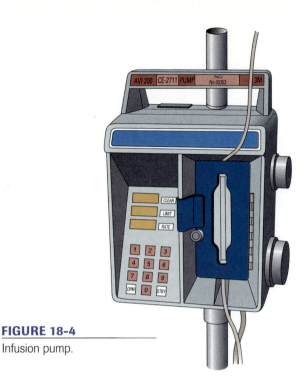

FIGURE 18-4

Infusion pump.

The nursing assistant should understand the basic operation of the infusion pump so that the charge nurse can be notified immediately if the pump is not operating properly. On the infusion pump there is a drip chamber; you can tell if the fluid is flowing by looking at the drops in this chamber. If no fluid is dripping, notify the charge nurse immediately (Figure 18-4).

The nursing assistant is *never* permitted to adjust the infusion pump or to adjust the clamp on the tubing. The nursing assistant is never responsible for starting or maintaining IV infusions.

The IV site is usually covered with a transparent dressing to stabilize the needle or catheter, as well as to provide a barrier to disease-causing bacteria. The dressing should be kept clean and dry; notify the charge nurse if the dressing is soiled or if the dressing is dislodged or missing.

The patient with an IV requires the same good nursing care as every other patient. Don't allow your concern about dislodging the tubing to cause you to

---

Nursing Assistant Responsibilities When Caring for a Patient with an IV Infusion

The role of the nursing assistant in providing care to a patient with an intravenous line or Port-a-cath is primarily one of providing care in such a way as to avoid any pulling or tension on the tubing or catheter and to protect the site from possible infection.

Other responsibilities include reporting any of the following observations to the charge nurse:

- Alarm ringing on the pump
- Noticeable changes in rate of flow or near-empty bag or bottle
- Drainage from the IV site
- Redness, swelling, or formation of a red streak at the IV or Port-a-cath site
- Difficulty breathing
- Signs of fever
- Fluid or blood leaking onto the bed or floor

CARE OF THE PATIENT WITH AN IV

- Wash hands thoroughly before providing care.
- Reassure the patient that you have been instructed in the proper care of the patient with an IV.
- Observe the patient carefully and often.
- Report your observations referenced above.
- Do not take the blood pressure on the arm with the IV.
- Do not get the site or dressing wet during bathing or showering; obtain specific directions from the licensed nurse.

- *Never* reconnect any tubing that has become disconnected. Once disconnected it is contaminated and must be replaced by the licensed nurse in order to prevent serious and possibly life-threatening infections.
- Report any mistakes that you may make so that prompt corrective action can be taken.

PROCEDURE

Changing the Clothing of a Resident with an IV

Beginning Steps

Note: If a pump or rate-controlled device is attached to the IV, ask the charge nurse to assist you. The nurse will have to disconnect the tubing from the pump and reconnect when you have finished changing the gown.

1. Wash your hands.
2. Identify the resident (Figure 18-5).

FIGURE 18-5

Identify the resident.

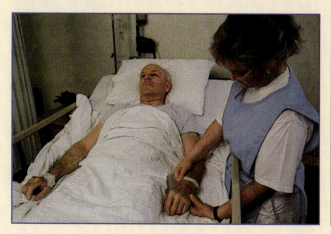

3. Explain what you are going to do.
4. Assist the patient to select clothing if appropriate.
5. Provide privacy.

Steps

6. Remove the gown or shirt from the arm without the IV.
7. When the IV is in the arm, move the gown carefully down the arm containing the IV, carefully sliding it over the site and off the hand. Bring the gown over the tubing.
8. When the IV is located elsewhere, protect the site and dressing from pulling or dislodging.
9. Remove the IV bottle or bag from the pole and slide the gown over it. *Do not lower the bag below the level of the patient's arm.*
10. Replace the bottle or bag on the pole.
11. Put on the new gown or shirt by beginning with the arm with the IV. Remove the bottle or bag from the pole and slide the clothing over the bag and tubing, being very careful not to lower the bag below the patient's arm.
12. Put the other arm through the sleeve.
13. Tie or button garment as indicated.

Ending Steps

14. Make the resident comfortable when dressing is completed and double-check to be sure that the rate of flow has not been changed or stopped.

PROVIDING CARE TO A PATIENT WITH A PATIENT-CONTROLLED ANALGESIC PUMP

Some patients will have a **patient-controlled analgesic (PCA) pump** attached to tubing and a needle/catheter that is inserted into the subcutaneous tissue, generally in the arm (see Figure 18-6). The pump allows the patient to receive a continuous dosage of pain medication, which is ordered by the physician. In addition, the patient is able to self-administer intermittent dosages as needed. The amount of drug that can be self-administered is also ordered by the physician. The ability to self-administer allows the patient to control pain during periods of increased activity or periods of acute pain. The pump has a locking mechanism that prevents overdosing.

- If the pump is not working properly it will make a beeping sound, which should be reported to the licensed nurse immediately. The nursing assistant should also notice if there is any evidence of swelling or drainage at the in-

sertion site. Report any complaints of increased pain to the licensed nurse immediately.
- The nursing assistant must be very careful not to dislodge the needle or catheter. Make sure when you move the patient that you also move the pump. The patient should not lay on the tubing and the tubing should not be kinked or caught in the bed rails when engaged or released. Check the patient frequently to ensure that the pump is in place and working properly.
- The pump should not get wet and is most often placed in a plastic bag and sealed during bathing or showering. The pump should never be submerged.
- It is *never* the responsibility of the nursing assistant to make any adjustments to the pump, this is the responsibility of the licensed nurse. Check the approved plan of care and clarify any questions.

patient-controlled analgesic (PCA) pump pain control managed by the resident

FIGURE 18-6

An analgesic pump.

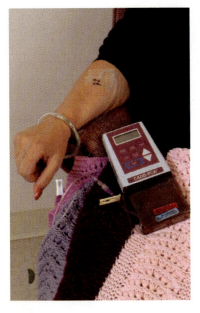

avoid providing necessary care to the patient. Ask for assistance if you are unsure of how to proceed safely!

Because nursing assistants generally spend more time providing direct patient care than other members of the health care team, they are in the best position to observe and report changes in the patient's condition before serious complications can occur. It is very important that you report *all observations* immediately so that the licensed nurse can further assess the patients condition. The nursing assistant should not try to diagnose (decide what the problem is), but should accurately report all observations.

Subacute units will have respiratory therapists available to meet the special needs of their postoperative patients as well as patients with impaired respiratory function. Special equipment may be used to administer oxygen by intermittent positive pressure breathing (IPPB) or continuous positive airway pressure (CPAP).

Respiratory therapists will provide the respiratory treatments and provide information to the physician. The responsibility of the nursing assistant is to follow the plan of care, as well as to observe and report changes in the patient's condition to the licensed nurse. Refer to Chapter 12, The Respiratory System, and review the section on oxygen therapy.

Patients in subacute units may have many different kinds of complex medical problems, including special postoperative care that is dictated by the type of surgical procedure performed. Each patient's care must be individually planned and provided according to the physicians orders and the approved plan of care. Some patients may have their mobility limited or require special positioning devices; others may not be able to bathe or shower; some may have food or fluid intake restrictions. It is absolutely essential that the nursing assistant follow the written plan of care and work under the direct supervision of a licensed nurse. Check with the licensed nurse at the beginning of each shift to obtain a report and to verify that

PROVIDING CARE TO PATIENTS WITH COMPLEX MEDICAL NEEDS, INCLUDING THE POSTSURGICAL PATIENT

The role of the nursing assistant in the subacute unit is primarily one of monitoring vital signs and observing and reporting changes in condition to the licensed nurse. With the exception of bathing and other activities of daily living (ADLs), most of the procedures are carried out by therapists or licensed nurses.

The care is designed to ensure:

- Adequate respiratory, circulatory, and neurological function
- Maintenance of normal body temperature
- Prevention of infection
- Control of pain and other distressing symptoms
- Protection from harm and injury

The tasks of monitoring, observing, and reporting become more important. These tasks include:

- Taking and recording vital signs including pain
- Checking for changes in neurological signs
- Measuring and recording fluid intake and output
- Calculating and recording percentage of food consumed

Other tasks include observing and reporting:

- Signs of circulatory impairment or shock, such as decreased blood pressure; increased pulse rate; or pale, clammy skin
- Signs of respiratory distress, such as changes in respiratory rate, difficulty breathing (dyspnea), changes in skin color to blue or gray (cyanosis), or sharp or stabbing pains in the chest
- Changes in neurological status, including changes in level of alertness or responsiveness, motor strength or symmetry, pupil size or reaction to light, or decreasing pulse with increasing blood pressure
- Signs of peripheral circulatory impairment, such as pale, cold extremities; pain; or absence of pulses
- Signs of infection, including redness, heat, drainage, swelling, foul odor, or elevated body temperature
- Signs of urinary retention, including inability to void or urinate, distended bladder, or complaints of pain or discomfort
- Signs of intestinal obstruction, including complaints of abdominal pain, nausea and vomiting, difficulty having a bowel movement, presence of impaction, and abdominal distention
- Signs of pneumonia, including presence of cough, congestion, fever, difficulty breathing, wheezing, or gurgling or rattling sounds in the chest
- Signs of bleeding, drainage, or infection
- Signs of circulatory impairment when there is a cast including numbness, tingling, pain, swelling, and discoloration

the plan of care is current (Figure 18-7). Never attempt to provide care if you are unsure about how to provide care safely; always seek assistance from the licensed nurse.

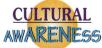 Because many of the patients on a subacute unit may be in serious or critical condition, the family may come to the facility in large numbers and may stay for a long time. In some cultures, the entire family surrounds their family member and remains with them until they die, are discharged, or are much improved. It is important to recognize that this is part of their beliefs and to accommodate them as much as possible. Be courteous. Provide extra chairs, if necessary. Show them where the bathrooms and sitting areas are located. If beverages are available, tell them where they can find them. Allow them to help you care for the patient as long

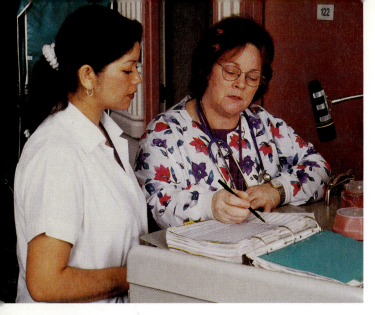

FIGURE 18-7

increased intracranial pressure   pressure inside the skull is increased because something is taking up space (hemorrhage, tumor, swelling of the brain)

as you have the permission of the patient. Remember to respect the privacy of the patient and other patients in the room.

CARING FOR PATIENTS WITH HEAD AND BRAIN INJURIES

Brain injuries are often the result of vehicle or industrial accidents, falls, sports injuries, or diseases such as a CVA (cerebrovascular accident) or brain tumor, as well as some types of metabolic disorders.

Some injuries may be considered minor and cause loss of consciousness or brief disorientation. Other brain injuries cause permanent damage and may result in paralysis, mental retardation, respiratory problems, seizures, loss of bowel and bladder control, and even irreversible coma. Some injuries occur as a result of brain hemorrhage or lack of blood flow to the brain (see Chapter 11, The Nervous System).

One of the most serious complications resulting from an acute brain injury is the development of **increased intracranial pressure** (the pressure exerted within the skull by the brain, cerebral blood, and cerebrospinal fluid). The most common reasons for pressure increases within the skull are due to hemorrhage and swelling of the brain tissue as a result of trauma or disease. Permanent brain injury and brain death can result from excessive intracranial pressure. In a head injury, changes often occur very rapidly and immediate emergency measures are necessary. Always report changes in condition to the licensed nurse immediately.

Many subacute units care for patients with an altered level of consciousness; terms such as subconscious, unconscious, unresponsive in a coma, or in a persistent vegetative state are used to describe this type of patient. Review Chapter 11 for nursing care of the patient with impaired consciousness. The nursing assistant has to be especially alert for changes in condition because these patients are unable to make their needs known. Many changes may be subtle and not obvious; the nursing assistant who has been providing care is often the first to notice changes in condition.

Patients with head injuries may have their fluids restricted or be given diuretics in order to decrease the swelling of the brain, or they may require special positioning or activity limitations. The approved plan of care should provide the nursing assistant with the necessary information to provide safe care. Always verify the plan of care with the licensed nurse to ensure that it is accurate.

Guidelines

PROVIDING CARE TO PATIENTS WITH BRAIN INJURIES

The responsibilities of the nursing assistant when caring for a patient with a brain injury include reporting to the licensed nurses any observed changes in:

- Level of consciousness (patient is less alert, disoriented, or less responsive)

- Symptoms including headache, dizziness, or blurred vision
- ADL skills, including balance, strength, and ability
- Pupil size or reactivity to light
- Vital signs
- Speech

COMPLEX WOUND CARE

Wound care or care of serious pressure sores has always been of great concern for those providing care to elderly debilitated or chronically ill patients. The basic principles of skin care and the prevention and treatment of pressure sores are outlined in Chapter 6, The Integumentary System. Take time to review this chapter thoroughly. The subacute unit provides specialized equipment and services for those patients who have serious wounds, wounds that are slow in healing or do not heal at all. Other members of the health care team may be involved in direct care. Physical therapists may provide whirlpool and debridement services. Many facilities employ or have a wound and ostomy specialist who will assess the wound and make recommendations to the physician for specialized treatment.

A **wound** is a disruption in the continuity and regulatory processes of tissue cells; wound healing is designed to restore that continuity. However, wound healing does not always restore cellular function.

Wounds are classified by the mechanism that caused the injury:

- *Incised wound*—made by a clean cut of a sharp instrument
- *Contused wound*—made by blunt force or pressure, which may not break the skin but produces considerable deep tissue damage (a pressure sore is this type of wound)
- *Lacerated wound*—made by an object that tears the tissue, resulting in jagged, irregular edges in the wound
- *Puncture wound*—made by a pointed instrument such as a bullet or ice pick

Wounds may heal by being surgically closed and dressed; this is called **first intention healing.** Other wounds may be left open and heal from the inside out; this is called **second intention healing** and is used when the wound is very large or has become infected (Figure 18-8).

wound   a disruption in the continuity and regulatory processes of tissue cells

first intention healing
surgical closure of a wound

second intention healing
wound heals from the inside out

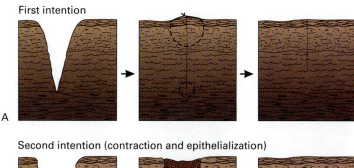

First intention

A

Second intention (contraction and epithelialization)

B

C

FIGURE 18-8

Classification of wound healing. (A) First intention: A clean incision is made with primary closure; there is minimal scarring. (B and C) Second intention: The wound is left open so that granulation can occur; a large scar results (B), or the wound is initially left open and later closed when there is no further evidence of infection (C).

PROVIDING CARE TO PATIENTS WITH WOUNDS WITH SUCTION DEVICES

The nursing assistant should make sure the resident is not lying on tubing attached to any suction device and check to ensure that the tubing is not kinked or disconnected. The nursing assistant should never raise the suction container above the insertion site and should not empty the drainage device. Observe the amount and type of drainage in the container and report your observations to the licensed nurse.

Some wounds may have significant drainage, and a catheter will be inserted and attached to a suction device to remove the excess drainage.

The subacute unit that specializes in wound care must have a very capable team of health care professionals to accomplish wound healing. Factors that promote wound healing include:

- Adequate nutrition and hydration
- Absence of pressure to enhance circulation
- Good skin hygiene and infection control practices
- Good underlying physiological health
- Good underlying psychological health

THE PATIENT WITH A TRACHEOSTOMY

A tracheostomy is a surgical procedure by which an opening is made into the trachea to provide the patient with an artificial airway (Figure 18-9). A tracheostomy tube is inserted into the opening and held in place by an inflatable cuff inside the trachea and by cotton twill ties tied loosely around the outside of the neck.

FIGURE 18-9

A tracheostomy provides an artificial airway.

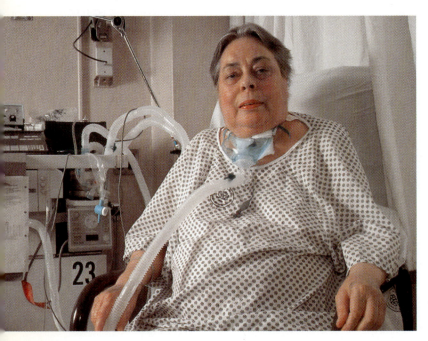

Tracheostomies are performed by a physician in respiratory emergencies and when the need for artificial ventilation is prolonged beyond a couple of weeks. Some tracheostomies are temporary and some become permanent. The patient must learn to live with the need for daily tracheostomy care.

Suctioning, referred to as tracheobronchial suctioning, is only done by a licensed nurse. Sterile suctioning equipment is kept at the bedside for immediate use (Figure 18-10). The nursing assistant must be sure not to touch the sterile suction catheter and to provide care in such a way as to prevent infection around the tracheostomy area. Follow your facility's procedures for cleaning the suction equipment.

If the trach tube appears dislodged or if any of the following signs of respiratory distress are present, the licensed nurse should be notified immediately:

PROVIDING CARE TO A PATIENT WITH A TRACHEOSTOMY

When you think of the tracheostomy as the patient's only airway, you can understand how important it is to keep it open and free of secretions. A new tracheostomy produces more secretions, so frequent suctioning by a licensed nurse may be necessary. It is important to the keep the area around the tracheostomy clean, dry, and free of infection. The constant moisture from the secretions and the irritation resulting from the need for frequent suctioning make the tracheostomy site a primary target for bacterial invasion. Some physicians use a small dressing around the tracheal opening, which is changed frequently; others prefer to keep the area open to the air and as dry as possible.

- Difficulty in breathing (dyspnea)
- Rattling sounds
- Bubbling secretions or blood coming from tracheostomy site
- Blue, gray, or ashen color to the skin (cyanosis)
- Rate of breathing increases or decreases

Some patient's may be receiving respiratory therapy treatments and some may have oxygen administered via their tracheostomy tube. Be sure to get specific directions from your charge nurse before showering or bathing the patient with a tracheostomy. The plan of care should be reviewed each shift to ensure that care is provided according to the physicians orders and the interdisciplinary team's recommendations.

INTENSIVE REHABILITATION SERVICES IN THE SUBACUTE UNIT

The nursing assistant will work directly with the therapy teams to assist patients in reaching their rehabilitation goals. The patient's plan of care will reflect the specific therapy goals to be achieved as well as detail what each member of the interdisciplinary team is supposed to do to assist the patient in achieving the goal. Always clarify your responsibilities with both the licensed nurse and the therapist if you have questions.

Review Chapter 17, The Restorative Nursing Assistant, and be sure you understand the basic rehabilitation principles. The subacute unit offers a very different rehabilitation program than that found in the typical nursing care center. The rehab team is usually three or four times larger and rehabilitation team meetings may be held daily.

Many patients are planning to go home and are only in the facility long enough to achieve their therapy goals. The nursing assistant is an important member of the rehabilitation team!

FIGURE 18-10

Suction machine.

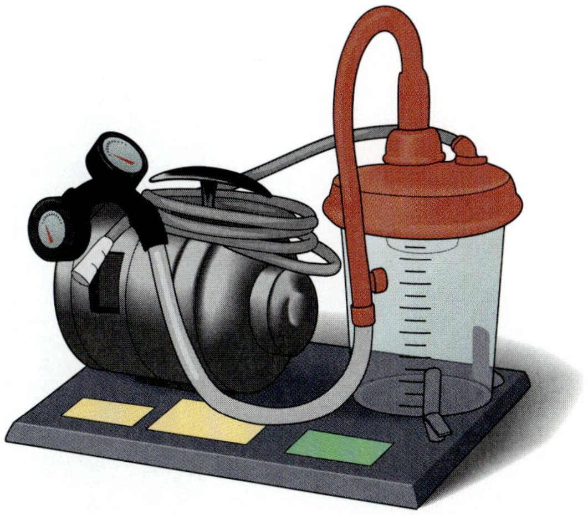

SECTION 3 Basic Emergency Care

OBJECTIVES
What You Will Learn

When you have completed this section, you will be able to:

- State the goal of providing first aid
- Complete the following sentence—when checking for life-threatening injuries, do so without _____

the victim because a _____ _____ _____ may be made worse during emergency treatment

- Identify six major changes in respiratory function that would signal a respiratory emergency exists

- From a given list, select those statements which are true related to complete airway obstruction and the Heimlich maneuver

- List the three signs of cardiac arrest

KEY TERMS

apnea
artificial ventilation
bag valve mask

biological death
clinical death
Heimlich maneuver
spontaneous breathing

sternum
stridor
tongue–jaw lift

Knowing what to do in an emergency may mean the difference between life and death for someone, whether you are at home, at work, or on the highway. Community-sponsored programs provided by the American Red Cross and the American Heart Association offer instruction in basic emergency care and disaster preparedness. These courses will prepare you to give safe care in many emergency situations.

Outside the long-term care facility, the Emergency Medical Services team, generally paramedics, in your local community will respond to a 911 call (Figure 18-11). In the facility the licensed nurse will initiate and direct appropriate emergency procedures. Always follow the directions of the licensed nurse in any emergency situation.

Every emergency is different and some basic principles apply. Remember that the goal of providing first aid is to prevent death and further injury.

- Call for help and have someone initiate the emergency 911 while you remain with the victim if possible.
- Do not attempt to perform procedures unless you are sure you can do so safely.

FIGURE 18-11

Emergency care.

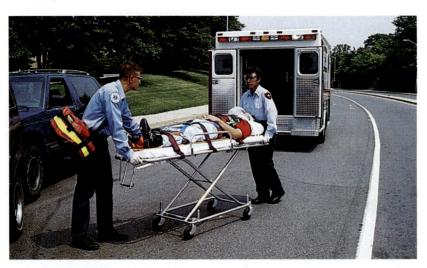

- Remain calm and check for life-threatening problems without moving the victim; a spinal cord injury may be made worse during emergency treatment. Keep the head and neck in a straight line.
- If the victim is in cardiac arrest, start cardiopulmonary resuscitation (CPR) immediately even if you could worsen existing injuries.
  —Check airway
  —Check breathing
  —Check pulse
  —Observe for hemorrhage
  —Observe for obvious fractures
- Perform necessary emergency measures or first aid. If the victim is conscious, reassure and explain what you are doing.
- Inform emergency personnel of the type of emergency and condition of the victim.
- Do not give food or fluids.
- Keep the victim warm; use whatever is available.

RESPIRATORY EMERGENCIES

As a nursing assistant, you must be alert for signs of a respiratory emergency and take immediate action to report the emergency and start appropriate life-saving measures.

The following conditions can signal a respiratory emergency:

- No chest movements or uneven chest movements.
- No exchange of air can be heard or felt at the mouth or nose.
- Breathing is very difficult.
- Skin, lips, and nailbeds are blue, gray, or ashen color.
- Breathing is too fast or too slow (below 8 or above 30 breaths per minute).
- Respirations become very shallow or noisy; there may be periods of **apnea** (no breathing)

These conditions require immediate attention; call for help and begin mouth-to-mouth breathing, following the step-by-step procedures described in the text. The facility emergency equipment will contain disposable airways, a pocket mask, and a ventilating device, usually called a **bag valve mask.** Use of a protective device is necessary as a barrier to protect both you and your resident from transferring any communicable diseases (Figure 18-12). Use of the airway or face pocket mask eliminates the need to place the mouth directly in contact with the patient. The ambu bag will have a face mask attached that will fit directly over the mouth and nose of the patient. Squeezing the bag forces air into the patient's lungs. The mask must be positioned to provide a tight fit over the nose and mouth. The patient's head must be positioned to allow air to enter. The positioning is the same for direct mouth-to-mouth ventilation. *If the patient does not begin breathing again, is unresponsive, and has no carotid pulse, cardiac arrest has occurred.*

MOUTH-TO-MOUTH VENTILATION

This procedure is very efficient in providing **artificial ventilation** (rescue breathing). It can be done by one person without any special equipment. This

apnea   absence of breathing

bag valve mask   a ventilator bag

artificial ventilation   rescue breathing

FIGURE 18-12
Barrier mask.

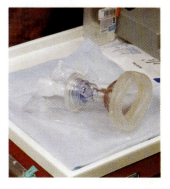

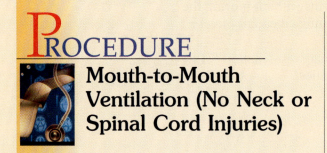

Mouth-to-Mouth Ventilation (No Neck or Spinal Cord Injuries)

1. *Open the airway*—by properly positioning the resident on his or her back using the head-tilt or chin-lift maneuver. Place one hand on the forehead and apply pressure to tilt the head back. Place the fingers of the other hand under the resident's chin and lift the chin forward with your fingers.

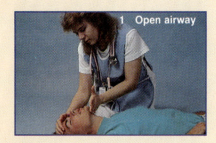

2. *Look, listen, and feel*—while maintaining the proper head tilt and determine whether the resident is breathing by: *Looking* for chest movements—are they present, are they even? *Listening* for air flowing into and out of resident's mouth and nose. Notice any unusual sounds (gurgling, snoring). *Feeling* for air exchange at the resident's mouth and nose. Take at least 3 to 5 seconds to accurately determine whether or not the resident is breathing.

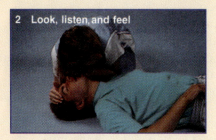

3. *Ventilate*—by maintaining the maximum head tilt and pinching the resident's nose closed with the thumb and forefinger of the same hand you are using to hold the resident's forehead. Open your mouth wide and take a deep breath in. Place your open mouth around the mouth of the resident, making a tight seal with your lips against the resident's face. Ventilate the resident by exhaling slowly into the resident's mouth until you can see the chest rise and feel resistance to the flow of your breath. The ventilation should take 1½ to 2 seconds. If the first attempt fails, reposition the head and try again.

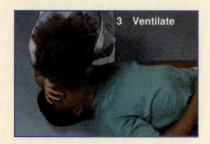

4. *Allow passive exhale*—by breaking contact with the resident's mouth and allowing air to flow from the lungs. Quickly take another deep breath and begin again until resident begins breathing independently **(spontaneous breathing).** Deliver repeated breaths to the adult at the rate of one breath every 5 seconds or 12 breaths per minute. Check to see if the resident has started breathing.

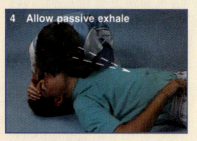

spontaneous breathing
in mouth-to-mouth ventilation, the point at which the victim begins to breathe independently

procedure would have to be modified if there were any indication the resident had sustained neck or spinal cord injuries (Figure 18-13).

You will know that you are performing these procedures correctly when you are able to:

- *Feel* resistance to your ventilations as the resident's lungs expand
- *See* the chest rise and fall
- *Hear/feel* air leaving the resident's airway as the chest falls

FIGURE 18-13

Mouth-to-mouth ventilation with pocket face mask. One breath every 5 seconds equals 12 breaths per minute.

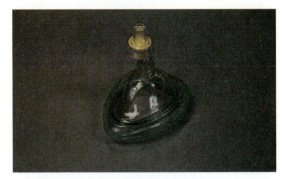

a. Pocket face mask with one-way value.

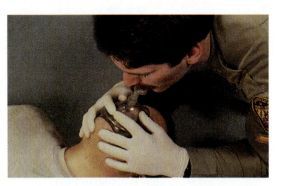

b. Providing breaths with a pocket face mask.

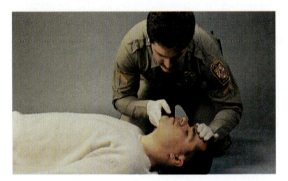

c. Open the airway.

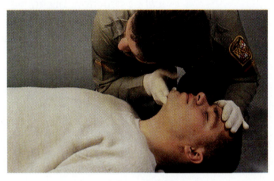

d. Look, listen, and feel for air exchange.

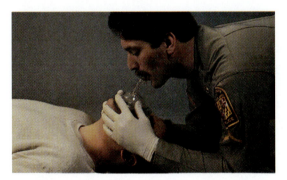

e. Breathe out into mask, watching for the chest rise.

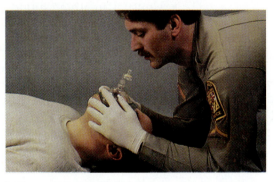

f. Allow passive exhalation, watching for the chest to fall.

AIRWAY OBSTRUCTION

Another common respiratory emergency is airway obstruction. Airway obstruction can occur under many different circumstances (Figure 18-14):

- *Obstruction by the tongue*—The tongue falls back to block off the throat. This can occur when for any reason the resident's head flexes forward, as in the case of sudden unconsciousness or even when too large a pillow is placed under the head.
- *Tissue damage*—This occurs following accidents or injuries in which the soft tissues of the neck and throat are crushed or punctured, resulting in swelling of these tissues and blockage of the airway.

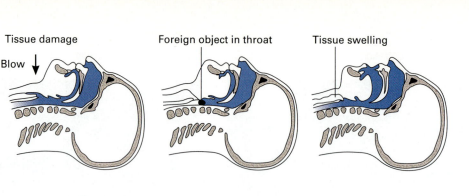

Tongue in the back of throat   Tissue damage   Foreign object in throat   Tissue swelling

Blow ↓

FIGURE 18-14

Various types of airway obstruction.

- *Diseases*—Some respiratory infections and chronic conditions (e.g., asthma) can cause tissue swelling and/or muscle spasms that will lead to airway obstruction.
- *Obstruction by foreign objects*—This type of obstruction, also called mechanical obstruction, occurs when any object or substance blocks the airway. This could occur with food, toys, or dentures as well as blood or vomitus, which could pool in the back of the throat.

The most frequent cause of airway obstruction in adults is choking on meat or other large, poorly chewed pieces of food. Many elderly residents experience difficulty in swallowing due to aging and disease. If the airway is obstructed down in the lower airway passages, there is usually very little that can be done. However, upper airway obstructions can often be removed with a few simple procedures.

SIGNS OF PARTIAL AIRWAY OBSTRUCTION

- Unusual breathing sounds
- Snoring, often caused by the tongue obstructing the back of the throat
- Gurgling, often caused by a foreign object or fluid in the airway
- Crowing, often caused by spasm of the larynx (voicebox), producing a high-pitched sound that is called **stridor**
- Wheezing, usually due to tissue swelling in the lower air passages (*Note:* Wheezing that is not severe does not generally result in airway obstruction.)

stridor a high-pitched sound produced during airway obstruction

When there is only partial airway obstruction, the resident may be capable of either good or poor air exchange.

If a conscious resident appears to have a partial airway obstruction, have the resident cough. A strong, forceful cough indicates that enough air is being exchanged. Encourage the resident to continue coughing in hopes that any foreign object will be dislodged and expelled. Do not interfere with resident's attempts to expel the foreign object.

If the resident cannot cough or the cough is very weak, begin to treat the resident as though *complete airway obstruction is present!*

COMPLETE AIRWAY OBSTRUCTION

Complete airway obstruction is recognized in a conscious resident when:

- A person is suddenly unable to speak or cough.
- A person grasps his or her neck and opens the mouth in an effort to indicate an inability to breathe (Figure 18-15).

Prompt action is required before the resident loses consciousness!

CORRECTING AIRWAY OBSTRUCTION

In recent years, the procedure known as the Heimlich maneuver included the use of back blows when partial or complete airway obstruction was present. However, back blows are no longer recommended for children or adults with complete airway obstruction. This previously taught technique is recommended only for infants who can be placed in a head-down position when the back blows are delivered.

The following procedures are for use with adults. They are not recommended for infants, very small children, pregnant women, or for anyone who has had recent chest or abdominal surgery. Special procedures for infants, very small children, and pregnant women are available from the American Red Cross and the American Heart Association.

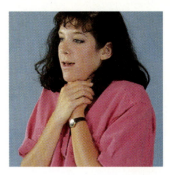

FIGURE 18-15
Universal sign of choking.

PROCEDURE

Correcting Airway Obstructions

1. Determine if there is *complete obstruction* or partial obstruction that must be treated as complete obstruction. Be certain to ask the conscious resident "Are you choking?"; "Can you speak?" Look, listen, and feel for the signs of complete obstruction or poor exchange. Quickly tell the resident you are going to help.

2. Give repeated abdominal thrusts until the object is expelled or the victim becomes unresponsive. The application of these thrusts is known as the **Heimlich maneuver.**

   • Position yourself behind the resident if the resident is standing or sitting.
   • Slide your arm under the resident's armpits, wrapping both of your arms around the waist (Figure 18-16).

   • Make a fist and place thumb side of this fist against the midline of the resident's abdomen, just above the navel. Keep your fist below the resident's rib cage, taking extra caution to avoid the area just below the breastbone **(sternum).**

   Grasp your fist with your free hand and apply pressure as an inward and upward thrust. This should press your fist into the resident's abdomen. Deliver quick, separate, *rapid inward and upward thrusts* (Figure 18-17). Repeat and continue the thrusts until the object is expelled, or the resident becomes unconscious. If the resident becomes unconscious call for help immediately. If the resident is lying down, you should:
   • Check the airway.
   • Check for breathing and check the circulation.
   • Place the resident on his back.
   • Kneel astride the resident at the level of the hips.
   • Position the heel of one hand on the resident's abdomen at the midline, between the navel and the rib cage. Your fingers should point toward the resident's chest. Keep your hand below the resident's rib cage, avoiding the area just below the breastbone.
   • Place your free hand over the positioned hand and put your shoulders directly over the resident's abdomen.
   • Press your hands inward and toward the resident's diaphragm, as if you are trying to push toward the resident's upper back (Figure 18-18).

FIGURE 18-16

Slip your arm under the resident's armpits.

FIGURE 18-17

Apply pressure as an inward and upward thrust.

FIGURE 18-18

Press your hands inward and toward the diaphragm.

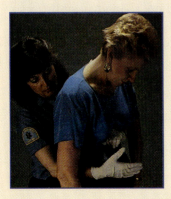

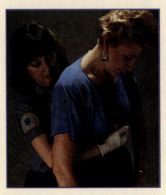

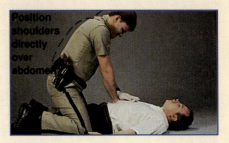

PROCEDURE

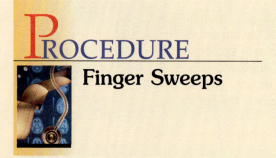

Finger Sweeps

Do not perform finger sweeps unless the object is visable.

1. Place resident on his or her back.
2. Cross your thumb under your index finger. Use one hand to steady the resident's forehead while you place your thumb against the resident's upper teeth and forefinger on lower teeth.
3. Force open the resident's mouth by uncrossing your thumb and index finger. Once the mouth is open, hold the resident's lower jaw and tongue so that the mouth cannot close. This is known as the **tongue–jaw lift** (Figure 18-19).
4. Release your grasp on the resident's forehead and use the forefinger of the free hand to sweep the resident's mouth, using your finger as a hook to capture any foreign materials. If you need to grasp an object, try to do so using your first and second fingers. You may need to turn the resident's head to one side in order to sweep an object from the mouth (Figure 18-20). If during your attempts to clear the airway of obstruction the resident becomes unconscious, you must then combine the procedures of:

- Attempting to ventilate
- Providing abdominal thrusts
- Performing finger sweeps
- Reattempting ventilation

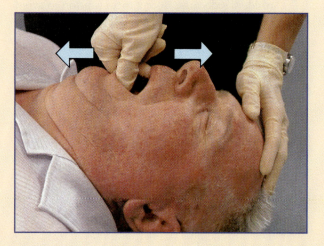

FIGURE 18-19
The tongue–jaw lift.

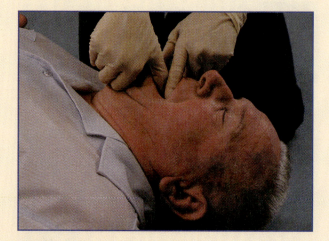

FIGURE 18-20
Finger sweeps.

Heimlich maneuver application of abdominal thrusts during airway obstruction

sternum breastbone

tongue–jaw lift in finger sweep procedures, forcing open the mouth and holding the lower jaw and tongue so that the mouth cannot close

You must assess the total situation quickly and determine whether or not complete or partial airway obstruction is present. Follow the steps below for correcting airway obstruction.

FINGER SWEEPS

You can use your fingers to remove a foreign object from a resident's airway once the object has been partially or completely dislodged. Only use finger sweeps when you can see the object. Be very careful not to inadvertently push the object back down the resident's throat. Also be alert so that the resident does not bite down on your fingers. *Note:* the tongue–jaw lift is used to open the airway when spinal cord injuries are suspected.

CARDIAC EMERGENCIES

Cardiac arrest means the heart has stopped, and cardiopulmonary resuscitation (CPR) *must be started immediately. Cardio* refers to heart and *pulmonary* refers to the lungs.

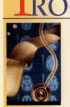

PROCEDURE

Airway Obstruction (Combined Procedures)

1. Position resident so that he is lying on his back.
2. Use the tongue–jaw lift to open mouth and perform finger sweeps.
3. Attempt to open the resident's airway using the head-tilt, chin-lift maneuver.
4. Pinch the resident's nostrils closed with the hand you are using to hold the forehead. Give *two ade-* *quate ventilations* as described in mouth-to-mouth ventilation procedure (Figure 18-21). If your attempt to ventilate fails, you should reposition the head and attempt to ventilate again. If still unsuccessful . . .
5. Perform *five* abdominal thrusts in rapid succession (Figure 18-22). If this fails . . .
6. Repeat the sequence of:
   - Finger sweeps (if object is visible) (Figure 18-23)
   - Attempting to ventilate, reposition and attempt to ventilate again (Figure 18-24)
   - Providing abdominal thrusts
7. You *must continue* these efforts until the obstruction is cleared and the resident's airway is open.

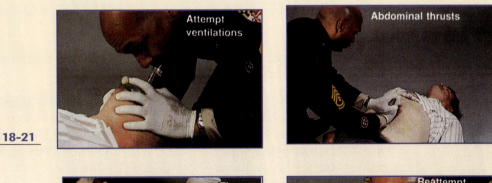

Attempt ventilations

FIGURE 18-21

Abdominal thrusts

FIGURE 18-22

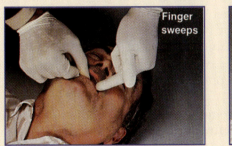

Finger sweeps

FIGURE 18-23

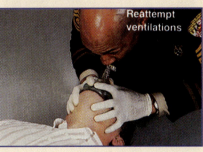

Reattempt ventilations

FIGURE 18-24

All the functions of the cardiovascular system depend on the heart pumping the blood in a constant, one-directional flow. When, for any reason, this process is interrupted, a serious cardiac emergency exists. There is an important relationship between breathing, circulation, and certain brain activity.

- If breathing stops, the blood being circulated to the brain will not contain enough oxygen, and the brain will send a signal to the heart; it will soon stop pumping.
- When the heart stops pumping, breathing stops almost instantly.
- If the centers in the brain that control breathing and cardiac function are damaged, heart and lung action will soon stop.

The activities of the heart, lungs, and brain are interdependent—if one fails, they all will fail (Figure 18-25).

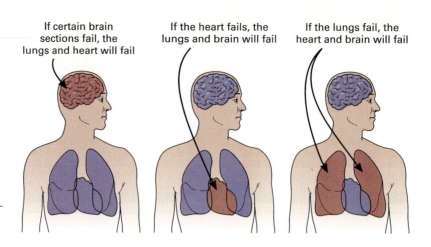

If certain brain sections fail, the lungs and heart will fail

If the heart fails, the lungs and brain will fail

If the lungs fail, the heart and brain will fail

FIGURE 18-25

Interdependence of the activities of the heart, lungs, and brain.

Whenever you read about basic life support, you will see reference made to the ABCs of emergency care. ABC stands for:

A = airway
B = breathing
C = circulation

CARDIOPULMONARY RESUSCITATION

clinical death cessation of breathing and heartbeat

biological death occurs when vital activity in the cells of the body stops

Cardiopulmonary resuscitation is an emergency procedure used to restore circulation and oxygenation when heart, lung, and/or certain brain functions have stopped. Check the carotid pulse by placing the index and middle fingers on the patient's trachea (windpipe); then slide your fingertips to the side of the neck nearest you, just under the jaw bone (Figure 18-26). Check for the carotid pulse on yourself so that you are familiar with its location.

When performing CPR, you must continue to keep an open airway and breathe for the victim. Your breaths provide oxygen for the blood. In addition, you must circulate the oxygenated blood to the vital organs of the body. During CPR the increased pressure in the chest cavity forces the blood into circulation (Figure 18-27).

FIGURE 18-26

Signs of cardiac arrest: unresponsiveness, lack of breathing, lack of pulse.

It is important to remember that when someone stops breathing and the heart stops pumping, **clinical death** results. Within just 4 to 6 minutes, lethal changes begin to take place in the brain, and generally within 10 minutes **biological death** will occur as the brain and other body cells start to die. For these reasons, quick action to call 911 and to start CPR on someone who is in cardiac arrest is essential. *Start CPR immediately* even if you could worsen existing injuries, for without CPR the victim will quickly go from clinical death to biological death.

The following procedure is a step-by-step outline for performing one-rescuer CPR. The procedures covered here follow the recommendations of the American Heart Association (AHA). Your instructor will inform you of any recent changes made by the AHA. This

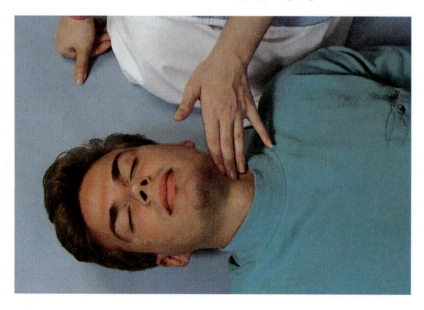

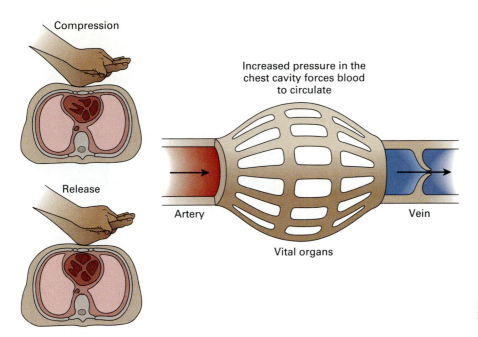

Compression

Release

Increased pressure in the
chest cavity forces blood
to circulate

Artery

Vein

Vital organs

FIGURE 18-27

The mechanics of CPR.

procedure should be learned exactly as presented. Extensive research by the
AHA has determined that the procedures presented here are the most efficient in saving lives of victims in cardiac arrest.

Note: There are slightly different techniques to be used on infants and small
children under the age of 8. For an average-sized child 8 years and older, the
adult techniques presented here can be used. The variations to be used on infants and small children are not represented in this book; however, specific
information is available through the American Red Cross and the American
Heart Association.

ONE-RESCUER CPR

Because CPR is a lifesaving procedure, it is essential that the rescuer understand exactly how to perform these procedures correctly. Therefore, it is recommended that these procedures be taught by an instructor certified by the
American Heart Association and/or the American Red Cross.

TWO-RESCUER CPR

The procedure for two-rescuer CPR varies slightly in that one rescuer delivers
the ventilations and the second person delivers chest compressions. In two-
rescuer CPR:

- Compressions are 15 every 10 seconds, or a rate of 100 compressions per
  minute.
- Provide two ventilations every 15 compressions, or 10 to 12 per minute.
- The person giving ventilations checks the carotid pulse.
- The person doing compressions counts out loud the two to 15 cycles.
- Check for carotid pulse after the first minute.

Emergency situations are sudden, unexpected events, when we are well prepared to handle emergencies we can do so with confidence and skill. The best
way to be prepared is to be knowledgeable. A first-aid course that provides actual practice in performing emergency procedures is especially valuable.

PROCEDURE

One-Rescuer CPR

1. *Establish unresponsiveness* (Figure 18-28). Gently shake the victim and ask, "Are you okay?" If the victim is unresponsive, immediately *call or have someone call 911.*

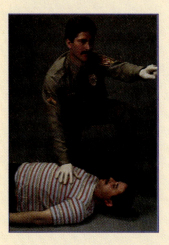

FIGURE 18-28
Establish unresponsiveness.

2. *Properly position the victim and yourself.* Place the victim on a flat firm surface face up. Kneel beside at chest level with your knees pointing in toward the patient's chest (Figure 18-29).

FIGURE 18-29
Properly position the victim and yourself.

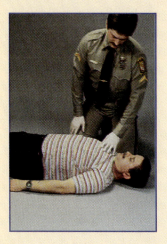

3. *Establish an open airway.* Use the head-tilt, chin-lift method to ensure an open airway (Figure 18-30).

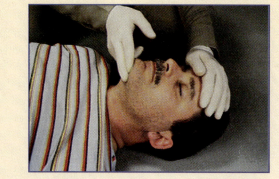

FIGURE 18-30
Establish an open airway using head-tilt, chin-lift method.

4. *Check for breathing—look, listen, and feel* for air exchange (Figure 18-31). This should take 5 to 10 seconds.

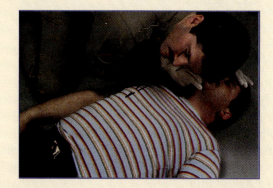

FIGURE 18-31
Check for breathing.

5. *Provide two adequate breaths* (Figure 18-32). Use the procedure outlined for mouth-to-mouth ventilation.

FIGURE 18-32
Provide two adequate breaths.

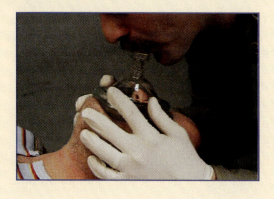

PROCEDURE
continued

6. If necessary, *clear the airway.* Use the techniques of manual thrusts, finger sweeps, and ventilations described previously.

7. *Establish cardiac arrest.* Check for circulation by feeling for a carotid pulse (Figure 18-33). This should take 5 to 10 seconds. If a carotid pulse is present but no breathing is present, give one breath every 5 seconds. If there is no carotid pulse, start CPR.

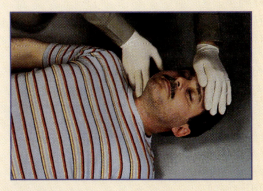

FIGURE 18-33

Check for circulation by feeling for a carotid pulse.

8. *Find the compression site.* Slide your index and middle fingers along the lower edge of the ribs until you locate the notch where the ribs join the breastbone (Figures 18-34 through 18-36).

FIGURE 18-34

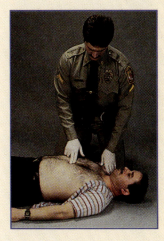

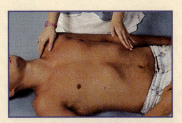

FIGURE 18-35

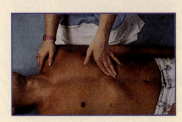

FIGURE 18-36

9. *Position your hands for delivering compressions.* Place your hand closest to the victim's head along the middle of the chest (Figures 18-37 and 18-38). Next move the hand used to locate the compression site. Place it on top of the hand positioned on the breastbone (Figure 18-39). The heels of both hands should now be parallel to one another, with your fingers pointing straight away from your body. The fingers may be interlocked or extended, or you may grasp the wrist of the hand placed at the compression site. *Your fingers must be kept off the victim's chest.*

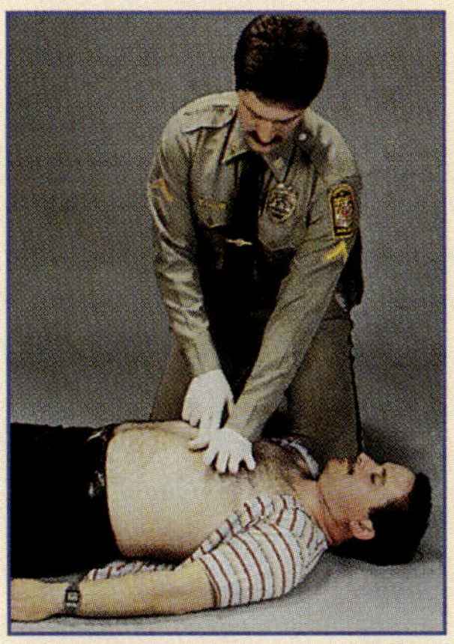

FIGURE 18-37

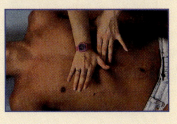

FIGURE 18-38

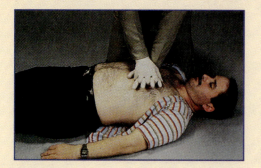

FIGURE 18-39

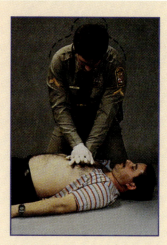

FIGURE 18-40

10. *Deliver 15 chest compressions*—keep your arms straight, elbows locked, and shoulders directly over the compression site (Figure 18-40). Bend at the waist when delivering compressions to utilize your upper body weight. *Remember:*
    - *Deliver compressions directly over the CPR compression site.* (Figure 18-41)
    - *Compress the victim's breastbone 1½ to 2 inches.*
    - *Deliver compressions at a rate of 100 per minute,* counting "One, two, three, four. . . ."
    - Release pressure completely to allow the heart to refill. Each release should take the same amount of time as the compression. *Remember, do not take your hands off the victim's chest.*
    - *Deliver 15 compressions, then . . .*

11. *Provide two breaths*—Ventilations are provided at the rate of *two adequate breaths every 15 compressions.* Do this at a rate of one ventilation every 1½ to 2 seconds. CPR compressions should not be interrupted for more than 10 seconds.

12. *Continue CPR*—Deliver 15 compressions at the rate of 100 per minute, followed by two ventilations. Continue the cycle for 1 minute.

13. *Check for a carotid pulse*—After 1 minute of CPR, check for a carotid pulse. *Remember: Do not* interrupt CPR for more than 10 seconds in order to check for pulse. *If there is a pulse, stop CPR.* If the victim has a pulse but is not breathing, provide

breaths at the rate of one breath every 5 seconds. If there is no pulse, deliver two breaths and. . . .

14. *Continue CPR*—Check for a carotid pulse every few minutes. Provide CPR until:
    - Victim regains a pulse
    - Another trained person can take over for you
    - You are physically unable to continue

FIGURE 18-41
Locating the CPR compression site.

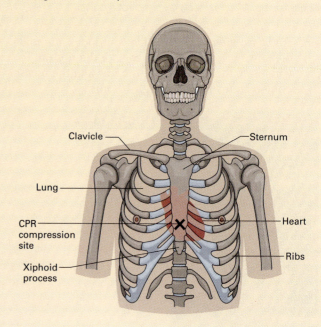

Clavicle   Sternum

Lung

CPR compression site   Heart

Xiphoid process   Ribs

Always consider how the emergency event affects other patients and residents of the facility. Remove patients from the immediate area and provide comfort and support.

Because these are lifesaving procedures, it is essential that you learn them by memory in order to be prepared at all times to provide the *ABCs of emergency care!*

PROCEDURE

Two-Rescuer CPR

NOTE: Assess for spontaneous breathing and pulse at the end of the first minute, and then every few minutes thereafter.

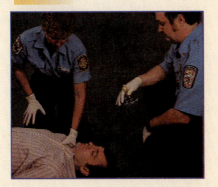

1. Determine unresponsiveness. Reposition resident.

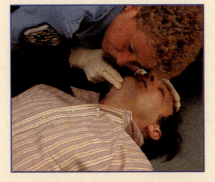

2. Open the airway and look, listen, and feel (5–10 sec.).

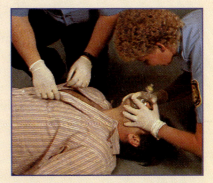

3. Ventilate twice (1½–2 sec./ventilation).

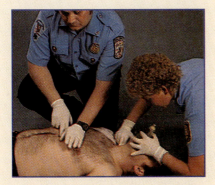

4. Determine pulselessness. Locate CPR compression site.

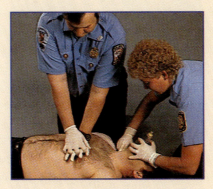

5. Say "no pulse." Begin compressions.

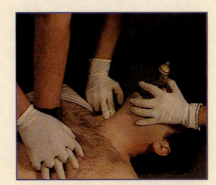

6. Check compression effectiveness. Deliver 15 compressions in 10 seconds (rate = 100/minute).

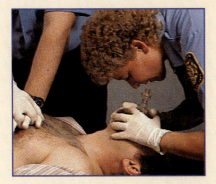

7. Ventilation once. (1½–2 sec./ventilation) Stop for ventilation.

Continue with one ventilation every five compressions.

8. Continue with one ventilation every five compressions.

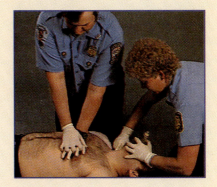

9. After four cycles, reassess breathing and pulse. No pulse—ventilate and say "continue CPR." Pulse—say "stop CPR."

SUMMARY This chapter has provided you with the opportunity to learn many new skills. The residents or patients who you care for in a subacute setting usually demand more care. They are less stable and more likely to change while in the subacute unit. The skills demanded of you include more thorough observation and reporting, enhanced technical skills, and working with limitations imposed by medical devices and equipment. Patients are often anxious and fearful and in the early stages of adjusting to their illness or injury. This means your ability to form a positive relationship may be more difficult. You'll need to focus on developing trust in you as a caregiver based on keeping your promises and demonstrating competence in the care you give. Never perform a procedure for the first time without supervision. Ask for help when needed, and if you make a mistake, report it immediately. This kind of nursing will be filled with opportunities to learn about new conditions or diseases as well as new treatments and procedures. Take advantage by asking questions and by seeking additional information in books and other publications.

OBRA HIGHLIGHTS

Many of the patients cared for in a subacute unit are addressed in the OBRA regulations as residents with "special needs." The regulation states: "The facility must ensure that residents receive proper treatment and care for the following special services:

• Injections
• Parenteral and enteral fluids
• Colostomy, ureterostomy, or ileostomy care
• Tracheostomy care
• Tracheal suctioning
• Respiratory care
• Foot care
• Prostheses."

Although much of the care listed is provided by the licensed nurse or by therapists, the nursing assistant has an important role in assuring proper care for the residents with special needs.

SELF STUDY

Choose the best answer for each question or statement.

1. Which of the following is true of a sub-acute unit?
   a. It provides a less costly alternative to continued hospitalization.
   b. The care is provided in a conventional long-term care nursing facility.
   c. The nursing assistants working in this unit have the same training as those working in long-term care.
   d. The residents admitted to this unit remain there until they are transferred to the long-term care facility.

2. An intensive rehabilitation program offered in a subacute unit differs from those offered in a hospital because
   a. only physical therapy and occupational therapy are offered
   b. the patient participates in therapies only 3 hours a day
   c. the pace and amount of therapy is adapted to the patient's tolerance
   d. all of the above

3. Which of the following services would *not* be offered in a subacute unit?
   a. intravenous therapy
   b. hospice care
   c. care of patient on a ventilator
   d. complex wound care

4. What is the purpose of a Port-a-cath?
   a. allows intravenous fluids or medications to be given without inserting a new IV each time
   b. allows the patient to be more mobile because he or she is not continuously connected to an IV bag
   c. allows access directly to the bloodstream for giving medications
   d. all of the above

5. Mrs. Suhani has an IV connected to a pump. Which of the following actions should the nursing assistant take?
   a. Slow the rate of infusion while she is taking a bath to prevent edema.
   b. Report to the licensed nurse observations of redness or swelling at the IV insertion site.
   c. Hang a new bag of fluid when the existing bag is empty.

d. Put a new dressing over the IV site if the old one becomes soiled or wet.

6. Mrs. Suhani's IV is easily dislodged. You have been cautioned by the nurse to be very careful while giving her care. Which of the following guidelines should you follow?
   a. Give complete personal care and ask for help if you are unsure of how to proceed.
   b. Bathe all areas except the arm with the IV and do not change the patient's gown.
   c. Disconnect the IV from the tubing during the bath and reconnect it afterwards.
   d. Ask another nursing assistant to bathe the side of the patient containing the IV.

7. After her morning care, the pump connected to Mrs. Suhani's IV begins to alarm. What should you do?
   a. Push the button to silence the alarm, and notify the licensed nurse that the alarm is ringing.
   b. Check the tubing, bag, and IV site for problems. If you see no problems, silence the alarm and see if it goes off again.
   c. Check for possible problems, then notify the licensed nurse immediately about the alarm and report your observations.
   d. Silence the alarm, then reset the rate to 5 drops per minute less than the current setting. The alarm often sounds if the IV is going too fast.

8. When you change the clothing of a patient with an IV in the left arm, which of the following steps should you take?
   a. Remove the IV bag or bottle from the pole and place it below the level of the patient's arm.
   b. Take the gown off of the left arm, then take the IV bag or bottle through the sleeve of the gown.
   c. Keep the IV bag or bottle below the level of the left arm during the entire procedure.
   d. Undress and dress the left arm first, then undress and dress the right arm.

9. What is the purpose of a PCA pump?
   a. It allows the patient to control the amount of insulin he is given each hour.
   b. It allows the patient to have a continuous dose of cancer medications at all times.

c. It blocks the feeling of pain by stimulating nerve endings with mild electrical shocks.

d. It allows the patient to give himself IV pain medication when it is needed most.

10. Which of the following is true of increased intracranial pressure?

a. It is a serious complication resulting from an acute brain injury.

b. It is pressure on the brain due to bleeding and swelling inside the skull.

c. It can cause permanent brain injury or even death.

d. All of these are true.

11. Which of the following observations about a patient with a serious brain injury should be reported to the nurse immediately?

a. The patient complains of tiredness and requests to take a nap.

b. The patient is disoriented to time and place, but was oriented earlier in the day.

c. The patient's blood pressure was 132/76 earlier and is now 130/70.

d. The patient is able to ambulate more steadily today than she could yesterday.

12. Which of these factors is necessary to promote wound healing?

a. adequate nutrition and hydration

b. antibiotic ointments or salves

c. bandages and dressings that keep out moisture

d. All of these are necessary.

13. Mr. Irving has an abdominal wound with a suction device in place. Which of the following actions should you take regarding his suction device?

a. Check to be sure that the tubing is not kinked or disconnected.

b. Raise the suction container higher than the wound to drain the tubing.

c. Empty the suction container at the end of the shift and record the amount.

d. Pin the suction container to the sheet to prevent it from being pulled accidentally.

14. Mr. Irving also has a tracheostomy in his throat. What is your responsibility regarding his tracheostomy?

a. Clean the sterile suction catheter in alcohol after it is used.

b. Wash around the tracheostomy with hydrogen peroxide and water.

c. Suction inside the tracheostomy if bubbles are present around the site.

d. Notify the nurse immediately if his respiratory rate increases or decreases.

15. Which of these observations would indicate a respiratory emergency?

a. a patient who complains of feeling short of breath

b. a patient whose lips and nailbeds are gray or an ashen color

c. a patient who coughs repeatedly without bringing up mucus

d. all of the above

16. If a patient's breathing stops, what effect will that have on the heart?

a. The patient's heart will stop beating almost instantly.

b. The patient's heart will stop beating when the brain gets the message that oxygen is low and sends a signal to the heart.

c. The patient's brain will be damaged from lack of oxygen and that will cause the heart to stop.

d. The patient's heartbeat will slow but not stop unless the patient also suffers a heart attack.

Getting CONNECTED
Multimedia Extension Activities

www.prenhall.com/will-black

Use the above address to access the free, interactive Companion Website created for this textbook. Hear the pronounciation of the key terms in the chapter. Get instant feedback to a variety of chapter-related questions. Link to other interesting sites.

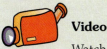

Video

Watch the section on handling infectious waste of the *Infection Control* video from the Care Provider Skills series.

CASE STUDY

You have been assigned to work in the new subacute section of your facility. You have been assigned to 18-year-old Sara James, who is an auto accident victim. She has some wounds on her back and legs and is receiving IV therapy to prevent infection. Because she will be receiving fluids for a long time, a Port-a-cath was implanted in the hospital.

1. One of your primary responsibilities in caring for Sara is to observe and report your observations. Which of the following conditions should you be watching for?
    a. infection
    b. increased intracranial pressure
    c. bowel obstruction
    d. kidney stones
2. You notice when you bathe her that Sara has a strange odor that wasn't there yesterday. You
    a. use extra baby powder when you complete her bath
    b. ask her mother to bring in deodorant
    c. ignore it
    d. report it to the nurse since one of her wounds might be infected
3. On your way to help serve trays in the dining room, you pass a resident sitting in her wheelchair with her lunch tray in front of her. She is holding her hand around her throat and waving frantically. You
    a. perform the Heimlich maneuver
    b. call 911
    c. report to the dining room and tell her CNA that she needs help
    d. report to the charge nurse immediately
4. The resident stops breathing. You don't feel a pulse. Your first priority is
    a. draw the curtain to provide privacy
    b. call for help
    c. establish an airway
    d. get the emergency cart

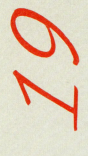

Chapter 19

END-OF-LIFE CARE

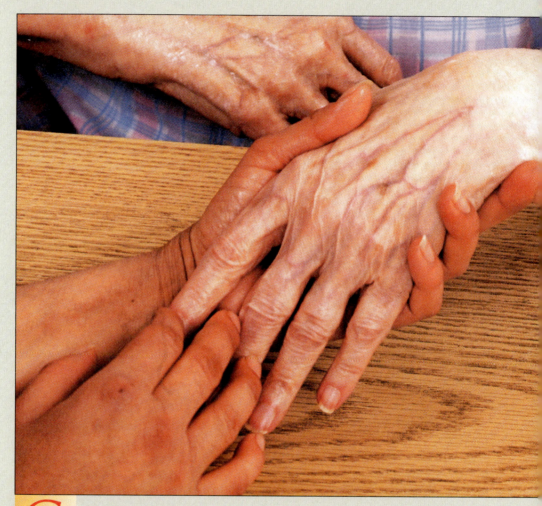

CARING TIP

The nursing assistant knows on a deep level the value of "presence" and touch and is comfortable sitting in silence and holding the hand of the dying resident.

Neva Babcock, BSN, RNC, CDONA, CIC
Performance Improvement/Infection Control Director
St. Thomas More Nursing and Rehab Center
Hyattsville, Maryland

SECTION 1 End of Life

END OF LIFE

There is some disagreement about the period of time called the *end of life.* Because it is so difficult to predict the time when a resident will die, the end of life is usually considered the last year or 6 months. Although predicting the end of life has been studied and measurements developed, they continue to be unreliable. Two persons with the same disease are very different from each other in many ways. These differences change the course of the disease and serve as a source of surprise to the physician. Some people seem to live longer because they have a positive outlook on life. Others may have unfinished business that seems to prevent them from dying when expected. Of course, there are differences in age, general health, and other diseases that will determine life expectancy. For purposes of determining when a person is eligible for hospice care, the U.S. Congress set a period of 6 months. It was thought that it would be easier to determine **prognosis** (outlook) 6 months before the death. Most health care professionals would say the closer to death a person is, the easier it is to predict. In other words, it is easier to tell if death is hours away than days away and easier to tell if death is days away than weeks away and so on.

Chronic illness is a disease or condition that is not curable nor is it considered terminal. Chronic illness is defined as any impairment or deviation from normal that is permanent; causes some disability; and often requires special training of the patient to manage the condition and a long period of care. It may be compared to an **acute illness,** which has a short course and from which there is usually a full recovery or an abrupt termination in death. Most diseases fall into the category of chronic illnesses. Some conditions begin as acute and linger to become chronic. Eighty percent of persons over 65 are said to have one or more chronic illnesses. Even cancer is now considered to be a kind of illness that people live with for many years. Recent studies show that about 20 percent of the predictable deaths (not accidents, homicides, or suicides) occur in a nursing home.

Each chronic disease has a history and a course of events. Diseases are staged according to the severity of symptoms and the likelihood of causing death. Some of the symptoms allow the physician to predict that the chronic disease is now terminal. Residents in the end stages of their diseases need special care. You have already learned about many diseases in their earlier stages. This chapter deals with the end stage of some of the common diseases and the special needs of the residents in those stages. In the next section, we will deal with cancer in all of its stages, including end stages.

prognosis   a prediction of the outcome of an illness

chronic illness   an illness that lasts a long time

acute illness   an illness of short duration

END-STAGE DEMENTIA

The resident with dementia is in the end stages of the disease when she is bed-bound and unable to speak coherently or to make needs known. The resident has problems with eating and with swallowing. Usually, the cause of death will be from pneumonia or other infection. The facility plan of care must be directed toward:

- Anticipating needs
- Creating a pleasant environment
- Preventing skin breakdown and other complications of inactivity
- Supporting the family
- Providing comfort and caring

Because this resident is unable to communicate, the nursing assistant must observe for behaviors indicating the presence of pain or discomfort and report to the charge nurse so that the pain can be treated appropriately. Remember, if it hurts in someone who can say it hurts, it hurts in the resident with dementia.

END-STAGE LUNG DISEASE

End-stage lung disease includes diseases like chronic obstructive pulmonary disease (COPD) and emphysema. Symptoms include shortness of breath, weakness and fatigue, anxiety, edema of the lower extremities. The resident usually is receiving oxygen, keeps the head of the bed elevated, and is dependent in activities of daily living (ADL). A common position is sitting on the side of the bed, leaning forward over the over-bed table or pillows. Every breath requires great effort. The shortness of breath may be so severe that the resident has difficulty speaking and eating. Weight loss is common due to both loss of appetite and severe fatigue. The resident is usually very anxious, fearful, and demanding. The struggle to breathe may make the resident create reasons for the nursing assistant to stay in the room. The call light may be used often for what may seem like unimportant reasons. The care of this resident must include:

- Reducing anxiety and fear
- Consistent staff to care for the resident
- Saving energy by doing all ADL for the resident
- Slowing down the care, particularly feeding
- Rest periods
- Scheduling activities
- Anticipating needs
- Doing things the resident's way

END-STAGE CARDIOVASCULAR OR HEART DISEASE

There is great variation in symptoms and progression depending on specific disease. Usually fatigue, shortness of breath, peripheral edema, weight gain, loss of appetite, nausea, anxiety, and restlessness occur. Some may have chest pain. The plan of care is much like that for the resident with end-stage lung disease. Remember what you learned about how the heart and lungs work together. The heart patient may have symptoms that come and go. You may be less aware of the symptoms than with the patient with lung disease. Your care plan will include making focused observations about the resident's plan and circulation such as the skin color around the lips and fingernail beds. Any reports of chest pain must be reported immediately. Some who have poor circulation to the feet and legs may have severe pain and nonhealing wounds. The feet and toes may become black from lack of circulation. These areas need to be handled gently and protected from the pressure of the bed linens and from being bumped against the side rails or other objects. Although a person in the end stages probably would not be appropriate for surgery and amputation, the wounds must be treated in as comfortable a way as possible.

The care plan includes:

- Observing and reporting signs of pain, respiratory distress, and injury
- Treating extremities gently
- Providing for pressure relief and cushioning of the feet
- Protecting from injury
- Performing ADL for the resident to conserve energy

END-STAGE RENAL/KIDNEY DISEASE

End-stage renal/kidney disease may follow an acute illness or may be the result of a long period of treatment, including kidney dialysis, use of many medications, and special diets. The signs of advanced renal disease include anemia, uremia, bone pain, pathologic fractures, muscle weakness, severe **pruritus** (itching), congestive heart failure, hypertension, decreased urine output, and mental changes called *uremic encephalopathy*. The resident usually slips into a coma and dies. Death from renal failure is not believed to be painful due to natural anesthesia brought about by the accumulation of toxic wastes. The plan of care for the nursing assistant must include:

pruritus   itching

- Observing and monitoring urine output
- Protecting from infection by following Standard Precautions
- Excellent skin care
- Gentle turning and repositioning
- Following fluid or diet restrictions if still in place

END-STAGE LIVER DISEASE

End-stage liver disease may result from diseases like cirrhosis of the liver or cancer of the liver. Signs of advanced liver disease include tendency for bleeding, weight loss, nausea, loss of appetite, fatigue, and **ascites,** or accumulation of fluid in the **abdomen.** There may be shortness of breath due to the ascites. Edema in the extremities, jaundice, itching of the skin, and mental changes and pain are also common. The person usually slips into a coma before death. However, uncontrolled bleeding may also occur. The bleeding usually comes from the gastrointestinal tract. Your plan of care will include:

ascites   an abnormal collection of fluid in the abdomen

abdomen   region of the body between the chest and the pelvis

- Excellent skin care
- Positioning for comfortable breathing
- Pain management

- Help with all ADL
- Serving small portions of favorite foods
- Creating a caring and comfortable environment
- Family support

GENERAL SYMPTOMS

The following are general symptoms experienced by most residents who have reached the end of life. They exist regardless of diagnosis.

ANOREXIA AND WEIGHT LOSS

cachexia ill health with malnutrition and severe weight loss

Loss of appetite and weight loss are symptoms present in over 65 percent of dying residents regardless of diagnosis. About 20 percent of these residents experience gross weight loss **(cachexia).** Sometimes, the loss of appetite is due to changes in taste because of treatments; other times, it may be a reflection of the morale of the resident, and at times it is because of the lack of physical activity with a decreased need for food. Even though the weight loss may be unavoidable, certain actions can be taken to slow the process.

- Conditions of the mouth such as thrush need to be treated.
- Constipation needs to be managed.
- Nausea must be treated.
- Favorite foods should be offered, with the diet unrestricted.
- Frequent small feedings attractively served may help.
- Provide a pleasant environment that is clean and orderly. The resident should be pain-free, clean and well groomed, and comfortably positioned (Figure 19-1).
- Some medications may be given to increase the appetite.

The nurse will help the family understand that loss of appetite is a natural course of the dying process. It is important not to force the resident to eat. Usually, things such as feeding tubes are avoided because they only serve to prolong the dying, cause discomfort, and do not restore well-being.

Consequences of weight loss have implications for the care of the resident. Weight loss places the resident at greater risk for skin breakdown. Aggressive caring is needed to prevent pressure ulcers. Good skin care involves:

FIGURE 19-1

Encourage the resident to eat.

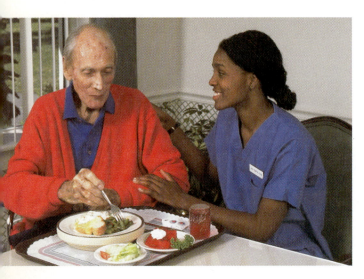

- Keeping the skin clean and dry
- Using lotions to lubricate
- Repositioning to reduce pressure
- Pressure reducing devices such as alternating pressure mattresses and pads or other types of cushioning

Residents who have dentures may have a problem with improper fit because of weight loss. Often, they can be relined, or sometimes denture adhesives may be helpful.

When one's body changes drastically, it is not unusual to have a disturbance in body image. A helpful approach is (1) assisting the resident to choose clothing that fits or does not accentuate the weight loss and

(2) assuring good grooming and dress. The family may want to purchase smaller clothing. It is best not to emphasize weight loss by commenting on it to the resident or to the family.

What should the nursing assistant do when the resident has a loss of appetite?

- Report any changes in appetite to the charge nurse.
- Help prepare the resident for mealtimes.
- Report any family comments or concerns to the charge nurse for follow-up.
- Protect from injury to the skin and provide good skin care.
- Take time when feeding the resident.
- Offer as much choice as possible.

FATIGUE AND WEAKNESS

Almost all residents with advanced disease complain of weakness and fatigue. There is no drug that restores strength. Blood transfusions do not help. Sometimes, mild exercise can help, especially if fatigue is due to spending too much time in bed.

When fatigue is due to depression, the depression needs to be treated. More often, residents need to learn energy conservation strategies and to allow others to help them.

The nursing assistant plays a crucial role in helping residents save their energy for those things only they can do. By helping with bathing, grooming, dressing, and all personal care, residents may have more energy to spend time with family and friends and doing things they enjoy. In a rehabilitation setting, the staff would be encouraging residents to do as much as possible for themselves. With a terminally ill resident, that probably is not important. Other things the nursing assistant can do for residents to preserve their energy include:

- Scheduling care with rest periods
- Avoiding excessively tiring activities
- Paying attention and allowing rest when signs of fatigue are present
- Helping the family to recognize the resident's need for rest

LOSS OF ABILITY TO PERFORM ADL

Some or all of the independence in ADL may be lost when one is terminally ill. The nursing assistant plays an important role in stepping in to perform many or all of these tasks when a resident loses his or her ability to be independent.

It is important to provide care in a matter-of-fact way that doesn't blame or criticize residents for their lack of ability to care for themselves. As you provide care and assistance in ADL, give residents as much control as possible. For example, ask residents what they want to wear versus you choosing the clothing. Think of as many ways as you can to give choice about each activity you are performing. Sometimes, the only choice may be "yes" or "no," or "now" or "later," but that is still a choice. Be aware that this represents a significant loss to residents and often to their families.

SADNESS, GRIEF, AND DEPRESSION

Most terminally ill residents experience emotional reactions to the process of dying and the losses that accompany the natural course of their disease. You have learned about the way Dr. Elisabeth Kübler-Ross described certain phases that are often, but not always, experienced.

- *Shock and denial*—It is important not to insist that residents admit that they are dying. Denial protects residents until they are able to accept more. However, we do not lie to residents either. The evidence of denial may be shown by residents' reluctance to sign a Do Not Resuscitate request or in their avoidance of making final arrangements or plans. They may continue drugs or treatments that are not considered beneficial any longer. The nursing assistant needs to do lots of listening, let the rest of the staff members know what is happening with the resident, but avoid supporting the denial by agreeing with the resident. For example, if the resident says "I know I am going to get well," a good response might be to say nothing or say "Wouldn't that be wonderful," "What would you do should that happen?," or "What will you do if that doesn't happen?"

- *Anger*—Once the resident can no longer deny the truth of his condition, he may become angry. This is the time when the resident may question all his beliefs—particularly in a higher power. They may ask "Why me?" Needless to say, there is no right answer. Sometimes, it is helpful just to say "It must seem very unfair to you" or "I wish I knew the answer." The key for the nursing assistant is not to take the resident's anger personally. Sometimes, the anger may seem like criticism or it may be directed at you. Keep in mind that it is probably anger about being ill and anger about dying. Do your best not to become hurt, defensive, or argumentative. Just listen and allow the resident to express his or her anger.

- *Depression* is one of the hardest responses to deal with. This may be difficult for family and friends as well. If the resident withdraws and doesn't converse with visitors, they may not return. Depression is an overwhelming sadness that keeps residents from functioning in a normal way. They seem to find no enjoyment in their life. They often have sleeping and eating problems. It is important to accept residents where they are, to be kind but firm, and to avoid trying to "cheer up" the depressed resident. This is a time for carrying out your caregiving in a quiet, calm manner. Make a special effort to spend a few minutes a day with the resident just "hanging out." You will show your caring and support without saying anything.

- *Bargaining* may not be apparent to staff, family, and friends because it often is between the resident and their higher power. Bargaining is a process of thinking that one behavior can be traded for something like a longer life or a pain-free life. For example, the dying resident may say in a prayer "God, if you will let me live to my daughter's wedding, I will be ready to go." You may notice from time to time that a resident surprised the entire staff by living longer than anyone expected has appeared to have been "waiting" for a particular event.

- *Acceptance* is defined as the acknowledgment of the reality. Acceptance does not mean that the resident likes what is happening, only that they are able to admit that it is true. When residents achieve this acceptance, they often want to talk about death, about their wishes, their fears, and their concerns. It is important to encourage this conversation. Some family and friends may tend to say, "Oh, don't talk like that" or "I don't want to talk about it" or "That is too depressing, lets talk about something else." The facility staff can serve as role models by being willing to listen and, if necessary, to write things down. Let the rest of the staff know when the resident begins talking about his or her death so that they too can listen and assist in making arrangements if necessary. Sometimes, the resident may want to complete some "unfinished business" and may need help from the staff to do so.

These phases serve as guides to the ways people usually deal with grief and loss. While they are not absolute, they help us make the distinction between normal and abnormal grief. They also give us some guidance in how we can be most helpful to the resident.

FEAR AND ANXIETY

Dying residents may experience fear and anxiety at times. The staff helps them express their fears and deal with each one as it arises. Common fears include:

- Fear of abandonment
- Fear of dying alone
- Fear of pain
- Fear of loss of control
- Fear of the unknown
- Fear of being a burden to the family

Most of the help comes by allowing residents to voice their fears. Sometimes, reassurance can be given, but not always. We can, for example, say that we will work with them to see that they are not in pain, or we will allow them to control as long as they can. We can't promise that they won't be alone at the time of death or assure them that we know what death is like. Sometimes, their spiritual advisor or minister can be helpful in these cases. Be sure you let the other staff know when you have reason to believe the resident is fearful or anxious.

CONFUSION

Often, near the end of life, residents are confused. They don't know the day, the place, or who various people are. They may hallucinate and see people who no one else can see. This could be a result of their disease and its impact on the function of their brain, such as in acquired immune deficiency syndrome (AIDS), cancer of the brain, or cardiovascular or respiratory disease that decreases the oxygen to the brain.

The main concerns at this time are for safety. The resident is at much higher risk for falls and other types of injury. This time requires substantial patience on the part of the staff, family, and friends.

Because one never knows what is understood, it is important to patiently explain everything you are doing before you do it. Talk residents through every procedure. Remind them of who you are, and assure them you are there to help. Call them by name—usually, the first name gets a better response. Try to put structure and routine into your activities with residents. They do better with consistency, not variety and change! Slow down everything you are doing to give the resident time to process.

Remove dangerous substances and objects from the immediate area. Keep the environment simple and free of distractions. Limit the amount of noise to

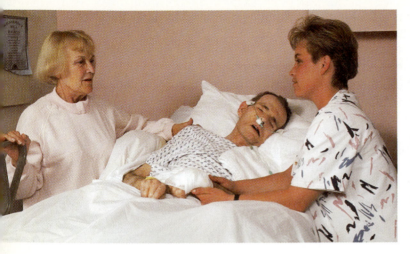

FIGURE 19-2

Explain that sleeping is normal.

the degree that you can. Avoid having private conversations with other staff or family within earshot of the resident. Be cautious in the presence of residents so that you never say anything you wouldn't want them to hear and understand.

SEDATION

While not normally distressing to the resident, sedation may be distressing to the family and friends. As a person gets closer to death, he or she may sleep a significant part of the time. This may frustrate others because they want the resident with them as long as possible (Figure 19-2). They may complain that the resident is sleeping his or her life away, or they may blame the medications used to control the pain.

They should be encouraged to discuss this with the charge nurse. Help them understand that this is normal and give them ideas on what they can do. For example, it is very helpful to sit quietly by the bedside and hold the hand of the resident. Residents and family may want to limit the number of visitors to have more private time for those closest to the resident. The staff should perform their roles quietly and with minimal disruption. Discuss changes in the plan of care with the charge nurse. Certain tasks may no longer be appropriate.

SECTION 2 Culture and End-of-Life Care

OBJECTIVES
What You Will Learn

When you have completed this section, you will be able to:

• List some of the ways culture affects the way a person dies

• Describe the responsibility of the nursing assistant related to cultural issues

• Explain the difference between stereotyping and cultural awareness

KEY TERMS　　　　　ethnocentrism　　　　　stereotype

CULTURAL AWARENESS The United States is a population that is made up of many different nationalities, ethnic groups, and religions. At this time, one in three Americans are members of an ethnically diverse cultural group, and by the year 2050, the nonwhite population in the United States will triple due to birth and immigration.

This diversity has created a wonderful strength and richness to our national heritage. The complexities of multiculturalism has also presented us with challenges, and never more so than in caring for people at the end of life. Most cultures have very specific views regarding dying, death, funeral, and burial and have developed religious or spiritual practices around them.

It is your responsibility to learn more about other cultures to better understand their values and belief systems. In this way, end-of-life care can be provided with respect, honor, and dignity according to their traditions.

One of the dangers in becoming knowledgable about another culture is that this information can then be used to **stereotype** a person or persons. Generalization begins with an assumption about a group but leads to seeking further information whether the assumption fits the person. When stereotyping, one makes an assumption about a person based on group membership without bothering to learn whether the individual fits that assumption. It is always important to remember that regardless of one's background, each person is still an individual and may not always follow the norm expected of him. There may be many reasons for this deviation, such as length of time the person has been in the United States, his age when he came here, level of education, social or economic class, and his own desire to assimilate.

stereotype a generalization

Ethnocentrism is the view that one's culture's way of doing things is the right and natural way and all others are inferior, unnatural, or barbaric. Most humans are ethnocentric. Anthropologists, on the other hand, look at behavior from a broader, more worldly viewpoint.

ethnocentrism belief that one's own race or group is superior to all others

Time orientation varies in different cultures. In looking at the past, present, or future, an individual culture will tend to emphasize one over the others. For example, Chinese, British, and Austrian cultures have a past orientation. This often occurs in cultures that were a major or dominant civilization at one time in history. Hispanics and African Americans tend to have a present-time orientation, while middle-class white American culture tends to be future oriented.

Cultures also vary in social structure. American culture is organized according to a model of equality. Theoretically, everyone is equal. In reality, things may operate differently, but we hold equality as our ideal. Some cultures are based on a hierarchical model in which status is based on characteristics such as age, sex, and occupation. Status differences are important as those commanding higher respect may also have influence over health care decision making.

Family of orientation is the family one is born into, which is composed of parents, brothers, and sisters. The family of procreation is the one a person marries into and includes spouse and children. Some cultures emphasize one over the other, and this can result in differing sets of loyalties.

Americans usually believe that germs cause disease; however, other cultures do not share that belief. Instead, they may believe causes of disease to be from upset body balance, soul loss, soul theft, spirit possession, breach of taboo, and object intrusion.

In order to develop cultural competency, you must begin by knowing your own attitude, beliefs, and practices that are developed from your heritage and past experiences. In end-of-life care, particular attention needs to be paid to the areas of illness, pain, death and dying, and belief in an afterlife. To be more aware of your own beliefs, ask yourself these questions:

- To what extent do you believe in life after death?
- How appropriate is it for children to attend funerals?
- To what extent do you believe in reincarnation?
- If you could choose, when would you die?
- What kind of death would you prefer?
- How do you feel about an autopsy being done on your body?
- Are you willing to be an organ donor?
- How do you want your body disposed of after death?
- What is your experience of participating in rituals to remember the dead?

Most people are eager to share knowledge about their beliefs, values, and customs with others, and they will appreciate your interest. You may start by asking some basic questions, such as:

- Where was the resident born? If an immigrant, how long has the resident lived in this country?
- What is the resident's ethnic affiliation, and how strong is his or her ethnic identity?
- Who are the major support people in the resident's life—family members, friends? Does the resident have strong ties to his or her ethnic community?
- What are the primary and secondary languages, speaking and reading ability?
- What is the resident's religion/philosophy, its importance in daily life, and current practices?
- What are the resident's food preferences and prohibitions?
- What are the health and illness beliefs and practices?
- What are the customs and beliefs around such transitions as birth, illness, and death?

Understanding culture requires knowledge of how an individual defines his or her heritage. Factors to consider are how long the individual has lived in the United States, geographic location, rural or urban setting, and family influences.

It has been noted that the wealthy in a culture are more likely to move away from their communities of origin and become less traditional in their beliefs and practices. The poor, on the other hand, are more likely to follow traditional practices.

Different religions and religious denominations shape spirituality in different ways. The more traditional the religious experience, the more conservative will be the attitudes, beliefs, and values. They hold onto the old ways of relating to death, dying, and funeral rites.

Communication of all types is the primary way culture is transmitted. It is important to be aware that there are significant contrasts within "minority" groups. Essential elements that must be studied include language volume (silence), use of touch, content of speech, emotional tone, and gestures, stance, and eye behavior. If there is one commonality in grief among cultures, it is the importance of crying as a grieving strategy. Grief is expressed across various cultures in differing ways and can be seen in both verbal and nonverbal communication.

Space is another cultural difference. Space refers to the distance needed in personal relationships. Spatial requirements vary among individuals of different cultures. Physical touching is accepted in some groups and taboo in others. Need for space serves four functions: (1) security, (2) privacy, (3) autonomy, and (4) expression of self-identity. Cultural practices related to space and the person who is dying vary dramatically. In some cultures (e.g., Buddhist), quietness and privacy for meditation is important. On the other hand, for a Moslem who is dying, it is considered important for another person of the same faith to be close to bedside and recite appropriate verses from the Koran so that these are the last words heard by the person.

For many cultural groups, the family is the single most important social organization, although the view of the family varies significantly between groups. In some cultures the extended family is the center of concern. This often requires consultation with the entire group before decisions can be made. Also important are gender role issues—is this a male- or female-dominated culture?

Social position is also a significant factor to consider in grief expressions. The mourning of death corresponds to age, sex, and socioeconomic status.

Research shows that people do differ biologically according to race, gender, and age. Persons from different cultures may vary biologically in ways such as racial–anatomical characteristics, growth and development patterns, body systems, skin and hair, physiology, mucous membranes, disease prevalence, and resistance to disease. It is important for health professionals to be aware of these differences if appropriate treatment and intervention is to occur.

In end-of-life care, we are dealing with one of life's greatest transitions—the death experience. This area is rich in the development of specific rituals, customs, and beliefs centering on illness, the dying process, the deathbed scene, and the grieving process. In this regard, nursing assistants providing end-of-life care need to be aware of the variey of responses that may be encountered, which may be quite different from their own.

For example, we may believe we know what dying, death, and life are about and when death has occurred. In some cultures, however, people are counted dead when most Americans would consider them alive, or people are considered dead that we would see as merely ill. It is important never to assume anything when it comes to cultural variables!

In the area of loss, we see grief responses that in our culture might be deemed inappropriate but is quite normal for that ethnic group. These responses include *muted grief,* in which emotional control is highly prized; *excessive grief,* in which bereavement continues for expected, long periods of time; and *violent grief,* in which anger and aggression are part of the mourning process.

Communication becomes a key factor when you are trying to learn more about a resident and family with a culture different than your own. Language barriers and nonverbal communication pose special challenges. When speaking to people for whom English is a second language, make sure you ask them to repeat or rephrase themselves if you did not understand what they were saying to you. If they use a word or phrase you are not familiar with, ask them to explain it to you. Be careful when you speak that you choose words that will be clearly understood and not misinterpreted. It is important for the facility staff to discover specific cultural issues in order to provide respectful care to the dying resident. Some of these questions include:

- Who is allowed to provide personal care? (Some cultures would not allow a member of the opposite sex to provide care.)
- Does the resident/family have any special customs the staff should follow?
- Are there customs unique to their culture and/or religion that we need to know and respect?
- What is the resident's/caregiver's understanding about medication?
- Are there specific customs regarding death that the facility staff needs to know beforehand?

There are many examples of cultural differences that show why these types of questions are important. For example, in the Chinese culture, traditional healing practices include using herbal preparations that are usually given once. Therefore, getting a resident to take medication on an intermittent basis could be difficult. In the Japanese culture, the number "four" means death, so getting medication taken QID (four times a day) could be problematic. Many cultures believe talking about funeral plans brings bad luck. Some believe that dying at home is preferred; others fear death at home and transfer the resident to a facility.

GENERAL GUIDELINES

- Develop an awareness of your own culture and values.
- Identify your strengths and limitations in dealing with someone from a different culture.
- Increase your knowledge about other cultures with which you will be involved.

Cultural diversity is complex and wide ranged even within a single ethnic group. It is important for you to learn as much as possible about the cultural groups you will most likely be working with and develop a good knowledge base. You can then utilize this information, but always keep in mind that every resident and family are unique in their own way. Do not put them into a certain stereotype, but rather see them as the individuals they really are.

SECTION 3   Food and Fluids at the End of Life

OBJECTIVES
What You Will Learn

When you have completed this section, you will be able to:

- Define key terms related to food/nutrition and fluids/hydration at the end of life
- Describe the benefits and burdens of artificial nutrition and hydration
- Match ethical principles with their correct definitions
- Explore the process of decision making regarding artificial nutrition and hydration

KEY TERMS

artificial hydration
artificial nutrition

bioethics
enterally

ethicist
total parenteral nutrition (TPN)

FOOD AND FLUIDS

Issues about whether to force-feed a dying resident have been the subject of legal, ethical, and emotional discussions with the public and with health care professionals across the country. Few issues cause so much conflict in our beliefs and values. In this section, we will explore the issues from a legal, medical, and ethical perspective.

Some of the important terminology includes:

artificial nutrition providing food and nourishment by means other than by mouth

enterally by means of the gastrointestinal tract

total parenteral nutrition (TPN) provision of nutrition directly into the circulation rather than through the digestive system

artificial hydration providing liquids by means other than by mouth

- **Artificial nutrition** is supplying the body with foodlike material by artificial means. Nutrients may be provided **enterally** (through the gastrointestinal tract via a tube that is inserted through the nose (nasogastric or NG tube), directly into the stomach (gastrostomy or G tube), or into the intestines (jejunostomy or J tube). Nutrients may also be supplied through the circulatory system by placing a tube in a vein or directly into the heart. This is called **total parenteral nutrition (TPN).** TPN is used when the gastrointestinal tract is not able to absorb and utilize nutrition in a normal manner. The formula is complex, requiring the considerable clinical expertise of a pharmacist, physician, and dietitian, as well as frequent laboratory monitoring. The resident is at risk for infection and usually requires considerable equipment to administer the solution.
- **Artificial hydration** is provision of fluids through an intravenous (IV) access to a vein. The fluids do not provide needed nutrition but prevent de-

hydration. The IV line is used for medication administration also. There is debate in the medical community about use of IVs for dying residents.

The normal course of most terminal illnesses leads to a gradual decline in appetite and consequent weight loss. As the body is "shutting down," the need for food decreases. Food is the fuel that the body needs to restore energy and rebuild body tissues. When the body is no longer repairing and restoring, the amount of food needed is sharply decreased.

One helpful analogy is that of fuel in a car. Suppose it is your habit to buy gas once a week on Thursdays, and you stop driving the car. What will happen if you continue to buy gas every Thursday? The gas will overflow. If you continue to feed residents who are not using their intake, they will be "overfilled." Decreasing their intake is a natural part of the dying process.

One key role of the facility staff is to help the resident and family to understand the dying process. The purpose of food for the dying resident is for pleasure, not nutrition. Normally, the diet is changed to allow the resident to eat what he wants, when he wants it.

CULTURAL AWARENESS Food is an important aspect of most cultures. We use food to show our caring and nurturing. Food is part of celebrations and rituals. One of the often-quoted passages from the Christian religious point of view is that there is an obligation to "feed the hungry and to give drink to the thirsty." Because of this, when one either chooses not to eat or is no longer able to eat, the family may be very distressed. They may push the resident to eat, causing friction and discomfort within the family. You may also feel uncomfortable with allowing a resident to choose not to eat. It may take some thoughtful discussion and study to resolve your own personal conflict with the resident's rights.

There may come a time when the family believes that the resident should be fed through a tube or be given IV fluids because of a decline in the amount the resident is taking in. It has been established in the U.S. Supreme Court that competent adults have the right to refuse any unwanted medical treatment. When the resident is no longer capable of making these decisions, the family often becomes the decision maker. It is difficult for them to decide not to do everything possible to keep the resident alive. Of course, the artificial nutrition does not change the outcome or cure residents, but it probably does extend their live. **Ethicists** (those who study and examine what is right and what is wrong) make the point that providing artificial nutrition and hydration is like any other medical intervention and thus can be refused. Furthermore, they remind us that artificial nutrition is nothing at all like eating. There is no taste, no pleasure; there is nothing social or nurturing.

ethicist person who is expert in moral issues

Although the facility staff may help educate the family about the medical, legal, and ethical elements of decision making, it is never appropriate to impose our own beliefs on the resident and family.

ETHICAL DECISION MAKING

Decision making at the end of life follows certain common ethical principles. These principles have been described in the literature in the field of bioethics. **Bioethics** refers to health care ethics as a subset of broader ethical concepts. The most common principles include:

bioethics a field of study of the moral values that relate to health care

- *Autonomy—self-determination.* The right to make decisions about ourselves and what is best for us is a highly valued principle of ethics. This, however, is not true in all cultures. In addition, the law supports the ethical principle of self-determination. The courts have established that any adult capable of decision making has the legal right to accept or refuse any medical intervention. According to ethical practices, artificial nutrition and hydration are medical interventions that may both legally and ethically be refused.

- *Veracity—truth telling.* Health care professionals have a duty to tell residents the truth related to the legal concept of informed consent, which requires truth telling so that the resident's decision making is based on accurate information.
- *Nonmaleficence—to do no harm.* Health care professionals do not intentionally harm those in their care. Part of the Hippocratic Oath taken by physicians is to "do no harm."
- *Beneficence—to do good for others.* It is not sufficient for health care professionals to do no harm; they are required to do good for those in their care.
- *Justice—fair and equal treatment of all.* Health care professionals have an obligation to give residents and their families what is due them and to use resources wisely and fairly.

The principles are not ranked in any way. In other words, each is equally important. When two or more of these principles come into conflict, a dilemma exists. Some facilities have an ethics committee that reviews cases and discusses solutions. In others, the facility interdisciplinary team serves as the body that conducts the review and discussion. Many long-term care (LTC) facilities have policies to serve as guidelines to staff, residents, and family. These guidelines explore the principles and provide a basis for decision making. The literature is rich with articles on the subjects of artificial nutrition and hydration in the terminally ill.

Some important points for staff to know in addition to the principles described here include:

- Residents and their legally authorized representatives have the right to refuse unwanted medical intervention.
- Artificially supplied nutrition and hydration are medical interventions.
- Being fed through a tube is nothing like eating. There is no taste, enjoyment, or psychological pleasure.
- There are risks and burdens to being fed or hydrated artificially.
- Those who are not artificially fed and hydrated have reported they are *not* uncomfortable. The only complaint is dry mouth, which can be managed with good oral hygiene and use of moisturizing agents.
- Terminally ill residents who are not eating do not "starve to death." The cause of death is their end-stage disease or an infection like pneumonia.

BENEFITS OF ARTIFICIAL NUTRITION/HYDRATION

Providing food and fluids through artificial means may prolong the life of the resident or, when used temporarily following an episode of nausea and vomiting, may actually provide comfort. The intravenous line or the tube may provide a route for medication administration when the resident is unable to swallow. At times, family members may be comforted by the fact that "something" is being done for the resident or "everything possible" is being provided for the resident.

Those who are not ready to face the impending death may attempt to postpone by continuing treatment. They may believe that artificial nutrition and hydration are basic and that the resident is "eating," with all of the attendant pleasure and satisfaction of a meal.

BURDENS OF ARTIFICIAL NUTRITION

The burdens of artificial nutrition are greatest with an NG tube. The tube is inserted through the nose and passed down to the stomach. The resident may experience gagging and may develop a sore throat. The appearance of a tube coming from the resident's nose may cause family and friends to avoid contact for fear of dislodging the tube. Residents, in their confusion or delirium, may pull the tube out because it bothers them. A decision may then be made to use hand restraints. They must have the head of the bed elevated to 45 degrees during and for about 1 hour after feedings. Many are fed continuously, requiring the head of bed to be elevated at *all* times. This increases pressure on the skin of the coccyx and buttocks, increasing the risk of pressure ulcer development. Should the tube become dislodged, the resident may aspirate the feedings into the lungs, causing a type of pneumonia. In addition, some residents feel uncomfortable because the stomach is overfilled with the feeding formula. If they are receiving more fluid and nutrients than their body requires, they may appear bloated, with their skin tight and shiny. This skin breaks down easily and increases the risk of sores.

Tubes inserted into the stomach through a minor surgical procedure (gastrostomy or G tubes) are less burdensome. The tube comes out through the skin on the abdomen and is less comfortable than an NG tube. However, it still may become dislodged. The risk of aspiration is minimal when compared to an NG tube. The problems with discomfort due to overfeeding are the same as with NG tubes. A jejunal feeding tube, or J tube, is similar to a G tube except that it is inserted into the upper portion of the intestines or jejunum. There may be additional problems with absorption of the formula, leading to either diarrhea or constipation.

For fluids provided through the intravenous route, there is some discomfort when the needle or catheter is inserted. There is also risk of infection, hemorrhage, dislodgment, and fluid accumulation in the surrounding tissues. If excessive amounts of fluid are provided, there may be swelling and respiratory difficulty. The frequency of urination increases, which may either increase the activity of toileting or the need for skin care and hygiene if the resident is incontinent. There is a need for additional equipment and the involvement of medical technology in the care of the resident.

BENEFITS OF NOT EATING OR DRINKING

Benefits include freedom from discomfort from being overfilled with food and fluid, easier breathing, less need for urination, and, according to many, a feeling of euphoria along with enhanced pain relief. Additional cessation of eating and drinking is a natural part of the dying process. Recent research on residents who stopped eating and drinking indicated that the only discomfort experienced was that of dry mouth. Good oral hygiene and use of special moisturizers for lips and mouth can prevent dry mouth.

It is important to note that food and fluids are always offered to residents because they can change their minds at any time. Offering fluids usually includes the following:

1. Find out what fluids the resident prefers.
2. Be sure you know the proper way to offer fluids to this resident (cup, straw, etc.). Check with the nurse or care plan if necessary.

3. Position the resident so that he or she is upright. Never give fluids to residents lying flat in bed.
4. Be cautious with hot liquids.
5. Offer the fluids slowly and in small quantities.
6. Observe for choking and report any changes or difficulties to the charge nurse.

In health care, the terms we use in talking about caring for residents at the end of life may influence both residents and families who must make decisions about a dying loved one's care. Treatment may be unnecessarily stopped or inappropriately prolonged. And when the resident dies, families or friends may be left feeling guilty about the decision they made. Consider some of the words we use in caring for dying residents and think about how we might use better terms to serve residents and families making difficult choices.

- *Feeding tube.* This mechanism for providing artificial nutrition does not "feed" a resident as described earlier. Chemical sustenance, not "food," is being mechanically administered to keep the body functioning (not necessarily the same thing as keeping the resident "alive"), just as a ventilator allows artificial respiration, not "breathing."
  To speak of food or water is to convey an image of warmth, caring, and nurturing. We think of feeding a baby or holding a cup to the resident's mouth to provide nourishment. It is easy to understand why a family would be unwilliing to remove what is called a "feeding tube." Who would "take food away" from a loved one? But the family might be willing to withhold or withdraw artificial nutrition and hydration if it were described in a more accurate way.
- *No CPR.* In most facilities, these words signify a do-not-resuscitate (DNR) decision—in other words, no artificial ventilation or chest compressions to restart the heart. Many residents, families, and even physicians are reluctant to agree to this status because they fear that it means stopping all treatment or doing nothing. They may believe that we abandon the resident and watch as the resident struggles, writhes, and eventually dies. The truth is that we never "do nothing" or "stop treatment." Instead, we change the goal of treatment from cure to comfort, maintaining all the appropriate safety, comfort, and dignity measures. For this reason, some facilities use terms like *Comfort Code.* This is a better description of what kind of care will be provided if their loved one begins to die. Rather than stating what is not done; it describes what will be done.
- *Futile treatment.* For some people, a treatment may be futile if it is unlikely to restore quality of life to what it was prior to illness. But others will prefer living without a limb or kidney to dying. We must always assess the wishes of the resident and family, and address the issue of futility in terms of their definitions of life, especially the way they define *quality* of life.
  Whether a treatment is futile depends on the individual resident and his medical condition. For some patients with pneumonia or in a respiratory crisis, a ventilator may be a standard treatment, with recovery expected. For a resident with end-stage chronic obstructive pulmonary disease or end-stage congestive heart failure, however, that same treatment may be futile. Similar distinctions can be made for treatments ranging from antibiotics to organ transplant.
- *Hope.* Some people may confuse hope with optimism. In illness, optimism means that you believe that the individual will recover regardless of the

facts. Optimism focuses on cheering up the resident. Hope, on the other hand, accepts the facts and focuses on living until death. Hope can acknowledge not just the possibility of death, but its inevitability. Hope can change to focus on reconciliation, peace, and comfort. Optimism would focus on "getting well" or living longer.

To be fair to the residents and families, it is necessary to recognize how what we say influences what we do. What we say also influences what others do and how they feel. There is a saying that states, "People will forget what you said. People will forget what you did, but people will never forget how you made them feel."

SECTION 4 The Dying Resident

OBJECTIVES
What You Will Learn

When you have completed this section, you will be able to:

- Identify the goals of hospice care

- Insert in the "grief wheel" the appropriate emotions that are present in each phase of the grieving process
- Participate in a simulated grief experience

- Answer questions regarding policies for care of the dying resident in your facility

KEY TERMS

bereaved
Cheyne–Stokes breathing

death
dying

grief process
hospice

There are cultural and religious beliefs about death and dying that profoundly affect our reaction to it. **Dying** is the process of decline in body functions that results in death. **Death** is the final cessation of all vital functions in a person. There are many mysteries and fears associated with death. It has only been in recent years that the subject is openly discussed on television and in movies, books, and magazines. The number of people dying of AIDS brought the process of death and dying into the public eye more than ever before. In the past, many people died without ever being told about their terminal condition. Physicians and families tried to "protect" the dying person from the truth about his or her condition. Research has confirmed, however, that almost always the dying person knows the truth. In recent years, this is changing and patients are given accurate information and are being permitted to control their lives during the dying process. This trend is reflected in the Dying Person's Bill of Rights (Figure 19-3, next page).

Special programs and organizations are available in most areas to give support to those with limited life expectancy. Volunteer programs, organizations such as Make Today Count, and the National Hospice Organization are making a big difference in improving the quality of life for people who are dying and their families.

dying the process of decline in body functions that results in death

death the final cessation of all vital functions

HOSPICE CARE

Hospice care is designed to meet the unique needs of the dying resident as well as his or her family or loved ones. Hundreds of years ago the word **hospice** referred to a place in the mountains of Switzerland where the monks took

hospice a program of care for residents who have a limited life expectancy

FIGURE 19-3

The dying person's bill of rights.

The Dying Person's Bill of Rights

As we face death, what are our rights as human beings? This bill of rights was created at a workshop on "The Terminally Ill Patient and the Helping Person," sponsored by the Southwestern Michigan Insurance Education Council and conducted by Amelia J. Barbus.

- I have the right to be treated as a living human being until I die.
- I have the right to maintain a sense of hopefulness, however changing its focus may be.
- I have the right to be cared for by those who can maintain a sense of hopefulness, however changing this might be.
- I have the right to express my feelings and emotions about my approaching death in my own way.
- I have the right to participate in decisions concerning my care.
- I have the right to expect continuing medical and nursing attention even though "cure" goals must be changed to "comfort" goals.
- I have the right not to die alone.
- I have the right to be free from pain.
- I have the right to have my questions answered honestly.
- I have the right not to be deceived.
- I have the right to have help from and for my family in accepting my death.
- I have the right to die in peace and dignity.
- I have the right to retain my individuality and not be judged for my decisions which may be contrary to beliefs of others.
- I have the right to discuss and enlarge my religious and/or spiritual experiences, whatever these may mean to others.
- I have the right to expect that the sanctity of the human body will be respected after death.
- I have the right to be cared for by caring, sensitive, knowledgeable people who will attempt to understand my needs and will be able to gain some satisfaction in helping me face my death.

FIGURE 19-4

The community hospice.

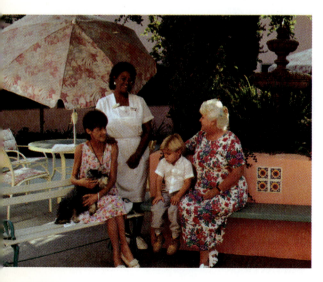

care of sick or weary travelers. Gradually, these places of respite became places for taking care of the sick and dying. In the early 1900s, the first British hospice, St. Joseph's, was opened and a prominent British physician, Dr. Cicely Saunders, championed the cause of the terminally ill. The first hospice program in the United States, Hospice of Connecticut, was opened in 1974, and the number of hospice programs in the United States has grown from a handful in the early 1970s to more than 1,800 (Figure 19-4).

In the past few years, hospice providers have become important partners with the long-term care facility in providing care to terminally ill residents and their families. Those persons who have been diagnosed with a terminal illness with a life expectancy of 6 months or less and who have decided to seek palliative (comfort) versus curative care are eligible for hospice services.

Hospice care can be provided wherever the terminally ill person resides, at home, in a care center, at a residential care center, or in a special hospice inpatient unit (Figure 19-5). Hospice care is provided through an interdisciplinary team, which provides all care and services (Figure 19-6).

The goals of hospice care include:

- Keeping the dying person comfortable through pain control and symptom management
- Allowing the resident and/or loved ones as much control as possible over the circumstances of dying
- Supporting family and loved ones following the death through the bereavement period (to be **bereaved** means to be left desolate by death)
- Providing the resident with the highest quality of life when the quantity of life is limited.

Most long-term care facilities contract with hospice providers for hospice care and services. Hospice care is paid for through Medicare, Medicaid, and most private insurance programs.

The hospice interdisciplinary team is responsible under the Medicare and Medicaid guidelines to "professionally" manage the care of the hospice resident that is related to the terminal illness. The long-term care facility is responsible to assist in carrying out the hospice plan of care and to provide daily care and services.

Hospice team members provide much of the direct care of the resident and provide supportive services for the family or loved ones. The nursing assistant will work with members of the hospice interdisciplinary team to meet the special needs of residents with a limited life expectancy. The resident's plan of care will specify how this care will be carried out and by whom. Regardless of how care is provided for the terminally ill resident, it must be done with knowledge, sensitivity, and concern for the rights of the dying person.

It is estimated that in long-term care facilities in the United States between 5 to 10 percent of the residents are in a terminal phase. The nursing assistant has a unique opportunity to assist those terminally ill residents in his or her care to die with dignity in a supportive environment.

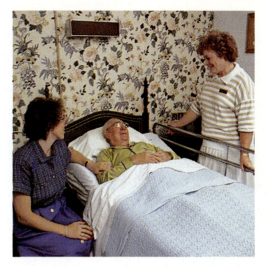

FIGURE 19-5

Hospice unit.

bereaved   to be left desolate by death

STAGES OF DYING

Generally, people who are dying react in similar ways. Dr. Elisabeth Kübler-Ross identified the phases or stages that she observed in her work with the dying (Figure 19-7, see page 483). Although individuals do not necessarily proceed in an orderly fashion from one stage to another, some people seem to follow a pattern. These stages occur when any major loss is experienced—loss of a job, loss of a husband or wife through divorce or death, or even loss of a treasured possession.

The dying person may remain in any of the various stages or may go back to an earlier stage or go forward to the next (Figure 19-8, see page 483). The role of the health care worker is to accept the person wherever he or she happens to be.

PROVIDING CARE FOR THE DYING RESIDENT

Research has shown that most people realize or sense in some way when they are dying. They often will ask the physician to confirm their suspicions, and they may also question you. Information of this nature should come only from the physician. The role of the nursing assistant is one of listening rather than talking. Listening without inserting any of your own experiences or the experiences of others is helpful. It is never appropriate to say "I understand how you feel," because we really are not able to put ourselves in the place of

THE HOSPICE CIRCLE OF CARE

COMMUNITY HOSPICE CARE

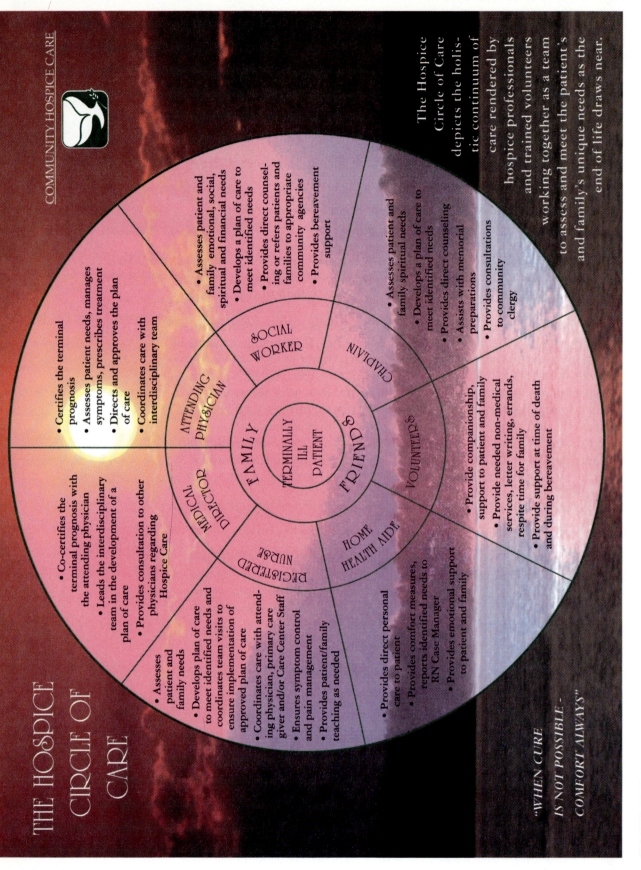

The Hospice Circle of Care depicts the holistic continuum of care rendered by hospice professionals and trained volunteers working together as a team to assess and meet the patient's and family's unique needs as the end of life draws near.

"WHEN CURE IS NOT POSSIBLE - COMFORT ALWAYS"

ATTENDING PHYSICIAN
- Certifies the terminal prognosis
- Assesses patient needs, manages symptoms, prescribes treatment
- Directs and approves the plan of care
- Coordinates care with interdisciplinary team

MEDICAL DIRECTOR
- Co-certifies the terminal prognosis with the attending physician
- Leads the interdisciplinary team in the development of a plan of care
- Provides consultation to other physicians regarding Hospice Care

REGISTERED NURSE
- Assesses patient and family needs
- Develops plan of care to meet identified needs and coordinates team visits to ensure implementation of approved plan of care
- Coordinates care with attending physician, primary care giver and/or Care Center Staff
- Ensures symptom control and pain management
- Provides patient/family teaching as needed

HOME HEALTH AIDE
- Provides direct personal care to patient
- Provides comfort measures, reports identified needs to RN Case Manager
- Provides emotional support to patient and family

SOCIAL WORKER
- Assesses patient and family emotional, social, spiritual and financial needs
- Develops a plan of care to meet identified needs
- Provides direct counseling or refers patients and families to appropriate community agencies
- Provides bereavement support

CHAPLAIN
- Assesses patient and family spiritual needs
- Develops a plan of care to meet identified needs
- Provides direct counseling
- Assists with memorial preparations
- Provides consultations to community clergy

VOLUNTEERS
- Provide companionship, support to patient and family
- Provide needed non-medical services, letter writing, errands, respite time for family
- Provide support at time of death and during bereavement

FAMILY

TERMINALLY ILL PATIENT

FRIENDS

FIGURE 19-6

The Hospice Circle of Care (Courtesy of Community Hospice Care at Riverside)

a person who is dying. It does help to say "I'm here, I will help in whatever way I can." You don't have to have the answers; just the fact that you are there and listening can be a great source of comfort to the dying resident.

Here are some guidelines for communication with residents who have limited life expectancy and their families or loved ones:

- Remember that dying residents need to be treated like living people; talk to and with them normally.
- Avoid whispering. Speak in your normal voice to the resident as well as to others in the room.
- Don't say things you wouldn't want the resident to hear. The dying person's hearing is usually one of the last senses to fail.
- Continue to talk to and touch the resident. Encourage the family to do the same.
- Respect the need for spiritual support. Learn the policy in your facility concerning religious observances and requirements at the time of death. For example, if a Roman Catholic resident wishes to see a priest and appears to be close to death, a priest should be called. Because the body of an Orthodox Jewish resident should not be touched after death until the rabbi of proper religious authority arrives, it is important to straighten the resident's limbs before death occurs.
- Be sincere and offer support and assistance without assuming control. The dying resident needs to remain in control of his or her own life and the circumstances of his or her environment as much as possible.
- Allow residents and/or family members to express their grief openly—remember, crying is a natural reaction to los.
- Create an atmosphere of comfort and let dying residents set the pace in their communication about dying and related matters.
- Allow residents to deal with their death according to their own needs and value system. Do not confuse your needs or impose your values on the dying resident.

When a person enters the final stage of the dying process, two different dynamics are at work, which are closely interrelated and interdependent. On the physical plane, the body begins the final process of shutting down, which will end when all the physical systems cease to function. Usually, this is an orderly and undramatic progressive series of physical changes that are not medical emergencies requiring invasive interventions. These physical changes are a normal, natural way in which the body prepares itself to stop and the most appropriate kinds of responses are comfort-enhancing measures.

The other dynamic of the dying process is at work on the emotional–spiritual–mental plane and is a different kind of process. The "spirit" of the dying person begins the final process of release from the body, its immediate environment, and all attachments. This release also tends to follow its own priorities, which may include the resolution of whatever is unfinished of a practical nature and reception of permission to "let go" from family members. These events are the normal, natural way in which the spirit prepares to move from this existence into the next dimension of life. The most appropriate kinds of responses

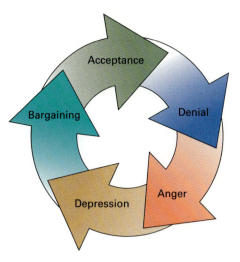

FIGURE 19-7
Stages of dying.

FIGURE 19-8
Losing friends and loved ones is one difficult aspect of growing older.

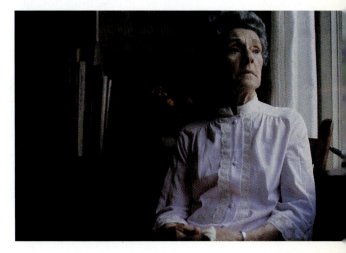

to the emotional–spiritual–mental changes are those that support and encourage this release and transition.

When a person's body is ready to cease functioning, but the person is still unresolved or unreconciled over some important issue or with some significant relationship, he or she may tend to linger even though uncomfortable or debilitated in order to finish whatever needs finishing. On the other hand, when a person is emotionally–spiritually–mentally resolved and ready for this release, but his or her body has not completed its final physical process, the person will continue to live until the physical "shutdown" is completed.

The following signs and symptoms of impending death are to help you understand and know what to expect. Keep in mind that not all of these will occur with every person or in this particular sequence.

PHYSICAL SIGNS AND SYMPTOMS

The resident's hands and arms, feet, and then legs may be increasingly cool to the touch, and at the same time the color of the skin may change. The underside of the body may become darker, and the skin becomes mottled. This is a normal indication that the circulation of blood is decreasing to the body's extremities and being reserved for the most vital organs. Keep the resident warm with a blanket, but do not use an electric one.

The resident may spend an increasing amount of time sleeping and appear to be uncommunicative or unresponsive and at times be difficult to arouse. This normal change is due in part to changes in the metabolism of the body. An appropriate intervention would be to sit with the resident and hold his or her hand, speaking softly and naturally.

The resident may seem to be confused about the time, place, and identity of people surrounding him or her, including close and familiar people. This is also due in part to the metabolism changes. Identify yourself by name before you speak, rather than ask the resident to guess who you are. Speak softly, clearly, and truthfully when you need to communicate something important for the resident's comfort, such as "I'm going to wash your face now," and explain the reason for the communication, such as "so you'll be more comfortable."

The resident may lose control of urine and/or bowel matter as the muscles in that area begin to relax. Make every effort to keep the resident clean and comfortable.

The resident may have gurgling sounds coming from his or her chest as though marbles were rolling around inside—these sounds may become very loud. This normal change is due to the decrease of fluid intake and inability to cough up normal secretions. Suctioning usually only increases the secretions and causes sharp discomfort. Gently turn the resident's head to the side and allow gravity to drain the secretions. You may also gently wipe the mouth with a moist cloth. The sound of the congestion does not indicate the onset of severe or new pain.

The resident may make restless and repetitive motions, such as pulling at bed linen or clothing. This often happens and is due in part to the decrease in oxygen circulation to the brain and to metabolism changes. Do not interfere with or try to restrain such motions. To have a calming effect, speak in a quiet, natural way; lightly massage the forehead; read to the resident; or play some soothing music.

The resident may have a decrease in appetite and thirst, wanting little or no food or fluid. The body will naturally begin to conserve energy, which is expended on these tasks. Do not try to force food or drink into the resident. To do this only makes the resident much more uncomfortable. Small chips of ice, frozen Gatorade, or juice may be refreshing in the mouth. Oral care may keep the mouth and lips moist and comfortable. A cool, moist washcloth on the forehead may also increase physical comfort.

The resident's urine output normally decreases and may become tea colored—referred to as *concentrated urine.* This is due to the decreased fluid intake as well as decrease in circulation through the kidneys.

The resident's regular breathing pattern may change with the onset of a different breathing pace. A particular pattern consists of breathing irregularly (i.e., shallow breaths with periods of no breathing of 5 to 30 seconds and up to a full minute). This is called **Cheyne–Stokes breathing.** The resident may also experience periods of rapid, shallow, pantlike breathing. These patterns are very common and indicate decrease in circulation in the internal organs. Elevating the head and/or turning the resident on his or her side may bring comfort. Hold his or her hand and speak gently.

EMOTIONAL–SPIRITUAL–MENTAL SIGNS AND SYMPTOMS

The resident may seem unresponsive, withdrawn, or in a comatoselike state. This indicates preparation for release, a detaching from surroundings and relationships and a beginning of letting go. Because hearing remains all the way to the end, speak to the resident in your normal tone of voice and identify yourself by name when you speak.

The resident may speak or claim to have spoken to persons who have already died, or to see or have seen places not presently accessible or visible to you. This does not indicate a hallucination or a drug reaction. The resident is beginning to detach from his life and is being prepared for the transition so it will not be frightening. Do not contradict, explain away, belittle, or argue about what the resident claims to have seen or heard. Just because you cannot see or hear it does not mean it is not real to the resident. Affirm his or her experiences. They are normal and common. If they frighten the resident, explain to him or her that they are normal.

Cheyne–Stokes breathing a kind of breathing that can be observed when a resident is near death. The breathing is slow and shallow at first followed by faster and deeper breathing which reaches a peak, then stops completely. The pattern then repeats until breathing stops completely.

CARE OF THE DYING RESIDENT

- Keep the room well ventilated and lighted as usual. Because the dying resident's eyesight may be failing, a dark room may be frightening.
- Change the resident's position at least every 2 hours, and more often if necessary, to ensure comfort and to prevent skin breakdown.
- The dying resident may lose control of bowel and bladder and soil the bed often. Keep the resident clean at all times. Take steps necessary to keep the room as odor free as possible.
- Change the bedding whenever necessary to prevent skin irritation and to increase comfort.
- The resident may be given softer food in smaller amounts than usual or may refuse food. Liquids are given as long as the ability to swallow remains. This helps to keep the mouth moist.

- The resident approaching death needs special mouth care. If the mouth is dry, use an applicator with glycerine (or other lubricant) to swab the mouth and lips to keep the mouth moist with toothettes mositened with water. When there are a lot of secretions in the mouth, tell the charge nurse, who may use suction to remove the material.
- If the resident has dentures, ask your charge nurse if you should leave them in or take them out. If you remove the dentures, place them in a denture cup with the resident's name on the cover.
- A resident's nostrils may also become dry and encrusted. If you notice dryness, clean the nostrils with cotton swabs moistened slightly with glycerine (or other lubricant).

Guidelines

The resident may perform repetitive and restless tasks. This may in part indicate that something is still unresolved or unfinished and is disturbing him or her and preventing him or her from letting go.

The resident may want to be with only very few people or even just one person. This is a sign of preparation for release and an affirmation of whom the support is most needed from in order to make the appropriate transition. Help family members to understand that if they are not part of this inner circle at the end, it does not mean they are not loved or are unimportant but that they have already fulfilled their tasks and it is time to say good-bye.

The resident may make a seemingly out-of-character or illogical statement, gesture, or request. This indicates that he or she is ready to say good-bye and is testing to see if the family is ready to let him or her go.

A dying person will normally try to hold on—even though it brings prolonged discomfort—in order to be sure that those who are going to be left behind will be all right. Help the family to give permission to their loved one to let go. They may use words like "We'll be okay, Mom" or "I'm going to be all right, Dad."

When the resident is ready to die and the family is able to let go, then it is the time to say good-bye. Saying good-bye is the final gift of love, for it achieves closure and makes the final release possible. Tears are a normal and natural part of saying good-bye. Suggest to the family that they lie on the bed with the resident and hold him or her, or take the resident's hand and say what they need to say. It may be as simple as saying "I love you" or it may include recounting favorite memories, places, and activities they shared. It may include saying "I'm sorry." One experienced hospice nurse stated that dying persons have five tasks to accomplish before they die. They need to say in their own way and in their own words:

"Forgive me for . . ."
"I forgive you for . . ."
"Thank you for . . ."
"I love you."
"Good-bye."

CARE OF THE BODY AFTER DEATH

The body *must* always be treated with dignity and respect after death. Usually, any roommates are taken out of the room, or the privacy curtains are drawn. You will be instructed about whether or not the family will be viewing the body before you begin physical preparation of the body.

Although procedures vary with the individual facility, there are some general guidelines:

• There is no laughing or joking while caring for the body after death.
• Providing privacy and treating the body with respect are essential.
• The body is carefully bathed.
• All tubings and dressings are removed.
• Clean dressings are applied if indicated.
• Dentures are placed in the mouth.
• Limbs are straightened.

Some facilities have special kits used to prepare the body. Preparations vary from simple to complex. In many facilities, the mortuary arrives promptly and completes some of the preparations, including identification and positioning.

Other residents will ask about the resident who died. The current thinking is that they should be informed of the death openly and honestly. The custom of closing all doors to the resident's room when the body is removed is questionable since the other residents usually know that this means that someone has died. They also watch how the deaths of others are handled, knowing that their own death will be dealt with in the same way. Most people wish to be remembered and to have their death acknowledged and mourned.

Many LTC and hospice facilities conduct brief memorial services for those who have died or pause for a moment before a meal to remember that person. The terms used in discussing death give some indication of the degree of comfort the person has with death. The correct term is *died* or *expired.*

THE FAMILY AND GRIEVING

After death, attention is focused on the family or friends of the resident. They may need someone to listen or perhaps provide coffee and a place to sit and talk. Your support comes not from trying to say "the right thing" but from listening to what the family has to say. A wonderful quote by Doug Manning emphasizes this point: "The ear is the most powerful part of the human body. People are healed by the laying on of ears."

Family and friends will experience the **grief process** in much the same way the dying resident did, even though the death may have been expected (Figure 19-9). The grief process is characterized by many different emotions experienced by people following a loss.

The way someone dies and the relationship to the person mourning the loss influences the length of time spent in each phase. People in the "shock phase" can be compared to someone under anesthesia; they are "numb." You can be most helpful to the person in the denial–shock phase by just listening— let the person know you want to listen and that you will take time to listen.

Denial is the part of grieving that deals with "It can't be true" or "No, he is not really gone" kinds of feelings. Losing a loved one is such a loss that it is natural to deny the truth. In some ways, denial allows people to protect themselves temporarily from the pain and hurt their loss brings until they are better prepared to handle it.

Anger is part of the protest, a reaction most commonly seen once the reality of the death has been faced. Anger may be toward God or toward medical science, other family members, or even directed toward those who have provided care. If this occurs, never try to argue or defend; allow the person to talk and encourage him or her to speak to the licensed nurse. Be sure to report any angry behavior to your charge nurse. Anger is a feeling that will not last, and most often people begin to defuse their own anger as they see things more clearly. Sometimes, people use their anger constructively to address issues that might have contributed to the death of their loved ones. A good example of this is MADD (Mothers Against Drunk Drivers), an organization designed to bring about constructive changes in laws related to drunk driving. MADD was founded by a mother whose daughter was killed by a drunk driver.

During the disorganization phase, depression and withdrawal occur as the mourner faces an emptiness that feels like it will never go away. There is a clear realization that the loved one will *never* return. Where anger and

grief process emotions experienced by people following a loss

FIGURE 19-9

Stages of grief.

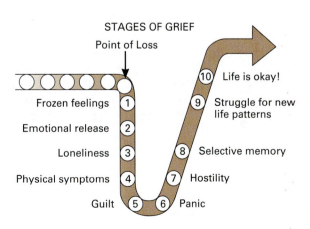

STAGES OF GRIEF

Point of Loss

1 Frozen feelings
2 Emotional release
3 Loneliness
4 Physical symptoms
5 Guilt
6 Panic
7 Hostility
8 Selective memory
9 Struggle for new life patterns
10 Life is okay!

pain once were are now feelings of aimlessness and loneliness. Frequently, during this phase, people may lose or reduce contacts with family and friends. Sometimes, it helps to drop a note, letting the person know that someone is thinking of him or her or to call with "I just wanted to call and let you know I was thinking of you." Many times, during a prolonged illness and death, facility staff can go a long way to helping people through their grieving and back toward a meaningful life in spite of their loss. In the final phase, reorganization, a philosophical acceptance of the death comes, and the individual begins to find new interests, increases socialization, and gradually returns to the mainstream of life and society.

As you provide care to the dying resident and support family members as they grieve, you must be aware of how your own feelings and attitudes toward death will influence how you are in providing care. For this reason, special training as well as selected reading materials are encouraged.

SUMMARY

End-of-life care is a subject on the minds of many Americans. We have come to recognize that this is an important time in one's life, and we are beginning to acknowledge it and to talk about it. This means that those who are privileged to provide care need to be experts.

This chapter has included information about care of residents who are at the end of their lives. You had an opportunity to learn about various common diseases as well as the symptoms most dying residents face. Tips on how to provide care were included. You had the opportunity to learn how culture affects the way people die and how you can use the information to be a better nursing assistant. The importance of learning about your own cultural beliefs and the beliefs and practices of other cultures was presented, along with ways to increase your cultural awareness. Tough issues that come up, including providing food and fluids at the end of life, were discussed from a legal, medical, and ethical point of view. Basics of ethics and decision making were provided, along with some ways of looking at the decisions from different points of view.

You have learned how important it is to provide compassionate and comprehensive care to the resident who is dying, and you have learned what that care includes.

OBRA HIGHLIGHTS

In 1991, a law called the Patient Self-Determination Act was implemented. This law was part of the Omnibus Budge Reconciliation Act for 1990. This law ensures that competent adults can make decisions about their health care. They can choose to accept or refuse any medical treatment. They can also make their wishes known in advance by writing them down. In most states, they can name someone to make decisions for them if they become unable to do so. In caring for dying residents, you may be aware that they have refused medical intervention. It is important for you to recognize that this is their right and to honor that right whether you personally agree or not.

SELF STUDY

Choose the best answer for each question or statement.

1. Who receives care from hospice?
   a. residents with a terminal disease who have 6 months or less to live
   b. residents with a terminal disease who are seeking not a cure but comfort
   c. the families and loved ones of residents receiving hospice care
   d. all of the above

2. What are the goals of hospice care?
   a. to keep the resident alert until death occurs so the family and resident can say good-bye
   b. to provide support for family members until death of the resident occurs
   c. to allow the resident and family to have control over the circumstances of death
   d. to keep the resident as active as possible for as long as he or she is physically able to be active

3. A resident has been diagnosed with a terminal illness. He keeps asking why this is happening to him. He tells you that he has always tried to be good and do what is right, so he doesn't understand why he has this disease. Which stage of dying is he experiencing?
   a. denial
   b. anger
   c. bargaining
   d. depression

4. Mrs. Herrera is very near death. Her family has not arrived at the long-term care facility yet. What should the nursing assistant do?
   a. Stay with her until the family arrives so she will not be alone.
   b. Close the door to her room so she will have privacy.
   c. Avoid going into her room so she will not be disturbed by staff.
   d. Ensure that other residents and staff are very quiet when near her room.

5. Mr. Morganstern is terminally ill. He sometimes talks with you about his impending death. What should you do when he talks about death?
   a. Tell him not to talk about dying because he is going to be around for a long time yet.
   b. Tell him about a relative of yours who died from a similar illness.
   c. Tell him that you will help in any way that you can, then listen as he talks.
   d. Tell him that you understand how he feels.

6. Mr. Morganstern is slipping in and out of consciousness. His family is in the room with him. His daughter is crying and sobbing at his bedside. You need to go into his room to make his bed. What should you do?
   a. Enter the room quietly and speak to the family, not to the resident.
   b. Speak in whispers to the family about what you need to do.
   c. Encourage his daughter to leave the room until she can pull herself together.
   d. Talk to him and touch him, and encourage the family to do the same.

7. Mr. Morganstern is no longer able to eat or drink fluids. His skin and mouth are becoming very dry. What will you do?
   a. Discuss his condition with the nurse so a feeding tube or IVs can be used to provide hydration.
   b. Give frequent oral and skin care; provide Vaseline or a wet cloth so the family can moisten his lips.
   c. Offer food and fluids every hour during your shift; instruct the family to notify you if he awakens enough to take water.
   d. Force a little water or other fluid into his mouth using a syringe every time you are in the room, making sure that he swallows the liquid.

8. You are assigned to care for Mr. Morganstern's body after death. Which of the following guidelines should you follow?
   a. Bathe the body carefully.
   b. Remove all tubes and dressings.
   c. Place his dentures in his mouth.
   d. All of these actions should be followed.

9. After Mr. Morganstern dies, one of the other residents asks you how he is doing. How will you answer?
   a. "He's not doing very well."
   b. "He's going to be in a better place."
   c. "I'm sorry, he died last night."
   d. "Let's go to the dining room for lunch."

10. When you care for a resident who is receiving chemotherapy for cancer treatment, she complains of itching skin. Which of the following should you do for her?

a. Use a good-smelling lotion on the itchy area.

b. Rub the area firmly with gentle pressure to reduce the itching.

c. Keep the area clean.

d. all of the above

11. In what order does a dying resident pass through the stages of dying?

a. anger, bargaining, denial, depression, then acceptance

b. no particular order is followed, and the resident may go back to a previous stage

c. denial, anger, bargaining, depression, then acceptance

d. alternates between denial and anger for a time, then progresses to acceptance

12. Mrs. Cannelli has been diagnosed with cancer. She tells you that she has prayed to live long enough to see her grandchild, whose birth is due in 6 months. She tells you she has promised to say her rosary everyday so she can live for 6 more months. Mrs. Cannelli is probably in which stage of dying?

a. anger

b. denial

c. bargaining

d. acceptance

13. Mrs. Cannelli later becomes depressed about her illness. She is very withdrawn and won't eat or talk. When you speak to her, she answers with only nods or does not answer at all. What should you do?

a. Insist that she talk to you about how she is feeling.

b. Give her good care and tell her you are available if she wants you for anything.

c. Tell her that she will never get better if she doesn't try harder to improve.

d. Spend little time with her so she can work out her feelings without being disturbed.

14. Which of the following would indicate that death is near?

a. The resident's hands and feet become cold to touch.

b. The resident perspires heavily, even though the body feels cold.

c. The pulse becomes rapid, weak, and irregular.

d. All of these indicate impending death.

15. When a resident has cancer, what has happened to the behavior of normal cells?

a. They grow more rapidly than normal.

b. They divide more rapidly than normal.

c. They move differently than normal.

d. All of these occur in cancer cells.

16. Another name for a cancerous tumor is a

a. malignant tumor

b. benign tumor

c. lymphatic tumor

d. T cell tumor

Chapter Review

Getting C O N N E C T E D
Multimedia Extension Activities

 www.prenhall.com/will-black

Use the above address to access the free, interactive Companion Website created for this textbook. Hear the pronunciation of the key terms in the chapter. Get instant feedback to a variety of chaper-related questions. Link to other interesting sites.

 Video

Watch the section on communication in the video *Age-Specific Competencies* and the section on the patient's right to refuse care in the video *Patient's Rights*, both from the Care Provider Skills series.

CASE STUDY

Mrs. Jones is 90 years old. She is dying from the end stages of heart disease. She has almost stopped eating. She does eat soup and crackers and drinks tea. Her daughter Sara is 70 years old and visits her mother daily. She seems distressed about her mother's weight loss.

1. Because of her illness, her symptoms will probably include
   a. pain, pressure ulcers, and dementia
   b. fatigue, loss of appetite, and shortness of breath
   c. bleeding tendencies, jaundice, and ascites
   d. decreased urine output, pruritus, and pain
2. Your role as the daughter and mother decide about a tube feeding is to
   a. listen and notify the nurse of the concerns
   b. tell the daughter that she should just "let go"
   c. notify the administrator since the daughter must authorize the tube
   d. explain that if she were your mother, you'd insist on force feeding her
3. If the daughter decides she does not want her mother fed by tube. You disagree. Your role is to
   a. Give her excellent care with special emphasis on oral hygiene.
   b. Attempt to convince her that you are right.
   c. Refuse to care for Mrs. Jones.
   d. Avoid spending any more time than necessary with her.
4. Your care of Mrs. Jones will primarily include
   a. keeping her active and independent
   b. providing excellent skin care and reporting signs of bleeding or pain
   c. recording intake and output
   d. assuring rest, pacing activities, and helping with all ADL

Chapter 20

THE CERTIFIED NURSING ASSISTANT

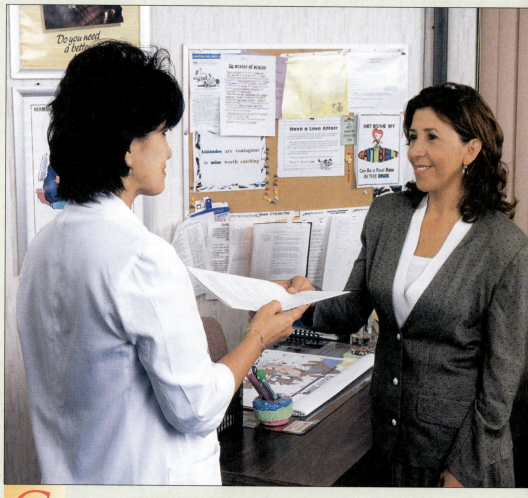

CARING TIP

The caring nursing assistant knows that his or her career is more than "just a job" and that it demands a commitment to truly care for the whole person who is much more than the sum total of all their body systems. The exceptional nursing assistant sees his or her career as a calling to care.

Neva Babcock, BSN, RNC, CDONA, CIC
Performance Improvement/Infection Control Director
St. Thomas More Nursing and Rehab Center
Hyattsville, Maryland

SECTION 1 Becoming Certified

- Describe the requirements for becoming certified
- List five suggestions for effective studying
- Create a study plan
- Give three test-taking tips
- Successfully complete a sample test

KEY TERMS

active study

competency

multiple choice questions

BECOMING A CERTIFIED NURSING ASSISTANT

In 1987, the U.S. Congress required that nursing assistants working in long-term care (LTC) facilities be trained and certified. A nurse aide is not permitted to work for more than 4 months without being enrolled in a nurse aide training and competency evaluation program. Some states are more strict and require that the nurse aide *complete* the training and competency evaluation within four months. Be sure to verify the rules for your state. The goal of the regulations was to improve the quality of services given to residents of nursing facilities by nurse aides. The nurse aides are expected to help residents to keep their independence and to demonstrate sensitivity to residents' needs. The nurse aide must have skills in observation and documentation. To become certified, the nursing assistant must complete a nurse aide training program and demonstrate competency using both written or oral examinations and demonstration of skills. **Competency** according to the regulations means a successful demonstration of the knowledge and skills that a nurse aide will be expected to perform in his or her duties as a nurse aide. Congress also directed each state to create a Nurse Aide Registry, which includes identification of individuals who have successfully completed and passed the nurse aide training and competency evaluation program with a score of 75 percent or above. The registry also records *confirmed* claims of resident neglect, abuse, or theft of resident property by a nurse aide in a nursing facility. If the nurse aide disputes the findings, this information is also entered into the registry.

competency   a skill or ability that can be demonstrated

This book includes the material needed to pass both the written and the skill demonstration portion of the competency examination. The knowledge and experience of your instructor, and your efforts to learn the material and practice the skills, place success within your reach. This chapter will help prepare you by exploring study skills and preparation for both examinations. Knowledge, skills, and a positive attitude will ensure your success!

Although there is some variation from state to state, the training program must be at least 75 hours in length. The regulations further list the topics that must be taught. Some but not all of the topics included are:

- Communication
- Infection control
- Safety and emergency procedures
- Respecting residents' rights
- Promoting residents' independence
- Basic nursing skills

Basic nursing skills include:

- Caring for the resident's environment
- Taking and recording vital signs
- Recognizing abnormal signs and symptoms of common diseases and conditions
- Personal care skills such as bathing, dressing, and grooming
- Restorative and rehabilitation services
- Dealing with different behaviors
- Care of possessions
- Privacy, confidentiality
- Protection from abuse, mistreatment, or neglect

A review of the Table of Contents of this book will give you an idea of the information required. The skill portion of the training includes those skills you will be performing in your role as a nurse aide/nursing assistant. This book contains step-by-step procedures of all of the required skills. The instructor must keep records that show the skills expected to be learned, the dates you have performed the skills, and whether the performance was satisfactory or unsatisfactory.

The training program may be offered by a school or by a skilled nursing facility (Figure 20-1). Each program must be approved. The instructors must be qualified to teach the program. It is important to know that you are receiving training from an approved program with a qualified instructor. Some skilled nursing faiclities can lose their program approval if they are found in violation of the regulations. Be sure to check out the program before enrolling.

Once your training is complete, your competency must be evaluated. The competency evaluation consists of two parts. One is a written examination administered by state-approved organizations. You may have to go to a high school, vocational school, or the American Red Cross to take the examination. The examination is given on a scheduled basis and monitored to ensure security. It is then scored by an organization approved by the state. The examination may be given orally under certain circumstances. Ask your instructor about the reasons the examination might be given orally. The examination consists of about 50 multiple choice questions. In the section on test-taking skills, you will learn more about the test. This book includes questions at the end of each chapter, which can provide you with an idea of the kinds of questions you might be asked and an opportunity to practice.

FIGURE 20-1

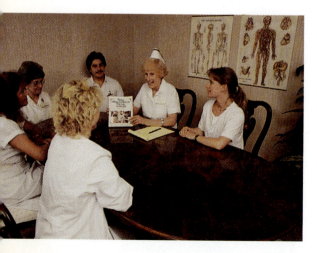

The second part is a skill demonstration, which is performed in a facility or a laboratory setting. It must be given and evaluated by a registered nurse. You will be tested on those skills that you are expected to perform in your job. Usually, you will be given five tasks chosen at random. Some examples of the kinds of skills you may be tested on include handwashing, taking vital signs, bathing, making a bed, weighing, providing range-of-motion exercises, or feeding a dependent resident. You will be expected to:

- Schedule the examination in advance
- Pay a fee to take the examination (cash, cashier's check, or money order)
- Arrive on time
- Follow all instructions

Should you fail the examination, you may retake the examination two additional times for a maximum of three times. If there is a period of time when you are not working for 24 months in a row, you will have to establish your competency again.

PREPARING FOR THE SKILL EVALUATION

The best way to prepare for the skill demonstration is to review the procedures in the text and to practice the skills on a daily basis while you are in the training program. Every time you perform a skill, follow the steps described. Ask a nurse or your fellow students to observe you. If necessary, practice on your family members. In almost every procedure you can think of, there are certain common elements. Preparation or beginning steps involve activities including:

- Gathering equipment and supplies
- Washing your hands
- Identifying the resident
- Explaining what you are going to do
- Providing privacy
- Putting on gloves

You then carry out the procedure with both *safety* and infection control in mind. Ending steps usually include:

- Making the resident comfortable
- Placing the call signal within reach
- Cleaning up
- Returning supplies and equipment to their proper place
- Reporting important observations
- Documenting or charting what you have done

PREPARING FOR THE WRITTEN COMPETENCY EXAMINATION

Your preparation begins when you enroll in a nurse aide or nurse assistant training program. Throughout the course of study and evaluation, keep your goal in mind. You decided that you wanted to become a certified nursing assistant. This is either a career choice or a step on the way to another career in health care. You may be exploring whether this is the path you want to take. Whatever your goal, successful completion of the class is necessary. Write down your goal so you can post it in an area where you will see it every day.

STUDY SKILLS

You will have to study in order to complete your training successfully. Everything cannot be learned in the classroom. Although you may not have homework assignments, you will have to read the textbook, complete learning activities, and study your class notes. You will be learning a new language—the language of health care. Review the Glossary in this book and you will see many new words and definitions. You'll be learning how the body works—a subject that can be difficult to grasp. Changes in the body as a result of aging may be new to you. You'll also learn about many diseases and conditions and how to provide the right care. You'll learn a great deal about people and how they behave, as well as how you can best respond to their behavior. No one is born knowing how to study. Study skills can be learned, however. Take the time to review the following study skills and implement those that will work for you. You may have good study skills already but may simply need a refresher. You may recognize that you have never had good study skills, or you may not have studied for many years. Perhaps there is some new information that will help you. Some of the skills included are for use in the classroom and at home. Examples are scheduling, listening, reading and comprehension, note taking, and good health habits.

Planning your studying begins with choosing a time and place. Each person has a time of day when they are most able to think and to learn. For some, it is in the morning, others at night. Choose a time when you are "at your best." This time should be about an hour in length and allow for few or no interruptions. You'll also need a place to study (Figure 20-2). Usually, a quiet place is best rather than in the midst of family activities or in front of the television. The place you choose as your study place needs to have a comfortable temperature and adequate lighting. A room is nice but not necessary. Even a corner of a room will do. You need to be comfortable but not *too* comfortable. As a rule, studying while lying on a bed or couch is too comfortable. You will probably fall asleep. Some people study better away from home, for example, at a library or at work either before or after your job. You may study with a friend who has a quieter place. Ask your family or friends to help you by not disturbing you during your study time. If you have young children, it may be difficult for them to understand. You may want to trade child care time with another student to provide your quiet time. Perhaps the study time can be after they go to bed or before they get up in the morning. Older children or adults can understand the importance of allowing you uninterrupted time to study. It may help to try different things and see what works best for you. As a general rule, try to minimize distractions and maximize your energy. Write down your schedule on a calendar. Consider this an appointment to study that is as important as your other appointments. Make a commitment and stick to it! If you miss one appointment, reschedule it rather than simply not doing it. Include in your schedule time for breaks and time for rest and relaxation. It is always better to study for a short time on a daily basis than to set aside one day every week.

Studying is an active process that requires effort. To learn, you must engage in **active study.** Active study means that you will be doing more than listening and reading. In order to do the work of learning, you must have energy. It is important to take care of your physical, mental, and emotional health. That means having the proper amount of rest and exercise. It means eating foods that are described in the Food Guide Pyramid in Chapter 9. You cannot study well if you are tired or hungry, if your eyes burn, or if you are sick. Mental health also requires rest. In other words, plan for some time to do things that you find renewing and restoring. For example, allow time to be alone, to pamper yourself, or to have fun. Build these kinds of activities into your study schedule and include them in your plan. Some people enjoy a movie, listening to music, time with friends, walking, reading, dancing, sports, arts and crafts, or puzzles and games.

active study a method of preparing for an examination or test that involves activity other than reading

FIGURE 20-2

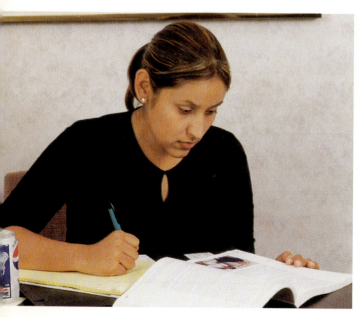

LISTENING AND READING SKILLS

You will need to develop your listening and reading skills to become competent in the knowledge required to be a certified nursing assistant. Listening is an active process. In a classroom setting, you can improve your listening by sitting as close to the instructor as you can. Those who sit in the back of the room are often distracted by everyone sitting between them and the instructor. Concentrate on what the instructor is saying. Give your full attention to the instructor to reduce distractions. Sit up straight in your chair. Do not "slouch." Pay attention to the instructor's body language, tone of voice, and gestures. If your mind starts to wonder, bring your attention back to the instructor by keeping your eyes on her at all times. Practice your listening at every opportunity such as attending church or watching a speech on television. Work at listening and you will discover that you improve with time.

Reading with understanding is also a skill. This book is designed to make your studying easier. Each chapter begins with learning objectives. The learning objectives tell you the most important information included in that section. For example, in the beginning of this section of Chapter 20, it says:

Objectives/What You Will learn

When you have completed this section, you will be able to;

- Describe the requirements for becoming certified
- List five suggestions for effective studying
- Create a study plan
- Give three test-taking tips
- Successfully complete a sample test

When you begin each section of a chapter, review all of the objectives. They serve as a preview of the contents of that section. Then as you read the chapter, look for the content related to each of the objectives. For example, in this section, you would look for the requirements for becoming certified and either underline or highlight, or write notes as you read them. The next part of each section that is very helpful in your learning is the list of key terms. These are the new words you'll be learning in this particular section. These same terms are shown in bold print and are defined in the margin. They are also listed in alphabetical order in the Glossary at the back of the book. You will be unable to understand the important parts of the chapter if you don't understand the key terms. Other helpful tools are the photographs, illustrations, charts, and diagrams. There is a saying that "a picture is worth a thousand words." This text has over 500 illustrations all in place to help you learn. Pay special attention to studying the photos and art because they communicate information without words. Each chapter ends with a summary. This summary is designed to reinforce or remind you of the most important information included in the chapter. Pay special attention to the chapter summary. There is also a case study at the end of each chapter. The case study is designed to help you apply the knowledge gained in the particular chapter. It means you must read the information and answer the questions about it. The case study is drawn from the important points in that chapter. Although other textbooks may not be designed in this same way, the same principles apply to improving your reading and comprehension.

1. Scan the chapter to get an overview.
2. Look for new terms, look them up, and write them down.

3. Study any illustrations.
4. Identify the key ideas and write them down.
5. Read the summary or write your own summary.

NOTE-TAKING SKILLS

Note taking is another useful study skill. Notes are taken when listening to the instructor and when reading your textbook. Because learning requires repetition of information, it is necessary to write it and review it several times. Note taking is writing down the key points that you need to remember. You need to write only those things that you don't already know. It is important to listen to the instructor for clues about what he thinks is important. In a book, you will learn more when you write down the key points rather than underlining or highlighting. If you highlight as you read, you often find yourself highlighting everything! Taking notes means you write down only selected information. You don't need complete sentences or to worry about spelling and grammar. Spelling is important only if you are writing new terms. Use drawings and diagrams to increase your understanding. For example, in Chapter 10, to help you understand dehydration, there is an illustration of a scale with more fluids leaving the body than coming in. It would be helpful in your notes on dehydration to draw a diagram of the scale. When marked with three words—*in, out,* and *dehydration*—you have a simple way to remember a very important concept. Another example is in Chapter 6. There is a diagram of a blood vessel to show what happens when heat and cold are applied. Heat opens the vessel and cold constricts it. Your notes could include a drawing showing a blood vessel that is larger or more open and the word *heat,* and a narrower or constricted vessel and the word *cold.* Because this is such an important principle, you must include it in your notes and learn it. During your reading about a particular disease, you may think of a resident or even a family member who has had that disease. Write that person's name in your notes so it will help you recall. Make note of the way that person is different from the way the disease is described. You can see now that taking notes is a thoughtful process.

Taking notes in class is more complex. You will have to listen and write down key information provided by the instructor. If you have read your textbook before class, you have an advantage. You will know what is in the book and need not write that down. You will write only key information that is not contained in your book. Reading the material in advance also allows you to ask questions about anything you don't understand. Although you must look at your instructor, listen, and pay attention, certain notes will need to be made. Make them brief and simple, using some of the abbreviations you learned in Chapter 4. Not only will your note taking be faster, you will learn the abbreviations faster. You may also use > (greater than or more than) and < (less than). Arrows can be used to show increase ($\uparrow$) and decrease ($\downarrow$). The symbols for female ($\female$) and male ($\male$) may come in handy in your notes. You may even use "☺" for some key ideas.

Remember: Don't write down everything!

TAKING THE TEST

You have prepared for this test throughout your course of study. Now, you need a positive attitude and some basic information about how to take a multiple choice test. There are many books written on how to take a test. You probably won't need a whole book, but the reason there are so many is that taking a test is a skill that can be learned. Many learners, especially adult learners, are fearful of taking tests. You may be among that group. The best way to overcome fear is to act. Actions you can take include learning as much as you can about the test, preparing for it, and changing your mental attitude about it. One way to learn about it is to ask your friends or co-workers who have taken the test to tell you about their experience. Next, learn about multiple choice examinations in general. You know that there will be about 50 multiple choice questions on the test. **Multiple choice questions** are test questions that provide a selection of answers. The student chooses the correct answer from those provided. Most standardized tests are multiple choice because they are easy to score by machine and they are objective rather than subjective. Because of wide use, there are standard ways they are written. There is usually a background statement, which provides the information to assist in answering the question, then the stem, which asks question, followed by the choices for answers. There are usually four choices of answers. It is most important to read the question carefully. Watch for terms like *not,* because this may change the meaning of the question. Other principles include:

multiple choice questions
a test question that provides a selection of answers; the student is to choose the correct answer from those provided

1. Scan the entire test first to help you feel more confident.
2. Don't assume anything not included in the question.
3. Look for the best answer, not the perfect answer.
4. Read every answer even if you think the first choice is correct.
5. Eliminate the wrong answers to narrow your choices in case you have to guess.
6. Look for key words in the question.
7. If two choices are similar, it may not be either one.
8. If two choices are opposite, one of them is probably the correct answer.
9. If three choices are similar, the correct answer is probably the fourth choice.
10. The answer is usually wrong if it says *all, always, never, none,* or *every.*
11. Often, the choice that is the longest is the correct answer.
12. Don't be afraid to change an answer if you have a good reason. When guessing, your first impulse is probably correct.

Practice these tips as you answer the questions at the end of each chapter. By the time you are ready for the test, you will have 20 chapters of practice! Review the following examples and apply the techniques listed.

George Green is 78 years old and has resided in the facility for about 6 months. He has been diagnosed with cirrhosis of the liver due to chronic alcohol abuse. He is on a low-fat diet. (Background statement)

1. Some of the foods that are not permitted on a low-fat diet include (Stem) (Choices)
   a. fruits and vegetables
   b. fish and chicken
   c. bacon and eggs
   d. sugar, fruit juice, and cake
2. Mr. Green wants to eat in bed instead of going to the dining room. When serving him, it is important that the nursing assistant
   a. position him in bed sitting at a 90-degree angle
   b. position him lying on his left side
   c. allow his food to cool before serving
   d. insist that he eat in the dining room

3. Mr. Green has a stroke and loses his ability to swallow. He has an advance directive that states that he does not wish to be fed by tube. Your responsibility to Mr. Green is to
   a. tell him he must have a tube or he won't get well
   b. give him excellent care in all ways but honor his wishes
   c. feed him with an oral syringe
   d. avoid contact with him
4. You notice it has been 4 days since Mr. Green had a bowel movement. You report this to the charge nurse. She asks if you believe the resident has a fecal impaction. The signs you would look for include
   a. chills and fever
   b. nausea and abdominal pain
   c. skin rash with itching
   d. burning pain upon urination

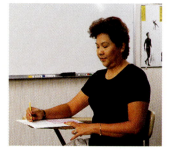

FIGURE 20-3

When the day for your scheduled test approaches (Figure 20-3), it is important to be prepared by getting enough rest. Arrive early. If you have never been to the test location, make a trip in advance so you will not get lost. Eat breakfast if the test is in the morning or lunch if it is in the afternoon. Avoid drinking lots of coffee or other caffeine-containing drinks. Usually, you are not allowed to bring textbooks or electronic devices into the room. By the same token, you are not permitted to take anything from the room. For machine-graded tests, usually a number 2 pencil is needed. Bring several that are already sharpened. Some people find it helpful to take some deep breaths and either take a few moments to relax or to say a prayer before the test begins. Use whatever strategy has helped you in similar situations. Keep in mind that if you don't pass, you can repeat the examination.

SECTION 2 Obtaining a Job as a Certified Nursing Assistant

OBJECTIVES
What You Will Learn

When you have completed this section, you will be able to:

- Describe the steps in the process of obtaining a job
- List four tips for completing an application
- Explain how to prepare for an interview
- Identify three common questions that you may be asked in an interview

KEY TERM   résumé

The job of a certified nursing assistant (CNA) is important and difficult. As more and more people are living longer lives, the need for skilled caregivers has increased. It is predicted that when the baby boomers (those born after World War II) are in need of long-term care, there may not be enough caregivers available. When you have a certificate that shows you have been trained and you have proven your competency, you are a valuable potential employee. As a rule, there are many jobs available. There is also flexibility because nursing assistants are needed 24 hours a day, 7 days a week. That means that you can probably find a job that can fit with your family and school responsibilities. For example, by working at night (usually 11 P.M. to 7 A.M.), you may be able to avoid child care costs or you may be able to continue going to school. You and your spouse may work different shifts in order to ensure that one of you is at home with your children. As a rule, you can't expect every weekend and holiday off. Usually, these days off are highly prized and must be shared equally. Many LTC facilities assign the CNAs to work 4 days followed by 2 days off. When you begin looking for a job, have a plan in mind about what shift you prefer to work. If that shift is not available, would you be willing to work an alternate shift until there is an opening? When an LTC facility has job openings, they usually advertise in three ways. First, they tell their employees that there is a position available. Word of mouth can be an effective way to find good staff. Next, they may post a sign outside their facility. They realize that people working close to home have a better record of attendance and keep their jobs longer. Finally, they may advertise in the newspaper. With this in mind, you can look for the right facility for you. Often, the right facility is the one where you received your training. You are probably comfortable there and the staff has observed the quality of your work and your work habits. Sometimes, the right facility is the one where a friend, relative, or acquaintence works. Be sure that the facility does not have a policy forbidding employment of relatives if that is the case. The right facility may be the one close to your home. Check out those facilities that you are considering. Find out if they have a reputation for providing good care. What do current and former employees say about how they were treated? It is important to be associated with a facility that provides good care and treats their employees with respect. Once you have chosen a facility or two where you would like to work, the next step is to call for an appointment. You may be asked to bring a résumé when you come or even to mail or fax it in advance. A **résumé** is a written document stating your qualifications for a job. It usually includes your education, certificates or credentials, special skills, and work history. Some include a list of references or refer to references that will be provided when requested. It is unusual for a nursing assistant to have a résumé, but it may help you to write one. It will give you practice and will provide you with information needed to complete an application. Also, because it is unusual, it will make you stand out when there are several applicants.

résumé a written document stating the individual's qualifications for a job; usually includes education, certificates or credentials, skills, and job history

JOB APPLICATION

You may pick up a job application at the facility and take it home to complete or you may complete it at the facility. Sometimes, the interview is immediate; other times, you will be called after review of your application. Bring your Social Security card, driver's license or official identification, your proof of citizenship or legal permission to live and work in this country, and your proof of certification. Some employers will ask for a current CPR card that shows you have been trained in cardiopulmonary resuscitation. Bring two pens with black or blue ink.

The application will ask for personal information such as name, address, telephone number, and whether you are authorized to work in the United States. You will be asked if you have been convicted of any crime. You are asked to provide your work history and a list of professional references with name and telephone number. Your education history is also requested, with dates and locations of your education and training. You may be asked to describe any additional special skills you bring to the job. Most applications ask you whether you are applying for full- or part-time employment and the shift you prefer. They may ask for your expectations for wages. They often ask about whether you know or are related to current employees and whether you have worked for the same organization in the past.

The keys to completing your application are:

1. Come prepared with the information that is required.
2. Print all responses so they can be easily read. Use ink.
3. Complete every line on the application.
4. Tell the truth. Most facilities have a policy that lying on an application is grounds for immediate termination.

THE JOB INTERVIEW

Your job interview gives the employer a chance to learn more about you and gives you a chance to learn more about the employer (Figure 20-4). Because the first impression is so important, prepare for your appointment. You must look your best. Your clothes, grooming, attitude, and posture are very revealing. Your clothes must fit well and be clean and pressed. Shoes must be clean and polished. Men should have had a haircut within 2 weeks. Nails need to be trimmed. Jewelry should be simple and minimal. Avoid excessive perfume and aftershave. Makeup should be simple and low-key. This is your opportunity to create a positive first impression. Plan to arrive 15 minutes before your appointment.

Most interviewers have a common set of questions that they ask. The following are some that you might expect. Think about how you will answer each of them. Write down the answers and discuss them with a friend or fellow student.

1. Why do you want to work at this facility?
2. Why should we choose to hire you?
3. What do you like about being a nurse assistant?
4. What don't you like about being a nurse assistant?
5. What are your greatest strengths?
6. What are your greatest weaknesses?
7. How would your last supervisor/instructor describe your strengths and weaknesses?
8. What would your former co-workers say about you?

FIGURE 20-4

The job interview.

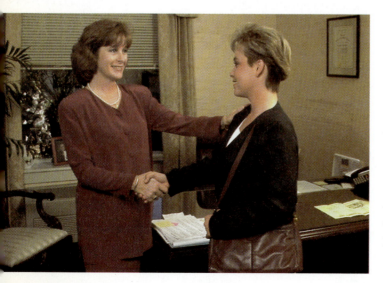

The interviewer may come out of his or her office to greet you or you may be invited in. In either case, offer to shake hands when you first meet. Listen carefully for the interviewer's name and use it in your conversation so you will remember it. People like to hear their own names. Be sure to use his or her last name, not the first name. Although every conversation begins with social comments about the weather or something you notice in the interviewer's office ("That is an unusual plant, what kind is it?"), keep these comments brief. Don't be afraid to talk about your good qualities. It is okay to provide open and honest feedback about your strengths and the skill that you bring to the job. It may be helpful to say "I have always been praised by my co-workers for _____" or "In my last evaluation, my supervisor said _____." This may be easier for you and seem less like bragging. Keep your answers as brief as possible. Many interviewers in an LTC facility have only 15 minutes to conduct your interview. Respect their time by sticking to the point of the interview. Show your energy and enthusiasm for this particular job. Pay attention to the interviewer. Use your listening skills. If you don't understand a question, ask for clarification rather than trying to "fake it." The interview also provides you with an opportunity to ask questions. You may want to ask about the facility's philosophy regarding continuing education for the staff. How many residents can you expect to be assigned to? Are there opportunities for increased responsibility (team leader, restorative nurse assistant, etc.)? Think about your questions in advance and write them down. You may refer to them during the interview. Usually, the interviewer will conclude the interview with a "thank you for coming" and some idea of when you will hear whether or not you have been given the job. Sometimes, you may be asked to return for a second interview, or you may even be hired on the spot. Before you leave, thank the interviewer for his or her time and conclude with a positive comment such as "I would really like to be part of this facility. I hope you'll consider me for the position," or "I look forward to hearing from you."

When you follow the guidelines to prepare for and participate in the hiring interview and you are sincere, enthusiastic, and genuine, you can be optimistic about your chances of being hired.

CONTINUING YOUR EDUCATION

Your learning doesn't end with obtaining your certification, nor does it end when you are hired. Education if a lifelong process that is just beginning when you pass the competency evaluation. Facilities will offer you regular opportunities to attend training classes. These classes are referred to as "in-service" education since they are provided on the job. Some states through their state laws specify the content of in-service education. They may also specify how many hours of training you must attend to keep your certification. It is your responsibility to attend the classes offered and to seek other opportunities to learn. You can continue your education in many ways. You can read books, articles, and newsletters. You can ask questions and observe others and how they do things. You can take correspondence courses in areas of interest. You can always learn from the other members of the interdisciplinary team by observing and asking them questions. If you have the right attitude, you will find that you learn from every experience with every resident you care for. You may have some bad experiences when things don't go the way they should. You will make mistakes. When you make a mistake, you will learn the most. You'll have good days and bad days, but you can learn every day.

SUMMARY This chapter is about you and your life as a certified nursing assistant. Although the content regarding study skills, test taking, and job seeking can be applied in other situations, it is designed to help you become certified and to obtain a job. The section on becoming certified includes how to listen, how to study, how to take notes, and how to plan for success. You have learned about test taking, particularly about multiple choice tests. Well-known principles and techniques have been included. Finally, you have a road map for finding and obtaining the job you want. Using these techniques will enhance your chance of getting that job.

SELF STUDY

Choose the best answer for each question or statement.

1. Which of the following is required for a person to become a certified nursing assistant?
   a. They must complete an approved nurse aide training program.
   b. They must demonstrate competency on a written or oral exam.
   c. They must demonstrate competency by demonstrating selected skills.
   d. They must do all of these things.

2. What information is available from the Nurse Aide Registry in each state?
   a. the names of individuals who have passed the certification exams
   b. a record of any arrests a nursing assistant has had
   c. a record of each nursing assistant's employment history
   d. all of the above

3. Which of the following is true of the written examination?
   a. It will be given at a long-term care facility.
   b. It will contain about 100 questions.
   c. It may be given orally under certain circumstances.
   d. It will contain multiple choice and true–false questions.

4. Lucy is getting ready to take her skills examination for her CNA. What does she need to take to the test with her?
   a. a set of sheets and a patient gown
   b. the cost of the test in cash or money order
   c. a personal check for the cost of the test
   d. paper and a number 2 pencil

5. What should you consider when you plan your study place and time?
   a. the time of day when you are at your best
   b. a place that is quiet with few interruptions
   c. a place that is somewhat comfortable
   d. all of these

6. What is meant by *active study*?
   a. using energy to learn

   b. listening to an instructor
   c. reading the textbook
   d. all of the above

7. When you listen to an instructor lecture, you should
   a. get in a comfortable position while you listen
   b. sit as close to the instructor as you can
   c. let your mind wander over the topics introduced
   d. read the textbook while the instructor speaks

8. What do the Learning Objectives in each chapter provide?
   a. an outline of the chapter contents
   b. the new terms that will appear in the chapter
   c. the most important information in the chapter
   d. a story drawn from the important points of the chapter

9. When you begin a new chapter and find new terms, what should you do?
   a. Try to guess what the term might mean.
   b. Scan over the terms and their meanings.
   c. Write them down only.
   d. Look up their meanings and write them down.

10. Why is studying the illustrations in a book chapter helpful to you?
    a. The illustrations communicate information without words.
    b. The illustrations are usually about the most important concepts.
    c. You will remember a picture longer than any other instruction.
    d. All of these are reasons illustrations are helpful.

11. When you are reading a textbook, you will learn key information best by
    a. highlighting or underlining new ideas
    b. writing down the key points
    c. taking notes on everything in the chapter
    d. reading the entire chapter several times

12. When you take notes during class, you should
    a. write down key information that is not in the book
    b. write down all information given by the instructor

c. write only information that you don't think you will remember

d. write only information that you don't understand

13. One way to make your notes brief and simple is to
   a. write only key words in your notes
   b. leave the vowels out of the words
   c. use medical abbreviations in your notes
   d. develop your own method of shorthand

14. One action you can take to prepare yourself for your certification examination is to
   a. read several different books about test taking
   b. try to guess what questions will be on the test
   c. spend one whole day per week studying for the test
   d. ask people who have taken the test what it was like

15. Which of the following strategies is helpful when answering the multiple-choice questions on the test?
   a. Look for the best answer, not the perfect answer.
   b. Look for key words in the question.
   c. Read every choice, even if you think the first one is correct.
   d. All of these strategies are helpful.

16. In a multiple choice question, three of the answers are wrong. What is one way to determine that an answer is wrong?
   a. If an answer is longer than the other choices, it is usually wrong.
   b. If an answer contains the words *all, always, never, none,* or *every,* it is usually wrong.
   c. If an answer is different from the other three choices, it is usually wrong.
   d. The first answer that comes to your mind is usually the wrong answer.

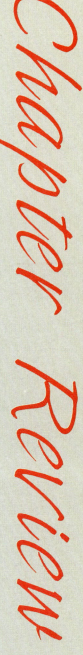

Getting C O N N E C T E D
Multimedia Extension Activities

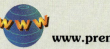 **www.prenhall.com/will-black**

Use the above address to access the free, interactive Companion Website created for this textbook. Hear the pronunciation of the key terms in the chapter. Get instant feedback to a variety of chapter-related questions. Link to other interesting sites.

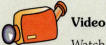 **Video**

Watch the *Focus on Professionalism* video from the Care Provider Skills series.

CASE STUDY

Sarah Sims has been taking the certification class with you. You are having a discussion about the upcoming competency evaluation. Sarah tells you she is terrified of the evaluation and isn't sure she will even show up.

1. She asks you if you have any suggestions to help her. You say
   a. "Give up now and stay home."
   b. "Everything will be all right. Don't worry."
   c. "You can still pass the test if you have the right attitude and if you study how to take a test."
   d. "Hire a tutor and start cramming now."

2. She asks you what will happen if she fails the test. You tell her
   a. "It doesn't matter. You can still work without it."
   b. "You can take the test two more times without repeating the course."
   c. "You must take the class again within 6 months of failing the test."
   d. "You only have one chance so you might as well give up now."

3. Sarah asks if she can borrow your notes to prepare for the evaluation. You tell her
   a. "Sarah, I'd love to share my notes with you."
   b. "I can't let you have them because I need them."
   c. "I don't think they would help you because I use a shorthand that is tailored to those things I need to remember. The notes wouldn't help anyone else."
   d. "Let's both borrow George's. He is a great student!"

4. Sarah plans to stay up all night before the test. She says black coffee will keep her awake. Using what you have learned, what do you think of her plan?
   a. Rest is more important to success than anything she learns at the last minute.
   b. It sounds like a great plan.
   c. It works for some people but not for me.
   d. It would work if she substituted diet cola for the coffee.

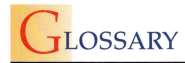

GLOSSARY

A

abdomen region of the body between the chest and the pelvis

abdominal respiration breathing using mostly the abdominal muscles

abduction to move an arm or leg away from the center of the body

absence seizures a type of seizure formerly called *petit mal* that involves numerous daily episodes in which the victim may stare vacantly for a few seconds, seeming to be out of contact with surroundings; occurs most often in children

accuracy factual or being correct

acetone by-product of the metabolism of fat; a type of ketone

acidosis a dangerous condition related to diabetes when toxic substances build up in the body

active study a method of preparing for an examination or test that involves activity other than reading

active treatment program plan including interdisciplinary evaluation and an individual plan of care with measurable goals and an integrated program of activities

activities of daily living (ADL) activities or tasks needed for daily living, such as eating, grooming, dressing, bathing, washing, and toileting

acute illness an illness of short duration

adduction to move an arm or leg toward the center of the body

adrenal glands two small glands located on top of each kidney; produce hormones that help the body react and adapt to stress

adult day care center provides meals and activities for the elderly who cannot or do not want to be alone during the day

advance directives written documents that allow an adult with decision-making capacity to write their preferences regarding medical care and treatment. Some documents allow them to name a person to make decisions for them if they are unable

advocates persons who represent residents or clients and act to protect their interests

age appropriate appropriate to the chronological age of a person

AIDS (acquired immune deficiency syndrome) a condition in which the body's immune system is damaged by attack from a virus (HIV)

airborne transmission passing on microorganisms through the air

alignment to put in a straight line

alimentary tract route taken by food as it passes from the mouth to the anus

alopecia loss of scalp and body hair

alveoli tiny air sacs in the lungs where oxygen enters the blood

Alzheimer's disease incurable disease affecting the brain that occurs predominantly in older adults and affects memory, thinking, and judgment

AM care assisting the resident with toileting needs, washing face and hands, providing oral hygiene, and preparing the resident for breakfast

ambulation walking or moving about in an upright position

ambulation device any apparatus to assist with walking; includes braces, canes, crutches, and walkers

amino acids the units of structure in proteins

amputation cutting off a body part, usually an arm or leg

anatomical position term of reference used when a person is standing facing you, with palms out and feet together

anatomy study of body parts, how the body is made, and what it is made of

anemia insufficient supply of red blood cells

aneurysm bulging out of the wall of an artery, creating a weakened area subject to rupture

angina pectoris acute chest pain caused by decreased blood supply to the heart

ankylosed condition in which joints become very stiff, unmovable, and frozen

aorta largest artery in the body

apathy lack of feeling or interest in things

aphasia loss of language or communication ability

apical pulse heartbeat measured at the apex of the heart

apnea absence of breathing

appendages attachments of the skin

appendix small projection of tissue located where the small and large intestines meet

arteries blood vessels that carry blood away from the heart

arterioles tiny arteries that carry blood from the large arteries to the capillaries

arteriosclerosis thickening and loss of elasticity in the arteries

artificial hydration providing liquids by means other than by mouth

artificial nutrition providing food and nourishment by means other than by mouth

artificial ventilation rescue breathing

ascites an abnormal collection of fluid in the abdomen

aseptic free of microorganisms

aspiration inhaling food or fluid into the lungs

assault threat or unsuccessful attempt to commit bodily harm

asthma a disease of the bronchi characterized by difficulty breathing, wheezing, and a sense of tightness or constriction in the chest due to spasm of the muscles

atherosclerosis clogging of the arteries with plaque and deposits of calcium or fat

atonic seizure a type of seizure with loss of tone in the muscles, leading to falling to the ground

atrium one of the two upper chambers of the heart

atrophy decreasing of muscle mass; wasting of muscle tissue

autism a disability related to lack of organization in the functioning of the brain

autoclaving sterilizing using superheated steam under pressure

autonomic dysreflexia in spinal cord–injured victims, a life-threatening condition that is caused by stimuli from the skin, the bowel, and the bladder

autonomic nervous system part of the nervous system that controls organs not under voluntary control

aversive unpleasant or painful

axillary in the armpit

B

backward chaining teaching the last step in a skill first, then the next to last, and so on

bacterium singular of bacteria, a type of microorganism

bag valve mask a ventilator bag

base of support foundation of an object or person

battery assault that is carried out, resulting in harm to another person

behaving courteously putting the needs of others before your own

behavior action that can be observed and measured

behavior modification a process of changing behavior patterns by eliminating useless behaviors and teaching or reinforcing useful ones

behavior shaping process of creating a new set of behaviors

benign prostatic hypertrophy noncancerous enlargement of the prostate gland

bereave to be left desolate by death

bile substance stored in the gallbladder that aids in the digestion of fats

bioethics a field of study of the moral values that relate to health care

biological death occurs when vital activity in the cells of the body stops

blood pressure measurable force of the blood against the walls of a blood vessel

blood pressure cuff common name for a sphygmomanometer

body language a form of communication that refers to facial expression, hand gestures, and body movement

body mechanics special ways of standing and moving one's body

Bowman's capsule part of the kidney containing the glomerules

brain syndrome signs or symptoms that indicate the presence of brain disease

bridging technique used to support areas above and below a designated area

bronchi two main branches of the windpipe

bulb portion of the thermometer that is placed in direct contact with the resident's body

bulbo-urethral glands exocrine glands located near the prostate in males

bursa small fluid-filled sac that allows one bone to move easily over another bone

bursitis inflammation of the fluid-filled sacs between bones, causing pain on movement

C

cachexia ill health with malnutrition and severe weight loss

calculi stones in the kidney or bladder

calibrated   marked with graduations, as on a thermometer or graduate

cancer   form of cellular disorder in which the normal mechanisms of the cell (that control rate of growth, cell division, and movement) are disrupted

capillaries   smallest blood vessels in the circulatory system; they nourish all body cells

carcinogen   substance known to cause cancer

carcinoma   a form of cancer found most often in the skin and the lining of hollow organisms and passageways

cardiac angioplasty   procedure used to open clogged coronary arteries

cardiac arrest   sudden cessation of the heartbeat

cardiac bypass surgery   procedure in which a blood vessel is removed from the leg to replace a portion of a coronary blood vessel that is clogged or blocked

cardiac muscle tissue   type of muscle in the heart that controls the heartbeat

cardiac pacemaker   part of the conduction system of the heart that creates the stimulus for the heart to beat

cardiovascular insufficiency   type of heart disease in which there is decreased blood supply to the major organs of the body

caring   compassion; understanding the fears, problems, and distress of another

cartilage   tough gristlelike substance that forms a pad at the end of or between bones

cataract   condition in which the lens becomes cloudy to the point of complete blindness

catastrophic reactions   sudden changes from baseline behavior that are socially unacceptable

cell   fundamental building block of all living organisms

cell membrane   rim or edge of the cell

Celsius (C)   measurement of temperature in which 0 degrees is the freezing point and 100 degrees is the boiling point for water

center of gravity   place where the bulk or mass of an object is centered

central line   catheter placed into the atrium of the heart

cerebellum   part of the brain that coordinates voluntary movement

cerebral palsy   a developmental disability caused by damage to the brain

cerebral vascular accident (CVA)   stroke

cerebrum   part of the brain responsible for thinking, learning, and memory

chart   written health or medical record, which is a legal document

chemotherapy   use of drugs or medications to treat disease

Cheyne–Stokes breathing   a kind of breathing that can be observed when a resident is near death. The breathing is slow and shallow at first, followed by faster and deeper breathing, which reaches a peak, then stops completely. The pattern then repeats until breathing stops completely

chromosomes   threadlike structures that carry genetic material

chronic illness   an illness that lasts a long time

chronic obstructive pulmonary disease (COPD)   emphysema, asthma, and chronic bronchitis, and problems related to these diseases

cilia   small hairlike projections of the respiratory passages

cirrhosis   inflammation of a tissue or organ, particularly the liver

clean   uncontaminated; free from known pathogenic organisms

clinical death   cessation of breathing and heartbeat

clitoris   primary female sex organ

clonic phase   stage of a convulsion in which the muscles jerk or spasm

closed urinary drainage system   method of collecting urine that prevents contamination as it is uninterrupted

code of ethics   rules of conduct for a particular group

colostomy   opening into the colon

coma   severe impairment of consciousness with absence of understandable speech, eye opening, and ability to follow instructions

communicable conditions   diseases and infections that spread from one person to another

communication   involves a sender, a message, and a receiver; may take place in speaking or writing, or without words through facial expressions, tone of voice, gestures, body position, and movement

competency   a skill or ability that can be demonstrated

complete airway obstruction   blocking of the airway so that no air passes through

complex partial seizure   a seizure with movement and sensory symptoms and a change in the level of consciousness

confidentiality   not revealing private information to others

congestive heart failure   inability of the heart to pump out all the blood returned to it from the veins

constipation   buildup of fecal material in the large intestine

contact transmission   passing on microorganisms by touch; may be touching of objects or an infected person

contaminated   not sterile; in contact with microorganisms

continuity   doing the same things in the same way

contracture   shortening of the muscles from inactivity

control   to stop or limit growth

convulsions   jerking of the muscles as they contract and relax

countertraction   exertion of pull in the opposite direction of traction

courteously   putting the needs of others before your own

cranium   bones of the head

crede   pressing on the area of the abdomen over the bladder to push the urine out

cross-infection   acquiring an infection from someone else

culture   specimen of body tissue or fluids kept under special laboratory conditions to detect the presence of microorganisms

culture   the thoughts, beliefs, and values of a social group

cure   correction or removal of a problem

cyanosis   blue or gray color of the skin, lips, and nailbeds, indicating lack of oxygen

cytoplasm   material surrounding the nucleus of a cell

D

death   the final cessation of all vital functions

debridement   removal of dead or unhealthy tissue

decubitus ulcers   tissue breakdown resulting from pressure or reduced blood flow (often called pressure sores or bed sores)

defamation of character   making false or damaging statements about another person that injure his or her reputation

defecation   process of eliminating waste material from the bowel

dehydration   condition in which fluid output is greater than fluid intake

demand pacemaker   a device used to stimulate the heart that senses the interval between the heart's natural beats and fires at a programmed interval

dementia   deprived of reason; mentally deteriorated

dermatologist   a physician who specializes in diseases of the skin

dermis   second layer of skin

developmental disability   a chronic condition related to or needing treatment similar to mental retardation

developmental model   a model of care that is based on the belief that human beings thrive only to the extent that they are allowed to develop

diabetes mellitus   disease in which the pancreas secretes insufficient amounts of insulin

diabetic coma   high blood sugar with presence of ketones in the urine

diabetic shock   very low blood sugar with symptoms of shock

dialysis   use of a machine that performs the base functions of the kidney

diaphragm   muscular organ that separates the chest and abdominal cavities

diarrhea   semifluid feces

diastolic pressure   pressure when the heart is relaxed (the lowest pressure)

diencephalon   area of the brain where control is exercised over body activities, such as regulation of body temperature and the endocrine glands

dirty   contaminated, used, or exposed to disease-producing organisms

disabled   limitation in the ability to function normally

discharge   long-time absence or permanent exit from an acute care hospital

disinfection   process of killing most microorganisms

dislocation   disruption of the normal alignment of bones where they form a joint

dorsiflexion   to flex the ankle (away from the sole of the foot)

douche   introduction of a cleansing solution into the vaginal canal with immediate return by gravity

droplet transmission   passing on microorganisms through droplets produced during activities like coughing, sneezing, and talking

dry application   application in which no water touches the skin

duodenum   first loop of the small intestine and most major area of digestion

dying   the processes of decline in body functions that results in death

dysphagia   difficulty in swallowing

dyspnea   difficult or labored breathing

E

edema   swelling of joints, tissue, or organs

ejaculated   released at the time the male experiences orgasm

electrocardiogram (EKG)   tracing of the heart's electrical conduction system

embolus   a blood clot that moves within the bloodstream

emesis   vomiting

emotional lability   overreaction of the emotions to a stimulus (e.g., crying or laughing inappropriately)

empathy   ability to put yourself in another's place and to see things as he or she sees them

emphysema   disease in which tiny bronchioles become plugged with mucus, making breathing difficult, especially during exhalation

encephalitis   inflammation of the brain

enema   introduction of fluid into the rectum and colon

enemas until clear   there is no solid fecal material present when the solution is expelled

enterally   by means of the gastrointestinal tract

environment   surroundings; all the factors that influence or affect the life of a person

environmental control   means of providing a safe environment that is as free as possible of pathogenic organisms

enzymes   digestive secretions

epidermis   outer layer of the skin

epiglottis   cartilage that covers the opening of the trachea when foods and fluids are swallowed

epilepsy   a disorder in the electrical functioning of the brain, resulting in seizures

erythema   redness of the skin

eschar   a slough produced after an injury (often called a scab)

estrogen   primary female sex hormone

ethicist   person who is expert in moral issues

ethnocentrism   belief that one's own race or group is superior to all others

euphoric   experiencing an exaggerated feeling of well-being

exacerbation   return or increase of symptoms

exocrine   secreting externally

exposure   contact with microorganisms

extension   to straighten an arm or leg

F

fading   a technique in behavior management in which the amount of guidance is decreased

Fahrenheit (F)   measurement of temperature in which 32 degrees is the freezing point and 212 degrees is the boiling point for water

fallopian tubes   tubes from the ovary to the uterus through which the ovum passes

false imprisonment   keeping or restraining a person without proper consent

fecal impaction   serious and painful condition in which feces remain in the S-shaped area of the colon and rectum, where they may block the intestinal passage

feces   solid human waste

feelings or emotions   outward expression of mood including happiness, grief, anger, etc.

fertile   able to become pregnant

fine motor skills   skills that require use of fine muscles such as those of the hands for writing, buttoning, eating

finger probes   manual removal of a foreign body by using the index finger

first intention healing   surgical closure of a wound

fixed-rate pacemaker   a device that emits a stimulus to contract the heart muscle at a set rate

flaccid   limp

flexion   to bend a joint (elbow, wrist, knee)

fluid balance   the individual takes in and eliminates about the same amount of fluid

fluid intake   total amount of fluid taken into the body over a given amount of time

fluid output   total amount of fluid eliminated from the body in a given amount of time

focal or Jacksonian seizure   type of seizure that affects only part of the body

follicles   roots of the hair

Food Guide Pyramid   a standard way of planning food intake. Good nutrition includes eating more from the bottom of the pyramid than from the top

force (pulse)   strength or power described as weak or bounding

force fluids   encourage fluid intake

formed elements   those parts of the blood that are not fluid (e.g., red blood cells and platelets)

forward chaining   complex skills broken down into specific steps and taught in the order in which they would normally be completed

fracture   breaking or cracking of a bone

frequency   the need to urinate often

functional life skills   skills necessary to allow an individual to function as independently as possible

G

gait belt   a belt placed around a patient's waist that allows better control over the center of gravity

gallstones   cholesterol crystals that settle out of the bile stored in the gallbladder

gangrene   a disease in which tissue dies and amputation is often necessary

gastritis   inflammation of the stomach caused by many different factors

gastrostomy tube   a tube is inserted directly into the stomach for purposes of providing food, water, and medications for a resident who is unable to swallow

gatch   handle or crank used to raise and lower the bed, head of bed, or foot of bed

genuineness   being yourself

GERD   gastroesophageal reflux disease—a condition with backflow of contents of the stomach into the esophagus, producing burning pain

glaucoma   increased pressure within the eye that can lead to blindness due to pressure on the optic nerve

glomerulus   a network of capillaries in the kidney that filters the blood

glucose   simple sugar to which food is converted

glycosuria   sugar in the urine

graduated guidance   a technique of behavior management in which the amount of assistance or prompting that is necessary is gradually decreased

grand mal seizure   type of seizure involving loss of consciousness and convulsions

gravity   attraction that the earth has for an object on or near its surface

grief process   emotions experienced by people following a loss

gross motor activities   involves use of the large muscles such as those used in walking, dancing, and swimming

gross negligence   person responsible shows so little care that it appears that he or she is indifferent to the welfare of others

H

Harris flush   return flow enema; irrigation of the rectum

health care plan   written guidelines for providing care

hearing aid   a mechanical device used to make certain sounds louder

heart   muscle that pumps blood through the vessels

Heimlich maneuver   application of abdominal thrusts during airway obstruction

hemiplegia   paralysis of one side of the body

hemispheres   halves

hemorrhage   bleeding

hemorrhoids   enlarged blood-filled vessels that surround the rectal area

heredity   traits we are born with

home health care agencies   businesses that provide health services to clients in the home

homeostasis   the body's attempt to keep its internal environment stable and in balance

hormone   fluid secreted by an endocrine gland

hospice   a program of care for residents who have a limited life expectancy

humidifier   water container through which oxygen is passed to reduce its drying effect

hydrated   having enough fluid

hyperactive   extremely, abnormally active

hyperextension   to move beyond the normal extension

hyperglycemia   high blood sugar

hypertension   high blood pressure

hypoglycemia   low blood sugar

hypotension   low blood pressure

hypothalamus   gland in the brain that controls body temperature and the function of the endocrine glands

hysterectomy   surgical removal of the uterus

I

ICFMR facility   a type of facility designed to provide care for the developmentally disabled or mentally retarded

ID   the interdisciplinary team that works with the developmentally disabled client

ileostomy   opening into the ileum

imbalance   lack of equality

immobilized   unable to move

impaired consciousness   the resident is not awake or alert; is unaware of and unable to react to the surroundings

implement   to carry out or accomplish a given plan

impotence   inability to engage in sexual intercourse

incidence   number of occurrences

incident report   written description of an accident involving resident, visitor, or staff member

incontinent   no control over bowel and bladder function

increased intercranial pressure   pressure inside the skull is increased because something is taking up space (hemorrhage, tumor, swelling of the brain)

individualized health care plan   plan of care tailored to reflect the individuality of each resident

indwelling catheter   tube inserted through the urethra into the bladder to drain urine into a collection bag

infarct   death of part of the heart muscle

infection   invasion of the body by a disease-producing organism

infectious objects   objects that have come in contact with a person who has an infection or communicable disease

inferior   toward the feet

inflammation   tissue reaction to disease or injury characterized by heat, redness, pain, and swelling

influenza   a contagious respiratory disease caused by a virus

informed consent   permission obtained from a resident to perform or withhold a medical procedure; must be voluntary and in writing

infusion   introduction of a fluid directly into a vein

insulin   hormone secreted by the pancreas

insulin shock   low blood sugar, usually from too much insulin or not enough food intake

intensive rehabilitation   services provided at a fast pace, often involving several kinds of therapy requiring 2 to 3 hours per day

interdisciplinary team   a group of health care workers from different professions who work together to provide care to residents

interests   those things we enjoy or care about

intramuscularly   injection into muscle

intravenously   injection into the vein

invasion   the process of taking over a part or function

invasion of privacy   when personal information is exposed publicly, violating an individual's right to privacy

IPPB   intermittent positive pressure breathing—a treatment providing oxygen under pressure to assist the resident to breathe more deeply. It often contains medication. The treatment is provided by respiratory therapist or licensed nurse

IPPs   the individual program plans used with developmentally disabled clients

I.Q.   intelligence quotient or score obtained on a standard test

irregular respiration   a change in the depth of breathing and an unsteady rate of rise and fall of the chest

isolation   to separate or set apart

isolation techniques   safety measure to prevent spread of communicable conditions

J

jaundice   a yellow coloring of skin and the white portion of the eye caused by the substance bilirubin, which is secreted by the liver

job description   describes the duties of a particular job category

joint   any connection between bones

K

ketonuria   presence of ketones in the urine

kidneys   two bean-shaped organs in the pelvis of the body that act as a filtration system to eliminate waste products

kyphosis   hunchback or forward curving of the spine

L

labored respirations   difficult breathing that may include gurgling, rattling, or wheezing sounds

lancet   sharp object used to prick the skin of a fingertip or earlobe to obtain a small sample of blood

larynx   voice box

laxative   medication that loosens the bowel contents and encourages evacuation

laxative suppository   a cone-shaped, easily melted mass inserted into the rectum to stimulate the bowel to empty

least restrictive alternative   a choice of treatment, activities, or living arrangement that minimally limits the freedom and independence of the individual

legal   according to the laws of the community, state, or nation

level of injury in spinal cord injury, the location of injury in relationship to the vertebrae that surround the cord

libel a written type of defamation of character

ligaments tough, white, fibrous cords that connect bone to bone

liver the largest gland of the body and one of its most complex organs; is part of the digestive system and performs about 500 functions

log rolling a technique of turning a patient

long-term care (LTC) facility a type of institution designed to provide care and services over a long period. Includes skilled nursing facility and rehabilitation centers. There is no age restriction

lymph fluid that surrounds the body cells

lymph vessels tiny capillary-like structures that collect lymph

M

mammary glands glandular tissue of the breast

manual thrusts series of rapid thrusts to the upper abdomen or chest that force air from the lungs

masturbation sexual self-stimulation apart from intercourse

MDS Coordinator title of the registered nurse responsible for completion of the resident assessment or MDS

medical subacute care for medically complex patients requiring specialized services

medical waste disposable items used by residents and any body discharges

medulla vital center in the brain that controls breathing, swallowing, and heartbeat

meningitis inflammation of membranes surrounding the brain

menopause the period of time when menstruation stops, ending reproductive ability and resulting in decreased hormone production

menstruation monthly shedding of the lining of the uterus

mental retardation a significantly subaverage general intellectual functioning existing with deficits in adaptive behavior

metabolism complex processes of the living cells in which oxygen is used and carbon dioxide is given off (called the work of the cell)

metastasize spread to other parts of the body

microorganisms tiny living things seen only with a microscope

midbrain part of the brain through which nerve impulses pass

midstream clean-catch urine specimen type of urine specimen obtained under clean conditions by collecting urine while it is being eliminated from the body

Minimum Data Set (MDS) a written, standardized assessment of all residents living in a skilled nursing facility

modeling a technique of behavior management in which the client is shown how to perform a task

moist application application in which water touches the skin

multiple choice question a test question that provides a selection of answers; the student is to choose the correct answer from those provided

multiple sclerosis chronic degenerative disease of the nervous system

muscular dystrophy a group of related muscle diseases that are progressively crippling due to weakness and atrophy of muscles

myelin insulating material that surrounds the nerve fibers

myocardial infarction heart attack in which part of the heart muscle dies

N

nasal cannulas tubes inserted into the nostrils to supply oxygen

nasogastric tube tube inserted through the nose and into the stomach

negligence failure to act as an average nursing assistant would act under the same circumstances

nephrons microscopic filtering units of the kidney

neurons specialized cells of the nervous system

nitroglycerin medication that, when placed under the tongue to dissolve, will act rapidly to increase blood flow to the heart

nocturia waking at night to urinate

nonpathogenic not capable of producing disease

normalization creating an atmosphere that is as close to normal as possible

NPO consuming nothing by mouth

nucleus part of the cell that directs growth of the cell and cell division

nursing care Kardex "nursing assistant information" record, which may be handwritten or printed from a computer

nutrition science of food and its actions or relationship to health

O

objective observations facts observed and not distorted by personal feelings

observation recognizing and noticing a fact or occurrence

obstruction blocking of the airway

occupied bed one with a resident in it

olfaction sense of smell

ombudsman an impartial person who investigates complaints and acts as an advocate for residents and/or families

Omnibus Budget Reconciliation Act (OBRA) a 1987 law passed by the U.S. Congress containing nursing home reform requirements

opportunistic infection occurs when organisms take advantage of a diseased immune system

oral in the mouth

oral hygiene care of the mouth, teeth, gums, and tongue

orally taken by mouth

organ body part in which two or more tissues work together to perform a particular function

organism any living thing

orientation ability to accurately describe person, place, and time

osteoarthritis disease characterized by deterioration of joint cartilage and formation of new bone at joint surfaces

osteocytes living cells of the bone

osteoporosis disease characterized by porous or chalk-like bones that fracture very easily

ostomy surgical opening made on the surface of the abdomen to release waste from the body

otologist a specialist in hearing

ova eggs

ovaries primary female reproductive organs

ovulation process in which an ovum is discharged from an ovary at regular intervals

P

pain an unpleasant sensory experience caused by actual or potential tissue damage

palliation to relieve symptoms

pancreas large gland located in the abdomen; secretes insulin and glucagon

paralysis loss of voluntary movement

paraplegic person with paralysis of the lower limbs

parasympathetic nervous system part of the autonomic nervous system that conserves energy

parathyroid glands two pairs of glands located within the thyroid that produce a hormone to help regulate the level of calcium and phosphorus in the body

parenterally through a tube inserted into a vein or into the atrium of the heart

partial airway obstruction incomplete blocking of the airway, allowing some air to pass through

partial bath bathing of only those areas of the body that require daily bathing to remain clean

partial seizures type of seizures in which the abnormal electrical discharge starts in one specific area of the brain

passive done for the patient by the nursing assistant

patient-controlled analgesic pump (PCA) a medical device that allows the patient to himself a measured dose of pain relieving medication; usually given intravenously or subcutaneously

pathogenic causing disease

penis primary male sex organ

perinatal during the birth process

perineal area in the female, the area between the vagina and the anus; in the male, the area between the scrotum and the anus

peripheral vascular disease poor circulation in the extremities

peristalsis rhythmic contractions that assist in moving food through the intestines

perpendicular at a right angle

petit mal seizure type of seizure common in children; does not include convulsions

philosophy search for a general understanding of values

physical needs basic human needs for food, water, oxygen, rest, exercise, and sex

physiology study of how the body functions, how all the body parts work independently and collectively

PICC line peripherally inserted central catheter—tubing inserted through a vein in the arm or leg that goes into the atrium of the heart. Used for administration of fluids, nutrition, or drugs

pituitary gland master gland of the body, which regulates metabolism

planning   devising a way of getting a job done

plantar flexion   extending the ankle (toward the sole of the foot)

plaque   substance that clogs arteries producing atherosclerosis

plasma   fluid portion of the blood

platelets   cells in the blood that are essential for clotting

PM care   assisting the resident with toileting needs, washing face and hands, giving bedtime nourishment, providing oral hygiene, dressing for bed, and giving a back rub

pneumonia   acute infection of the lung

podiatrist   a physician who specializes in treating the feet

policy   describes what is to be done

pons   part of the brain through which nerve impulses pass

Port-a-cath   a device implanted under the skin to give easy access to the veins for medication administration

postnatal   after birth

postural drainage   physical therapy in which the resident is positioned so that the upper trunk is lower than the rest of the body, forcing secretions from respiratory passages to be coughed up

postural support   soft protective device or restraint used to protect a resident from injury

prenatal   during pregnancy

presbyopia   condition in which the lens of the eye looses its ability to focus clearly due to loss of elasticity

pressure ulcer   an inflammation, sore, or ulcer of the skin over a bony prominence caused by shearing or pressure

procedure   description of how to do a task

procrastination   putting off doing something until some other time

prognosis   a prediction of the outcome of an illness

prolapse   protruding of the uterus into the vagina

prompting   a technique used in rehabilitation programs in which the staff verbally reminds the resident what to do next

pronation   turning palms down

proprioception   knowledge and awareness of the position of one's body parts in space

prostate gland   a firm muscular gland that encircles the male's urethra like a donut

prosthesis   artificial replacement for a body part such as a limb or eye

protoplasm   essential living matter of all animal and plant cells

pruritus   itching

psychomotor seizure   type of seizure that results in temporary impairment of consciousness and abnormal behavior

psychosocial   an individual's mental or emotional processes in combination with his or her ability to interact and relate with others

pulmonic   a valve in the heart between the right ventricle and the pulmonary artery

pulse   the rhythmic expansion and contraction of the arteries, which can be measured to show how fast the heart is beating

pulse force   weak or bounding force of pulse beats

pulse rate   number of pulse beats per minute

pulse rhythm   regularity of the pulse beats

purulent material   liquid inflammation product containing cells and other fluid

Q

quadriplegic   person with paralysis of all four extremities

quality of life   a concept that includes all the aspects that make life worth living; best defined by the individual himself

QMRP   the qualified mental retardation professional who heads the interdisciplinary team for developmentally disabled clients

R

radial deviation   toward the thumb side of the hand

radial pulse   pulse felt at the inner aspect of the wrist (radial artery)

radiation therapy   use of high-energy rays to stop cancer cells from growing and multiplying

range of motion   extent to which a joint can be moved before causing pain

reagent   substance used in a chemical reaction to determine the presence of another substance

reality orientation   technique for reducing and eliminating disorientation

rectal   in the rectum

rectum   lowest section of the large intestine adjacent to the outside of the body

reduction   setting a bone in proper position for healing

reflex   automatic response to stimulation

reflux   return flow of urine back into the bladder from a drainage bag

rehabilitation   the restoration of the individual to the fullest physical, mental, social, vocational, and economic capacity of which he or she is capable

rehabilitation philosophy   understanding that promotes independence and recognizes the accomplishment of small, simple goals

reinfection   being infected a second time

reinforcer   a reward

reminiscence   the act or habit of thinking about or relating to past experiences

remission   lessening or disappearance of disease symptoms

renal artery   artery that supplies blood to the kidneys

renal pelvis   part of the kidney that serves as a funnel for urine coming from the kidney into the ureter

Resident Assessment Protocols (RAPs)   in-depth focused assessments on specific aspects of care such as risk for falls or tube feeding

resident's rights   those aspects of care that the resident in a facility is entitled to have honored. There is a specific and detailed list identified in the regulations

respect   recognition of the worth of another person

respiration   process of inhaling and exhaling

restraint   device that holds back or limits movements; used in reference to postural support or soft protective devices

résumé   a written document stating the individual's qualifications for a job; usually includes education, certificates or credentials, skills, and job history

rheumatoid arthritis   disease characterized by painful, stiff, swollen red joints that eventually become deformed

role   part one plays in relationship to others

rotation   to move a joint in a circular motion around its axis

rounds, making   going to each resident to determine briefly whether they have any immediate needs

S

salivary glands   glands that produce saliva to moisten the mouth and begin the digestion of food

sarcoma   a form of cancer found most often in bone, muscle, cartilage, and lymph systems

scabies   a disease caused by mites that burrow under the skin

scoliosis   S-shaped curving of the spine

scrotum   sac outside the male containing the testes

second intention healing   wound heals from the inside out

security needs   basic human needs for physical safety, shelter, and protection

seizure   overreaction of brain cells; a sudden attack

self-fulfillment   basic human need to reach the highest potential and to accomplish one's life goals

semen   fluid expelled through the penis during ejaculation; contains sperm, water, and nutrients

sensory deprivation   loss or lack of stimulation from the environment

sensory-motor activities   activities designed to improve the thinking of the client

sensory neurons   specialized type of nerve cell

septum   tissue that divides the heart into right and left chambers

setting priorities   looking at all things that need to be done and putting them in the order of importance

sexuality   quality of being male or female

sexually transmitted disease   a disease passed on from one person to another through vaginal, rectal, or oral sex

shadowing   a technique of behavior management in which the staff member's hands are kept within one inch of the client's hands while he or she performs a task

shallow respiration   breathing with only the upper part of the lungs

shaping   a behavior modification technique used to create a new set of behaviors

shearing   force that occurs when skin moves one way while bone and tissue under the skin move another way

sick role   behavior associated with being sick; dependence, weakness, control by others, decreased responsibility, and uselessness

sigmoid colon   lower portion of the large intestine which curves in an 'S' shape

slander   a verbal type of defamation of character

smooth muscle tissue   involuntary muscle tissue

social needs   basic human need for approval and acceptance

sodium chloride   table salt

spasm   involuntary contraction of muscle

spasticity tightening of the muscle with short jerking movements

sperm male reproductive cells released upon ejaculation

sphincter type of muscle that contracts to close a body opening

sphygmomanometer instrument used to measure blood pressure; can be either aneroid (measurer watches a calibrated dial) or mercury type (measurer watches a column of mercury)

spinal cord long cable of nerves that extends from below the medulla to the second or third lumbar vertebra

spiritual needs need to find meaning in life

spontaneous breathing in mouth-to-mouth ventilation, the point at which the victim begins to breathe independently

spontaneous combustion ignition of burnable materials caused by a chemical reaction

sprain stretched or torn ligaments or tendons

sputum mucus from the lungs, usually mixed with saliva

Standard Precautions a system of precautions to be used in the care of all residents in order to prevent the spread of disease

standards what is acceptable and unacceptable to us

Staphylococcus type of harmful bacteria commonly found in health care institutions; treated by antibiotic drugs

stasis stoppage of flow

stasis ulcers open wounds or sores on the legs caused by stoppage of blood flow

status needs basic human needs for recognition and respect

stem (thermometer) long narrow portion of a thermometer, opposite from the bulb

stereotype a generalization

sterile free from all microorganisms

sterilization process of killing all microorganisms

sternum breastbone

stertorous respirations abnormal noises like snoring when breathing

stethoscope instrument that picks up sound when placed against part of the body

stimulus action or agent that causes a response in an organ or organism

stoma an opening

stool solid waste material discharged from the body through the rectum and anus; feces, excreta, excrement, bowel movement, fecal material

Streptococcus type of harmful bacteria commonly found in health care institutions; treated by antibiotic drugs

stretch receptors nerve cells in the wall of the bladder that send a message to the brain when the bladder is full

striated muscle tissue type of voluntary muscle tissue

stridor a high-pitched sound produced during airway obstruction

subacute care a kind of care that is less than provided in an acute care hospital but more than normally provided in a long-term care facility

subjective observations individual judgments based on personal feelings

superior toward the head

supination to turn palms up

suppository cone-shaped semisolid medicated substance inserted into the rectum

surgery a process of removing or cutting out tissue from the body

sweat glands glands that produce moisture to cool the body and excrete waste products

sympathetic nervous system part of the autonomic nervous system that controls response to stress

systolic pressure pressure created when the heart is contracting; highest pressure

T

tact ability to say or do the right thing at the right time

tendons elastic cordlike structures that connect muscles to bone

terminal illness serious illness providing life expectancy of six months or less in the end stage of the illness

testes primary male reproductive organs that produce sperm

testosterone male hormone related to sexual activity and reproduction

therapeutic pertaining to or effective in treatment of disease

thrombosis the condition of having a blood clot

thrombus blood clot

thymus gland two-lobe ductless gland believed to play a role in the immune system of the body

thyroid gland   largest of the endocrine glands; regulates growth and metabolic rate

tissue   group of the same type of cells functioning in the same way

tongue–jaw lift   in finger sweep procedures, forcing open the mouth and holding the lower jaw and tongue so that the mouth cannot close

tonic–clonic seizures   previously called *grand mal*. The limbs first become stiff and rigid and breathing stops. The jaws are clenched and the tongue or lips may be bitten. The tonic phase is followed by the clonic phase in which the body is shaken by violent, rhythmic jerking of the limbs. The person loses consciousness and may be confused and sleepy for an hour or two afterwards

tonic seizure   a type of seizure in which stiffening of the body is the predominant feature; may or may not be followed by loss of consciousness

total parenteral nutrition   provision of nutrition directly into the circulation rather than through the digestive system

touch   form of communication that conveys friendliness and affection

toxins   waste products released by disease-producing organisms

trachea   windpipe; the passage that conveys air from the larynx to the bronchi

tracheostomy   an opening into the trachea

traction   exertion of "pull" by means of weights

transfer   to move from one place to another

transfer belt   belt placed around the resident's waist to provide a "handle" to hold during transfer

transmission-based precautions   a group of infection control methods based on the way a particular disease is spread

transurethral surgery   a procedure that removes some of the prostate tissue

tricuspid valve   valve between the right atrium and right ventricle of the heart

triggered pacemaker   a device that senses cardiac events and delivers its pacing stimulus based on what is needed

trochanter roll   a rolled towel or blanket

tuberculosis   an infectious disease that commonly attacks the lungs and is usually spread by contact with the sputum of an infected person

tympanic membrane   thin membrane inside the ear that vibrates when struck by sound waves; the eardrum

U

ulcer   break in the skin creating an open wound

ulnar deviation   away from the thumb side of the hand

unconscious   unaware of the surrounding environment

unoccupied bed   a bed with no one in it

ureterostomy   opening into one of the ureters

ureters   tubes that extend from the kidneys to the bladder through which urine passes

urethra   tube from the bladder to the outside of the body

urgency   an immediate need to urinate

urinary incontinence   inability to control urination

urination   the process of emptying the bladder of its contents

uterus   womb

V

vaginal irrigation or douche   introduction of solution into the vaginal canal with immediate return by gravity

vaginitis   inflammation of the tissue of the vagina

validation therapy   a method of helping residents with dementia by supporting their feelings rather than reminding them of the day, time, and place

values   what we consider to be most important

varicose veins   swollen (distended) veins especially prominent in the leg caused by lack of exercise, prolonged standing, and loss of elasticity associated with aging

veins   blood vessels that carry blood back to the heart

ventricle   one of two small cavities in the heart

ventricles   thick muscular walls of the heart

venules   very tiny veins that carry blood back to the heart

vertebrae   bones of the spine

vertebral column   column of bones of the spine through which the spinal cord passes; spine; backbone

villi   small fingerlike projections of the duodenum that absorb digested food particles and release them into the bloodstream

virus   microorganisms that can cause infection and disease

vital signs   temperature, pulse, blood pressure, and respiration

vulvitis   inflammation of the vulva

W

warmth demonstrating concern and affection

well role behaviors associated with being well (i.e., independence, increased responsibility, usefulness, control, and decision making)

wound a disruption in the continuity and regulatory processes of tissue cells

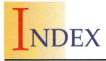

INDEX